GULF WAR and HEALTH

VOLUME 11

Generational Health Effects of Serving in the Gulf War

Committee on Gulf War and Health, Volume 11:
Generational Health Effects of Serving in the Gulf War

Board on Population Health and Public Health Practice

Health and Medicine Division

A Consensus Study Report of

The National Academies of
SCIENCES · ENGINEERING · MEDICINE

THE NATIONAL ACADEMIES PRESS
Washington, DC
www.nap.edu

THE NATIONAL ACADEMIES PRESS 500 Fifth Street, NW Washington, DC 20001

This activity was supported by Contract Number VA701-16-C-0029 between the National Academy of Sciences and the Department of Veterans Affairs. Any opinions, findings, conclusions, or recommendations expressed in this publication do not necessarily reflect the views of any organization or agency that provided support for the project.

International Standard Book Number-13: 978-0-309-47823-6
International Standard Book Number-10: 0-309-47823-5
Digital Object Identifier: https://doi.org/10.17226/25162

Additional copies of this publication are available for sale from the National Academies Press, 500 Fifth Street, NW, Keck 360, Washington, DC 20001; (800) 624-6242 or (202) 334-3313; http://www.nap.edu.

Printed in the United States of America

Suggested citation: National Academies of Sciences, Engineering, and Medicine. 2018. *Gulf War and health, volume 11: Generational health effects of serving in the Gulf War*. Washington, DC: The National Academies Press. doi: https://doi.org/10.17226/25162.

The National Academies of
SCIENCES • ENGINEERING • MEDICINE

The **National Academy of Sciences** was established in 1863 by an Act of Congress, signed by President Lincoln, as a private, nongovernmental institution to advise the nation on issues related to science and technology. Members are elected by their peers for outstanding contributions to research. Dr. Marcia McNutt is president.

The **National Academy of Engineering** was established in 1964 under the charter of the National Academy of Sciences to bring the practices of engineering to advising the nation. Members are elected by their peers for extraordinary contributions to engineering. Dr. C. D. Mote, Jr., is president.

The **National Academy of Medicine** (formerly the Institute of Medicine) was established in 1970 under the charter of the National Academy of Sciences to advise the nation on medical and health issues. Members are elected by their peers for distinguished contributions to medicine and health. Dr. Victor J. Dzau is president.

The three Academies work together as the **National Academies of Sciences, Engineering, and Medicine** to provide independent, objective analysis and advice to the nation and conduct other activities to solve complex problems and inform public policy decisions. The National Academies also encourage education and research, recognize outstanding contributions to knowledge, and increase public understanding in matters of science, engineering, and medicine.

Learn more about the National Academies of Sciences, Engineering, and Medicine at **www.nationalacademies.org.**

The National Academies of
SCIENCES • ENGINEERING • MEDICINE

Consensus Study Reports published by the National Academies of Sciences, Engineering, and Medicine document the evidence-based consensus on the study's statement of task by an authoring committee of experts. Reports typically include findings, conclusions, and recommendations based on information gathered by the committee and the committee's deliberations. Each report has been subjected to a rigorous and independent peer-review process, and it represents the position of the National Academies on the statement of task.

Proceedings published by the National Academies of Sciences, Engineering, and Medicine chronicle the presentations and discussions at a workshop, symposium, or other event convened by the National Academies. The statements and opinions contained in proceedings are those of the participants and are not endorsed by other participants, the planning committee, or the National Academies.

For information about other products and activities of the National Academies, please visit www.nationalacademies.org/about/whatwedo.

COMMITTEE ON GULF WAR AND HEALTH, VOLUME 11: GENERATIONAL HEALTH EFFECTS OF SERVING IN THE GULF WAR

KENNETH S. RAMOS (*Chair*), Associate Vice President for Precision Health Sciences, Professor of Medicine and Director, Center for Applied Genetics and Genomic Medicine, University of Arizona Health Sciences

TRACY L. BALE, Professor and Director, Center for Epigenetic Research in Child Health and Brain Development, University of Maryland School of Medicine

JOHN R. BALMES, Professor of Medicine, University of California, San Francisco

BRENDA ESKENAZI, Jennifer and Brian Maxwell Professor of Maternal and Child Health and Epidemiology, Director, Center for Environmental Research and Children's Health, University of California, Berkeley

ELAINE M. FAUSTMAN, Professor and Director, Institute for Risk Analysis and Risk Communication, Department of Environmental and Occupational Health Sciences, University of Washington

MARI S. GOLUB, California National Primate Research Center, University of California, Davis

RAFAEL A. IRIZARRY, Professor of Biostatistics, Dana-Farber Cancer Institute, Harvard University

TAMARRA JAMES-TODD, Mark and Catherine Winkler Assistant Professor of Environmental Reproductive and Perinatal Epidemiology, Harvard T.H. Chan School of Public Health

STEPHEN A. KRAWETZ, Associate Director, C.S. Mott Center for Human Growth and Development, Charlotte B. Failing Professor of Fetal Therapy and Diagnosis, Department of Obstetrics and Gynecology, Center for Molecular Medicine and Genetics, Wayne State University

LINDA A. McCAULEY, Dean, Nell Hodgson Woodruff School of Nursing, Emory University

JACOB D. McDONALD, Senior Scientist, Vice President, Chief Science Officer, Lovelace Respiratory Research Institute

DYLAN S. SMALL, Professor, Department of Statistics, The Wharton School, University of Pennsylvania

JACQUETTA TRASLER, Senior Scientist, Research Institute of the McGill University Health Centre, James McGill Professor in Pediatrics, Human Genetics, and Pharmacology and Therapeutics, McGill University

CHERYL LYN WALKER, Director, Center for Precision Environmental Health, Professor, Department of Molecular and Cell Biology and Medicine, Baylor College of Medicine

CAROL S. WOOD, Staff Scientist, Toxicology and Hazard Assessment Group, Environmental Sciences Division, Oak Ridge National Laboratory

ROBERT O. WRIGHT, Ethel H. Wise Professor of Pediatrics, Chair, Department of Environmental Medicine and Public Health, Icahn School of Medicine at Mount Sinai

Study Staff

ROBERTA WEDGE, Study Director

CARY HAVER, Program Officer

T. CHERI BANKS, Associate Program Officer

PAMELA RAMEY-McCRAY, Senior Program Assistant

ROSE MARIE MARTINEZ, Senior Board Director, Board on Population Health and Public Health Practice

Reviewers

This report has been reviewed in draft form by individuals chosen for their diverse perspectives and technical expertise. The purpose of this independent review is to provide candid and critical comments that will assist the institution in making its published report as sound as possible and to ensure that the report meets institutional standards for objectivity, evidence, and responsiveness to the study charge. The review comments and draft manuscript remain confidential to protect the integrity of the deliberative process. We wish to thank the following individuals for their review of this report:

Bruce A. Barron, University of Rochester Medical Center
Joseph Braun, Brown University
Dana C. Dolinoy, University of Michigan School of Public Health
Seth Eisen, Washington University School of Medicine
David Korn, Harvard Medical School
Nancy E. Lane, University of California, Davis, School of Medicine
Germaine Buck Louis, George Mason University
Donald R. Mattison, Risk Sciences International, Ottawa
Reza J. Rasoulpour, Dow AgroSciences
Laura N. Vandenberg, University of Massachusetts

Although the reviewers listed above have provided many constructive comments and suggestions, they were not asked to endorse the conclusions or recommendations, nor did they see the final draft of the report before its release. The review of this report was overseen by **Nancy F. Woods,** University of Washington, and **Maryellen L. Giger,** The University of Chicago. They were responsible for making certain that an independent examination of this report was carried out in accordance with institutional procedures and that all review comments were carefully considered. Responsibility for the final content of this report rests entirely with the authoring committee and the institution.

Preface

Veterans of the 1990–1991 Gulf War and the Post-9/11 conflicts in Iraq and Afghanistan were exposed to a variety of biological, chemical, radiological, psychosocial, and physical stressors during their deployments. Over the past 20 years the National Academies of Sciences, Engineering, and Medicine (the National Academies) has convened more than 10 committees of experts to assess the health effects that might be linked to those exposures. Some of the health effects identified by past committees include post-traumatic stress disorder, other mental health disorders, Gulf War illness, respiratory effects, and self-reported sexual dysfunction. Veterans' concerns regarding the impacts of deployment-related exposures on their health have grown to include potential adverse effects on the health of their children and grandchildren. These concerns now increasingly involve female veterans, as more women join the military and are deployed to war zones and areas that pose potential hazards. The committee notes that veterans' harmful exposures are not restricted to deployment; such exposures may occur during military service in general or even outside of active duty (for example, exposure to trichloroethylene in contaminated drinking water at Camp Lejeune). As such, the need for data and knowledge to protect the health of the children and grandchildren of veterans who may have experienced harmful exposures during deployment has become urgent.

The exposure of male and female veterans to toxicants during their deployments may pose unknown risks to their future children, whether conceived during or after deployment. Harmful exposures may affect germ cells in both men and women and compromise the reproductive health of veterans and the future health of their children. For female veterans who may be deployed before they are aware they are pregnant, there may also be a risk to the developing fetus. The impact of exposures experienced during these periods on the developing embryo is largely unknown. Given these inherent risks, and in light of several public reports linking a parent's or even a grandparent's exposure to a toxicant to negative health outcomes in their descendants, veterans' concerns about generational effects continue to escalate. While the public reporting of generational effects has garnered considerable attention, the scientific evidence to support those links is not compelling at this time.

To address these gaps in data and knowledge, the Department of Veterans Affairs (VA) requested this eleventh update of the *Gulf War and Health* series of reports. This volume addresses two major tasks: evaluating the scientific and medical literature on reproductive and developmental effects and health outcomes associated with Gulf War and Post-9/11 exposures, and determining those research areas requiring further scientific study on potential health effects in the descendants of veterans of any era.

To accomplish these tasks, the National Academies established a committee of 16 members representing a broad range of areas of scientific and medical expertise. Its work was informed by two public meetings at which the committee heard from key stakeholders, including veterans, veterans' service organizations, research scientists, and representatives from VA, the Department of Defense, and other governmental organizations that are also attempting to determine what, if any, generational health effects may result from a veteran's exposures prior to or during pregnancy. The committee completed a comprehensive evaluation of relevant literature and integrated its findings with the large amounts of data on reproductive and developmental health outcomes reviewed in previous updates. The synthesis of the evidence was then used to craft a path forward for VA to address veteran concerns related to multigenerational health effects, particularly as they relate to veterans' children conceived during and after deployment, their grandchildren, and even future generations.

The Volume 11 committee thanks those who presented valuable information to the committee, including Fred Tyson, National Institute of Environmental Health Sciences; Vicki Walker, National Toxicology Program; Antonia Calafat, Centers for Disease Control and Prevention; John Greally, Albert Einstein School of Medicine; Colleen Baird, U.S. Army Public Health Command; R. Loren Erickson, Peter Rumm, and Aaron Schneiderman, Department of Veterans Affairs; and the many veterans who shared their deployment experiences with the committee. The committee is most grateful to Roberta Wedge, our outstanding study director, who helped us navigate through the report process and ensured that progress was made at all times. The committee is also indebted to Cary Haver and Cheri Banks for their hard work in support of committee functions and to Pam Ramey-McCray for her graceful administrative support of our activities. The committee acknowledges the expert assistance provided by Daniel Bearss of the National Academies Research Center helping to create and execute a detailed literature search strategy and for fact-checking the lengthy and sometimes complicated chapters included in the volume. A heartfelt thank-you to my fellow committee members for their collegiality, insights, hard work, thoughtfulness, and outstanding service over the past 2 years.

The committee is optimistic that the recommendations contained in this report will help answer many of the critical questions facing VA and the nation as a whole regarding the complex interactions between genes, environment, and lifestyle that may influence health outcomes across multiple generations. The report also provides specific guidance on the development of a health monitoring research program that can help gather the data required to evaluate generational effects and to establish a path forward in continuing to meet our responsibility to veterans of all conflicts.

Kenneth S. Ramos, *Chair*
Committee on Gulf War and Health, Volume 11: Generational Health Effects of Serving in the Gulf War

Contents

Acronyms and Abbreviations

αGSU	glycoprotein hormone α-subunit
γ-HCH	gamma-hexachlorocyclohexane (lindane)
ΣDAP	sum of DAP
1-N	1-naphthol
1-OHNa	1-hydroxynaphthalene
1-OHP	1-hydroxypyrene
2-MMA	2-methoxyacetic acid
2-OHF	2-hydroxyfluorene
2-OHNa	2-hydroxynapthalene
4-OHPh	4-hydroxyphenanthrene
9-OHFlu	9-hydroxyfluorene
9-OHPh	9-hydroxyphenanthrene
AChE	acetylcholinesterase
ADHD	attention deficit–hyperactivity disorder
AHLTA	Armed Forces Health Longitudinal Technology Application system (of DoD)
AhR	aryl hydrocarbon receptor
ALL	acute lymphoblastic leukemia
AMH	anti-Müllerian hormone
AML	acute myeloid leukemia
APC	adenomatous polyposis coli
aPR	adjusted prevalence ratio
ASD	autism spectrum disorder
ATSDR	Agency for Toxic Substances and Disease Registry
AVA	anthrax vaccine absorbed

BaP	benzo[a]pyrene
BASC	Behavior Assessment System for Children
BDNF	brain-derived neurotrophic factor
BMI	body mass index
BN-1MN	binucleated cells with one micronucleus
BNBAS	Brazelton Neonatal Behavioral Assessment Scale
BPA	3-phenoxybenzoic acid
BRIEF	Behavior Rating Inventory of Executive Functioning
BSID-II	Bayley Scales of Infant Development II
BTEX	benzene-toluene-ethylbenzene-xylene
BuChE	butyrylcholinesterase
CARC	chemical agent-resistant coating
CBCL	Child Behavior Checklist
CCCEH	Columbia Center for Children's Environmental Health (study)
CD3+	cluster of differentiation 3
CD4+	cluster of differentiation 4
CD19+	cluster of differentiation 19
CDCCA	cis-3-(2,2- dichlorovinyl)-2,2-dimethylcyclopropane carboxylic acid
CHAMACOS	Center for the Health Assessment of Mothers and Children of Salinas (study)
CHARGE	Childhood Autism Risks from Genetics and Environment (study)
ChE	cholinesterase
CHEAR	Children's Health Exposure Analysis Resource (of NIEHS)
CI	confidence interval
CIA	Central Intelligence Agency
CO	carbon monoxide
CO_2	carbon dioxide
CPF	chlorpyrifos
CpG	cytosine-adjacent-to-guanine (sites in the human genome)
CPT-II	Conners' Continuous Performance Test-II
Cr6	hexavalent chromium
CYP1A1	cytochrome P450 1A1
CYP2E1	cytochrome P450 2E1
DAG	directed acyclic graph
DAP	dialkylphosphate
DBCA	cis-2,2-dibromovinyl-2,2-dimethylcyclopropane-carboxylic acid
DCA	dichloroacetate
DEDTP	diethyldithiophosphate
DEP	diethylphosphate
DETP	diethylthiophosphate
DFI	DNA fragmentation index
DLA	Defense Logistics Agency
DLC	dioxin-like chemical
DMDC	Defense Manpower Data Center
DMDTP	dimethyldithiophosphate
DMP	dimethylphosphate

DMSS	Defense Medical Surveillance System
DMTP	dimethylthiophosphate
DNA	deoxyribonucleic acid
DNAm	DNA methylation
DNMT	DNA methyltransferase
DNMT3B	DNA methyltransferase 3 beta
DoD	Department of Defense
DOEHRS	Defense Occupational and Environmental Health Readiness System
DOHaD	developmental origins of health and disease
DSM-IV	*Diagnostic and Statistical Manual of Mental Disorders*, Fourth Edition
DU	depleted uranium
E2	estradiol
EAA	ethoxyacetic acid
ECHA	European Chemicals Agency
EGBE	ethylene glycol monobutyl ether (2-butoxyethanol)
EGEE	ethylene glycol monoethyl ether (2-ethoxythanol)
EGMBE	ethylene glycol monobutyl ether (2-butoxyethanol)
EGME	ethylene glycol monomethyl ether (2-methoxyethanol)
EHR	electronic health record
ELEMENT	Early Life Exposures in Mexico to Environmental Toxicants (study)
EPA	U.S. Environmental Protection Agency
EU	enriched uranium
FAI	free androgen index
FDA	Food and Drug Administration
FeNO	fractional exhaled nitric oxide
FSH	follicle-stimulating hormone
FT4/FT3	free thyroxin/triiodothyronine ratio
FT4	free thyroxine
FVC	forced vital capacity
GD	gestational day
GnRH	gonadotropin-releasing hormone
GSTM1	glutathione S-transferase mu 1 (M1)
GSTT1	glutathione S-transferase theta 1 (T1)
GWAS	genome-wide association study
H_2S	hydrogen sulfide
Hmlh1	human mutL homolog 1
HMRP	health monitoring and research program
HOME	Health Outcomes and Measures of the Environment (study)
HR	hazard ratio
HRMS	high-resolution mass spectrometry
HSD11B2	11β-hydroxysteroid dehydrogenase type 2

IARC	International Agency for Research on Cancer
ICM	inner cellular mass
IDR	incidence density ratio
IFNγ	interferon gamma
IGC	immature germ cell
IgE	immunoglobulin E
ILER	individual longitudinal exposure record
IOM	Institute of Medicine
iPSC	induced pluripotent stem cell
IQR	interquartile range
IRIS	Integrated Risk Information System
IRR	incidence rate ratio
JBB	Joint Base Balad
JP-4	jet fuel 4
JP-5	jet fuel 5
JP-8	jet fuel 8
KIDS	Kinder Infant Development Scale
LBW	low birth weight
LEP	leptin
LH	luteinizing hormone
md	mean difference
MDA	malathion dicarboxylic acid
MDI	mental development index
MGMT	methyl guanine methyl transferase
MHS	Military Health System
MilCo	Millennium Cohort (DoD study)
miRNA	microribonucleic acid
MLH1	mutL homolog 1
mRNA	messenger ribonucleic acid
Mt. Sinai	Mount Sinai Children's Environmental Health Cohort Study
mtDNA	mitochondrial DNA
MVP	Million Veteran Program (VA study)
NAS	National Academy of Sciences
NBDPS	National Birth Defects Prevention Study
NBNA	Neonatal Behavioral Neurological Assessment
ncRNA	noncoding RNA
NHL	non-Hodgkin's lymphoma
NIEHS	National Institute of Environmental Health Sciences
NIH	National Institutes of Health
NK	natural killer (cell)
NMDA	N-methyl-D-aspartate
NO	nitrogen oxide

NO_2	nitrogen dioxide
NRC	National Research Council
NTD	neural tube defect
O_3	ozone
OEF	Operation Enduring Freedom
OIF	Operation Iraqi Freedom
OND	Operation New Dawn
OP	organophosphate
OR	odds ratio
OSAGWI	Office of the Special Assistant for Gulf War Illnesses
PAH	polycyclic aromatic hydrocarbon
PB	pyridostigmine bromide
PBA	3-phenoxybenzoic acid
PCDD	polychlorinated dibenzo-p-dioxin
PCDF	polychlorinated dibenzofuran
PCE	tetrachloroethylene (perchloroethylene)
PCOS	polycystic ovary syndrome
PDI	psychomotor development index
PGC	primordial germ cell
piRNA	Piwi-interacting RNA
PM	particulate matter
PND	postnatal day
PNET	pancreatic neuroendocrine tumor
PON1	paraoxonase 1
PR	progesterone receptor
PROGRESS	Programming Research in Obesity, Growth, Environment and Social Stressors
PTB	preterm birth
RNA	ribonucleic acid
ROS	reactive oxygen species
RR	relative risk
SDQ	Strengths and Difficulties Questionnaire
SES	socioeconomic status
SGA	small for gestational age
SHBG	sex hormone binding globulin
SIR	standardized incidence ratio
SM	sulfur mustard
SO_2	sulfur dioxide
sRR	summary relative risk
SRS	Social Responsiveness Scale
SSVS	stochastic search variable selection
TBDD	2,3,7,8-tetrabromodibenzo-p-dioxin
TBG	thyroxin-binding globulin

TCA	trichloroacetate
TCDD	2,3,7,8-tetrachlorodibenzodioxin
TCE	trichloroethylene
TCPy	trichloro-2-pyridinol
TDCCA	trans-3-(2,2-dichlorovinyl)-2,2-dimethylcyclopropane carboxylic acid
TDG	thymine DNA glycosylase
TDM	tail distributed moment
TET2	Tet methylcytosine dioxygenase 2
TGCT	testicular germ cell tumor
THREE	Tracking Health Related to Environmental Exposures
tRNA	transfer RNA fragment
TSH	thyroid-stimulating hormone
TTP	time to pregnancy
VA	Department of Veterans Affairs
VAERS	Vaccine Adverse Event Reporting System
VAO	*Veterans and Agent Orange*
VHEMBE	Venda Health Examination of Mothers, Babies and Their Environment
VISTA	Veterans Information Systems and Technology Architecture (of VA)
VOC	volatile organic compound
VSO	veterans service organization
WBC	white blood cell
WHO	World Health Organization
WISC-IV	Weschler Intelligence Scale for Children, 4th edition
WPPSI-III	Weschler Preschool and Primary Scales of Intelligence-III
XIST	X-inactive specific transcript

Summary

In response to the invasion of Kuwait by Iraq in August 1990, the United States led a coalition of 34 countries in Operation Desert Shield in the Persian Gulf. This was followed by Operation Desert Storm, which began in January 1991 with an air offensive and a 4-day ground war; the war ended with a cease-fire in April 1991. Almost 700,000 U.S. troops were deployed to the Persian Gulf region during the height of the buildup.

The U.S. military engaged in further conflicts in the Middle East following the terrorist attacks of September 11, 2001. Operation Enduring Freedom began in October 2001 with troops stationed in and around Afghanistan. Operation Iraqi Freedom began in March 2003 with the invasion of Iraq, and it ended on August 31, 2010. Operation New Dawn, whose goal was to reduce the number of U.S. military personnel in Iraq, was initiated in September 2010 and ended in December 2011. The U.S. military mission in Iraq ended in 2011; the U.S. mission in Afghanistan continues.

In any war, the service members who deploy to theaters of conflict may be exposed to many hazardous agents and situations, some intentional and many unknown. Some of the exposures may be to chemicals that are, or were, used in civilian life, such as pesticides and fuels, but the duration or frequency of those exposures may be different in the deployment situations. Other potential deployment exposures are chemical and biological agents, mandatory vaccines, oil-well-fire smoke, dust, high ambient temperatures and heat stress, depleted uranium (DU), and pyridostigmine bromide (PB), a prophylactic agent against nerve agent exposure. Veterans who served in the 1990–1991 Gulf War, Post-9/11, and Vietnam conflicts, among others, were subject to a variety of exposures during deployment that have been associated with health effects in veterans and other exposed populations.

In 1998, in response to the health concerns of Gulf War veterans, Congress passed two laws: P.L. 105-277, the Persian Gulf War Veterans Act, and P.L. 105-368, the Veterans Programs Enhancement Act. Those laws directed the Secretary of Veterans Affairs to enter into a contract with the National Academy of Sciences (NAS) to review and evaluate the scientific and medical literature regarding associations between illness and exposure to the toxic agents, environmental and wartime hazards, and preventive medicines and vaccines associated with Gulf War service. Since the legislation, the National Academies of Sciences, Engineering, and Medicine (the National Academies) has prepared more than 10 reports focused on the health of Gulf War veterans.

Veterans' concerns regarding the impact of deployment exposures on their health have grown to include concerns about whether their exposures might adversely affect the health of their children and, possibly, their grandchildren. The National Academies report *Veterans and Agent Orange, Update 2014* examined the potential for such generational effects and recommended areas of research that might elucidate the biological mechanisms associated with them, specifically, the investigation of environmentally induced epigenetic mechanisms and biomarkers of effect.

This *Gulf War and Health, Volume 11* report provides guidance to the Department of Veterans Affairs (VA) on addressing those research recommendations for all veterans. The report also focuses on the assessment of the available evidence on the reproductive effects related to exposures that may have occurred during the Gulf War and Post-9/11conflicts as well as on the health of veterans' children. Finally, the report examines the mechanisms, methods, and feasibility issues of potential research approaches for determining if there are health effects in the children or grandchildren of veterans of any era related to their parents' or grandparents' deployment exposures.

CHARGE TO THE COMMITTEE

The full statement of task for the Gulf War and Health, Volume 11 committee is presented in Box S-1.

THE COMMITTEE'S APPROACH

The Volume 11 committee began its deliberations with public meetings to hear from representatives of VA, academic researchers, interested veterans, and veterans' service organizations and to gather information from representatives of the National Institute for Environmental Health Sciences and its affiliated National Toxicology Program, the Centers for Disease Control and Prevention, and the Department of Defense (DoD). That input helped the committee understand VA's needs, appreciate the veterans' concerns, and be cognizant of complementary efforts already under way at other organizations.

The public meetings helped the committee develop an approach to identify what exposures a veteran might have experienced (e.g., lifestyle, toxicants, stress), how those exposures might be assessed (e.g., how to deal with the variability of exposures and multiple exposures), and what factors might influence the transmission of effects from parent to offspring (e.g., the concentration and timing of the exposure). The committee then considered what reproductive, developmental, and generational effects were already associated with the Gulf War toxicants and what data and knowledge gaps needed to be addressed to understand those effects. These data and information were then used to develop approaches for studying and monitoring potential health problems related to veterans' deployments and their impact on children and grandchildren. The committee's approach to its tasks was driven by the literature as well as by the committee's expertise.

Identification of the Literature

The Volume 11 committee began its work with extensive searches of the scientific literature using five databases: Embase, Medline, Scopus, Proquest, and PubMed. The specific searches targeted (1) studies of the health of Gulf War or Post-9/11 veterans published since the last update, without regard for specific toxicants or outcomes; (2) studies that looked at reproductive effects associated with any

BOX S-1
Statement of Task

An ad hoc committee of the National Academies of Sciences, Engineering, and Medicine will conduct a study to assess the current research available on possible generational health effects that may be the result of exposures experienced by Veterans of the 1990–1991 Gulf War and the Post-9/11 wars during their deployments. The committee will consider which toxicants, including but not limited to burning oil wells, pesticides, nerve agents, prophylactic agents, depleted uranium, and vaccines, are known to be associated with pathophysiological and reproductive, developmental, and teratogenic effects across the lifecourse in parents, offspring, and second-generation offspring.

In addition, the committee will also assess areas requiring further scientific study on the descendants of Veterans with toxic exposures. Finally, the committee will further assess the scope and methodology required to conduct research on such descendants to identify current or possible health effects in the Veterans' descendants, including but not limited to:

- Cellular pathophysiology studies associated with the long-term generational health effects of the toxicants of concern (among these, the committee should consider studies in laboratory animals and other models);
- Multigenerational effects of the toxicants of concern in various animal species, if such effects have not already been well-established;
- The feasibility of conducting a long-term epidemiologic study to assess the generational health effects of Veterans and the resources (technological, logistical) that would need to be available to support such research;
- Develop a framework for monitoring and studying generational health effects over time, including post-exposure assessments, initial screening of Veterans and their descendants, the frequency and duration of such screenings;
- Based upon a careful assessment of available laboratory technologies, establish a process for what is to be included in the screening including biomarkers and early symptoms;
- The number of Veterans and their descendants who should be part of such a study(ies); and
- The appropriate federal agency(ies), e.g., the Department of Defense, the Department of Veterans Affairs, the Department of Health and Human Services, or other organization(s) or collaborative consortia that would be best suited to coordinate and/or conduct the research and screenings on an ongoing basis.

toxicants of concern; and (3) studies of developmental or other health outcomes in children or grandchildren associated with parental exposures to those toxicants. The searches included studies carried out in both human populations and animal and cellular models. The searches retrieved more than 80,000 publications that had appeared through January 2018. To help manage the large volume of data, the committee relied upon existing reviews of epidemiologic and toxicologic data published by authoritative bodies, including prior National Academies committees, the U.S. Environmental Protection Agency, and the Agency for Toxic Substances and Disease Registry.

The paucity of studies on reproductive or developmental effects specific to veterans' exposures during deployment necessitated the identification of populations—mostly occupationally and environmentally exposed cohorts—that had exposures to some of the same toxicants experienced by Gulf War and Post-9/11 veterans. The committee was unable to determine how relevant the exposures in these nonveteran studies are to those experienced by deployed veterans in terms of the exposure magnitude, duration, frequency, mixtures and co-exposures, and population characteristics such as gender, age, ethnicity, and lifestyle. A few studies in veterans were specific to deployment exposures such as studies of the effects of DU. Studies were categorized as reporting reproductive (including adverse pregnancy outcomes), developmental, genetic, or epigenetic effects (see Box S-2).

Categories of Association

The committee determined that it would follow the evaluation processes established by previous Gulf War and Health and other National Academies committees, including the categories of association used by those committees to draw its conclusions regarding the strength of the association between an exposure and various reproductive or developmental health effects. The five categories of association described below have gained wide acceptance by Congress, government agencies (particularly VA), researchers, and veterans groups. They present a common message: the validity of an association is likely to vary to the extent to which common sources of spurious associations can be ruled out as the reason for the observed association. Accordingly, the criteria for each category express a degree of confidence based on the extent to which sources of error were reduced. The committee discussed the evidence and reached consensus on the categorization of the evidence for each toxicant from experimental studies.

Sufficient Evidence of a Causal Relationship

Evidence is sufficient to conclude that a causal relationship exists between being exposed to a toxicant and a reproductive or developmental effect in humans. The evidence fulfills the criteria for sufficient evidence of a causal association in which chance, bias, and confounding can be ruled out with reasonable confidence. The association is supported by a consideration of the consistency of association and biologic plausibility from experimental studies.

Sufficient Evidence of an Association

Evidence suggests an association, in that a positive association has been observed between an exposure and a reproductive or developmental effect in humans; however, there is some doubt as to the influence of chance, bias, and confounding. Experimental animal and cellular studies either supported or diminished the committee's decision in making these associations.

Limited/Suggestive Evidence of an Association

Some evidence of an association between exposure and a reproductive or developmental effect in humans exists, but this is limited by the presence of substantial doubt regarding chance, bias, and confounding. The evidence in experimental animal or cellular models was used to strengthen, or weaken the associations between exposure and effect.

BOX S-2
Effects and Health Outcomes Identified in the Literature

Reproductive effects: any effect on the ability to reproduce

- Effects on male reproduction, including changes in sperm parameters and reproductive hormones, infertility, time to pregnancy;
- Effects on female reproduction, including effects on menstrual cycle, endometriosis, infertility, time to pregnancy, changes in reproductive hormones;
- Adverse pregnancy outcomes, including
  - Maternal health, such as gestational diabetes, gestational hypertension, and inflammation during pregnancy; and
  - Birth outcomes, such as preterm birth, birth weight or size, spontaneous abortion, and still birth.

Developmental effects: any adverse health effects in children or offspring of any age, including reproductive effects

- Neurodevelopmental deficits, including measures of cognition (IQ, attention, motor skills, etc.), autism spectrum disorders, attention deficit disorders;
- Respiratory effects, including respiratory symptoms (e.g., wheezing), lung function, asthma, respiratory infections;
- Childhood cancers;
- Birth defects;
- Immune outcomes: eczema, dermatomyositis;
- Obesity and metabolism; and
- Growth.

Epigenetic and genetic effects, including

- Markers of DNA oxidative stress;
- DNA methylation in maternal blood, umbilical cord blood, placenta, or peripheral blood lymphocytes, sperm;
- mRNA expression;
- Histone modifications; and
- Mitochondrial DNA content in umbilical cord blood.

Inadequate/Insufficient Evidence to Determine Whether an Association Exists

The available studies are of insufficient quantity, quality, validity, consistency, or statistical power to permit a conclusion regarding the presence or absence of an association between an exposure and a reproductive or developmental effect in humans. Evidence in experimental animal studies may have provided additional support for these assessments, but, in the absence of human data, it was not used to strengthen the categorization of the association. In some cases, the body of evidence is too small to permit conclusions, such as when there are no available studies to validate or corroborate the findings of a single study. In other cases, there is evidence from human or animal studies, but the heterogeneity of exposures, outcomes, and methods leads to inconsistent findings that preclude the committee from identifying an association between exposure and effect.

Limited/Suggestive Evidence of No Association

There are several adequate studies, covering the full range of levels of exposure that humans are known to encounter, that are consistent in not showing an association between an exposure and a reproductive or developmental effect. A conclusion of no association is inevitably limited to the conditions, levels of exposure, and length of observation covered by the available studies. In addition, the possibility of a very small increase in risk at the levels of exposure studied can never be excluded. Experimental animal studies were examined to support such findings.

FINDINGS AND CONCLUSIONS

The committee organized the toxicants of concern into four groups: deployment-related exposures, pesticides, combustion products and fuels, and solvents. Deployment-related exposures included deployment itself, vaccines, chemical warfare agents, infectious diseases, DU, hexavalent chromium, and PB. The committee's conclusions for each toxicant of concern are listed in Box S-3 (reproductive effects, adverse pregnancy outcomes, and developmental effects). No toxicant had sufficient evidence of a causal association between exposure and reproductive or developmental effects, nor did any toxicant have limited/suggestive evidence of no association between exposure and reproductive or developmental effects.

The committee emphasizes the need to interpret the conclusions in this report and any future research within the broader context of both the veterans' and their descendants' exposures over the course of their lives. Exposures across the lifecourse, beginning in utero, can have an impact on health, including that of future children. Those exposures, such as nutritional exposure and exposure to toxicants, may interact with one another and be influenced by the genetic and epigenetic background of cells. Such changes are being studied, but at present there is insufficient evidence to link any deployment exposures to epigenetic[1] effects.

Animal Studies

The committee made its decisions concerning associations between deployment exposures and reproductive and developmental effects primarily on the basis of human data, using animal and cellular data to provide additional support. For some toxicants, however, the animal data were robust, but the lack of human data precluded the committee from assigning a category of association that reflected a stronger level of association. These toxicants include the following:

- Depleted uranium and reproductive effects in males;
- Lindane and reproductive effects in males and developmental effects in offspring;
- Toluene and developmental effects in offspring;

[1] *Genetics* is the study of deoxyribonucleic acid (DNA) and the genes it encodes, sometimes referred to as the genome when referencing the totality of the DNA (and all the genes) of an organism. *Epigenetics* is the study of processes that cause heritable changes in gene expression without changing DNA sequence. The epigenome is composed of chemical modifications made to DNA and the histone proteins that make up chromatin. "Heritable" in this context can refer to inheritance not only between parents and offspring (generational or meiotic inheritance of epigenetic alterations) but also between parent and daughter cells.

- Xylenes and developmental effects in offspring;
- Trichloroethylene and reproductive effects in females; and
- Dioxins and reproductive effects in males and females.

Although animal and cellular models permit defined exposures, they may lack temporal resolution since only specific points in time are considered, and they may not model the cumulative effects of exposures to mixtures that are observed in humans. In addition, adsorption, distribution, metabolism, and excretion processes and organ systems can vary widely among humans and other species, and effects seen in one species might not be seen in another. Because of these species differences, the committee cautions that even robust animal data must be interpreted with caution.

HEALTH MONITORING AND RESEARCH PROGRAM

To help determine if veterans' descendants are at risk for health effects resulting from the veterans' exposures during deployment, the committee has proposed creating a health monitoring and research program (HMRP) with three arms: monitoring the health of veterans and their descendants over time; epidemiologic studies to examine groups of veterans and their descendants for health outcomes of concern; and basic and translational research to help address data and knowledge gaps. The HMRP might base some of its work upon the health effects identified for the deployment toxicants considered by the committee in this report, but it would need to be tailored to specific questions.

Potential epidemiologic studies may be nested within the HMRP, make use of the data collected by the HMRP, or identify cases among HMRP participants. In addition, researchers who are not affiliated with the HMRP may also conduct epidemiologic studies simultaneously. Epidemiologic studies might focus on a specific veteran cohort (e.g., veterans who served in Vietnam) or specific exposures (e.g., sarin) or examine specific outcomes in children and grandchildren (e.g., birth defects or neurodevelopment). The pathophysiologic research program, described later, would emphasize the use of basic research studies to help elucidate cellular processes that may be responsible for generational health effects.

The committee's framework for developing an HMRP begins with defining the program's scope. The program scope will guide the recruiting and enrolling of the HMRP participants—active-duty service members, reservists, veterans, and their descendants—now and in the future as well as the collection and maintenance of each participant's data. Establishing the program's scope and goals early in the process will provide not only the overarching framework for the program but also a platform to establish communication with veterans, their descendants, and collaborators, thus helping to promote clarity and transparency, prevent redundancies, and optimize the use of resources.

The committee suggests that pilot programs be conducted to determine the feasibility of collection strategies, to establish the linkages for appropriate use of data, to assess response rates among veterans and their descendants, or to test surveys or other data collection methods. Focus groups and other exploratory strategies can help identify the specific exposures, health effects, populations, datasets, and logistics that are most appropriate for the study and that best respond to VA's needs and veterans' concerns.

An HMRP that includes participant recruitment at enlistment will ensure that a sufficient sample size is available to observe small effects in veterans and provide a mechanism to contact dependents (partners and children). By enrolling all new recruits as they enter DoD using an opt-out approach, a baseline of health status, including information on lifestyle and environment as well as biological samples, can be established prior to deployment. This approach will also facilitate the tracking of exposures associated with each deployment or occupational assignment. As service members transition from DoD to VA, the follow-up will be challenging and will require concerted approaches and coordination to identify and

BOX S-3
Summary of Conclusions Regarding Categories of Association Between Gulf War Deployment Exposures and Reproductive Effects, Adverse Pregnancy Outcomes, or Developmental Effects

Sufficient Evidence of a Causal Relationship

- None

Sufficient Evidence of an Association

- Leishmaniasis infection during pregnancy and adverse pregnancy outcomes
- Hexavalent chromium and reproductive effects in men
- Prenatal exposure to hexavalent chromium and developmental effects
- Prenatal exposure to organophosphate pesticides and neurodevelopmental effects
- Carbamate pesticides and reproductive effects in men
- Prenatal exposure to particulate matter and adverse pregnancy outcomes—low birth weight and preterm birth
- Prenatal exposure to benzene and childhood leukemia

Limited/Suggestive Evidence of an Association

- Sulfur mustard and reproductive effects in men
- Hexavalent chromium and adverse pregnancy outcomes
- Organophosphate pesticides and reproductive effects in men
- Pyrethroid pesticides and reproductive effects in men
- Lindane and reproductive effects in women
- Prenatal exposure to pyrethroid pesticides and developmental effects
- Prenatal exposure to particulate matter and pregnancy-induced hypertensive disorders
- Prenatal exposure to particulate matter and respiratory or neurodevelopmental effects in children
- Polycyclic aromatic hydrocarbons and reproductive effects in men
- Prenatal exposure to polycyclic aromatic hydrocarbons and adverse birth outcomes—low birth weight and preterm birth, or developmental effects—birth defects, childhood cancer, neurodevelopmental effects, and respiratory outcomes in childhood
- Benzene and reproductive effects in men
- Trichloroethylene and reproductive effects in men, or adverse pregnancy outcomes
- Prenatal exposure to trichloroethylene and developmental effects
- Prenatal exposure to perchloroethylene and developmental effects
- Glycols and glycol ethers and reproductive effects in men
- Prenatal exposure to glycols or glycol ethers and birth defects

Inadequate/Insufficient Evidence to Determine Whether an Association Exists

- Deployment and reproductive or developmental effects
- Sarin/cyclosarin and reproductive or developmental effects
- Sulfur mustard and reproductive effects in women, adverse pregnancy outcomes, or developmental effects
- Leishmaniasis and reproductive or developmental effects
- Anthrax vaccination and reproductive or developmental effects
- Depleted uranium and reproductive or developmental effects
- Pyridostigmine bromide and reproductive or developmental effects
- Hexavalent chromium and reproductive effects in women
- Organophosphate pesticides and reproductive effects in women, or adverse pregnancy outcomes
- Prenatal exposure to organophosphate pesticides and other developmental effects (other than neurodevelopmental effects)
- Carbamate pesticides and reproductive effects in women, or adverse pregnancy outcomes
- Prenatal exposure to carbamates and developmental effects
- Pyrethroid pesticides and reproductive effects in women, or adverse pregnancy outcomes
- Lindane and reproductive effect in men or developmental effects
- DEET and reproductive or developmental effects
- Particulate matter and reproductive effects in men and women
- Prenatal exposure to particulate matter and other developmental effects (other than respiratory and neurodevelopmental effects)
- Polycyclic aromatic hydrocarbons and reproductive effects in women
- Prenatal polycyclic aromatic hydrocarbons exposure and other developmental effects (other than birth defects, childhood cancer, neurodevelopmental effects, and respiratory outcomes in childhood)
- Polychlorinated dibenzodioxins and polychlorinated dibenzofurans and reproductive or developmental effects
- Exhaust and reproductive or developmental effects
- Fuels and reproductive or developmental effects
- Benzene and reproductive effects in women, or adverse pregnancy outcomes
- Prenatal exposure to benzene and other developmental effects in children (other than childhood leukemia)
- Toluene and reproductive or developmental effects
- Xylenes and reproductive or developmental effects
- Trichloroethylene and reproductive effects in women
- Perchloroethylene and reproductive effects in men and women, or adverse pregnancy outcomes
- Glycols and glycol ethers and reproductive effects in women, or adverse pregnancy outcomes
- Prenatal exposure to glycols or glycol ethers and any other developmental effects (other than birth defects)

Limited/Suggestive Evidence of No Association

- None

engage the veterans in the HMRP. Not all service members are eligible for care in VA, and thus not all are captured in the VA databases. Veterans who enter the VA health care system will be easier to identify, whereas veterans who do not enter the system may be difficult to locate and recruit.

The enrollment of active-duty service members' partners could begin with the partners' entry into the Military Health System/TRICARE system as beneficiaries, with follow-up being carried out for the duration of their eligibility for TRICARE. Partners may provide information on their own exposures that may affect the health of veterans' children and may also represent a valuable source of information about those children's health.

The recruitment and enrollment of, engagement with, and collection of data from veterans, partners, and the children themselves will be essential elements of the HMRP. Recruiting the children may begin with those who are born to an active-duty service member and covered under TRICARE so as to facilitate access to the child's health records. The recruitment and follow-up of older children will present additional feasibility and ethical challenges. All these populations will require appropriate participant consent, which may be modeled after existing long-term follow-up studies that collect data on children, including the National Health and Nutrition Examination Survey, the Environmental Influences on Child Health Outcomes program, or the Growing Up Today Study.

The analysis of biospecimens from HMRP participants will require the identification of appropriate sample collection and storage systems and equipment (e.g., laboratory facilities and biorepositories) as well as well-controlled and standardized protocols. For example, blood, urine, and semen samples should be collected from service members at their entry into the military, prior to each deployment, and after each deployment. After their separation from the military, veterans participating in the HMRP could provide additional samples on a periodic basis.

Deployment and occupational exposures may result in or contribute to a biological response that ultimately manifests itself as adverse health effects in the veteran or his or her descendants. The veterans' exposure to stressors (nutritional, psychological, biological, physical, and chemical) during preconception and in utero development may affect the health of their descendants. Although the committee suggests that biological samples be collected periodically from service members, individual validated measures of exposure are not available for veterans of any era, and the estimates of exposure often rely on self-reported information or military records of incidents of exposure.

When children are born following a parent's deployment, they too may be monitored during their lifecourse to determine what, if any, health effects they may experience, compared with children of veterans who were not deployed or other reference populations. Data collected directly from children can be used to document outcomes and assess the risk factors present throughout the children's lives, such as air pollution or occupational factors. Data collection may begin with the electronic health records (EHRs) of children born in the TRICARE system, including information in the DoD Birth and Infant Health Registry.

New methodologies and efficiencies are available for identifying the population to be sampled, issuing invitations, determining the what and how of data collection and analyses, using incentives for recruiting and retaining participants, and using reminders to increase response rates. As the collected data will be both electronic and biologic, adequate preparation to receive, catalog, and maintain multiple forms of information will be important. The data analysis will require linking databases and statistical software, particularly VA and DoD EHRs and other records, and potentially other databases (e.g., of the Centers for Medicare & Medicaid Services and state cancer registries).

Program management is a critical, integral, and continuous function of an HMRP. Addressing the many requirements and opportunities of an HMRP will require the identification of lead organizations to design and implement the program and studies. These may be VA, DoD, the National Institutes of

Health, or other organizations, such as academic research centers or consortia. Close coordination and collaboration among the program partners will be critical to increase efficiency, to avoid duplicate efforts, and for accountability. Different partners may have different strengths, including the availability of subject matter experts, access to relevant data or records, and strong information technology capabilities. Limitations might include a lack of legislative mandates to participate in the program, financial constraints, and a lack of familiarity with program data requirements, each of which can be addressed through a multi-organization, nationwide, collaborative effort among the participants. In particular, sufficient information technology capabilities, combined with linked medical records from DoD and VA and potentially from other participants, will be critical elements of these research efforts.

Publishing the program's results will ensure that veterans and their descendants are aware of the findings, positive or negative, that may affect their health and well-being. This dissemination to a broader audience, including researchers and the general public, can spur interest in the program and its activities. Finally, the HMRP needs to be evaluated on a continuing and regularly scheduled basis. Without an adequate review of all aspects of the program, resources may not be efficiently used, data collection and analysis may lag, and veterans and their descendants may be participating in a program that does not serve their needs.

The committee finds that it may be possible to implement parts of the proposed HMRP and hypothesis-driven studies by leveraging ongoing programs. The committee examined a number of ongoing research programs, including the VA-sponsored Million Veteran Program (MVP) and the DoD-sponsored Millennium Cohort (MilCo) and MilCo Family Study as well as the DoD Birth and Infant Health Registry and the DoD Serum Repository. Building on and coordinating among these existing health monitoring and epidemiologic research programs can reduce costs, expedite data collection, and provide access to already engaged study populations.

PATHOPHYSIOLOGIC STUDIES

While there is a growing base of human and animal evidence concerning the reproductive and developmental effects of many of the toxicants of concern to veterans and their descendants, there is a dearth of information on the specific effects of veterans' exposures on their children, grandchildren, and great-grandchildren. Furthermore, although targeted epidemiologic studies are being designed, it may be years or decades before the effects (if any) of parental exposures are evident in a future generation. Such studies may not capture rare events that occur only in a few descendants, as a result of a narrow range of exposures, or in those instances where specific genotypes interact with specific exposures. Basic and translational research in model systems—in vitro systems that use cells and tissues as well as whole animals—where both genetics and exposures can be controlled as well as generational animal studies that can be conducted in days or months provide powerful opportunities to assess biological plausibility, gain mechanistic insights, and address the complexities inherent in human studies. Such studies may detect subtle effects; follow genetic or epigenetic changes at the cellular and whole-animal levels, including effects on germ cells; assess impacts on reproductive function; and identify susceptible phenotypes.

The results of studies in model organisms need to be extrapolated to humans to enhance understanding of the reproductive, developmental, and generational effects of toxicant exposures across the exposure → effect → outcome pathway. Understanding the range of biological diversity across animal species—including humans—can help achieve this goal. For example, it has been shown that the gene for the aryl hydrocarbon receptor that mediates dioxin toxicity shows sensitivity differences among mouse strains; between rats, mice, and guinea pigs; and among humans. Knowledge about what those differences are makes it possible to estimate human risk from rodent studies.

Basic and translational research can also identify targets and mechanisms to help identify biomarkers of exposure, effect, and susceptibility for a toxicant or stressor; explore factors that underlie individual variation in response to an exposure, such as the impact of sex differences on response to a toxicant; and identify susceptible cell types (e.g., somatic cells, eggs, sperm) for specific exposures. Basic and translational research should include developing the following: fit-for-purpose models and reagents for generational studies; genetically engineered induced pluripotent stem cells; validated models (animal- and cell-based) that are most appropriate for studying specific exposures; and methods and databases for acquiring, curating, and analyzing the resulting datasets.

Studies should focus on deployment-specific exposures (single-agent or mixtures), although using surrogate exposures in reproductive or multigenerational studies may be adequate if that use is sufficiently responsive to research needs. Knowledge gaps to be addressed relate to the adverse reproductive effects in veterans and the developmental effects of these exposures in offspring, including details about windows of susceptibility, dose–response relationships, duration, and co-exposures (mixtures).

Both genetic and epigenetic alterations induced by environmental exposures can cause changes that result in reproductive, developmental, or generational effects. Although a few of the toxicants considered in this report are known to be reproductive or developmental toxicants or mutagens (e.g., benzene), there is little evidence that if a parent is exposed prior to the child's conception these toxicants affect germ cells in such a way as to cause developmental effects in offspring. What effects occur in parental germ cells, what happens after exposure ceases, and if and how lifecourse events compound epigenetic alterations are crucial knowledge gaps. Focused research on the transmission, persistence, gene *x* environment interactions, and modifiers (e.g., stress, diet) of genetic and epigenetic effects is necessary to understand the impact of deployment exposures on veterans and their descendants.

MOVING FORWARD

As the committee completed its review of the epidemiologic and toxicologic literature on the Gulf War and Post-9/11 toxicants of concern, a framework for an HMRP was developed and an agenda for basic and translational research on generational effects laid out. Several scientific priorities became evident during the course of the committee's deliberations. Addressing these priorities will be critical to implementing a functional and useful HMRP and a concrete agenda to answer questions about the reproductive, developmental, and generational health effects of deployment exposures. These priorities include the following:

- **The collection, storage, and maintenance of comprehensive baseline and longitudinal data and biospecimens from veterans, their partners, and their descendants;**
- **A detailed characterization and assessment of exposures during and after deployment; and**
- **The development, evaluation, standardization, and interoperability of biomarkers of exposure, susceptibility, and biological effects.**

The Volume 11 committee acknowledges that the creation of new large-scale HMRPs designed specifically to address the question of whether descendants of deployed veterans are at increased risk of adverse health effects will be an ambitious undertaking. Several important issues need to be addressed in order to optimize an HMRP, including the collection of complete and accessible health information on veterans as they enter the military and before and after deployments; developing better deployment and occupational exposure assessments based on environmental and biological sampling; and access to and the follow-up of partners, children, and grandchildren over time.

An integrated EHR system between DoD and VA (under development) not only will improve the transition of veterans from one health care system to another but also will provide access to longitudinal health data, particularly those related to reproductive and birth outcomes. Access to electronic health data will also be essential for the large number of veterans who receive care at ancillary facilities or outside the VA system.

The lack of exposure monitoring during deployments, whether at the individual or the military-unit level, precludes an adequate assessment of the nature, duration, and frequency of deployment exposures. This limitation is exacerbated by the lack of information on lifecourse exposures and on the toxicologic effects of complex chemical mixtures that are often encountered with environmental and occupational exposures. Importantly, the capture of health information on veterans' partners and their children and grandchildren from health systems that are often fractured and location-specific will pose unique challenges.

Implementing and maintaining an HMRP and a basic research agenda will require a consistent and committed funding stream. The costs of designing and conducting an HMRP for any veteran cohort will be considerable, as demonstrated by the cost of similar programs such as the National Children's Study and the All of Us Research Program. However, while the costs of an HMRP may be substantial, the costs of some of the underlying technologies—such as whole-genome sequencing—have plummeted, and the preemptive health program and research results may translate into significant cost savings for the nation.

There are numerous resource, methodologic, and organizational considerations that must be addressed across several governmental agencies—and, likely, private organizations as well—to implement a large-scale HMRP of the magnitude envisioned and recommended by the Volume 11 committee. Critical considerations include financial and human resource costs, the availability and expertise of adequately trained personnel, the time required for project completion, technologic competencies, ready access to well-curated data, the maintenance of confidential human health data, ethical considerations for investigations that include parents and children, and the implementation of appropriate health and risk communication strategies between and among organizations and veterans and their families. Given these considerations, the committee proposes that a practical and expedient approach to exploring generational health effects should leverage ongoing veteran's health research programs, such as the MVP and the MilCo study. In addition, the newly established partnership between MVP and All of Us may prove extremely useful. This approach would greatly benefit from past investments and take advantage of existing infrastructure to address some of the critical issues identified in this report. These programs have already enrolled large cohorts and are linked to a variety of large data sources, and some of them already have in place protocols for the collection of biological specimens and the participation of partners and children.

In conclusion, the committee commends the efforts of VA and Congress to address veterans' concerns about generational health effects. The path forward demands an understanding of certain critical issues that will define the success of the program. The committee believes that the results and deliverables that arise from studying generational effects will ultimately be rewarded with new knowledge of veterans' exposures, their reproductive health, and the health of their children and grandchildren. Importantly, the knowledge and understanding derived from these investments will be relevant to the health of all Americans now and for future generations.

1

Introduction

U.S. service members who deploy outside the United States may encounter chemical, biological, physiological, radiological, and psychological exposures they may never have experienced during military service in the United States or as civilians. These potential exposures include chemical warfare agents, vaccines for anthrax, vector-borne diseases such as malaria, extreme heat and cold, and the stresses of being in a war zone. Some of the exposures may be to chemicals that are, or were, used in civilian life, such pesticides and fuels, but the duration or frequency of those exposures may be different in deployment situations. Veterans who served in the Vietnam, 1990–1991 Gulf War, and Post-9/11 conflicts have a variety of health effects that are associated with their deployment exposures. In some cases, those health effects can be long-lasting and affect reproductive functions. Veterans are understandably concerned that their exposures during their deployments might have caused or might be the cause of adverse health effects in their children and possibly their grandchildren.

The National Academies of Sciences, Engineering, and Medicine's (the National Academies') *Veterans and Agent Orange: Update 2014* highlighted some of the areas of research that might shed light on the biological mechanisms associated with generational effects and also addressed issues related to the feasibility of research designed to investigate these concerns (NASEM, 2016a). Specifically, the report recommended that the Department of Veterans Affairs (VA) encourage the investigation of epigenetic[1] changes in somatic tissues, germ cells, and epigenetic changes that take place during gestation. The report also supports research to identify specific markers of environmentally induced epigenetic activity. Such research efforts may help elucidate the mechanisms responsible for adverse health effects in exposed individuals or their offspring. In part, the present report provides guidance to VA on how to address those research recommendations.

This *Gulf War and Health, Volume 11* report examines the long-term health consequences of military service in the Gulf War. While the previous 10 volumes focused on the health of Gulf War veterans, this

[1] *Epigenetics* is most commonly taken to refer to heritable changes in gene expression that do not result from change in actual gene sequences. ("Heritable" here can refer to inheritance not only between parents and offspring but also between parent and daughter cells.)

volume includes an assessment of reproductive effects related to exposures that may have occurred during the Post-9/11 conflicts as well as any effects on the health of any children born after both Gulf War and Post-9/11 exposures. This report also examines the mechanisms, methods, and feasibility issues of potential investigations intended to help determine if there are health effects in children or grandchildren of veterans, of any era, related to their parents' or grandparents' deployment exposures.

THE GULF WAR AND POST-9/11 CONFLICTS

In response to the invasion of Kuwait by Iraq in August 1990, the United States led a coalition of 34 countries, including the United Kingdom, Australia, Canada, France, and Denmark, in a buildup of forces in the Persian Gulf called Operation Desert Shield. This multinational effort was followed by Operation Desert Storm, which began in January 1991 and was over by the end of February. Over the course of the buildup and war, almost 700,000 U.S. troops were deployed to the Persian Gulf region, although by June 1991 only about 50,000 U.S. troops remained in the area. Although brief, with relatively few injuries and deaths among the coalition forces, the legacy of the war has been a large contingent of veterans who suffer from a number of health problems, particularly Gulf War illness,[2] which have persisted for more than 25 years (NASEM, 2016).

The U.S. military engaged in further conflicts in the Middle East following the terrorist attacks of September 11, 2001. Operation Enduring Freedom (OEF) began in October 2001, with troops stationed in and around Afghanistan for military and humanitarian purposes. Operation Iraqi Freedom (OIF) began in March 2003 as American-led coalition forces invaded Iraq, and it officially ended on August 31, 2010. Operation New Dawn (OND) was initiated on September 1, 2010, to reflect the changing mission of and reduction in U.S. military personnel in Iraq, and it officially ended on December 15, 2011. The U.S. military mission in Iraq ended in 2011; the U.S. mission in Afghanistan continues.

The operation of the 1990–1991 Gulf War reflected a number of changes from previous wars, particularly in the demographic composition of military personnel. Military personnel were, overall, men who were older than those who had participated in previous wars, with a mean age of 28 years (Joseph, 1997). There were also more women (almost 7%), parents, and activated members of the reserves and National Guard (about 17%, or 106,000), who were temporarily uprooted from their civilian lives (VA, 2011). As of 2014, more than 2.6 million service members have served in Iraq and Afghanistan, and almost half have deployed to the region more than once (VA, 2015). As of 2010, 15.5% of all military personnel and nearly one-fourth of Army reserves were women (Reynolds and Shendruk, 2018).

During the Gulf War and Post-9/11 conflicts, service members who were deployed to the theater of conflict were potentially exposed to hazardous agents and situations, both known and unknown, many of which were unique to those conflicts. Because Iraq had been known to use chemical and possibly biological agents against its own people and others, many Gulf War service members received mandatory vaccines to prevent anthrax and botulism. Pyridostigmine bromide (PB) was first used as a prophylaxis against potential nerve agent exposure in the Gulf War. Both the Gulf War and Post-9/11 conflicts included exposures to depleted uranium in munitions. Gulf War service members were also exposed to oil-well-fire smoke from the burning oil wells in Kuwait. Veterans of both the Gulf War and Post-9/11 conflicts were exposed to dust, dust storms, excessive heat, pesticides, chemical-agent-resistant coating paint, and diesel fuels, among other exposures. Military field operations also generated large quantities of waste; it has been estimated that 8–10 pounds of solid waste per person per day were generated

[2] Gulf War illness is characterized by persistent symptoms of fatigue, mood and cognition problems, musculoskeletal pain, sleep disturbance, and neurologic, respiratory, skin, and gastrointestinal problems (NASEM, 2016).

at the military bases in Iraq and Afghanistan, although this number varied depending on the base and its population (Faulkner, 2011). A wide variety of refuse was burned, from food and human waste to packaging and equipment, as well as materials abandoned by the enemy. Thus, the characterization of exposures and their associated health effects is complicated by the possible exposure to multiple chemical and biologic agents, repeated exposures to those agents, a dearth of environmental sampling data, and individual variability. While some of these exposures were documented in medical records or via air sampling, many were not.

LEGISLATIVE ACTIONS

In response to the growing concerns of Gulf War veterans about their health, Congress passed two laws in 1998: P.L. 105-277, the Persian Gulf War Veterans Act, and P.L. 105-368, the Veterans Programs Enhancement Act. The goals of these laws were to identify what health outcomes might be expected from the environmental agents to which veterans had been exposed during their deployments and to require VA to treat those health outcomes (see Box 1-1 for a list of the toxicants of concern). The laws directed the Secretary of Veterans Affairs to enter into a contract with the National Academy of Sciences (NAS, now part of the National Academies) to review and evaluate the scientific and medical literature regarding associations between illness and exposure to toxic agents, environmental or wartime hazards, or preventive medicines or vaccines associated with Gulf War service and to consider the NAS conclusions when making decisions about compensation.

The Persian Gulf War legislation directs the National Academies to study diverse biologic, radiologic, chemical, and physical agents. Exposures to some Gulf War agents have been extensively studied and characterized, primarily in occupational settings (for example, exposure to pesticides, solvents, and fuels). However, exposures to other agents have not been studied or characterized in human populations (for example, exposure to nerve agents or oil-well-fire smoke) (NASEM, 2016b).

In December 2016, Congress passed P.L. 114-315, also known as the Jeff Miller and Richard Blumenthal Veterans Health Care and Benefits Improvement Act of 2016; section 632 of that law again called on VA to contract with the National Academies to examine the "scientific research regarding the descendants of individuals and veterans with toxic exposure." The law requests that the National Academies conduct a review of the toxicologic and epidemiologic literature and areas needing further study relating to descendants of veterans with toxic exposures. It further asks for details regarding the scope, methodology, and feasibility of any future study and other agencies suited to conduct such research.

GULF WAR AND HEALTH AND RELATED REPORTS

The National Academies has previously prepared numerous studies on the health of Gulf War and other veterans, including Vietnam veterans. As a result of 1998 legislation, the National Academies has conducted more than 10 studies and updates in the *Gulf War and Health* series on veterans' exposures and the health effects associated with those exposures:

- *Volume 1: Depleted Uranium, Pyridostigmine Bromide, Sarin, and Vaccines* (IOM, 2000)
- *Volume 2: Insecticides and Solvents* (IOM, 2003)
- *Updated Literature Review of Sarin* (IOM, 2004)
- *Volume 3: Fuels, Combustion Products, and Propellants* (IOM, 2005)
- *Amyotrophic Lateral Sclerosis in Veterans: Review of the Scientific Literature* (IOM, 2006a)
- *Volume 4: Health Effects of Serving in the Gulf War* (IOM, 2006b)

BOX 1-1
Toxicants of Concern

Agents Specified in P.L. 105-368 and P.L. 105-277

(A) The following organophosphorous pesticides:
- (i) Chlorpyrifos.
- (ii) Diazinon.
- (iii) Dichlorvos.
- (iv) Malathion.

(B) The following carbamate pesticides:
- (i) Proxpur.
- (ii) Carbaryl.
- (iii) Methomyl.

(C) The carbamate pyridostigmine bromide used as nerve agent prophylaxis.

(D) The following chlorinated hydrocarbons and other pesticides and repellents:
- (i) Lindane.
- (ii) Pyrethrins.
- (iii) Permethrins.
- (iv) Rodenticides (bait).
- (v) Repellent (DEET).

(E) The following low-level nerve agents and precursor compounds at exposure levels below those which produce immediately apparent incapacitating symptoms:
- (i) Sarin.
- (ii) Tabun.

- *Volume 5: Infectious Diseases* (IOM, 2007)
- *Updated Literature Review of Depleted Uranium* (IOM, 2008a)
- *Volume 6: Physiologic, Psychologic, and Psychosocial Effects of Deployment-Related Stress* (IOM, 2008b)
- *Volume 7: Long-Term Consequences of Traumatic Brain Injury* (IOM, 2009)
- *Volume 8: Update of Health Effects of Serving in the Gulf War* (IOM, 2010)
- *Volume 9: Long-Term Effects of Blast Exposures* (IOM, 2014)
- *Volume 10: Update of Health Effects of Serving in the Gulf War, 2016* (NASEM, 2016b)

Beginning with volume 1 of the *Gulf War and Health* series, National Academies' committees developed a process for assessing the evidence for each study and reaching conclusions regarding the weight of the evidence for each exposure or environmental agent and possible health outcomes (see

(F) The following synthetic chemical compounds:
- (i) Mustard agents at levels below those which cause immediate blistering.
- (ii) Volatile organic compounds.
- (iii) Hydrazine.
- (iv) Red fuming nitric acid.
- (v) Solvents.

(G) The following sources of radiation:
- (i) Depleted uranium.
- (ii) Microwave radiation.
- (iii) Radio frequency radiation.

(H) The following environmental particulates and pollutants:
- (i) Hydrogen sulfide.
- (ii) Oil fire byproducts.
- (iii) Diesel heater fumes.
- (iv) Sand micro-particles.

(I) Diseases endemic to the region (including the following):
- (i) Leishmaniasis.
- (ii) Sandfly fever.
- (iii) Pathogenic Escherichia coli.
- (iv) Shigellosis.

(J) Time compressed administration of multiple live, attenuated, and toxoid vaccines.

Additional Toxicants of Concern

Resmethrin
Fuels
Combustion products (including particulate matter, polycyclic aromatic hydrocarbons, dioxin, and exhaust)
Hexavalent chromium

Chapter 2). Because each committee was composed of different experts and the exposures to be assessed varied for each report, each committee made slight modifications to the assessment process. Although the first three volumes of the *Gulf War and Health* series dealt with specific environmental agents, in 2005, VA requested that the National Academies appoint a committee to review the medical literature and to summarize what was known then about the current status of Gulf War veterans' health. The resulting report, volume 4, and two subsequent updates, volumes 8 and 10, summarized the overall health effects in veterans and noted which health outcomes were more evident in veterans who had deployed to the Persian Gulf region than in their nondeployed counterparts, irrespective of the specific exposures experienced by the deployed veterans. Volumes 6, 7, and 9 deviated from the rest of the series with a broader scope to include Post-9/11 veterans; volume 6 also included and addressed Vietnam veterans. All these efforts assessed reproductive effects in veterans and developmental effects in their children based on the evidence available at that time.

The National Academies has also produced other reports of relevance to this report beginning with four reports published after the 1990–1991 Gulf War, but prior to the Post-9/11 conflicts in Afghanistan and Iraq: *Health Consequences of Service During the Persian Gulf War: Recommendations for Research and Information Systems* (IOM, 1996); *Strategies to Protect the Health of Deployed U.S. Forces: Medical Surveillance, Record Keeping, and Risk Reduction* (IOM, 1999); *Strategies to Protect the Health of Deployed U.S. Forces: Analytical Framework for Assessing Risks* (NRC, 2000a); and *Strategies to Protect the Health of Deployed U.S. Forces: Assessing Health Risks to Deployed U.S. Forces, Workshop Proceedings* (NRC, 2000b). These studies provide a roadmap for DoD to identify and assess the potential health effects from the toxicants to which U.S. service members may be exposed during any deployment, including the use of environmental and biological sampling. In response to veterans' concerns about exposure to burn pits, *The Long-Term Health Consequences of Exposure to Burn Pits in Iraq and Afghanistan* report was released (IOM, 2011); this study built on the earlier *Review of the Department of Defense Enhanced Particulate Matter Surveillance Program Report* (NRC, 2010). Health effects for the several toxicants of concern—particularly trichloroethylene, tetrachloroethylene, and benzene—were also evaluated in *Contaminated Water Supplies at Camp Lejeune: Assessing Potential Health Effects* (NRC, 2009).

CHARGE TO THE COMMITTEE

In response to veterans' concerns about the health of their children and grandchildren as legislated in P.L. 114-315, VA asked the National Academies to examine the potential health effects of deployment-related exposures on veterans and on their children and grandchildren and to provide guidance on a path forward for research in this area. The committee's full statement of task is given in Box 1-2. The committee organized its approach to its statement into two tasks. Task 1 is an update of prior *Gulf War and Health* reports, but with a focus on the reproductive and developmental effects that might occur in, respectively, veterans and their offspring following exposure to the many agents listed in Box 1-1. Task 2 is the development of a framework for a health monitoring program as well as an approach to designing epidemiologic studies to identify any reproductive or developmental studies in veterans and their descendants. Task 2 also includes an in-depth discussion of potential cellular and animal pathophysiological studies that might provide important information to address the many data gaps identified throughout both tasks 1 and 2. The committee's approach to its statement of task is discussed in more detail in Chapter 2.

ORGANIZATION OF THE REPORT

Chapter 2 explains the committee's approach to the statement of task given in Box 1-2. It provides an overview of how the committee assessed exposures that might have been experienced by Gulf War and Post-9/11 veterans and how it evaluated the literature and came to its conclusions, along with a description of the categories of association that are used to determine the strength of an association between an exposure and a reproductive or developmental health effect. Chapter 3 provides background information on how environmental exposures can affect the genome and epigenome, explains how those changes may be transmitted to descendants, and gives context for this new and evolving field of research. Chapters 4 through 7 are updates of what is known about the reproductive and developmental effects that are associated with exposures to many of the toxicants listed in Box 1-1. Specifically, Chapter 4 examines deployment-related exposures, such as to chemical warfare agents and vaccines, as well as new studies comparing deployed versus nondeployed veterans; Chapter 5 focuses on exposures to

BOX 1-2
Statement of Task

An ad hoc committee of the National Academies of Sciences, Engineering, and Medicine will conduct a study to assess the current research available on possible generational health effects that may be the result of exposures experienced by veterans of the 1990–1991 Gulf War and the Post-9/11 wars during their deployments. The committee will consider which toxicants, including but not limited to burning oil wells, pesticides, nerve agents, prophylactic agents, depleted uranium, and vaccines, are known to be associated with pathophysiological and reproductive, developmental, and teratogenic effects across the lifecourse in parents, offspring, and second-generation offspring.

In addition, the committee will also assess areas requiring further scientific study on the descendants of veterans with toxic exposures. Finally, the committee will further assess the scope and methodology required to conduct research on such descendants to identify current or possible health effects in the veterans' descendants, including but not limited to:

- Cellular pathophysiology studies associated with the long-term generational health effects of the toxicants of concern (among these, the committee should consider studies in laboratory animals and other models);
- Multigenerational effects of the toxicants of concern in various animal species, if such effects have not already been well established;
- The feasibility of conducting a long-term epidemiologic study to assess the generational health effects of veterans and the resources (technological, logistical) that would need to be available to support such research;
- Develop a framework for monitoring and studying generational health effects over time, including post-exposure assessments, initial screening of veterans and their descendants, the frequency and duration of such screenings;
- Based upon a careful assessment of available laboratory technologies, establish a process for what is to be included in the screening, including biomarkers and early symptoms;
- The number of veterans and their descendants who should be part of such a study(ies); and
- The appropriate federal agency(ies), e.g., the Department of Defense, the Department of Veterans Affairs, the Department of Health and Human Services, or other organization(s) or collaborative consortia that would be best suited to coordinate and/or conduct the research and screenings on an ongoing basis.

pesticides, such as organophosphates and pyrethroids; Chapter 6 examines exposures to combustion products, such as particulate matter and dioxins, and fuels, including diesel and JP-8; and Chapter 7 focuses on exposures to solvents, such as benzene, trichloroethylene, and tetrachloroethylene. The committee's conclusions concerning the health effects of those exposures, which are based on the strength of the evidence described in these chapters, are summarized in Chapter 8, which also includes a brief discussion of epigenetics and what is being learned from human and animal studies in this area. Chapter 9 addresses the committee's second task of providing VA with a framework for a health monitoring research program to identify any health effects in the descendants of veterans that may be related to the veterans' deployment exposures. Chapter 10 describes the various basic research studies that might be conducted to elucidate the underlying genetic and epigenetic mechanisms of these health effects as well as other biological repercussions that are passed down from generation to generation. Chapter 11 provides a context and path forward to help VA and veterans identify and understand whether exposures experienced by veterans during their deployments may be affecting the health of their children, grandchildren, and future generations. Finally, short biographical sketches of the committee members may be found in Appendix A, while Appendix B provides a glossary of the technical terms used in this report.

REFERENCES

Faulkner, W.M. 2011. *Exposure to toxins produced by burn pits: Congressional data request and studies*. Memorandum for the Assistant Secretary of Defense for Health Affairs. Washington, DC: Joint Staff. March 28, 2011. Enclosure: ASD (HA) Memorandum, February 17, 2011. Response to ASD (HA) Request for Information.

IOM (Institute of Medicine). 1996. *Health consequences of service during the Persian Gulf War: Recommendations for research and information systems*. Washington, DC: National Academy Press.

IOM. 1999. *Strategies to protect the health of deployed U.S. forces: Medical surveillance, record keeping, and risk reduction*. Washington, DC: National Academy Press.

IOM. 2000. *Gulf War and health, volume 1: Depleted uranium, pyridostigmine bromide, sarin, vaccines*. Washington, DC: National Academy Press.

IOM. 2003. *Gulf War and health, volume 2: Insecticides and solvents*. Washington, DC: The National Academies Press.

IOM. 2004. *Gulf War and health: Updated literature review of sarin*. Washington, DC: The National Academies Press.

IOM. 2005. *Gulf War and health, volume 3: Fuels, combustion products, and propellants*. Washington, DC: The National Academies Press.

IOM. 2006a. *Amyotrophic lateral sclerosis in veterans: Review of the scientific literature*. Washington, DC: The National Academies Press.

IOM. 2006b. *Gulf War and health, volume 4: Health effects of serving in the Gulf War*. Washington, DC: The National Academies Press.

IOM. 2007. *Gulf War and health, volume 5: Infectious diseases*. Washington, DC: The National Academies Press.

IOM. 2008a. *Gulf War and health: Updated literature review of depleted uranium*. Washington, DC: The National Academies Press.

IOM. 2008b. *Gulf War and health, volume 6. Physiologic, psychologic, and psychosocial effects of deployment-related stress*. Washington, DC: The National Academies Press.

IOM. 2009. *Gulf War and health, volume 7: Long-term consequences of traumatic brain injury*. Washington, DC: The National Academies Press.

IOM. 2010. *Gulf War and health, volume 8: Update of health effects of serving in the Gulf War*. Washington, DC: The National Academies Press.

IOM. 2011. *The long-term health consequences of exposure to burn pits in Iraq and Afghanistan*. Washington, DC: The National Academies Press.

IOM. 2014. *Gulf War and health, volume 9: Long-term effects of blast exposures*. Washington, DC: The National Academies Press.

Joseph, S.C. 1997. A comprehensive clinical evaluation of 20,000 Persian Gulf War veterans. *Military Medicine* 162(3):149–155.

NASEM (National Academies of Sciences, Engineering, and Medicine). 2016a. *Veterans and Agent Orange: Update 2014*. Washington, DC: The National Academies Press.

NASEM. 2016b. *Gulf War and health, volume 10: Update of health effects of serving in the Gulf War*. Washington, DC: The National Academies Press.

NRC (National Research Council). 2000a. *Strategies to protect the health of deployed U.S. forces: Analytical framework for assessing risks*. Washington, DC: National Academy Press.

NRC. 2000b. *Strategies to protect the health of deployed U.S. forces: Assessing health risks to deployed U.S. forces, workshop proceedings*. Washington, DC: National Academy Press.

NRC. 2009. *Contaminated water supplies at Camp Lejeune: Assessing potential health effects*. Washington, DC: The National Academies Press.

NRC. 2010. *Review of the Department of Defense Enhanced Particulate Matter Surveillance Program report*. Washington, DC: The National Academies Press.

Reynolds, G.M., and A. Shendruk. 2018. Demographics of the U.S. Military. Washington, DC: Council on Foreign Relations. April 24. https://www.cfr.org/article/demographics-US-military (accessed July 27, 2018).

VA (Department of Veterans Affairs). 2011. Caring for Gulf War I veterans. Veterans Health Administration. http://www.publichealth.va.gov/docs/vhi/caring-for-gulf-war-veterans-vhi.pdf (accessed October 20, 2018).

VA. 2015. The scent of war: VA studies a legacy of dust, smoke, and burn pits and what it means for veterans. VA Research Currents, February 18. https://www.research.va.gov/currents/winter2015/winter2015-18.cfm (accessed July 27, 2018).

2

Committee's Approach

To address the statement of task given in P.L. 144-315, the National Academies of Sciences, Engineering, and Medicine (the National Academies) empaneled a multidisciplinary committee composed of 16 experts from the fields of toxicology, epidemiology, environmental health and occupational medicine, epigenetics, and statistics. The Volume 11 committee began its deliberations with an open public meeting held in Washington, DC, to hear from the Department of Veterans Affairs (VA), interested veterans and veterans' service organizations, and other stakeholders and to gather information from the National Institute for Environmental Health Sciences and the National Toxicology Program. That input helped the committee understand VA's needs, appreciate the veterans' concerns, and be cognizant of complementary efforts already under way.

Given the precedence set by *Volumes 6, 7,* and *9* in the *Gulf War and Health* series, the Volume 11 committee included military personnel who had served in the Gulf region after 1991, particularly those who had served after September 11, 2001 (Post-9/11 veterans), in its considerations. This decision was justified because of the overlap of many deployment-related exposures and the anticipated need to proactively address potential health effects in these groups. To understand the potential reproductive and developmental[1] effects that might occur in veterans and descendants as a result of deployments to the 1990–1991 Gulf War and the Post-9/11 conflicts, the Volume 11 committee divided its statement of task into two tasks with four activities:

Task 1:

- Assessment of the current research on possible generational health effects that may be the result of deployment exposures during the 1990–1991 Gulf War and Post-9/11 conflicts (see Chapters 4 through 7); and

[1] The committee considered "reproductive effects" to include changes in reproductive function that may affect fertility and the ability to carry a healthy child through to a term birth. "Developmental effects" is used to represent any outcomes in offspring observed at birth and across the lifecourse. See Box 2-1 for a list of effects.

Task 2:

- Development of a framework for monitoring the reproductive health of veterans and the health of their descendants (see Chapter 9);
- Determination of the feasibility of conducting an epidemiologic study on the reproductive and developmental effects of toxicants in veterans and their descendants and, if feasible, provision of guidance on the design of such a study (see Chapter 9); and
- Provision of guidance on what research should be conducted to address the data and knowledge gaps, including the use of animal and mechanistic studies (see Chapter 10).

The committee began its work on these tasks by developing an approach to identifying whom might be affected by deployment exposures (i.e., parents, children, grandchildren), what exposures a veteran might have experienced (e.g., lifestyle, toxicants, stress), the characteristics of those exposures (e.g., measuring exposure, the variability of exposures, multiple exposures), and what factors might influence the transmission of effects from parent to descendants (e.g., levels and timing of exposure). The committee then considered how to determine what reproductive and developmental effects may be associated with the toxicants listed in the Gulf War legislation (see Chapter 1, Box 1-1). This determination began with an extensive literature search and review using the evaluation processes established by previous Gulf War and Health committees. The evaluation process, including the categories of association used by the committee to draw its conclusions regarding the strength of the association between an exposure and any reproductive or developmental health effect, is described later in this chapter. The results of the committee's deliberations for deployment-related exposures, pesticides, combustion products, and solvents are given in Chapters 4 through 7 and summarized in Chapter 8.

The committee's approach to Task 2 was also driven by the literature as well as by the committee's expertise. Both the committee's framework for monitoring veteran and descendant populations for health effects and its guidance on conducting epidemiologic studies that might help link deployment exposures to health outcomes in descendants relied on literature describing studies that are gathering information on veterans' exposures (deployed and nondeployed) and cataloging their health effects during and after military service. Determining what research is necessary to understand how exposures may contribute to health effects in offspring and future generations was informed by the data reviewed in Chapters 4 through 7—including the genetic and epigenetic literature—that highlighted data and knowledge gaps. The transmission of effects from a veteran to his or her children and possibly grandchildren or great-grandchildren is called generational effects.

EXPOSURE CONSIDERATIONS

To understand the potential impact of deployment exposures on veterans and their descendants, the committee needed to consider any reproductive and developmental outcomes in the broader context of the veterans' genetic and epigenetic profiles and of their exposures to other stressors (biological, chemical, radiological, psychological, or physiological) they had experienced in their lives before, during, and after deployment. Prior *Gulf War and Health* volumes have examined the variety of deployment-related exposures (e.g., living conditions, threat of biological and chemical warfare) a veteran might experience in the Persian Gulf region (e.g., IOM, 2006) as well as in Iraq and Afghanistan (e.g., IOM, 2011). Deployment itself has been used as an exposure variable and stressor in several *Gulf War and Health* reports with deployed veterans being compared with veterans who remained in the United States or who were deployed elsewhere (e.g., Germany, Somalia, Bosnia [see IOM, 2006, 2010; NASEM, 2016]).

Gulf War and Health, Volume 6 found "that military personnel deployed to a war zone, even if direct combat was not experienced, have the potential for exposure to deployment-related stressors and that the emotional and physical reactions of military personnel to those stressors can vary widely" (IOM, 2008).

Veteran Exposures

Throughout life, a person is exposed to any number of external and internal events and agents, including environmental toxicants and those that are the result of lifestyle choices, that can interact with a person's genome and epigenome[2] to affect health and the occurrence of disease. The combined effects of genetic makeup, lifestyle, and environment, all of which may affect a person from conception to death, set the stage for a person's response to potentially harmful exposures. Veterans' exposure during deployment must be considered within the context of their lifetime exposure to adverse events (e.g., psychological and physical stress, accidents, diseases) and toxicants (e.g., drugs, cleaning products, pesticides). Nutrition, smoking, and stress are but a few of the factors that can affect a person's health. For example, if a veteran was a smoker before deployment and continued to smoke during and after deployment, that exposure may influence his or her response (susceptibility) to other toxicants experienced during deployment.

Military service itself—and not just deployment experiences—may also contribute to a veteran's exposures. As discussed in *Gulf War and Health, Volume 6*, on deployment-related stress, deployment to a war zone itself can be a stressor regardless of whether the service member engaged in direct combat. Stresses such as being away from family, seeing casualties, and poor living conditions are among the many factors that may result in or contribute to adverse health effects for deployed service members (IOM, 2008). Certain military occupational specialties that are engaged in prior to or after deployment may involve exposure to toxicants such as solvents for degreasing equipment and chemical-agent-resistant coating paint. These exposures may be compounded during deployment. For example, a mechanic may continue to use solvents for degreasing during deployment but might have additional exposures to mixtures of other toxicants, such as particulate matter from dust storms and combustion products in smoke from burn pits. Determining those additional exposures may be difficult given that the composition of the dust storm and what is disposed of in the pit may vary with time and location. Exposures during military training and those encountered in the civilian environment, such as cleaning products and various other products that are dependent upon lifestyle, hobbies, and social activities, may also affect a veteran's cumulative exposures and, ultimately, lead to health effects.

Assessing Deployment Exposures

Several important issues must be considered when evaluating the health impacts of stressors and toxicants in veteran populations. These issues include the route of exposure; the magnitude, duration, and frequency of the exposure; possible interactions between multiple single exposures; exposure to mixtures; and the time in the lifecourse at which the exposure occurs. Characterizing veteran exposures is difficult because of the almost complete lack of exposure information collected during U.S. deployments to the Gulf War or Post-9/11 conflicts (IOM, 2011) or to the Vietnam War. Nevertheless, as noted in the report *Strategies to Protect the Health of Deployed U.S. Forces: Analytical Framework for Assessing Risks*, "Many hazards are specific to military situations, military exposure factors can differ from those relevant to civilians, and stress and extreme environments can affect toxic responses" (NRC, 2000).

[2] See the glossary in Appendix B for definitions of terms.

Only rarely is environmental sampling conducted by the Department of Defense (DoD) that would help in determining or modeling the levels of a toxicant or toxicants to which veterans might be exposed. Although air or water models may be helpful for estimating exposure for an area, they cannot be used to assess individual exposures. What sampling is conducted tends to be only a snapshot at a given time and location and does not capture the totality of a veteran's exposure during deployment or even for a particular incident, such as the exposure to sarin gas that may have occurred with the demolition of the Khamisiyah munitions depot in Iraq (IOM, 2006). Furthermore, some veterans' exposures were specific to deployment to the 1990–1991 Gulf War or Post-9/11 conflicts (e.g., pyridostigmine bromide [PB], burn pits), although others were not (e.g., diesel and solvents).

Route of Exposure

The route of exposure can affect the dose of a toxicant a person receives. It is important to know whether the route of exposure for a veteran in a given situation is comparable to those examined in epidemiologic and occupational or animal studies. For example, if a veteran is typically exposed to a solvent by handling rags soaked in a solvent, but occupational studies show that most workers are exposed via inhalation, will these different routes of exposure affect the potential for reproductive outcomes differently? Additionally, there is the question of whether the doses and the routes of administration used in animal studies are relevant surrogates for human exposures and what extrapolations or uncertainty factors are necessary to compare animal and human exposures.

Multiple Exposures and Chemical Interactions

Gulf War and Post-9/11 veterans were, and continue to be, potentially exposed to numerous toxicants in the environment (co-exposures, e.g., dust and solvents) or together in the same exposure (mixtures, e.g., smoke from burn pits). These exposures include agents used as preventive measures (e.g., PB, vaccines, pesticides, and insecticides), hazards of the natural environment (e.g., sand and endemic infectious agents), job-specific toxicants (e.g., paints, solvents, and diesel fumes), war-related toxicants (e.g., depleted uranium and smoke from burn pits), hazards from cleanup operations (e.g., sarin and cyclosarin), persistent organic pollutants (e.g., lindane and dioxins), and numerous other stressors (e.g., smoking and physical or psychological stress). Thus, deployed veterans have exposures that vary by toxicant or stressor; the frequency, duration, and timing of the dose; individual response; and the theater of operation. The number and combination of toxicants to which a veteran might be exposed make it difficult to determine whether any specific agent or combination of agents is likely to result in reproductive effects in the veterans or developmental effects in their descendants. Adding to the complexity of assessing multiple exposures is that although Gulf War veterans for the most part experienced single deployments to the Persian Gulf area during the war, many Post-9/11 veterans have been deployed more than once and to different areas of southwest Asia, for instance, Iraq and Afghanistan. For extended conflicts in the future, multiple deployments may be common.

Addressing exposure to multiple toxicants has been a subject of much debate and research in the fields of toxicology, environmental and occupational health, and medicine. Although it is possible to assess the toxicity of some mixtures rather than assessing the toxicity of their individual constituents (Elhalwagy and Zaki, 2009), the interactions of toxicants are not, in general, well understood in either humans or animals. However, there are exceptions; for example, the toxic effects of some pesticide mixtures have been studied (Hernández et al., 2013, 2017). In animal studies of Gulf War illness, the effects of mixtures of pesticides and other agents such as PB have been studied (Abdel-Rahman et al., 2004).

Although many scientific studies evaluate the risks of adverse health effects caused by exposure to a single toxicant, the European Union, the U.S. Environmental Protection Agency (EPA), and the Agency for Toxic Substances and Disease Registry (ATSDR) have developed systematic approaches to evaluating multiple exposures (ATSDR, 2018; EPA, 1986, 2000; EU, 2011). Exposure to multiple agents or stressors may result in interactions that produce an effect that might not have occurred with exposure to a single toxicant, or the interactions might produce a greater, different, or lesser effect than would be caused by a single exposure. Simultaneous exposure to more than one agent might produce not only a variety of adverse effects and severity of those effects; protective or beneficial effects might also occur. Therefore, attributing an effect to one toxicant or a combination of toxicants is difficult, especially in situations where there are many different types of exposures (e.g., chemical, physical, biological). Prior National Academies committees have attempted to determine the toxicity of some mixtures to which veterans were exposed while deployed in southwest Asia. The 2011 IOM report *Long-Term Health Consequences of Exposure to Burn Pits in Iraq and Afghanistan* reviewed the air sampling done by the DoD and found numerous flaws in the sampling methodology that made it difficult to determine if military personnel stationed at bases with burn pits were likely to have an increased risk of health problems. The Volume 11 committee notes that burn pit emissions were only one poorly defined mixture to which service members might be exposed during their deployment. As a result, the committee did not evaluate all studies of occupational and environmental exposures to the many mixtures in the literature that included a toxicant of interest (such as benzene in the hydrocarbon mixture called BTEX [benzene-toluene-ethylbenzene-xylene]) but instead, generally restricted itself to examining studies that assessed the individual components of a mixture. This decision was made because, given the available information, the committee was unable to determine if a given mixture was analogous to mixtures that might have been present during deployment.

Timing of Exposure

The timing of exposure can refer to a number of different things: when the exposure occurred during a lifetime; when the exposure occurred relative to the manifestation of an effect; how long the exposure lasted (duration); and how frequently the exposure occurred. In this report, the committee focuses on the timing of exposure relative to conception or to a particular window of gamete, fetal, or child development and on the possible manifestation of effects in men, women, fetuses, or children. These effects include direct toxic effects on development and genetic or epigenetic effects.

Exposures that may lead to reproductive effects in men or women can occur at any time. Parental exposures that may affect the development of a fetus or child can occur before conception (during the development or maturation of the germ cell) or during pregnancy (prenatal). Developmental toxicity studies are generally limited to specific windows of development relative to conception and birth (shortly before conception through early life). The timing of exposure is particularly important for understanding inherited genetic and epigenetic effects (see Chapter 3 for more details).

There are only a few rare studies of human populations in which it has been possible to say with certainty when an exposure to a toxicant began and ended. Rather, most exposures are continuous or intermittent over extended periods of time: for example, living in a hot climate or polluted area or being a tobacco user. Other exposures may be infrequent or isolated, such as using a pesticide or an industrial accident. Deployment exposures, on the other hand, occur during a defined time frame of limited duration, usually many months.

Assessing the exposures of female service members poses some unique challenges. Female service members who are pregnant are precluded from being deployed (DoD, 2010). If female veterans are pregnant during deployment, they are removed from the theater of operation, so their exposures should be limited to preconception or early pregnancy (after the pregnancy is detected). This is not to say that a female veteran's military occupational specialty or other duties after she returns from deployment will not expose her to toxicants, but it might be difficult to determine whether any adverse pregnancy outcomes in a veteran or developmental effects in her children could be attributed specifically to her deployment exposures. Given different occupations and military assignments, it is possible for women to serve on active duty during later stages of pregnancy, but not to be deployed (DoD, 2007). An exception to a female service member's exposure to toxicants being limited to preconception or early pregnancy is her possible exposure during deployment to persistent organic pollutants such as lindane or dioxins. These chemicals may be taken up during deployment and stored in adipose tissue. However, should a woman become pregnant after deployment, these toxicants may be mobilized from the adipose tissue and enter the blood stream or milk of a pregnant or lactating woman, thus exposing her child during pregnancy and during lactation.

The Volume 11 committee found that studies that specifically assessed exposure prior to conception or early in the pregnancy were particularly useful, but they were also relatively rare. Because the timing of exposures in relation to a pregnancy is difficult to determine in epidemiologic studies, the committee took into account those studies where maternal exposures were assessed from preconception through birth (e.g., prenatal), including later in the pregnancy or at the time of birth, even though female veterans were not deployed late in pregnancy.

COMMITTEE'S REVIEW PROCESS

The approach and methods that the committee used to identify, select, and evaluate the scientific and medical literature on Gulf War and Post-9/11 exposures are, for the most part, the same as those used by previous Gulf War and Health committees. The committee also used a similar process to reach conclusions on the strength of the associations between those exposures and reproductive or developmental health effects. The Gulf War legislation was the primary source of the committee's list of possible toxicants (see Box 1-1), although the committee also considered additional toxicants such as fuels and combustion products, as described in the IOM report *Long-Term Health Consequences of Exposure to Burn Pits in Iraq and Afghanistan* (2011), a report of concern to Post-9/11 veterans. The committee was asked to assess hexavalent chromium at the request of VA. Exposures relevant to Vietnam veterans are discussed in the most recent update of the *Veterans and Agent Orange* series (NASEM, 2016b), although dioxins are also considered in this volume because dioxins are among the many combustion products measured in emissions from burn pits in Iraq and Afghanistan.

Identification of the Literature

The Volume 11 committee began its work by overseeing extensive searches of the scientific literature, including published articles, other reports, and government documents. Searches were conducted using five databases: Embase, Medline, Scopus, Proquest, and PubMed. The specific searches targeted studies of (1) the health of Gulf War or Post-9/11 veterans published since *Volume 10* without regard for specific toxicants or outcomes; (2) reproductive effects associated with any of the toxicants listed in Box 1-1; and (3) developmental or other health outcomes, including biomarkers of response, in children or grandchildren (F1 or F2) associated with the parental exposures to the toxicants of concern. Studies in both human populations and animal or cellular models were included. No publications that appeared before 1999 were considered in order to focus on data published since the *Gulf War and Health* series began.

The searches retrieved more than 29,000 publications on reproductive effects and more than 56,000 publications related to effects in offspring, which were published through January 2018. Publications that came to the committee's attention after January 2018 were included in the review where appropriate.

Because few studies on reproductive or developmental effects were specific to veterans' exposures during deployment, the committee decided to approach its review of the health effects by identifying populations that had exposures to the same toxicants as Gulf War and Post-9/11 veterans. For the studies of occupational and environmental cohorts, it is difficult to ascertain how comparable the deployment exposures are to those of the study cohorts in terms of exposure magnitude, duration, frequency, mixtures, and co-exposures and also in terms of population characteristics such as gender, age, ethnicity, and lifestyle. For example, several large cohort studies examined associations between environmental exposures to pesticides and particulate matter and developmental effects on children, such as neurodevelopmental deficits or asthma in childhood (Eskenazi et al., 2007; Tetreault et al., 2016). Those studies examined long-term, continuous exposures throughout the preconception, prenatal, and postnatal periods. These exposures may not accurately reflect exposures during only preconception or early pregnancy periods as experienced by female veterans who were pregnant in theater because late pregnancy and postnatal exposure windows can have a significant impact on development and child health. However, the committee took note of studies that reported trimester-specific exposure associations or that tried to control for effects related to postnatal exposures.

The committee realizes that considerable work is being done to study epigenetic effects in nonmammalian organisms such as fruit flies (*Drosophila*), zebrafish (*Danio rerio*), frogs (*Xenopus*), and roundworms (*Caenorhabditis elegans*). However, although studies of relevant exposures and reproductive and developmental effects in mammalian models such as rodents and rabbits were included in the review, nonmammalian models were excluded because their immediate relevance to human health is difficult to determine at this time.

In addition to identifying studies on distinct health outcomes such as infertility, birth outcomes, and diseases in offspring, the committee also included studies of biological markers that have been associated with the health outcomes of interest. These studies of biological markers were particularly informative in assessing the potential implications of an association between the exposures of interest and generational effects—for example, Guzick et al. (2001), Khatun et al. (2018), Ombelet et al. (2014), and Patel et al. (2017). The committee considered reproductive and developmental effects as reported in the literature, without a priori decisions on what would be included in each of those areas and regardless of whether it had been identified in an earlier volume of the *Gulf War and Health* series. Once the literature was screened and a list of effects was generated, the effects were then categorized as reproductive effects, including adverse pregnancy outcomes; developmental effects; and genetic and epigenetic effects, as described in Box 2-1. Because the effects varied somewhat depending on the toxicant, the description of the literature for each toxicant also varies. Although adverse pregnancy outcomes are described throughout this report as a subset of reproductive outcomes, conclusions about those outcomes are made separately, depending on the availability of data. The committee decided not to assess studies on menopause (other than early menopause) or reproductive cancers because they have little relevance for generational effects.

Studies that did not appear to be relevant, based on an assessment of their title and abstract, were deleted from further consideration. The inclusion and exclusion criteria used to select relevant studies are given in Box 2-2. The results were categorized by the toxicants of concern, and specific publication cutoff dates were applied to each exposure based on the latest relevant *Gulf War and Health* review or a review by another authoritative body such as EPA and ATSDR. Those committee members who had the most familiarity with a particular health outcome or area of expertise reviewed all screened titles

BOX 2-1
Effects and Health Outcomes Identified in the Literature

Reproductive effects: any effect on the ability to reproduce

- Effects on male reproduction, including changes in sperm parameters and reproductive hormones, infertility, time to pregnancy;
- Effects on female reproduction, including effects on menstrual cycle, endometriosis, infertility, time to pregnancy, changes in reproductive hormones;
- Adverse pregnancy outcomes, including
  - Maternal health, such as gestational diabetes, gestational hypertension, and inflammation during pregnancy; and
  - Birth outcomes, such as preterm birth, birth weight or size, spontaneous abortion, and still birth.

Developmental effects: any adverse health effects in children or offspring of any age, including reproductive effects

- Neurodevelopmental deficits, including measures of cognition (IQ, attention, motor skills, etc.), autism spectrum disorders, attention deficit disorders;
- Respiratory effects, including respiratory symptoms (e.g., wheezing), lung function, asthma, respiratory infections;
- Childhood cancers;
- Birth defects;
- Immune outcomes: eczema, dermatomyositis;
- Obesity and metabolism; and
- Growth.

Epigenetic and genetic effects, including

- Markers of DNA oxidative stress;
- DNA methylation in maternal blood, umbilical cord blood, placenta, or peripheral blood lymphocytes, sperm;
- mRNA expression;
- Histone modifications; and
- Mitochondrial DNA content in umbilical cord blood.

and abstracts in that area and identified papers for full text retrieval; titles and abstracts of more than 4,000 publications were reviewed.

Evaluation Process

The Volume 11 committee adopted a policy of using only literature that had been published in a peer-reviewed journal or rigorously peer-reviewed government reports or monographs. While the process of peer review by fellow professionals increases the likelihood that higher-quality studies will appear in the

BOX 2-2
Literature Search Inclusion and Exclusion Criteria

Inclusion:

- Epidemiologic or toxicologic studies
- Exposure of interest AND any reproductive or developmental effect or outcome (including health across the lifecourse)
- Exposure occurred before conception or during pregnancy
- Peer-reviewed

Exclusion:

- Toxicologic studies in nonmammalian species
- Pharmacokinetic studies
- Studies that only examined postnatal exposures
- Socioeconomic impacts and impacts on families
- Short-term or acute effects
- Studies on treatments, therapies, and rehabilitation
- Exposures as a result of substance abuse (e.g., alcohol and "huffing" solvents) or physical events (e.g., gunshot wounds)
- Studies of reproductive cancers and menopause
- Opinions and editorials

literature, it does not guarantee the validity or quality of any particular study or the generalizability of its findings. The committee did not collect original data nor did it perform any secondary data analysis.

For a study to be included in the committee's review, it had to meet specific criteria. It had to (1) have sufficient detail to demonstrate rigorous methodology (for example, it had a control or reference group and adjusted for confounders when needed); (2) have sufficient power to detect an effect; and (3) provide information regarding a persistent health outcome.

Small groups of committee members conducted a preliminary review of the relevant studies for each set of exposures to determine what, if any, relevant information the studies had on the health outcomes of interest. Each study was assigned to a committee member who reviewed it critically for its relevance and quality without preconceived ideas about the strength of the evidence regarding the association between an exposure and a reproductive or developmental health effect. The responsible committee member or members then presented the information from the preliminary screening and categorization to the full committee for discussion.

The information presented for each exposure included a review of the relevant prior *Gulf War and Health* volumes and their studies and conclusions, the populations used in any new studies, the methods for selecting and evaluating the populations, the study results, and the committee members' assessments of the strengths and limitations of the study. Because of the variability in the description of the reproductive and developmental effects considered in this report it was impossible for the committee to make a priori assumptions about the usefulness of any study.

Greater weight was given to studies that were conducted in a manner that reduced sources of error, bias, and confounding. More weight was given to studies in which there was an individual-level exposure assessment or biological assessment of exposure (e.g., urine analysis); in which specific exposures were associated with an occupational title or industry, such as when a job exposure matrix was used to categorize exposure; or in which an assessment was made by an industrial hygienist. Studies that had self-reported exposures were considered less rigorous. For greater detail about epidemiology, biases, confounders and other methodological background, see Chapter 2 of *Gulf War and Health, Volume 1* and *Volume 8* (IOM, 2000, 2010).

Given the amount of human and animal literature on the reproductive effects of these exposures, the committee also considered reviews from authoritative bodies, such as EPA and ATSDR or other reports from the National Academies. Those reviews follow systematic methodologies, summarize human and animal data for the purposes of identifying human health risks, and undergo rigorous review. The conclusions of these authoritative bodies are presented in this volume and were taken into account by the committee in the context of the time period when they were produced as well as the purpose and approach used by the authoritative bodies. The committee examined any literature that had been published since those reviews, had not been assessed in those reviews, or was of particular interest (such as multigenerational studies), but it relied on the totality of information to reach conclusions. Systematic reviews and meta-analyses in the published literature were also considered by the committee, but they were given no greater weight than any individual study.

After the studies were discussed in a plenary session, the responsible committee member or members drafted the text for that exposure and health outcome. Human and animal data were summarized by outcomes for each exposure. Data and units are presented as reported in the cited studies, except where otherwise noted.

The draft text was reviewed and discussed in further plenary sessions until all committee members reached a consensus on the description of the studies and the conclusions for each health outcome. After this language was agreed upon, the full committee assigned a category of association (discussed later in this chapter) based on the weight of the evidence and expert judgment. It should be noted that the committee did not use a formulaic approach in deciding the number of studies that would be necessary to assign a specific category of association. Rather, the committee's review consisted of a thoughtful, nuanced, and qualitative consideration of all of the studies as well as expert judgment, and this could not be accomplished by adherence to a narrowly prescribed formula of what data would be required for each category of association or for a particular health outcome. In its evaluation of the evidence, the committee considered a set of overarching concerns—specifically, statistical considerations, the availability of animal and mechanistic studies, the consistency of association, and biologic plausibility—when assigning a category of association to a particular exposure and adverse reproductive or developmental effect.

Statistical Considerations

The strength of an association between an exposure and an outcome is generally estimated quantitatively by using prevalence ratios, relative risks, odds ratios, hazard ratios, or correlation or regression coefficients, depending on the study design. These various measures of the strength of the association are generally referred to as *effect sizes*. A ratio greater than 1.0 indicates that the outcome variable has occurred more frequently in the exposed group than in the unexposed or control group, and a ratio less than 1.0 indicates that it has occurred less frequently. When the effect size is 1, there is no effect. For correlations (usually denoted with *r*) and regression coefficients (usually denoted with β), values greater than 0 indicate that the outcome variable increases with exposure and negative values indicate they decrease; when the effect size is 0, there is *no effect*.

Effect sizes are typically reported with a confidence interval (CI) to quantify random error. Statistical significance may be represented by a CI or a p-value. A p-value is defined as the probability of observing an effect size as large as or larger than the one observed when there is no effect. In the scientific literature, a result associated with a p-value less than 0.05 is generally referred to as *statistically significant*. There is a connection between p-value and 95% confidence intervals. Specifically, if the effect size associated with *no effect* (1 for ratios and 0 for correlation and regression coefficients) is not included in a 95% confidence interval, then the p-value is less than 0.05. If the 95% CI for a risk estimate (such as a risk ratio or odds ratio) includes 1.0, the association is not considered to be statistically significant.

Generally, the greater the effect size, the greater the likelihood that the exposure–disease association is causal and the lower the likelihood that it is due to undetected error, bias, or confounding. Measures of statistical significance, such as p-values, are not indicators of the strength of an association. Small increases in relative risks that are consistent among studies, however, might be evidence of an association, and some forms of extreme bias or confounding can produce a high relative risk. A study must have enough statistical power to be able to detect effects of a certain magnitude, which is especially important in identifying negative results. The committee reviewed the studies in this report with a consideration not only for uncertainty due to sampling variability, measurement error, and biological variability but also for the potential for bias and the authors' strategies for examining and limiting the effect of each of these on the study's findings. The committee gave less weight to studies that included only p-values or statements of statistical significance, but no CI. This is because, on their own, p-values provide no information of the effect sizes. With a large enough sample size, a p-value can be close to 0, even when the effect size is practically negligible. Common types of biases found in the Gulf War veteran literature are identified in Box 2-3 and discussed in greater detail in Chapter 9, Statistical Considerations. For greater detail about epidemiology, biases, confounders, and other methodological background, see Chapter 2 of *Gulf War and Health, Volume 8* (IOM, 2010).

In its assessment of the scientific literature, the committee was careful to consider the statistical approaches used in the studies it reviewed. In particular, the committee examined whether possible confounding effects were considered and appropriately accounted for when model-based approaches, such as multivariable linear regression, were used. Many of the studies also estimated a large number of associations and ran many statistical tests on a single dataset. For example, in many air pollution studies, the investigators compared multiple outcomes (i.e., a long list of birth defects including multiple levels of specificity from general to specific subcategories) and many measures of exposure (i.e., multiple pollutants and multiple estimates of exposure). In such cases, researchers are likely to find statistically significant associations at the $p<0.05$ level even by chance alone: that is, 5% of cases will appear to have an association just by chance alone when using $p<0.05$. There are ways to correct for multiple comparisons in studies, such as a Bonferroni correction (a statistical adjustment for multiple comparisons) which raises the standard of proof needed when an investigator examines a wide array of hypotheses simultaneously by proportionally decreasing the p-value used to evaluate associations.

Animal, Cellular, and Mechanistic Studies

Animal, cellular, and mechanistic studies were included in the committee's considerations because they provide valuable information on reproductive and developmental effects that may not be evident in human populations or that cannot ethically be studied, such as spontaneous abortion. Furthermore, in animal studies the route, dose, timing of exposure, and mixture or co-exposure composition may be controlled. Specific organ systems can also be examined before effects are clinically apparent and confounders can be carefully controlled.

BOX 2-3
Some Medical Research Biases in the Gulf War and Health Literature

Selection bias: Selection bias is a systematic error that occurs when the method of recruiting a study sample results in a sample that differs in some systematic way from the target population of the study. The findings of such a study may then potentially over- or underestimate the true association with the direction being dependent upon the form of selection bias. Selection bias can also occur in a prospective study when there are losses to follow-up that differ between the exposed and unexposed group. This may be due to a poor definition of the eligible population or a failure to obtain a random sample. Selection bias includes

- *Non-response bias*: Participants have, on average, a different exposure or disease status from non-participants.
- *Volunteer bias*: Participants who volunteer are more likely to have the exposure or disease of interest; this is a particular problem for registry studies that collect information on voluntary participants.
- *Healthy-warrior effect*: Veterans or personnel who were deployed may be healthier than those who were not deployed or than civilians; the selection of healthier people occurs at enlistment and separation (ill and injured personnel are more likely to leave the military).

Information or measurement bias: The misclassification of a participant's exposure or disease status may be based on the information collected by various methods (such as a mailed questionnaire, a telephone interview, record review, or a medical examination). This type of bias includes

- *Recall bias*: The presence of a disease influences participants' reflection and perception of possible causes and can make them likely to report more exposures than or different exposures from non-diseased participants.
- *Reporting bias*: Participants are more likely to report responses that they perceive as highly favorable or adverse.
- *Temporal ambiguity*: This occurs when it cannot be established that an exposure occurred before the onset of disease; it is common in cross-sectional assessments.

Confounding: This occurs when a risk factor for the disease that is also related to the exposure creates a spurious exposure–disease association; in other words, a risk factor may cause the exposed and non-exposed participants to have different background disease risks.

SOURCES: IOM, 2010, 2014a.

Experimental studies are of particular use for studying the generational effects of toxicants. Most laboratory animals reproduce rapidly, and thus generation effects in the F0 (parental), F1, F2, and F3 generations may be studied in a matter of months or a few years, compared with the decades-long maturation and reproductive cycle of humans.

Well-established experimental animal protocols exist that minimize the potential influence of co-exposures, control for background responses, and more clearly characterize dose–response relationships.

Still, experimental animal studies can be challenging to interpret because most studies evaluate a single strain of a species with a homogeneous genetic background, while humans have a large amount of genetic variability shaping their response to stressors, which makes comparisons problematic. There are also animal studies that have examined the impact of mixed exposures (mixtures and co-exposures), and the committee decided that such studies could help inform some of its deliberations. The committee reviewed mammalian toxicologic studies, as those were deemed most relevant for identifying agents of potential concern for humans. Therefore, the committee referred to experimental animal studies to help provide information on biologic plausibility and the specificity of effects and to fill in gaps where no human data were available.

Animal research may also focus on a toxicant's mechanism of action (i.e., how a toxicant exerts its deleterious effects at the cellular and molecular levels). Mechanism-of-action (or mechanistic) studies encompass a range of laboratory approaches with whole animals and in vitro systems using tissues or cells from humans or animals. In some cases, the committee used in vitro and/or mechanistic studies to support or enhance its understanding of the plausibility of the results observed in animal models if those models provided evidence of reproductive effects or processes that may lead to molecular or organ damage in fetuses or children. Some mechanistic studies also provided evidence of epigenetic changes that may have effects on cellular processes that might affect reproduction or produce developmental effects.

Consistency of Association

To conclude that an association is consistent requires that the exposure–effect relationship be found regularly in a variety of studies—for example, in more than one study population and with different study methods. However, consistency alone is not sufficient evidence of an association. The committee considered findings that were consistent in direction among different categories of studies to be supportive of an association. It did not require exactly the same magnitude of association to be present in different populations in order to conclude that there was a consistent association. A consistent association could occur when the results of most studies were positive and the differences in measured effects were within the range expected on the basis of sampling error, selection bias, misclassification, confounding, and differences in dose.

Thus, for a health effect to be associated with an agent, there had to be corroboration—that is, replication of findings among multiple studies and populations and under relevant conditions. The greater the degree to which an effect could be consistently reproduced, the more confidence the committee had that there was a true effect.

Biologic Plausibility

Biologic plausibility is based on knowledge of a biologic mechanism by which a toxicant can lead to a health effect. That knowledge is derived from mechanism-of-action or other types of studies—typically animal studies. Biologic plausibility is often difficult to establish and may not exist when an association is first documented. The extent to which all the data in a study are consistent and in line with a biologically plausible mechanism influences the weight attached to the results of that study, as does evidence that the mechanism is similar between the animal or animals under study and humans. This point is especially relevant for the transgenerational impacts that this committee evaluated.

CATEGORIES OF ASSOCIATION

The committee expressed its judgment of the available data clearly and precisely in the Synthesis and Conclusions section for each toxicant discussed in Chapters 4 through 7. It agreed to use the categories of association that have been established and used by previous Gulf War and Health committees and other National Academies committees (IOM, 2000, 2003, 2005, 2006, 2007, 2008, 2009, 2010). Those categories of association have gained wide acceptance by Congress, government agencies (particularly VA), researchers, and veterans groups.

The five categories below describe different levels of association and present a common message: the validity of an association is likely to vary in line with the extent to which common sources of spurious associations can be ruled out as the reason for the observed association. Accordingly, the criteria for each category express a degree of confidence based on the extent to which sources of error were reduced. The committee discussed the evidence and reached consensus on the categorization of the evidence for each toxicant.

Sufficient Evidence of a Causal Relationship

Evidence is sufficient to conclude that a causal relationship exists between being exposed to a toxicant and a reproductive or developmental effect in humans. The evidence fulfills the criteria for sufficient evidence of a causal association in which chance, bias, and confounding can be ruled out with reasonable confidence. The association is supported by a consideration of the consistency of association and biologic plausibility from experimental studies.

Sufficient Evidence of an Association

Evidence suggests an association, in that a positive association has been observed between an exposure and a reproductive or developmental effect in humans; however, there is some doubt as to the influence of chance, bias, and confounding. Experimental animal and cellular studies either supported or diminished the committee's decision in making these associations.

Limited/Suggestive Evidence of an Association

Some evidence of an association between exposure and a reproductive or developmental effect in humans exists, but this is limited by the presence of substantial doubt regarding chance, bias, and confounding. The evidence in experimental animal or cellular models was used to strengthen or weaken the associations between exposure and effect.

Inadequate/Insufficient Evidence to Determine Whether an Association Exists

The available studies are of insufficient quantity, quality, validity, consistency, or statistical power to permit a conclusion regarding the presence or absence of an association between an exposure and a reproductive or developmental effect in humans. Evidence in experimental animal studies may have provided additional support for these assessments, but, in the absence of human data, it was not used to strengthen the categorization of the association. In some cases, the body of evidence is too small to permit conclusions, such as when there are no available studies to validate or corroborate the findings of a single study. In other cases, there is evidence from human or animal studies, but the heterogeneity of exposures, outcomes, and methods leads to inconsistent findings that preclude the committee from identifying an association between exposure and effect.

Limited/Suggestive Evidence of No Association

There are several adequate studies, covering the full range of levels of exposure that humans are known to encounter, that are consistent in not showing an association between an exposure and a reproductive or developmental effect. A conclusion of no association is inevitably limited to the conditions, levels of exposure, and length of observation covered by the available studies. In addition, the possibility of a very small increase in risk at the levels of exposure studied can never be excluded. Experimental animal studies were examined to support such findings.

REFERENCES

Abdel-Rahman, A., S. Abou-Donia, E. El-Masry, A. Shetty, and M. Abou-Donia. 2004. Stress and combined exposure to low doses of pyridostigmine bromide, DEET, and permethrin produce neurochemical and neuropathological alterations in cerebral cortex, hippocampus, and cerebellum. *Journal of Toxicology and Environmental Health A* 67(2):163–192.

ATSDR (Agency for Toxic Substances and Disease Registry). 2018. *Framework for assessing health impacts of multiple chemicals and other stressors*. Atlanta, GA: U.S. Department of Health and Human Services, Public Health Service. https://www.atsdr.cdc.gov/interactionprofiles/ipga.html (accessed August 6, 2018).

DoD (Department of Defense). 2007. Guide to Female Soldier Readiness. U.S. Army Center for Health Promotion and Preventive Medicine Technical Guidance 281. January 23.

DoD. 2010. Department of Defense Instruction Number 6490.07: Deployment-Limiting Medical Conditions for Service Members and DoD Civilian Employees. Under Secretary of Defense for Personnel and Readiness. February 5, 2010.

Elhalwagy, M.E., and N. Zaki. 2009. Comparative study on pesticide mixture of organophosphorus and pyrethroid in commercial formulation. *Environmental Toxicology and Pharmacology* 28(2):219–224.

EPA (U.S. Environmental Protection Agency). 1986. Guidelines for the health risk assessment of chemical mixtures. EPA/630/R-98/002. September 24. *Federal Register* 51(185):34014–34025.

EPA. 2000. *Supplementary guidance for conducting health risk assessment of chemical mixtures*. EPA/630/R-00/002. Washington, DC: Risk Assessment Forum Technical Panel, Environmental Protection Agency.

Eskenazi, B., A.R. Marks, A. Bradman, K. Harley, D.B. Barr, C. Johnson, N. Morga, and N.P. Jewell. 2007. Organophosphate pesticide exposure and neurodevelopment in young Mexican-American children. *Environmental Health Perspectives* 115(5):792–798.

EU (European Union). 2011. *Toxicity and assessment of chemical mixtures*. Brussels: Scientific Committee on Health and Environmental Risks, Scientific Committee on Emerging and Newly Identified Health Risks, and Scientific Committee on Consumer Safety, European Commission. http://ec.europa.eu/health/scientific_committees/environmental_risks/docs/scher_o_155.pdf (accessed August 6, 2018).

Guzick, D.S., J.W. Overstreet, P. Factor-Litvak, C.K. Brazil, S.T. Nakajima, C. Coutifaris, S.A. Carson, P. Cisneros, M.P. Steinkampf, J.A. Hill, D. Xu, and D.L. Vogel, for the National Cooperative Reproductive Medicine Network. 2001. Sperm morphology, motility, and concentration in fertile and infertile men. *New England Journal of Medicine* 345(19):1388–1393.

Hernández, A.F., F. Gil, and M. Lacasaña. 2017. Toxicological interactions of pesticide mixtures: An update. *Archives of Toxicology* 91(10):3211–3223.

Hernández A.F., T. Parrón, A.M. Tsatsakis, M. Requena, R. Alarcón, and O. López-Guarnido. 2013. Toxic effects of pesticide mixtures at a molecular level: Their relevance to human health. *Toxicology* 307:136–145.

IOM (Institute of Medicine). 2000. *Gulf War and health, volume 1. Depleted uranium, pyridostigmine bromide, sarin, and vaccines*. Washington, DC: National Academy Press.

IOM. 2003. *Gulf War and health, volume 2: Insecticides and solvents*. Washington, DC: The National Academies Press.

IOM. 2005. *Gulf War and health, volume 3: Fuels, combustion products, and propellants*. Washington, DC: The National Academies Press.

IOM. 2006. *Gulf War and health, volume 4: Health effects of serving in the Gulf War*. Washington, DC: The National Academies Press.

IOM. 2007. *Gulf War and health, volume 5: Infectious diseases*. Washington, DC: The National Academies Press.

IOM. 2008. *Gulf War and health, volume 6: Physiologic, psychologic, and psychosocial effects of deployment-related stress*. Washington, DC: The National Academies Press.

IOM. 2009. *Gulf War and health, volume 7: Long-term consequences of traumatic brain injury*. Washington, DC: The National Academies Press.

IOM. 2010. *Gulf War and health, volume 8: Update of health effects of serving in the Gulf War*. Washington, DC: The National Academies Press.

IOM. 2011. *Long-term health consequences of exposure to burn pits in Iraq and Afghanistan*. Washington, DC: The National Academies Press.

Khatun A., M.S. Rahman, and M.G. Pang. 2018. Clinical assessment of the male fertility. *Obstetrics & Gynecology Science* 61(2):179–191.

NASEM (National Academies of Sciences, Engineering, and Medicine). 2016a. *Gulf War and health, volume 10: Update of health effects of serving in the Gulf War*. Washington, DC: The National Academies Press.

NASEM. 2016b. *Veterans and Agent Orange: Update 2014*. Washington, DC: The National Academies Press.

NRC (National Research Council). 2000. *Strategies to protect the health of deployed U.S. forces: Analytical framework for assessing risks*. Washington, DC: National Academy Press.

Ombelet, W., N. Dhont, A. Thijssen, E. Bosmans, and T. Kruger. 2014. Semen quality and prediction of IUI success in male subfertility: A systematic review. *Reproductive BioMedicine Online* 28(3):300–309.

Patel, A.S., J.Y. Leong, and R. Ramasamy. 2017. Prediction of male infertility by the World Health Organization laboratory manual for assessment of semen analysis: A systematic review. *Arab Journal of Urology* 16(1):96–102.

Tetreault, L.F., M. Doucet, P. Gamache, M. Fournier, A. Brand, T. Kosatsky, and A. Smargiassi. 2016. Childhood exposure to ambient air pollutants and the onset of asthma: An administrative cohort study in Quebec. *Environmental Health Perspectives* 124(8):1276–1282.

3

Introduction to the Study of Generational Effects

The transmission of health effects to his or her children, grandchildren, and subsequent generations resulting from a veteran's exposures is referred to as generational inheritance. A basic knowledge of both genetics[1] and a newer field—epigenetics[2]—is necessary to appreciate the potential biological mechanisms underlying heritable effects across generations. The potential impact of deployment exposures on veterans and their descendants must be considered in the broader context of a veteran's genome and epigenome as well as of exposures to other stressors (biological, chemical, psychological, radiological, or physiological) before, during, and after deployment that can also have genetic and epigenetic effects. This chapter describes how environmental exposures can affect the genome and epigenome, explains how those changes can be transmitted to children and subsequent generations, and provides a brief background on the evolving field of generational health effects. The committee cautions, however, that not all adverse effects on reproduction or fetal development are the result of genetic or epigenetic mechanisms: during gestation, on the developing embryo and fetus.

A more detailed description of the concepts of genetics and epigenetics as they apply to deployment-related exposures is presented below. Both genetic and epigenetic mechanisms have emerged as possible mediators of exposure-related impacts on the health of veterans and subsequent generations. As such, the committee's review of the literature included studies on genetic and epigenetic effects in its assessment of deployment exposures, and these studies are described in chapters 4 through 7. The committee recognizes that the principles of genetics and epigenetics can be complicated areas of study and that the information summarized in this chapter is at times highly technical and contains terminology that may not be familiar to all readers. A glossary of the key terms used in this report is presented in Appendix B.

---

[1] *Genetics* is the study of DNA and the genes it encodes, sometimes referred to as the genome when referencing the totality of the DNA (and all the genes) of an organism.

[2] *Epigenetics* is the study of processes that cause heritable changes in gene expression without changing the DNA sequence. The epigenome is comprised of chemical modifications made to DNA and the histone proteins that make up chromatin. "Heritable" in this context can refer to inheritance not only between parents and offspring (generational or meiotic inheritance of epigenetic alterations) but also between parent and daughter cells (mitotic inheritance).

HERITABLE TARGETS FOR DEPLOYMENT-RELATED EXPOSURES

According to current knowledge, the main biological targets for deployment-related exposures that could potentially mediate heritable effects across generations are the genome (and ribonucleic acid [RNA] linked to the genome), mitochondrial DNA, and the epigenome.

The Genome

The human genome encodes the genetic information necessary for human development in DNA molecules, and, with a few exceptions, all cells in the body contain an exact copy of this genome. Except for identical twins and triplets, everyone has a unique genome, which remains relatively stable throughout a lifetime. Human cells contain both nuclear and mitochondrial DNA, which together carry the instructions (referred to as the genetic "code") for making all the proteins within a human cell. Nuclear DNA is organized into chromosomes, which are made up of chromatin, a term used to describe DNA packaged with its associated proteins (see Figure 3-1). It has been estimated that the nuclear genome encodes in total about 20,000 genes, which through a number of different mechanisms give rise to the more than 6 million types of proteins needed by cells to function (Ponomarenko et al., 2016).

The human genome has 23 pairs of chromosomes (46 total chromosomes). Every individual inherits one set of 23 chromosomes from its mother and another 23 from its father. The sperm and the egg (the mature male and female germ cells, also called gametes) have only one set of 23 chromosomes each. These germ cells are thus different from other cells in the body, which are called somatic cells. Each copy of a gene is called an allele, and we inherit two alleles of every gene, one from each parent. The

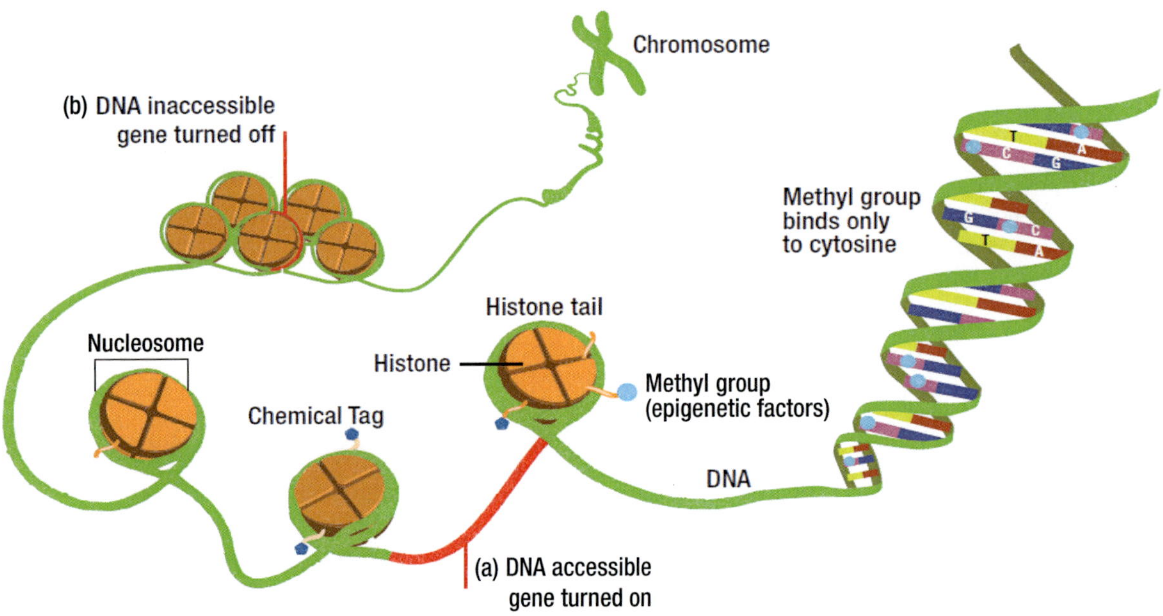

FIGURE 3-1 Chromatin structure. DNA is assembled with histone proteins into chromatin structures called nucleosomes. Nucleosomes form the basic packing unit for chromatin when it is condensed into chromosomes, and they also regulate chromatin structure and gene expression. Open chromatin lacking nucleosomes exposes DNA for gene expression (a), while tight nucleosome packing closes chromatin and silences gene expression (b). Both DNA and histone proteins are targets for epigenetic marks (e.g., methyl groups) that regulate chromatin structure and gene expression.
SOURCE: NHGRI, 2016.

exceptions are the sex chromosomes, X and Y, where genes contained on the male Y chromosome are only inherited from the father. When the sperm and the egg (oocyte) unite, the new cell that is formed, called a zygote, combines the chromosomes from each parent. As a result of this combination, the newly formed zygote carries characteristics inherited from each parent, with the exception of mitochondrial DNA (mtDNA), which is inherited solely from the mother. The unique features of mitochondria and their DNA are discussed further below.

The building blocks of DNA are the *bases* that make up the genome: adenine, thymine, cytosine, and guanine (A, T, C, G). Errors in copying genes and gene rearrangements can occur during the course of cell replication, and individual DNA bases can mutate, either spontaneously or after exposure to DNA-damaging agents. Throughout the course of hundreds of thousands of years, mutations have accumulated in the human genome that have given rise to the phenotypic variations now seen among humans.

Mutations in DNA can occur for many reasons, including environmental exposures such as ultraviolet light and chemical carcinogens. However, if these exposures are limited to somatic cells and no mutations occur in the sperm or the oocyte, the mutations will not be passed to future generations. While some mutations are benign, others can be lethal or change the DNA in ways that give rise to or alter susceptibility to disease. The latter types of mutations can cause birth defects and diseases such as cystic fibrosis, leukemias, hemochromatosis, and sickle cell anemia. Some DNA mutations may even be beneficial and protective against diseases, such as by conferring resistance to malaria or to viral infections (Williams, 2016). Because some mutations are only harmful when present in both alleles, carriers of harmful mutations on only one allele can lead healthy lives but may pass the mutated allele to their offspring. In the latter case, if both parents are healthy carriers of one copy of the same disease-causing mutation, the offspring has a 25% chance of inheriting two mutation-carrying alleles and becoming affected. Mutations may also be acquired during the formation of the gametes or of the zygote, resulting in new mutations that the offspring genome carries but that are absent in either parent.

While genetics focuses on DNA and mutations as mechanisms of inheritance and disease, the field of epigenetics focuses on mechanisms that can cause diseases that are not dependent upon DNA mutations. Like DNA mutations, some epigenetic alterations may be transmitted across cell divisions (i.e., from mother to daughter cells) and generations (i.e., from parent to offspring). The modifications associated with epigenetic inheritance can affect both the DNA itself, as happens with DNA methylation, and also the histone proteins, which together with DNA constitute a nucleosome, the structural unit of chromatin (see Figure 3-1).

The transmission of heritable traits to future generations in response to environmental exposures of the parent or parents aligns with the so-called Barker hypothesis, also known as the developmental origins of health and disease (DOHaD) (Skogen and Overland, 2012). DOHaD hypothesizes that early life events can influence health and disease susceptibility for the entire life of an individual. Thus, in addition to DNA mutations and small variations in DNA sequence within populations (polymorphisms), environmental exposures and life experiences may also affect an individual's susceptibility to disease. For example, both famine-influenced and obesity-influenced nutrition in utero has been associated with disease in adulthood, including type-2 diabetes and cardiovascular mortality (Langley-Evans, 2014). The diversity of the human genome may contribute to differences in susceptibility to environmental and occupational exposures. The immediate effects of those differences may be an accelerated or diminished response to harmful exposures, such as the hostile environment of a war zone. Only when environmental and lifestyle factors as well as genetic and epigenetic variation are appropriately considered will it be possible to fully understand the impact of deployment-related exposures on generational health.

The Mitochondrial Genome

In addition to changes in the nuclear genome and epigenome discussed above, environmentally driven changes in mtDNA represent another potential mechanism for environmental inheritance. Mitochondria are the energy powerhouses of cells, and they possess a genome that is distinct from that of the nucleus. The mitochondrial genome encodes 37 genes that give rise to 13 proteins crucial to cellular bioenergetic functions. A unique feature of mtDNA is that it is transmitted to subsequent generations exclusively through the maternal lineage. When mtDNA is damaged by mutations, maternally inherited disorders, termed mitochondrial encephalomyopathies, may occur. Because there are multiple copies of mtDNA, mitochondrial diseases arise when a significant proportion of affected mitochondria carry a mutation that can then be passed to the offspring. Mitochondria are extremely sensitive to environmental sources of oxidative stress because, unlike nuclear DNA, mtDNA lacks histones and DNA repair mechanisms (Kucej et al., 2008).

The Epigenome

By definition, epigenetic modifications influence the chromatin structure and gene expression without altering the underlying sequence of DNA (Barbara and Abdilla, 2017). The epigenome refers to the entire collection of epigenetic modifications of chromatin, which are sometimes called epigenetic marks. The main epigenetic marks are the methylation of DNA and histone modifications (Murr, 2010; Robertson, 2005). Small RNAs that interact directly with DNA to modulate its function also function as epigenetic modulators and play a role in epigenetic inheritance. A large number of proteins make up the epigenetic machinery that adds, removes, or acts on epigenetic marks. This machinery modifies chromatin in ways that change genome structure and function—for example, modifying how DNA is condensed into chromosomes—and determines when genes are expressed or silenced (Atlasi and Stunnenberg, 2017; Youn, 2017). The inheritance of epigenetic changes is a mechanism (in addition to DNA mutation) by which traits can be passed from parent to children—in this case, without changes in the sequence of DNA. Additional details on the epigenome are provided below.

Unlike the genome, which is mostly static and unique to each individual, the epigenome is dynamic and changes during the course of development, across the passage of time, and from one cell type to another. In fact, the way that multiple cell types and diverse tissues in the human body originate from a single cell is accounted for almost entirely by differences in the epigenome. While each person has only one genome, each cell type of the body has its own epigenome, which can change over time in response to the internal and external environment. Thus, epigenomes are considerably more malleable than genomes and as a result are inherently more vulnerable to environmental exposures. The timing of exposure is also important (described below), and development is a time of rapid changes in the epigenome, as the zygote rapidly transitions from the sperm and egg epigenomes to the new epigenomic programming that will direct the development of all cells and tissues of the body. Thus, the epigenome of developing germ cells in the embryo and fetus is quite susceptible to environmental exposures (Fraser and Lin, 2016; Xu and Xie, 2018).

Some epigenetic modifications to DNA and histones as well as modifiers such as noncoding RNAs (ncRNAs) can interact and reinforce or negate each other to influence patterns of gene expression. This means that an exposure affecting one type of epigenetic factor could also influence (reinforce or negate) another type of epigenetic factor. For example, when somatic cells are exposed to benz(a)pyrene, the initial effect is an inhibition of repressive histone marks at selective sites in the genome, along with the promotion of activating histone marks at other sites; these initial epigenetic alterations in turn affect DNA methylation (i.e., they inhibit DNA methylation), with the overall result being an increased expression of affected genes (Teneng et al., 2011). Thus, while an exposure may initially lead to an effect on one type of epigenetic factor (e.g., histone modification), generational effects caused by that exposure could be mediated by a different type of epigenetic factor, such as DNA methylation.

The epigenetic machinery—the enzymes that "read, write, and erase" epigenetic marks—controls DNA methylation, histone marks, ncRNAs, and chromatin-remodeling proteins and is essential for the proper installation and maintenance of epigenetic functions. There are several pathways by which environmental exposures can affect the epigenome, resulting in effects that persist long after the exposure ceases—or even across generations (Walker, 2016). For example, toxicants such as endocrine disruptors can activate signaling pathways within the cell that change the activity of the epigenetic machinery and alter patterns of epigenetic marks. This reprogramming of the epigenome can alter gene expression in the progeny of exposed cells or individuals (Uzumcu et al., 2012). Other variations in the epigenome may result either from DNA mutations that directly affect the genes encoding components of the epigenetic machinery and alter epigenetic control or else from a modulation of regulatory control that compromises the functionality of the epigenetic machinery (Ramos et al., 2018). The environment may also influence the availability of cofactors needed for normal epigenetic processes to occur, such as the iron or oxygen needed for demethylase "erasers" or dietary folate that provides methyl groups for both DNA and histone methylation (Crider et al., 2012; Walker, 2016). In addition to epigenetic "readers, writers, and erasers," many other proteins can associate with chromatin, including those that change chromatin structure to influence gene expression. The activity of these chromatin remodelers can also be influenced by environmental exposures (Bariar et al., 2013; Biswas and Rao, 2018). While these proteins may not themselves be considered part of the epigenome, they can influence epigenetic marks and thus change the epigenome in ways that are heritable. Examples of these types of proteins would be the high-mobility group proteins and the SWI/SNF ATPases that modulate chromatin structure (Hepp et al., 2014).

Epigenetic patterns vary from one cell type to another, and virtually all tissues have mixed cell populations. Therefore, when a sample of mixed cell types is analyzed, care must be taken to determine that the changes in both DNA and histone methyl marks are due to changes in the epigenome and not simply to changes in the relative cell populations in the sample. This cell heterogeneity may complicate the interpretation of the effects of exposures. For example, Jaffe and Irizarry (2014) reported cell composition changes across age in whole blood and demonstrated that cellular composition can explain much of the observed variability in the measured DNA methylation. This implies that if an exposure such as $PM_{2.5}$ changes the cell composition of blood—for example, because of an immune response without any changes in methylation patterns themselves—changes in the methylation profile of blood can be observed even when no methylation changes have occurred in any cell. Future studies will need to eliminate or account for this type of confounder. This limitation applies to both human and animal studies that use tissue-based sampling. Methods to address this issue with single-cell approaches are being developed (Angermueller et al., 2016; Karemaker and Vermeulen, 2018).

DNA Methylation

DNA methylation is of interest because of the numerous examples of diseases caused by an increase in methylation (that is, hypermethylation) associated with the suppression of gene expression as well as by a loss of methylation (that is, hypomethylation) associated with increases in gene expression. Because genes are expressed differently in each cell type, gene-specific methylation patterns are one way to specify a cellular response. DNA methylation can be modified (both increased and decreased) in response to the environment. Altered DNA methylation patterns can then be copied and passed on to daughter cells during cell division, allowing the transmission of altered methylation patterns to daughter cells, which is termed mitotic inheritance. Modified DNA methylation caused by an environmental exposure can also occur in germ cells and be passed on to future generations. This is termed meiotic inheritance and can lead to generational effects.

Depending on the timing of the exposure during development, DNA methylation changes can profoundly affect germ cells (Ly et al., 2015; Wu et al., 2015). DNA methylation is also involved in genomic imprinting, an important process that occurs during gametogenesis and early embryogenesis when gene expression patterns are established in a parent-of-origin-dependent manner, directing genes to be expressed solely from DNA inherited from the mother or from the father (McEwen and Ferguson-Smith, 2010). Imprinted genes are a classic example of genes that are marked in a sex-specific manner in the male or female germ line, often by DNA methylation, such that only one of the parental genes will be expressed in the offspring (with the gene from the other parent being methylated and therefore silenced). The methylated imprinted gene in the sperm or egg is thus inherited by the offspring and represents an example of how epigenetic changes in germ cells can be "remembered" and passed on to the next generation. The methylation silencing of the maternal or paternal gene in genomic imprinting is critical for normal development, as dysregulation of this process can result in a number of disorders, including Angelman, Prader-Willi, and Beckwith-Weidemann syndromes (Butler, 2009). Experimental studies show that toxicants' effects on the germ cell's epigenome can result in long-lasting marks on the chromatin which remain through cell divisions and across generations and which can affect health (Wei et al., 2015).

DNA methylation can occur at approximately 28 million cytosine-adjacent-to-guanine (CpG) sites in the human genome. While other DNA bases can also be methylated, CpG methylation is by far the most prevalent and best understood mechanism for how DNA methylation regulates gene expression; however, non-CpG methylation and hydroxymethylation are emerging marks of interest (Jang et al., 2017). The precise location of DNA methylation at CpG sites provides context for how methylation affects gene expression. Both global (genome-wide) changes and site-specific effects that are more nuanced and only affect small regions of the genome (e.g., specific genes) can be influenced by the environment.

Histones and Other Chromatin-Associated Proteins

In the cell nucleus, DNA wraps around eight histones (two each of the core histones 2a, 2b, 3, and 4) to form the nucleosome and thus chromatin. Another histone (histone 1) links proteins between nucleosomes (see Figure 3-1). Histones are subject to several types of chemical modifications, including methylation, acetylation, sumoylation, and phosphorylation, and they can participate in both the activation and the repression of gene expression. Importantly, as is the case with DNA methylation patterns, patterns of epigenetic histone marks, specifically methyl marks, can be both mitotically and meiotically inherited. Thus, exposures that alter histone methyl marks could potentially cause generational health effects. Indeed, alterations in histone marks exhibit a much greater dynamic range in terms of their effects on gene expression than changes in DNA methylation (Anonymous, 2015). At the cellular level, alterations in histone methylation can result in changes in gene expression that can be both quantitative (i.e., high versus low levels of transcription) as well as qualitative (i.e., is a gene expressed or not), whereas alterations in DNA methylation primarily result in qualitative changes in gene expression—for example, gene silencing caused by increased promoter methylation.

Noncoding RNAs

There are at least 48 different noncoding classes of RNAs in addition to the protein-coding messenger RNAs (mRNAs) in the human genome. These ncRNAs vary in size from 20–30 nucleotides in length for the small ncRNAs to longer than 200 nucleotides for the long ncRNAs. They participate in a wide array of cellular processes, from protein synthesis to epigenetic regulation and inheritance. Although examples can be found throughout the plant and animal kingdoms, this report focuses on using rodent models to inform and contrast with what is known about humans. For example, X-inactive specific transcript, a long ncRNA, is a major effector of X-chromosome inactivation. Various small ncRNAs, such as microRNAs (miRNAs) which act as scaffolds for histone and DNA methyltransferases, also participate in the epigenetic regulation of the genome in many species (Holoch and Moazed, 2015), along with transfer RNA fragments and Piwi-interacting RNAs which limit the action of transposable elements to protect the integrity of the genome (Julinano et al., 2011; Schorn et al., 2017).

Given their important functions in human germ cells, miRNAs are particularly relevant to the study of generational inheritance. While acting directly at the epigenetic level, miRNAs can also act as post-transcriptional regulators of gene expression in mammals (Virant-Klun et al., 2016). Through complementary base pairing, the miRNA can specifically destabilize and silence mRNA and modulate gene expression without altering the DNA sequence. For example, miRNAs, such as mir-181c, affect DNA methylation at fertilization by regulating DNA methyltransferase, which affects embryo pluripotency (Xu et al., 2013).

In males, epigenetic inheritance is thought to be mediated, in part, by a wide spectrum of sperm RNAs that are delivered at fertilization. The sperm RNAs are likely to participate in early embryonic development until the point of zygotic genome activation (Sendler et al., 2013; Yuan et al., 2016). From a mechanistic standpoint, sperm RNAs may have immediate effects in the zygote: extending calcium oscillations in the embryo to signal fertilization, early cell-fate decisions, genome restructuring through interaction with repetitive elements, or direct modification of the genome (Jodar et al., 2017). Similarly, various types of short and long noncoding RNAs are present in oocytes (Svoboda, 2017). Evidence is emerging that oocyte-derived miRNAs can influence gene expression in early embryos (Eckersley-Maslin et al., 2018).

Paternal exposures to toxicants can affect sperm RNA, and this may explain the patterns of paternal inheritance. Mouse models have shown that sperm RNAs can be affected by psychological and physiological factors, with the altered RNAs being passed to offspring (Yeshurun and Hannan, 2018). In the context of transgenerational inheritance, mouse sperm RNAs appear to have the capacity to be integrated into an offspring's genome, although at a very low rate (Spadafora, 2016). The influence of paternal diet and age on mouse sperm RNAs is well documented. For example, paternal obesity can lead to an increased risk of metabolic disease in the offspring, irrespective of maternal body weight (Sharma and Rando, 2017). This parallels changes in patterns of DNA methylation and levels of various sperm RNAs. In contrast to these recent studies in males, little is known at this point regarding the role of female, small ncRNAs in the intergenerational inheritance of effects (Clarke and Vieux, 2015).

PARADIGMS OF INHERITANCE

This report uses two terms to describe paradigms of generational inheritance: "intergenerational" and "transgenerational." Whether the effects of parental exposures on offspring are considered "inter" or "trans" generational is determined by the timing of the exposure relative to conception and by whether the exposure has a direct or an indirect effect on the health of descendants (see Figure 3-2).

In the upper panel in Figure 3-2, men and nonpregnant women (i.e., the F0 generation) may be exposed to harmful agents, but the exposure ends before conception, and subsequent generations are not

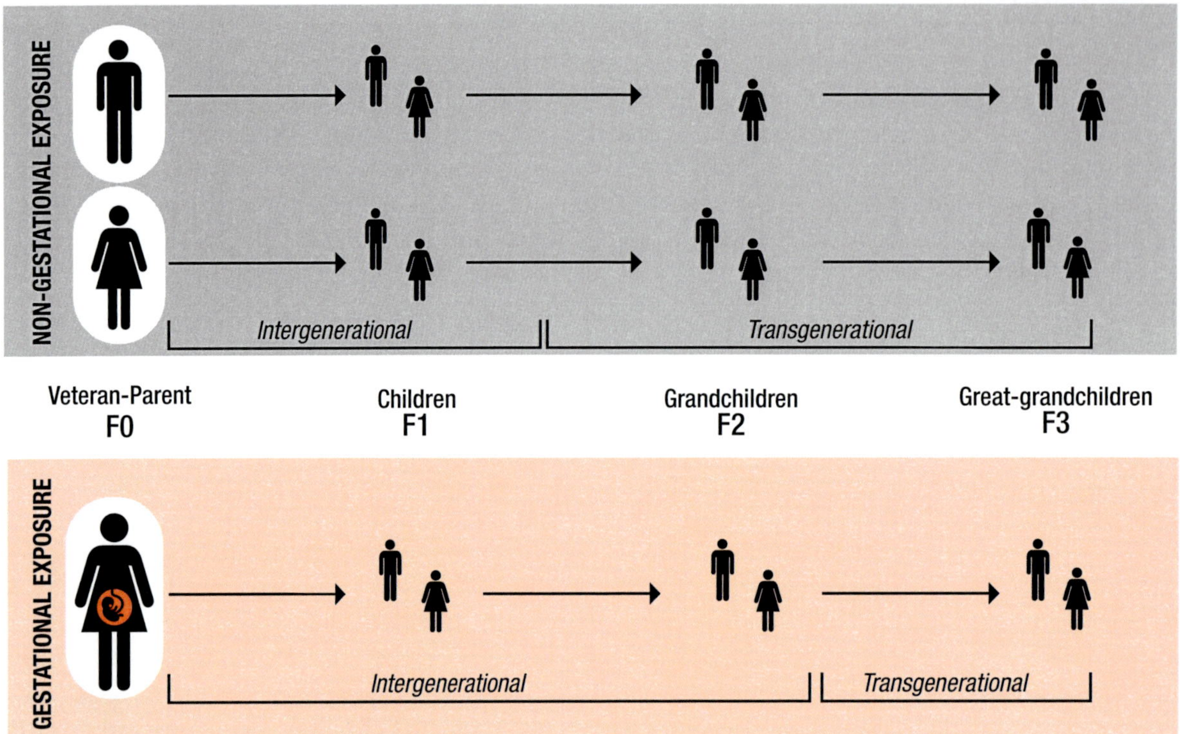

FIGURE 3-2 Comparison of intergenerational and transgenerational effects. The upper panel shows that intergenerational effects occur in the children (F1) of exposed men and exposed nonpregnant women (F0) and that transgenerational effects occur in grandchildren (F2) and great-grandchildren (F3) of the same F0 generation. The lower panel shows that for pregnant women with exposures (F0), intergenerational effects occur in their children (F1) and grandchildren (F2), whereas transgenerational effects occur in their great-grandchildren (F3).

directly exposed. However, if a male or female veteran's germ cells are exposed to a toxicant, his or her children, the F1 generation, may be considered to have been exposed as well via the exposed gametes giving rise to what is called an intergenerational effect. The observed effect in the F1 generation may be due to genetic or epigenetic changes or both. The effects that are then passed on to the children of the veteran's children—that is, the grandchildren, the F2 generation, who were not exposed to the toxicant directly or via the germ cells—are called transgenerational effects.

When a pregnant woman is exposed to a toxicant (the lower panel in Figure 3-2), three generations are directly exposed: the mother (F0), her fetus (the F1 generation), and the germ cells of the developing fetus. Because fetal germ cells give rise to the F2 generation, that generation is also considered to have been exposed. In Figure 3-3, effects of the maternal exposure observed in the children and grandchildren (F1 and F2 generations) constitute intergenerational effects, while effects observed in the great-grandchildren—that is, the F3 generation, the first generation to not have been exposed directly or via germ cells—are considered to be transgenerational effects.

These differences in direct and indirect exposure to a toxicant as well as the timing of that exposure represent important variables to be considered in evaluating and interpreting the results of studies designed to examine reproductive, developmental, and intergenerational and transgenerational effects. These variables are discussed in the following sections and in subsequent chapters.

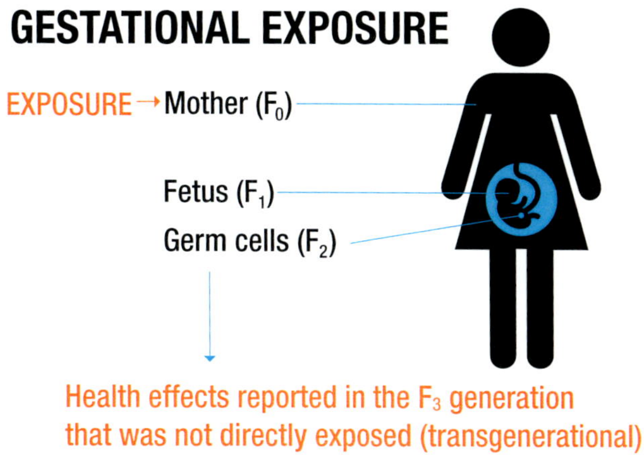

FIGURE 3-3 Gestational exposure paradigm. When a pregnant woman is exposed, three generations are directly affected by the exposure: the mother (F0), her fetus (the F1 generation), and the germ cells of the developing fetus. Consequently, the effects of gestational exposures on children and grandchildren (F1 and F2) are considered to be intergenerational effects, while effects observed in the great-grandchildren—that is, the F3 generation, the first generation to not have been exposed directly or via germ cells—are considered to be transgenerational effects.
SOURCE: NTP, 2018.

TIMING OF EXPOSURES AND OUTCOMES

Exposures that lead to reproductive effects in men or women can occur at any time. Parental exposures that may affect the development of an embryo, a fetus, or a child can occur before conception (during the development or maturation of germ cells or gametes) (see Figure 3-4) or during pregnancy (see Figure 3-5). The timing of exposure is particularly important to understanding whether genetic or epigenetic effects can be inherited. Mechanistically, the timing of exposure and of effects on genetic and epigenetic processes is important in the regulation of normal germ cell development (including the regulation of gene expression) and in the establishment of epigenetic marks that are passed onto the offspring at the time of fertilization.

One consideration with respect to evaluating exposure–disease associations in an intergenerational or transgenerational context is that certain exposures may have differing effects depending on when they occur prior to or across an individual's lifecourse. In fact, exposure during the preconception and prenatal time periods may be particularly important to consider, as these may be particularly vulnerable critical windows of growth and development with later life effects on chronic disease risk in the offspring. This concept of windows of vulnerability has led to the DOHaD hypothesis discussed earlier in the chapter. A critical period is defined as a specific window of time during which an exposure can affect development resulting in a subsequent risk of disease. In this hypothesis, the exposure only has an effect during a finite time period; for example, studies of vaginal epithelial changes in women born to mothers who used diethylstilbestrol during pregnancy indicate that unless diethylstilbestrol exposure was begun before the 18th week of gestation, the chance of vaginal epithelial changes in the female children was very small (Glaze, 1984). Thus, an exposure can have an irreversible effect on disease risk in the offspring and future generations later in life. In addition to critical periods, sensitive periods also have to be considered. A sensitive period is similar to a critical period in that exposure during this period of possibly rapid biological change can affect disease risk, but the impact of the exposure on disease risk can be altered outside of this time period (Kuh and Ben-Shlomo, 2004). Thus, effects caused by exposure during a sensitive period may be reversed or exacerbated by later life exposures.

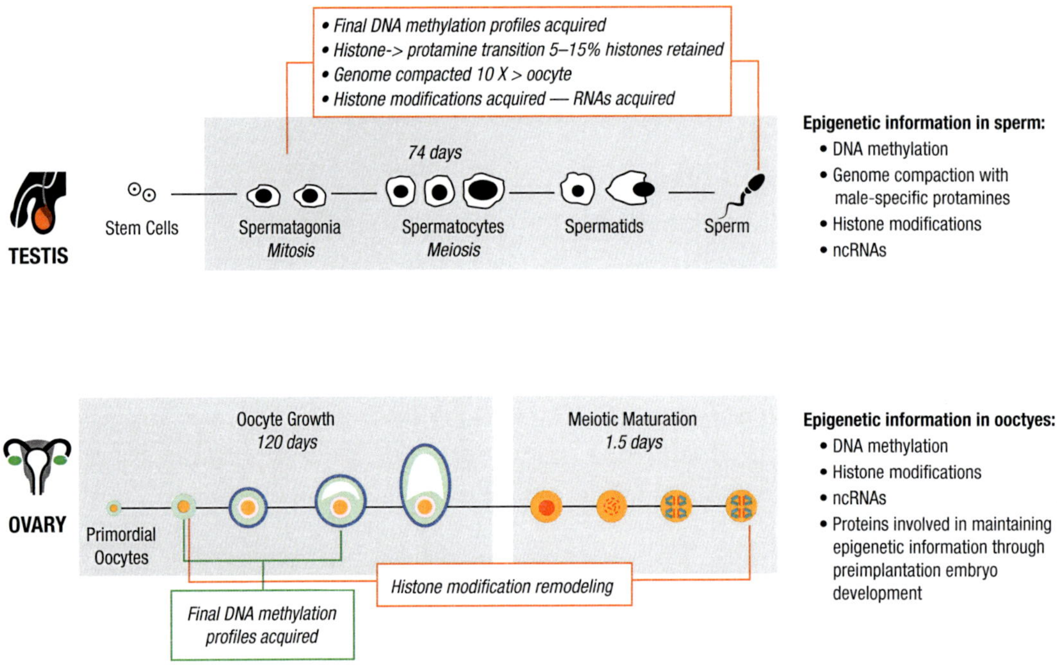

FIGURE 3-4 Key phases in the development of mature male (spermatozoa or sperm) or female (oocytes) germ cells that may be affected by toxicant exposures are shown in the top and bottom panels, respectively. Epigenetic remodeling of DNA methylation and histone marks take place during both male and female germ cell development. Sperm and oocytes contribute unique epigenetic information to the zygote (i.e., the fertilized oocyte) at the start of embryogenesis. For sperm, this epigenetic information includes DNA methylation, male-specific protamines, histone modifications to the 5–15% of histone that remain after chromatin remodeling and compaction in spermatids, and ncRNAs. For oocytes, along with sex-specific DNA methylation, histone modifications, and ncRNAs, there are also proteins present in the cytoplasm of the oocyte that are important for epigenetic events taking place in the early embryo in the first week of life.

These concepts come from the framework of lifecourse epidemiology. The World Health Organization (2000) has embraced a lifecourse epidemiology approach using conceptual models to evaluate exposure–disease questions; four models are discussed here. These different models should be considered when designing studies, as well as the appropriate statistical methods that could involve effect modification, and carefully considering confounding and other forms of potential bias.

One proposed model is the critical period model, which occurs when an exposure has an immutable effect on later life disease risk through alterations to the structure or function of organs, tissues, or body systems. For example, prenatal exposure to trichloroethylene has been associated with cardiac defects in children, and such defects may lead to heart problems later in the child's life (see Chapter 7 for a discussion of the developmental effects of trichloroethylene).

The second model is the critical period model with later effect modifiers. For this, an exposure has an effect on later life disease risk for the same reasons mentioned above, but later life exposures can alter the impact of the exposure. For example, a veteran's exposure to certain deployment toxicants might alter the metabolism of his or her children, and the metabolic alternations might affect the future development of metabolic diseases such as obesity and type 2 diabetes. However, a healthy diet and physical activity in childhood and early adulthood could act as effect modifiers to decrease the risk of developing these conditions in later life. In essence, these two lifecourse models are equivalent to the respective critical and sensitive periods discussed earlier.

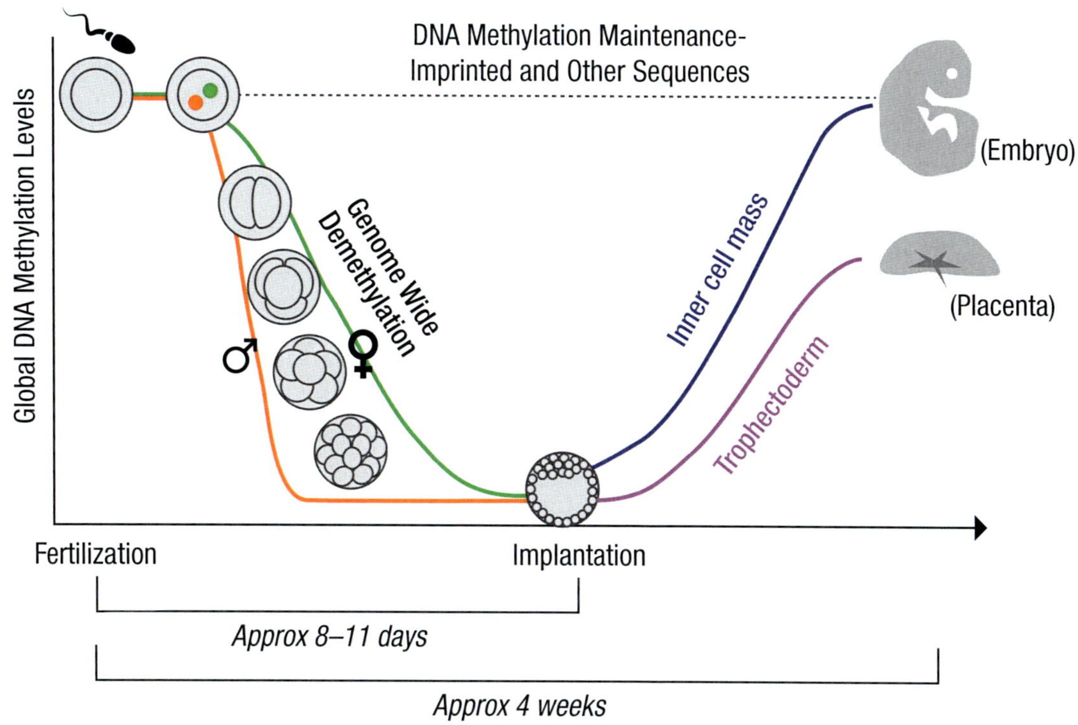

FIGURE 3-5 Schematic representation of post-fertilization epigenetic reprogramming of DNA methylation. Following fertilization, while most of the genome is demethylated and then remethylated after implantation, DNA methylation patterns on imprinted genes and some other sequences in the genome must be maintained during preimplantation development (dotted line). Imprinted genes carry sex-specific epigenetic marks that differ between sperm and oocytes and are key for the normal development and growth of the fetus. For clarity, sperm are depicted as much larger than their actual size in relation to the oocyte. SOURCE: Adapted from Trounson et al., 2013, with permission.

A third model is that of cumulative risk, where exposures are independent and uncorrelated. In the model, the accumulation of not just one, but multiple exposures could impact later life disease risk. For example, if a service member is exposed to a chemical both on the base and at a single time during a patrol, the two exposures are not correlated, but the exposures could interact synergistically or antagonistically to affect the risk of subsequent disease.

Finally, the fourth model is where exposures accumulate but are also correlated. In this case, the correlated exposures result in clustering or chains and pathways of risk. An example of this with respect to generational health effects is the establishment of a "warrior caste" where children and grandchildren of military parents serve in the military as well (Schafer, 2017). In these military families, exposures may be correlated or clustered resulting in disease risk accumulation that might affect multiple generations.

Toxic Insult to Sperm or Eggs Prior to Conception

Animal models and epidemiological studies have demonstrated a significant role of sex in the response of parental germ cells to toxicants. Because the timing of germ cell production and maturation is vastly different for men and for women (refer to Figure 3-4 for details), environmental exposures will produce different effects depending on whether the mother or the father was exposed and the timing of the exposure.

The primary reproductive organs are the testes in males and the ovaries in females, which are responsible for producing sperm and oocytes, respectively, and also hormones. In men, testosterone stimulation of the testis causes germ cells to develop from spermatogonia to spermatozoa, a process called spermatogenesis. Spermatogenesis takes about 74 days, with an additional 10 days or so for these cells to further mature as they pass through the epididymis (Amann et al., 2008; Heller et al., 1969) (Figure 3-4, top panel). The sperm cell epigenome undergoes a number of modifications during spermatogenesis, including changes in DNA methylation patterns and histone modifications, as part of an extensive chromatin remodeling process that occurs during male germ cell development.

At birth, females are thought to have about 1 million primordial germ cells (PGCs; oocytes). In response to hormonal stimulation beginning at puberty, individual oocytes within the ovary grow and differentiate within the follicles over a period of about 4 months prior to ovulation (Figure 3-4, bottom panel). Key epigenetic marks, such as DNA methylation and epigenetic marks on imprinted genes, are acquired during this growth phase, and exposure of the oocyte to toxicants during this time might adversely affect the viability of the oocyte, fetus, or child.

Male-Mediated Effects on Offspring Due to Fathers' Exposures

For men, the exposures of most concern are those that permanently affect the male germ line stem cells since these cells continue to produce the precursors of sperm throughout a man's life. Although small-scale studies (Robbins et al., 1997) found no genetic effects following a complete cycle of spermatogenesis subsequent to receiving chemotherapy for cancer, in larger studies, both genetic (e.g., Tempest et al., 2008) and epigenetic (e.g., Shnorhavorian et al., 2017) effects in sperm have been found to persist for years after treatment ended. The larger studies suggest that chemotherapy-induced abnormalities in male germ line stem cells have the potential to affect the children of these men.

After the stem cell phase, epigenetic changes can be incorporated into sperm in two main ways: at the time of the repackaging of DNA and through RNAs included with the sperm in semen. Key epigenetic modifications normally occur in male germ cells during the repackaging of chromatin. This genome compaction using protamines makes sperm chromatin unique. Protamine compaction reduces the genome size and, functionally, renders the sperm genome transcriptionally and translationally inert by condensing DNA to an almost crystalline form. This process is brought about as DNA exchanges its chromatin through a final wave of methylation, acetylation, and exchange of packaging proteins. At each stage of the compaction process, the genome and epigenome are susceptible to exposure-related modifications.

During epididymal transit, RNAs are added to the sperm (Jodar et al., 2017; Johnson et al., 2015). RNAs reach the epididymal fluid from multiple sites throughout the body (Cossetti et al., 2014) and then reside within the sperm (Johnson et al., 2015). The incorporation of RNAs with sperm from throughout the body provides a direct mechanism to epigenetically communicate exposures to gametes. For example, impacts on expression of sperm miRNAs have been identified in association with smoking (Marczylo et al., 2012), but it has not been established that those miRNAs are actually delivered by the sperm to the zygote. An understanding of the mechanisms by which epigenetic changes are incorporated into sperm is beginning to emerge, but much research is still needed to establish how these epigenetic changes are retained or recoded for the next and subsequent generations.

Female-Mediated Effects on Offspring Due to Mothers' Exposures

Unlike men, women are born with their full complement of germ cells (i.e., oocytes). Thus, exposures of women that affect oocytes that enter the reproductive cycle could result in abnormal reproductive outcomes and effects in the next generation. Studying the effects of toxic exposures on oocytes is challenging because of the small numbers of available cells and the difficulty in obtaining oocytes, even in animal models. There are several examples of intergenerational effects on the health of offspring following the exposure of females to high-fat or low-protein diets or to diabetic states (Clarke and Vieux, 2015). Several defects were identified in oocytes that could underlie the health effects of these maternal exposures in the offspring, including mitochondrial defects, lipid abnormalities, meiotic spindle abnormalities, and DNA methylation defects in imprinted genes. Other relevant studies of female-mediated effects via altered epigenetic marks or gene expression in the offspring have examined the effects of alcohol "binges" (VandeVoort et al., 2015), high dietary sugar intake (Chaffin et al., 2014), and maternal zinc deficiency (Tian and Diaz, 2012, 2013).

Toxic Insult to the Mother and Fetus

Exposure of a pregnant mother to a toxicant might adversely affect her developing embryo or fetus. Although the detection of a pregnancy in a deployed female service member is reason for her evacuation from a war zone, toxic exposures during the earliest period of gestation and before a pregnancy can pose a threat to the developing fetus.

During the first week of gestation, the zygote develops into the multicellular blastocyst, which implants into the uterus and goes on to develop into an embryo and portions of the placenta (see Figure 3-5). As noted earlier, an important phase of epigenetic reprogramming occurs at this time of development (i.e., between fertilization and implantation at about 1 week of pregnancy) during which most, but not all, of the epigenetic marks in the blastocyst cells are erased. This time is the beginning of embryonic stem cell differentiation, the process that ultimately decides the fate of individual cells (Messerschmidt et al., 2014). At this early blastocyst stage, various chemical, genetic, and cellular interactions determine if these earliest stem cells differentiate into the inner cellular mass (ICM) or into the trophectoderm. The trophectoderm is the outer covering of cells which eventually forms the placental interface between mother and fetus. The trophectoderm is necessary for successful embryonic development, as it transfers nutrients and oxygen from the mother to the developing fetus. The ICM is the bundle of cells that will eventually form the fetus itself. Stem cells in the ICM differentiate into organ systems, although some stem cells will remain to participate in tissue renewal and repair. Epigenetic patterns in both DNA and histone methylation are then reacquired in a cell- and tissue-specific manner as the embryo and placenta continue to develop (Developmental Biology Interactive, n.d.).

The reprogramming of epigenetic information in the first week of life has been shown in studies in mice to be particularly susceptible to the external environment (McGowan and Roth, 2015; Sunde et al., 2016). To emphasize the complexity of the challenge of understanding intergenerational effects, it should be noted that for epigenetic marks to have an effect on future generations they need to be malleable enough to be affected by a subtle environmental effect but, at the same time, stable enough to survive the reprogramming that occurs during the formation of the early embryo and the germ line and during development.

The window of exposure during pregnancy relative to the developmental stage of the embryo or fetus is critically important. The period of organogenesis that occurs within the first 3 months of the pregnancy follows a tightly orchestrated series of biochemical events that give rise to the different organ systems. Different organs develop at different times as a function of cell–cell and cell–matrix interactions which define the survival of the developing embryo (Chen et al., 2009; Hill, 2018). Therefore, exposures during this critical window can affect different organs depending not only on the nature of the exposure itself but also on the timing of the exposure. It is important to note that the ways in which certain organ systems, such as the nervous system and the lung, mature can extend the window of susceptibility (Rice and Barone, 2000; Shi et al., 2007).

Toxic Insult to Fetal Somatic Cells

In utero exposures of fetal somatic (non-germ-cell) tissues can cause birth defects or may affect the health of the child after birth or later in life, depending on the organ affected and the timing of the exposure. Post-fertilization growth and developmental trajectories occur at different rates for male and female offspring, and studies have shown that epigenetic changes reflect this by taking place differently in male and female offspring (Faulk and Dolinoy, 2011; Kanherkar et al., 2014). Furthermore, the placenta produces signals that are specific to the sex of the fetus, so exposures during pregnancy that affect the placenta can produce birth outcomes that are specific to fetal sex. Therefore, a maternal exposure can have very different impacts on pregnancy and fetal development for girls versus for boys.

Toxic Insult to the Germ Cells of the Fetus

A new area of concern is the potential generational effects associated with the exposure of fetal germ cells to toxicants during the mother's pregnancy. Both animal and human studies suggest that adverse health effects in the grandchildren can result from a woman's exposures while pregnant (i.e., an intergenerational effect) (Lane et al., 2014). In contrast to the effects on fetal somatic cells, exposures of the developing fetal reproductive organs can affect the future reproductive function of a child or may be passed on to the next generation. Fetal germ cells undergo a dramatic epigenetic reprogramming of DNA methylation and histone modifications during the first 16 weeks of pregnancy (see Figure 3-6). After the PGCs in the ovary of a female fetus enter their final mitotic phase, they quickly arrest until puberty (see Figure 3-6). At puberty, the oocytes gain epigenetic marks as they mature (see Figure 3-4). In comparison, PGCs in the testes of a male fetus gain epigenetic marks before birth (see Figure 3-6) and undergo meiosis at puberty (see Figure 3-4). That is, epigenetic marks are gained in male germ cells in the fetal period, whereas epigenetic marks are gained in female germ cells as adults. These relationships are important because the genome/epigenome is most vulnerable to environmental exposures when it is undergoing mitosis.

Timing of Outcomes

The consequences of deployment on the health of a veteran's descendants (generational effects) can be viewed within the framework of the DOHaD hypothesis that early life experiences can program the pathologies of old age (Xin et al., 2015). Epigenetic modifications are thought to be largely responsible for DOHaD "reprogramming," whereby the developing epigenome is "reprogrammed" by environmental exposures in a way that persists for the life of the individual and can result in adverse health effects in adulthood. Prenatal insults, such as malnutrition and stress, can lead to an increase in common metabolic and cardiovascular diseases in adulthood (Barker, 2004). Similarly, in some cases adverse childhood outcomes, such as cancer and neurodevelopmental effects, are thought to be related to prenatal exposures to toxicants, such as, respectively, benzene and organophosphate pesticides. Other exposures, such as to endocrine-disrupting chemicals which mimic the biological actions of endogenous hormones, have been found to have later life effects on adult metabolic function in mice (La Merrill et al., 2014) and also behavioral and neurological outcomes in both humans and animals (Gore et al., 2015). Other adult diseases thought to originate from developmental exposures include impaired reproductive capability

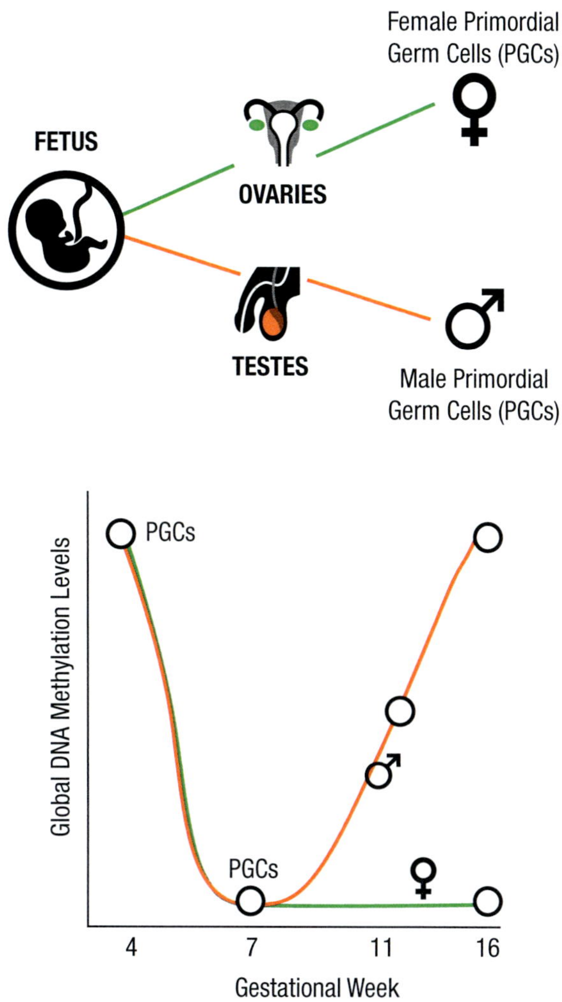

FIGURE 3-6 Primordial germ cell (PGC) reprogramming. (top) An exposure during pregnancy can affect the fetus and the germ cells developing in the fetus' ovaries or testes. (bottom) PGCs are subject to reprogramming, such as DNA methylation, in the first few weeks of pregnancy, when most epigenetic marks are erased, as shown by decreased global DNA methylation levels. After the epigenetic marks are erased, beginning at about gestational week 7, there is a sex-specific reacquisition of epigenetic marks. In male fetuses, PGCs are methylated (i.e., reprogrammed) between gestational weeks 7 and 16, but in female fetuses, the PGCs are not methylated until after birth at the time of oocyte growth (see Figure 3-4).

in animals (Gore, 2008; Ho et al., 2017) and mental illness in humans and animals (Guintivano and Kaminsky, 2016).

Early life development and pubertal onset are also maturation periods which can trigger the manifestation of latent effects of developmental reprogramming and can be significant factors in disease presentation. For instance, neurodevelopmental disorders such as autism, attention deficit and hyperactivity disorder, and early-onset schizophrenia have a profound sex bias, with an increased incidence of presentation in males, supporting the concept that vulnerabilities and resiliencies to preconception or prenatal insults may be unique to the sex of the fetus (Kern et al., 2017; McCarthy, 2016; Waddell and McCarthy, 2012; Werling, 2016).

EPIDEMIOLOGIC GENERATIONAL AND EPIGENETIC STUDIES

The paucity of information about exposures associated with generational effects, combined with the current lack of understanding about male and female germ cell reprogramming, make it difficult to determine whether there is an increased risk of health effects among children or grandchildren. It is clear from the few epidemiological studies in which risk factors for generational health outcomes have been examined that much less is known about paternal exposures than about maternal exposures, as most of these studies have focused on maternal experiences during pregnancy. However, some epidemiological studies examining men exposed to the Swedish famines or to the Dutch "Hunger Winter" have attempted to identify periods of development where germ cells may be more susceptible to environmental stresses (Vansant et al., 2016).

In epidemiologic studies the interpretation of epigenetic patterns is complicated by disease status. Many studies use a case-control study design, where study participants are recruited based on disease status (i.e., cases versus controls), and samples are collected after disease development among the cases. In this scenario, any change in an epigenetic pattern among cases may have arisen *after* the disease onset in response to differences in treatments, diets, exercise, and metabolism. Therefore, it is difficult to distinguish between pre-disease epigenetic changes and those that are the result of such post-disease factors. Therefore, a better study design to assess the effects of an exposure on epigenetic changes and resulting disease would examine epigenetic patterns in tissue samples collected before disease onset. This design would ensure that epigenetic changes preceded the onset of the disease and were not a downstream consequence of the disease or treatment.

It is also important in epigenetic research to assess appropriate tissue samples. The most accessible human biospecimen for studying DNA methylation or histone biomarkers is blood, most commonly white blood cells, but these may not be the best target for studying the disease of interest. For example, the N-methyl-D-aspartate (NMDA) receptor is found in glutamatergic neurons in the brain and plays a key role in schizophrenia. The DNA methylation pattern of the NMDA receptor gene in white blood cells is different than the methylation pattern in the brain (Walton et al., 2016); therefore, white blood cells are poor surrogates for studying epigenetic changes affecting NMDA receptor function in schizophrenia. This highlights the need for appropriate tissue samples, but research may be hindered by the relative lack of access to human brain and other tissue.

Recent studies on the effects of parental exposures on genetic and epigenetic inheritance leading to generational health effects are intriguing and provide preliminary evidence of the potential for research in this area. Epigenetics provides a new mechanism that may help explain generational effects, and while the study of epigenetics has received much attention in the press, the field is still in its infancy. New and rapidly developing "omics"[3] technologies promise to elucidate biomarkers that may be used to follow exposure-related effects across generations and help establish what, if any, effects may be occurring in children and grandchildren. Omic technologies will be crucial for unraveling the mechanisms underlying such generational health effects.

ANIMAL MODELS

There are several advantages to using animal models for the study of generational effects. Most animal models have much shorter generation times (days to months rather than decades); have many physiological and molecular properties in common with humans; and, in comparison with human studies,

[3] *Omics* refers to the study of genomic, proteomic, metabolomic, and associated information to study biological function and response.

are relatively inexpensive. In addition, they can facilitate the study of the molecular basis for how chemical exposures cause generational effects. This is particularly true for studies in which the cells with the affected epigenome, including germ cells, might be hard to access or study in humans. For example, some cell types and tissues such as neurons or lung tissue are rarely available from humans. Animals—mice, in particular—are also useful for inter- and transgenerational studies because they reach sexual maturity quickly and have a short gestational age and reproductive cycle, which permits researchers to observe three or more generations within a year. An important caveat is that it is important to pay attention to differences between species in such factors as metabolism, susceptible developmental stages, and lifespans when considering the applicability of findings in animal models to humans.

In animal studies, transgenerational outcomes following maternal exposures have been examined more extensively than paternal modes of transmission. One important limitation is that there are few data on maternal exposures that occur *only* prior to pregnancy, as might be experienced by female service members exposed to toxicants or stressors prior to conceiving. In contrast, paternal studies (including those focused on stress) suggest that exposures experienced prior to mating can affect future offspring via germ cell reprogramming. For instance, recent animal models of paternal stress have shown a wide window of germ cell vulnerability across spermatogenesis and maturational periods. Recent paternal studies have examined the effects of social defeat, chronic stress, dietary challenges, endocrine disrupters, and conditioned fear on offspring (Chan et al., 2018). In the case of social defeat stress, the offspring from defeat-subjected fathers showed changes in behavioral and physiological stress reactivity (Dietz et al., 2011). Similarly, in a mouse model of conditioned fear stress, males exposed to a shock paired with a specific odor passed on this conditioning effect to their first- and second-generation offspring (Dias and Ressler, 2014). Studies in male mice exposed to chronic stress prior to mating also showed a significant epigenetic reprogramming of their germ cells. This reprogramming resulted in long-term changes in offspring brain development and in their stress reactivity throughout their lives (Rodgers et al., 2015).

SUMMARY

This chapter provides an overview of the genetic and epigenetic mechanisms that have emerged as possible mediators of exposure-related impacts on the health of veterans' children and grandchildren. For genetic mechanisms, a new environmentally mediated mutation could arise in a germ cell (sperm or oocyte), and this mutation could then be passed on to descendants. For epigenetic changes, the mechanisms are less clear. There is a growing body of research suggesting that health effects in descendants are not mediated by germ cell mutations and are therefore not directed by genetic mutations. These effects likely arise by environmentally mediated changes in the epigenome. The primary candidate mechanisms that have been implicated in the generational inheritance of health effects include changes in DNA methylation and histone modifications that regulate transcription and also changes in noncoding RNAs that regulate both transcription and translation. These mechanisms are a major focus of the field of epigenetics.

REFERENCES

Amann, R.P. 2008. The cycle of the seminiferous epithelium in humans: A need to revisit? *Journal of Andrology* 29(5):469–487.

Angermueller, C., S.J. Clark, H.J. Lee, I.C. Macaulay, M.J. Teng, T.X. Hu, F. Krueger, S. Smallwood, C.P. Ponting, T. Voet, G. Kelsey, O. Stegle, and W. Reik. 2016. Parallel single-cell sequencing links transcriptional and epigenetic heterogeneity. *Nature Methods* 13(3):229–232.

Anonymous. 2015. 2. Relationship between different epigenomic marks: DNA accessibility and methylation, histone marks, and RNA. *Nature* 14310. doi:10.1038/nature14310.

Atlasi, Y., and H.G. Stunnenberg. 2017. The interplay of epigenetic marks during stem cell differentiation and development. *Nature Reviews Genetics* 18:643–658.

Barbara, M. A., and Y. Abdilla. 2017. An Introduction to Epigenetics. *Neonatal Network* 36(3):124–128.

Bariar, B., C.G. Vestal, and C. Richardson. 2013. Long-term effects of chromatin remodeling and DNA damage in stem cells induced by environmental and dietary agents. *Journal of Environmental Pathology, Toxicology and Oncology : Official Organ of the International Society for Environmental Toxicology and Cancer* 32(4):307–327.

Barker, D.J.P. 2004. Developmental origins of adult health and disease. *Journal of Epidemiology and Community Health* 58:114–115.

Biswas, S., and C.M. Rao. 2018. Epigenetic tools (The Writers, The Readers and The Erasers) and their implications in cancer therapy. *European Journal of Pharmacology* 17:S0014-2999(18)30466-7. doi: 10.1016/j.ejphar.2018.08.021 [Epub ahead of print].

Butler, M.G. 2009. Genomic imprinting disorders in humans: A mini-review. *Journal of Assisted Reproduction and Genetics* 26(9–10):477–486.

Chaffin, C.L., K.E. Latham, N.R. Mtango, U. Midic, and C.A. VandeVoort. 2014. Dietary sugar in healthy female primates perturbs oocyte maturation and in vitro preimplantation embryo development. *Endocrinology* 155(7):2688–2695.

Chan, J.C., B.M. Nugent, and T.L. Bale. 2018. Parental advisory: Maternal and paternal stress can impact offspring neurodevelopment. *Biological Psychiatry* 83(10):886–894.

Chen, S., W. Fitzgerald, J. Zimmerberg, H.K. Kleinman, and L. Margolis. 2009. Cell–cell and cell–extracellular matrix interactions regulate embryonic stem cell differentiation. *Stem Cells* 25(3):553–561.

Clarke, H.J., and K.F. Vieux. 2015. Epigenetic inheritance through the female germ-line: The known, the unknown, and the possible. *Seminars in Cell and Developmental Biology* 43:106–116.

Cossetti, C., L. Lugini, L. Astrologo, I. Saggio, S. Fais, and C. Spadafora. 2014. Soma-to-germline transmission of RNA in mice xenografted with human tumour cells: Possible transport by exosomes. *PLOS ONE* 9(7):e101629.

Crider, K.S., T.P. Yang, R.J. Berry, and L.B. Bailey. 2012. Folate and DNA methylation: A review of molecular mechanisms and the evidence for folate's role. *Advances in Nutrition* 3(1):21–38.

Developmental Biology Interactive. n.d. *Embryonic stem cell differentiation and trophectoderm development in primates*. http://www.devbio.biology.gatech.edu/vertebrate-development/mammals-2/primates-embryonic-stem-cell-differentiation-and-trophectoderm-development/ (accessed July 11, 2018).

Dias, B.G., and K.J. Ressler. 2014. Parental olfactory experience influences behavior and neural structure in subsequent generations. *Nature Neuroscience* 17(1):89–96.

Dietz, D.M., Q. Laplant, E.L. Watts, G.E. Hodes, S.J. Russo, J. Feng, R.S. Oosting, V. Vialou, and E.J. Nestler. 2011. Paternal transmission of stress-induced pathologies. *Biological Psychiatry* 70(5):408–414.

Eckersley-Maslin, M. A., C. Alda-Catalinas, and W. Reik. 2018. Dynamics of the epigenetic landscape during the maternal-to-zygotic transition. *Nature Reviews Molecular Cell Biology* 19(7):436–450.

Faulk, C., and D.C. Dolinoy. 2011. Timing is everything: The when and how of environmentally induced changes in the epigenome of animals. *Epigenetics* 6(7):791–797.

Fraser, R., and C.J. Lin. 2016. Epigenetic reprogramming of the zygote in mice and men: on your marks, get set, go! *Reproduction* 152(6):R211–R222.

Glaze, G.M. 1984. Diethylstilbestrol exposure in utero: Review of literature. *Journal of the American Osteopathic Association* 83(6):435–438.

Gore, A.C. 2008. Developmental programming and endocrine disruptor effects on reproductive neuroendocrine systems. *Frontiers in Neuroendocrinology* 29(3):358–374.

Gore, A.C., V.A. Chappell, S.E. Fenton, J.A. Flaws, A. Nadal, G.S. Prins, J. Toppari, and R.T. Zoeller. 2015. The Endocrine Society's second scientific statement on endocrine-disrupting chemicals. *Endocrine Reviews* 36(6):593–602.

Guintivano, J., and Z. A. Kaminsky. 2016. Role of epigenetic factors in the development of mental illness throughout life. *Neuroscience Research* 102:56–66.

Heller, C.G., G.V. Heller, and M.J. Rowley. 1969. Human spermatogenesis: An estimate of the duration of each cell association and of each cell type. In C. Gual and F.J.G. Ebling (eds.). *Progress in Endocrinology (Proceedings of the Third International Congress of Endocrinology, Mexico)*. Amsterdam: Excerpta Medica. Pp. 1012–1018.

Hepp, M.I., V. Alarcon, A. Dutta, J.L. Workman, and J.L. Gutiérrez. 2014. Nucleosome remodeling by the SWI/SNF complex is enhanced by yeast high mobility group box (HMGB) proteins. *Biochimica et Biophysica Acta* 1839(9):764–772.

Hill, M.A. 2018. *Embryology: Timeline human development*. August 7. https://embryology.med.unsw.edu.au/embryology/index.php/Timeline_human_development (accessed August 8, 2018).

Ho, S.M., A. Cheong, M. Adgent, J. Veevers, A. Suen, N.C. Tam, Y.K. Leung, W.N. Jefferson, and C.J. Williams. 2017. Environmental factors, epigenetics, and developmental origin of reproductive disorders. *Reproductive Toxicology* 68:85–104.

Holoch, D., and D. Moazed. 2015. RNA-mediated epigenetic regulation of gene expression. *Nature Reviews Genetics* 16(2): 71–84.

Jaffe, A.E., and R.A. Irizarry. 2014. Accounting for cellular heterogeneity is critical in epigenome-wide association studies. *Genome Biology* 15(R31):1–9.

Jang, H.S., W.J. Shin, J.E. Lee, and J.T. Do. 2017. CpG and non-CpG methylation in epigenetic gene regulation and brain function. *Genes* 8(6):148.

Jodar, M., A. Soler-Ventura, and R. Oliva. 2017. Semen proteomics and male infertility. *Journal of Proteomics* 162:125–134.

Johnson, G.D., P. Mackie, M. Jodar, S. Moskovtsev, and S.A. Krawetz. 2015. Chromatin and extracellular vesicle associated sperm RNAs. *Nucleic Acids Research* 43(14):6847–6859.

Juliano, C., J. Wang, and H. Lin. 2011. Uniting germline and stem cells: The function of Piwi proteins and the piRNA pathway in diverse organisms. *Annual Review Genetics* 45:447–469.

Kanherkar, R.R., N. Bhatia-Dey, E. Makarev, and A.B. Csoka. 2014. Cellular reprogramming for understanding and treating human disease. *Frontiers in Cell and Developmental Biology* 2:67.

Karemaker, I.D., and M. Vermeulen. 2018. Single-cell DNA methylation profiling: Technologies and biological applications. *Trends in Biotechnology*. https://doi.org/10.1016/j.tibtech.2018.04.002.

Kern, J.K., D.A. Geier, K.G. Homme, P.G. King, G. Bjørklund, S. Chirumbolo, and M.R. Geier. 2017. Developmental neurotoxicants and the vulnerable male brain: A systematic review of suspected neurotoxicants that disproportionally affect males. *Acta Neurobiologiae Experimentalis Journal* 77(4):269–296.

Kucej, M., B. Kucejova, R. Subramanian, X.J. Chen, and R.A. Butow. 2008. Mitochondrial nucleoids undergo remodeling in response to metabolic cues. *Journal of Cell Science* 121(11):1861–1868.

Kuh, D., and Y. Ben-Shlomo. 2004. *A life course approach to chronic disease epidemiology*, 2nd Ed. New York: Oxford University Press.

La Merrill, M., E. Karey, E. Moshier, C. Lindtner, M.R. La Frano, J.W. Newman, and C. Buettner. 2014. Perinatal exposure of mice to the pesticide DDT impairs energy expenditure and metabolism in adult female offspring. *PLOS ONE* 9(7):1–10.

Lane, M., R.L. Robker, and S.A. Robertson. 2014. Parenting from before conception. *Science* 345(6198):756–760.

Langley-Evans, S.C. 2014. Nutrition in early life and the programming of adult disease: A review. *Journal of Human Nutrition and Dietetics* 28(Suppl 1):1–14.

Ly, L., D. Chan, and J. M. Trasler. 2015. Developmental windows of susceptibility for epigenetic inheritance through the male germline. *Seminars in Cell and Developmental Biology* 43:96–105.

Marczylo, E.L., A.A. Amoako, J.C. Konje, T.W. Gant, and T.H. Marczylo. 2012. Smoking induces differential miRNA expression in human spermatozoa: A potential transgenerational epigenetic concern? *Epigenetics* 7(5):432–439.

McCarthy, M.M. 2016. Sex differences in the developing brain as a source of inherent risk. *Dialogues in Clinical Neuroscience* 18(4):361–372.

McEwen, K.R., and A.C. Ferguson-Smith. 2010. Distinguishing epigenetic marks of developmental and imprinting regulation. *Epigenetics & Chromatin* 3:2.

McGowan, P.O., and T.L. Roth. 2015. Epigenetic pathways through which experiences become linked with biology. *Development and Psychopathology* 27(2):637–648.

Messerschmidt, D.M., B.B Knowles, and D. Solter. 2014. DNA methylation dynamics during epigenetic reprogramming in the germline and preimplantation embryos. *Genes & Development*. 28(8):812–828.

Murr, R. 2010. Interplay between different epigenetic modifications and mechanisms. *Advances in Genetics* 70:101–141.

NHGRI (National Human Genome Research Institute). 2016. *Epigenomics fact sheet*. https://www.genome.gov/27532724/epigenomics-fact-sheet/ (accessed July 23, 2018).

NTP (National Toxicology Program). 2018. *State of the Science Evaluation for Transgenerational Inheritance of Health Effects*. https://ntp.niehs.nih.gov/pubhealth/hat/selected/trans/index.html (accessed August 8, 2018).

Ponomarenko, E.A., E.V. Poverennaya, E.V. Ilgisonis, M.A. Pyatnitskiy, A.T. Kopylov, V.G. Zgoda, A.V. Lisitsa, and Alexander I. Archakov. 2016. The size of the human proteome: The width and depth. *International Journal of Analytical Chemistry* 2016:1–6. doi: 10.1155/2016/7436849.

Ramos, K.S., and P. Bojang. 2018. Long interspersed nuclear element (LINE-1/L1). In *Comprehensive Toxicology*, 3rd ed. Edited by C.A. McQueen. Waltham, MA: Elsevier. Pp. 626–643.

Rice, D., and S. Barone. 2000. Critical periods of vulnerability for the developing nervous system: Evidence from humans and animal models. *Environmental Health Perspectives* 108(Suppl 3):511–533.

Robbins, W.A., M. L. Meistrich, D. Moore, F.B. Hagemeister, H.U. Weier, M.J. Cassel, G. Wilson, B. Eskenazi, and A.J. Wyrobek. 1997. Chemotherapy induces transient sex chromosomal and autosomal aneuploidy in human sperm. *Nature Genetics* 16:74–78.

Robertson, K.D. 2005. DNA methylation and human disease. *Nature Reviews Genetics* 6(8):597–610.

Rodgers, A.B., C.P. Morgan, N.A. Leu, and T.L. Bale. 2015. Transgenerational epigenetic programming via sperm microRNA recapitulates effects of paternal stress. *Proceedings of the National Academy of Sciences* 112(44):13699–13704.

Schorn, A.J., M.J. Gutbrod, C. LeBlanc, and R. Martienssen. 2017. LTR-retrotransposon control by tRNA-derived small RNAs. *Cell* 170(1):61–71.

Sendler, E., G.D. Johnson, S. Mao, R.J. Goodrich, M.P. Diamond, R. Hauser, and S.A. Krawetz. 2013. Stability, delivery and functions of human sperm RNAs at fertilization. *Nucleic Acids Research* 41(7): 4104–4117.

Sharma, U., and O.J. Rando. 2017. Metabolic inputs into the epigenome. *Cell Metabolism* 25(3):544–558.

Shi, W., S. Bellusci, and D. Warburton. 2007. Lung development and adult lung diseases. *Chest* 132(2):651–656.

Shnorhavorian, M., S.M. Schwartz, B. Stansfeld, I. Sadler-Riggleman, D. Beck, and M.K. Skinner. 2017. Differential DNA methylation regions in adult human sperm following adolescent chemotherapy: Potential for epigenetic inheritance. *PLOS ONE* 12(2):1–18.

Skogen, J. C. and S. Overland. 2012. The fetal origins of adult disease: A narrative review of the epidemiological literature. *Journal of the Royal Society of Medicine Short Report* 3(8):59.

Spadafora, C. 2016. Soma to germline inheritance of extrachromosomal genetic information via a line-1 reverse transcriptase-based mechanism. *Bioessays* 38(8):726–733.

Sunde, A., D. Brison, J. Dumoulin, J. Harper, K. Lundin, M.C. Magli, E. Van den Abbeel, and A. Veiga. 2016. Time to take human embryo culture seriously. *Human Reproduction* 31(10):2174–2182.

Svoboda, P. 2017. Long and small noncoding RNAs during oocyte-to-embryo transition in mammals. *Biochemical Society Transactions* 45(5):1117–1124.

Tempest, H.G., E. Ko, P. Chan, B. Robaire, A. Rademaker, and R.H. Martin. 2008. Sperm aneuploidy frequencies analysed before and after chemotherapy in testicular cancer and Hodgkin's lymphoma patients. *Human Reproduction* 23(2):251–258.

Teneng, I., D.E. Montoya-Durango, J.L. Quertermous, M.E. Lacy, and K.S. Ramos. 2011. Reactivation of L1 retrotransposon by benzo(a)pyrene involves complex genetic and epigenetic regulation. *Epigenetics* 6(3):355–367.

Tian, X., and F.J. Diaz. 2012. Zinc depletion causes multiple defects in ovarian function during the periovulatory period in mice. *Endocrinology* 153(2):873–886.

Tian, X., and F.J. Diaz. 2013. Acute dietary zinc deficiency before conception compromises oocyte epigenetic programming and disrupts embryonic development. *Developmental Biology* 376(1):51–61.

Trounson, A., R. Gosden, and U. Eichenlaub-Ritter (Eds.). 2013. *Biology and pathology of the oocyte, role in fertility, medicine and nuclear reprograming*, 2nd Ed. Cambridge University Press.

Uzumcu, M., A.M. Zama, and E. Oruc. 2012. Epigenetic mechanisms in the actions of endocrine-disrupting chemicals: Gonadal effects and role in female reproduction. *Reproduction in Domestic Animals = Zuchthygiene* 47(0 4):338–347.

VandeVoort, C.A., K.N. Grimsrud, U. Midic, N. Mtango, and K.E. Latham. 2015. Transgenerational effects of binge drinking in a primate model: Implications for human health. *Fertility and Sterility* 103(2):560–569.

Vansant, G., S. Wallace, and L. Godderis. 2016. Effect of maternal and paternal nutrition on DNA methylation in the offspring: A systematic review of human and animal studies. *Advances in Obesity, Weight Management & Control* 4(4):00093.

Virant-Klun, I., A. Ståhlberg, M. Kubista, and T. Skutella. 2016. MicroRNAs: From female fertility, germ cells, and stem cells to cancer in humans. *Stem Cells International* 2016:3984937.

Waddell, J.M., and M. McCarthy. 2012. Sexual differentiation of the brain and ADHD: What is a sex difference in prevalence telling us? *Current Topics in Behavioral Neurosciences* 9:341–360.

Walker, C.L. 2016. Minireview: Epigenomic plasticity and vulnerability to EDC exposures. *Molecular Endocrinology* 30(8):848–855.

Walton, E., J. Hass, J. Liu, J.L. Roffman, R. Bernardoni, V. Roessner, M. Kirsch, G. Schackert, V. Calhoun, and S. Ehrlich. 2016. Correspondence of DNA methylation between blood and brain tissue and its application to schizophrenia research. *Schizophrenia Bulletin* 42(2):406–414.

Wei, Y., H. Schatten, and Q.Y. Sun. 2015. Environmental epigenetic inheritance through gametes and implications for human reproduction. *Human Reproduction Update* 21(2):194–208.

Werling, D.M. 2016. The role of sex-differential biology in risk for autism spectrum disorder. *Biology of Sex Differences* 7(58):1–18.

WHO (World Health Organization). 2000. The implications for training of embracing a life course approach to health. International Longevity Centre–UK. WHO/NMH/HPS/00.2.

Williams, S.C.P. 2016. News feature: Genetic mutations you want. *Proceedings of the National Academy of Sciences* 113(10):2554–2557.

Wu, H., R. Hauser, S.A. Krawetz, and J.R. Pilsner. 2015. Environmental susceptibility of the sperm epigenome during windows of male germ cell development. *Current Environmental Health Reports* 2(4):356–366.

Xin, F., M. Susiarjo, and M.S. Bartolomei. 2015. Multigenerational and transgenerational effects of endocrine disrupting chemicals: A role for altered epigenetic regulation? *Seminars in Cell & Developmental Biology* 43:66–75.

Xu, Q., and W. Xie. 2018. Epigenome in early mammalian development: inheritance, reprogramming and establishment. *Trends in Cell Biology* 28(3):237–253.

Xu, Z., J. Jiang, C. Xu, Y. Wang, L. Sun, X. Guo, and H. Liu. 2013. MicroRNA-181 regulates CARM1 and histone aginine methylation to promote differentiation of human embryonic stem cells. *PLOS ONE* 8(1):e53146.

Yeshurun, S., and A.J. Hannan. 2018. Transgenerational epigenetic influences of paternal environmental exposures on brain function and predisposition to psychiatric disorders. *Molecular Psychiatry* March 8. doi: 10.1038/s41380-018-0039-z.

Youn, H.K. 2017. Methylation and demethylation of DNA and histones in chromatin: The most complicated epigenetic marker. *Experimental & Molecular Medicine* 49:e321.

Yuan, S., A. Schuster, C. Tang, T. Yu, N. Ortogero, J. Bao, H. Zheng, and W.Yan. 2016. Sperm-borne miRNAs and endo-siRNAs are important for fertilization and preimplantation embryonic development. *Development* (Cambridge, England) 143(4):635–647.

4

Deployment-Related Exposures

Several of the agents of concern specified by the U.S. Congress in the Gulf War legislation (P.L. 105-368 and P.L. 105-277)[1] were not only used in the 1990–1991 Gulf War but are also applicable to exposures in the Post-9/11 conflicts in Iraq and Afghanistan. Many of them are not commonly encountered by service members stationed at military installations in the United States or by the U.S. general public. Those agents include the chemical warfare agents sarin, tabun, and mustard gas; infectious diseases endemic to Southwest Asia; several vaccinations (including those against anthrax and botulinum); depleted uranium (DU); pyridostigmine bromide (PB); and hexavalent chromium (Cr6). Exposures to these agents distinguish military personnel deployed to the Persian Gulf region from those who did not deploy to the Middle East. The health outcomes associated with exposure to these agents were reviewed by previous Gulf War and Health committees (IOM, 2000, 2005, 2008a). Deployment to a war zone itself has been associated with several adverse health reactions, as described in *Gulf War and Health, Volume 6* (IOM, 2008b). The potential impact of each of these exposures on the reproductive and developmental health of veterans and their descendants is considered in this chapter, beginning with the pervasive effect of deployment itself. The following sections review previous National Academies' reports, authoritative reviews, and new literature identified by the Volume 11 committee on deployment exposures and associated reproductive and developmental effects.

DEPLOYMENT

The committee uses the term "deployment" to refer to a military assignment or assignments leading to the collective and complex set of chemical, biological, radiological, and physiological exposures and psychological impacts that may be encountered in theater. Numerous studies have investigated the

[1] P.L. 105-368 Veterans Program Enhancement Act of 1998. Sec 1-101 Agreement with the National Academy of Sciences regarding the health consequences of veterans serving in the Persian Gulf. P.L. 105-277 was the emergency appropriations given to the National Academy of Sciences to study "exposure to toxic agents or wartime hazards." This was codified in Compensation for Disabilities Occurring in Persian Gulf War Veterans, 38 USC 1117.

potential health effects of deployment since 1993. These studies usually compare military personnel who deployed to the Persian Gulf theater of operations with those who deployed to other regions (for example, Bosnia or Somalia) or who remained in garrison in the United States. Four volumes of the *Gulf War and Health* series have reviewed the literature that compares the health status of these veteran populations as well as the available information on the many potential and variable exposures that may have occurred in theater (IOM, 2006b, 2008b, 2010; NASEM, 2016). Those reports found that there was inadequate/insufficient evidence for any reproductive or developmental effects (including birth defects, adverse pregnancy outcomes, fertility problems, or genitourinary conditions). One exception was found: several studies of different groups of veterans found that sexual difficulties were reported more frequently by male veterans who had deployed than by veterans who had not deployed. This finding led the Volume 10 committee to conclude that there was limited/suggestive evidence of an increased prevalence of self-reported sexual difficulties among Gulf War veterans (NASEM, 2016). Although the other reproductive and developmental effects had been reported in the literature, the evidence was limited by methodologic issues, inconsistent results, and sparse data.

The Volume 11 committee identified several new studies that examined reproductive and developmental health outcomes in veterans, but the results are inconclusive because of low response rates. Recent surveys by the Department of Veterans Affairs (VA) have collected information on the reproductive health of Gulf War and Post-9/11 era veterans. Although a 2012 survey of Gulf War veterans (with a 50% response rate) inquired about reproductive health for female veterans only, survey results published as of 2016 did not include the status of female or male veterans' reproductive health (Dursa et al., 2016). A 2009–2011 survey of 30,000 Operation Enduring Freedom (OEF) and Operation Iraqi Freedom (OIF) deployed and 30,000 nondeployed veterans who served between 2001 and 2008 asked respondents about infertility. There were 20,370 respondents, for a 34.3% response rate. Results indicated that infertility is a concern among both male (n=16,056) and female (n=4,314) veterans. Compared with men, female veterans had similar odds of a lifetime history of infertility (OR=1.07, 95% CI 0.94–1.20), but the actual risk of infertility associated with deployment was not determined (Katon et al., 2014a).

Reproductive Effects

There is a dearth of studies on the reproductive effects of deployment and deployment exposure on male and female veterans. Buller et al. (2007) reviewed gynecology visits at Camp Doha, Kuwait, from August 2003 through April 2004. Of the 1,737 visits, 77 had a positive pregnancy test, 77% of the pregnancies occurred in country, and 23% of the women had been pregnant when they arrived in country.

Reproductive Effects in Men and Women

One study using administrative data from VA examined gestational diabetes and hypertensive disorders of pregnancy among women who used maternity benefits. Compared with the general population of civilian women, Post-9/11 deployed women using VA maternity benefits (n=2,288) had a higher risk of gestational diabetes (standardized incidence ratio [SIR]=1.40, 95% CI 1.16–1.68) and hypertensive disorders (SIR=1.32, 95% CI 1.15–1.51) after controlling for maternal age and year of delivery. No comparisons were made between deployed and nondeployed women veterans (Katon et al., 2014b). The Volume 11 committee notes that although gestational diabetes and hypertensive disorders are endpoints that are possibly mediated through abnormalities in placental implantation, this effect was not considered in this study.

The Millennium Cohort Study is a longitudinal study initiated in 2001 by the Department of Defense (DoD) to assess the long-term health of service members from all military branches over an extended period. This study assessed miscarriages in 3,366 female veterans who deployed to Iraq and Afghanistan. Self-reported miscarriage, self-perceived impaired fecundity, combat exposures, and other lifestyle and health metrics and self-perceived reduced fertility was assessed by a questionnaire and documented for 11,183 female veterans (Ippolito et al., 2017). Women completed questionnaires in 2004–2006 and again in 2007–2008, and their deployment status, including combat exposure, was determined from personnel files. Neither deployment status, with or without combat exposure, nor days deployed nor life stressors were associated with a significantly increased risk of having a miscarriage (ORs ranged from 0.86 to 1.67; none were significant) or of having had self-perceived reduced fertility in the previous 3 years (ORs ranged from 0.86 to 1.24; none were significant).

No new studies on the effects of deployment on male reproduction were identified by the Volume 11 committee.

Adverse Pregnancy Outcomes

The Volume 11 committee identified a systematic review of the impacts of active-duty military service on the reproductive health of female service members and male and female veterans from around the world, although most of the 46 studies cited in the review were of U.S. women (Lawrence-Wood et al., 2016). There was insufficient evidence that military service had an effect on pregnancy outcomes, including preterm births and birth defects, although there was evidence that deployment was associated with ectopic pregnancies. The authors noted that the small number of studies limited any definitive conclusions. Military occupational exposures, whether during deployment or not, were associated with birth defects but not with fertility issues, ectopic pregnancy, or miscarriage, and the evidence was mixed for preterm births.

The association between adverse birth outcomes among U.S. Navy women and occupational and environmental exposures experienced by either the mother or the father was explored by Hourani and Hilton (2000). A mailed survey of active-duty women serving in the U.S. Navy who gave birth to a live infant between January and October 1993 in any of three large naval hospitals yielded a response rate of 56%. Women were asked about their own and their partners' exposures in the 3 months prior to conception and about adverse birth outcomes (low birth weight, preterm birth [<37 weeks], birth defects, fetal distress prior to or during delivery, and small for gestational age). Compared with civilian beneficiaries, active-duty women who self-reported exposure to petroleum products in the home were at an increased risk of having a low-birth-weight infant (<2,500 g; OR=2.4, 95% CI 1.3–6.56). Paternal exposure to pesticides at work and maternal exposure to heavy metals at work were both associated with an increased risk of having a preterm birth (<37 weeks; OR=2.6, 95% CI 1.28–5.43 and OR=2.2, 95% CI 1.11–4.47, respectively). Fetal distress and small for gestational age were not associated with any maternal or paternal exposures. Thus, more research should be conducted to see if there is an association between the exposures of interest and reproductive and developmental effects.

A study by Conlin et al. (2012) examined birth outcomes in children born to men and women veterans who had deployed within a 3-mile radius of a documented burn pit in Iraq. The authors used the DoD Birth and Infant Health Registry to identify live infants born to deployed men or women between 2004 and 2007. Infants born to deployed women with burn pit exposure were not at increased risk of being preterm (≤36 weeks; OR=1.09, 95% CI 0.86–1.37). The risk of preterm birth was not significantly associated with the length of the mother's exposure to the burn pit or to whether she became pregnant during deployment. Paternal exposure was not significantly associated with preterm births, regardless of the length or proximity of the father's exposure to a burn pit.

Katon et al. (2017) conducted a retrospective cohort study of Gulf War veterans in 2014. Using data from the National Health Study for a New Generation of U.S. Veterans from the years 2009–2011, samples from 30,000 veterans who were deployed or not deployed to OEF/OIF were examined to evaluate the types of pregnancy outcomes among women who served in OEF and OIF. Live births and pregnancies were reported (nondeployed n=1,295; deployed n=1,773), and among women who had deployed, conceptions and outcomes were classified as occurring before deployment, during deployment, or post-deployment. Only 79 women out of the 3,068 with at least one pregnancy (3%) reported more than five pregnancies. Outcomes included, but were not limited to, preterm birth, low birth weight, and macrosomia. Among the 2,276 pregnancies that resulted in live births, there were 191 preterm births, 153 low-birth-weight infants, and 272 macrosomic infants. After comparing women who were pregnant before deployment with nondeployed women or women who became pregnant after deployment, the researchers found that there was a significantly increased risk of preterm birth among the nondeployed (OR=2.16, 95% CI 1.25–3.72) but not among those who became pregnant after deployment (OR=1.90, 95% CI 0.90–4.02). There was no association between deployment and low birth weight or macrosomia. Thus, deployment was not associated with the three adverse pregnancy outcomes in this study.

Ryan et al. (2011) reported that, based on DoD Birth and Infant Health Registry data for 2002–2005, of 63,053 infants born to U.S. military women during that period, 2,941 infants were born to female service members who were deployed at some time during their first trimester of pregnancy. Compared with infants born to women who had deployed prior to or post-pregnancy, infants born to women who had deployed while pregnant were not at an increased risk of preterm birth (OR=1.13, 95% CI 0.97–1.32) or extreme preterm birth (≤28 weeks; OR=1.11, 95% CI 0.73–1.68). Women who were deployed during their first trimester of pregnancy were not at an increased risk of having an infant with a birth defect compared with women who had deployed at any time other than the first trimester (OR=1.14, 95% CI 0.93–1.40).

A study by Shaw et al. (2018) extracted data from the Stanford Military Data Repository on 12,877 deliveries to U.S. Army soldiers who had children between 2011 and 2014. The prevalence of spontaneous preterm birth was twice the rate among female soldiers who delivered within a 6-month period after returning from deployment than among women who had longer post-deployment intervals before delivery (OR=2.1, 95% CI 1.5–2.9). This finding was interpreted by the authors to suggest that women in service should postpone conception for longer than 6 months after returning from deployment.

Developmental Effects

The 2011 Institute of Medicine (IOM) committee that assessed the long-term health consequences of exposure to burn pits in Iraq and Afghanistan did not find any evidence for health effects in veterans who had been exposed during deployment. However, the committee referred to an earlier *Gulf War and Health* (IOM, 2005) report on combustion products from the burning of fuel that reported an association with (unspecified) reproductive effects. Further assessment of exposure to burn pits and birth outcomes was conducted by Conlin et al. (2012), who also used the DoD Birth and Infant Health Registry to identify live infants born to deployed men or women between 2004 and 2007. There was no increase in the risk of being diagnosed with a birth defect within the first year of life for infants born to active-duty women regardless of whether the women were within a 3-mile radius of a burn pit (OR=1.18, 95% CI 0.85–1.63), the cumulative deployment length, or whether they were pregnant while exposed. Nor was there an association between birth defects and paternal exposures to the burn pits.

The association between adverse birth outcomes among U.S. Navy women and occupational and environmental exposures for either the mother or the father was explored by Hourani and Hilton (2000).

Compared with the children of civilian beneficiaries, children born to active-duty women and whose fathers had exposure to chemicals other than pesticides, heavy metals, or petroleum products at home or at work were at an increased risk for birth defects (home OR=8.4, 95% CI 2.18–32.09, and work OR=3.4, 95% CI 1.35–8.82); maternal exposure was not associated with birth defects.

Synthesis and Conclusions

Reproductive Effects

Only two studies of female reproductive effects were identified by the committee. One study assessed the long-term health of service members who were deployed and found that there were no increased risks of having a miscarriage on the basis of military service or deployment alone. Only one study reported on self-perceived fertility, and it also found no association with deployment. There were no studies of male reproductive effects.

The Volume 11 committee identified five studies that examined the association between deployment of women and adverse pregnancy outcomes. Three of the studies found no significant association between deployment exposures and the risk of a female veteran having a preterm or low-birth-weight infant (Conlin et al., 2012; Katon et al., 2017; Ryan et al., 2011). One study found an association between exposure to petroleum products around the home and an increased risk of having a low-birth-weight infant among female U.S. Navy veterans compared with civilian beneficiaries, but the exposures were not related to deployment. Shaw at al. (2018) found an increase in the risk of preterm birth for women who gave birth within 6 months of returning from deployment compared with those who had a child later. None of the studies found an association between a father's deployment exposure and any adverse pregnancy outcomes. It is difficult to interpret these studies because of the variability in the duration and nature of the exposures and the outcomes that were assessed.

The Volume 11 committee concludes that there is inadequate/insufficient evidence to determine whether an association exists between deployment and reproductive effects in men or women, or with adverse pregnancy outcomes.

Developmental Effects

The Volume 11 committee identified two studies of developmental effects and deployment exposures. Conlin et al. (2012) found no association between mothers' or fathers' exposures to burn pits during deployment and birth defects in their children. A second study found an association between some parental environmental exposures and birth defects, but the exposures were not deployment-specific.

The Volume 11 committee concludes that there is inadequate/insufficient evidence to determine whether an association exists between deployment and developmental effects.

CHEMICAL WARFARE AGENTS

Several chemicals used for tactical purposes during the Gulf War were identified by P.L. 105-368 and P.L. 105-277, including the nerve agents sarin and tabun and the vesicant agent sulfur mustard. The Gulf War legislation specified chemical warfare agents that veterans may have been exposed to during their deployments to the Persian Gulf: that is, sarin/cyclosarin, tabun, and mustards. Because few data have been available for review regarding tabun, previous Gulf War and Health committees have not reviewed or made conclusions pertaining to it. No new information on possible exposures to tabun during the Gulf War or Post-9/11 conflicts is available. No literature on any reproductive or developmental health effects of tabun or sarin/cyclosarin were identified in the Volume 11 committee's literature search; new literature for other agents was examined. Background information was derived from earlier reviews of these agents as summarized in volumes 1 and 4 (IOM, 2000, 2006a). The studies used by the committee to reach its conclusions on chemical warfare agents are summarized in Table 4-1 at the end of this section.

Sarin/Cyclosarin

Sarin and cyclosarin are highly toxic nerve agents used for chemical warfare. These agents were first manufactured in 1937 in Germany for use as insecticides. However, they were not used in warfare until the Iran–Iraq conflict in the 1980s (IOM, 2000). Sarin is a member of a class of chemicals known as organophosphorus esters (or organophosphates), and it is structurally similar to the drug PB (IOM, 2000).

As reported in *Gulf War and Health, Volume 4* (IOM, 2006a), during a cease-fire period in March 1991, troops from the US 37th and 307th engineering battalions destroyed enemy munitions throughout the occupied areas of southern Iraq, including at a large storage complex at Khamisiyah, which contained more than 100 bunkers. Two sites in the complex—1 bunker and a pit—contained stacks of 122-mm rockets loaded with sarin and cyclosarin. When these were detonated, an estimated 371 kg of sarin and cyclosarin combined were released (Winkenwerder, 2002). U.S. troops performing the demolitions were unaware of the nerve agents because their detectors, sensitive only to lethal or near-lethal concentrations of nerve agents, did not sound any alarms before demolition. It was reported that soldiers who experienced high levels of exposure had symptoms such as tightness of the chest, watery eyes, and muscle twitching. If the estimated dose was less than what would be needed to generate visible effects, it was considered a "low exposure." The Central Intelligence Agency and DoD used models to estimate ground-level concentrations of sarin and cyclosarin as a function of distance and direction from the detonation sites and used those to estimate the extent of potential exposure of U.S. military personnel to the nerve agents. The models suggested that nearly 10,000 U.S. troops were potentially exposed to these nerve agents within a 25-km radius of Khamisiyah (CIA–DoD, 1997; IOM, 2000).

The effects of sarin and cyclosarin exposure during the Gulf War were reviewed in *Volume 1* and later updated in 2004 (IOM, 2000, 2004). The analyses centered on the mechanisms and effects of acetylcholinesterase inhibition and neurologic outcomes, and reproductive effects were reported in animal studies. Thus, neither committee made any conclusions regarding sarin/cyclosarin exposure and reproductive or developmental effects in humans (IOM, 2000, 2004). The Volume 1 committee concluded that although there was "sufficient" evidence that sarin is capable of causing acute-cholinergic syndrome within hours of exposure that resolves within months, there was "limited/suggestive" evidence that there is a relationship between sarin exposure and long-term health effects at the concentrations encountered in theater. Finally, at low doses of sarin not sufficient to cause acute-cholinergic signs and symptoms, there was "inadequate/insufficient" evidence to determine long-term health effects.

After a comprehensive literature search, the Volume 11 committee found no further specific information on exposures of Gulf War or Post-9/11 service members to sarin or cyclosarin during deployment or on any resulting health effects.

Synthesis and Conclusions

The Volume 1 committee did not find evidence for an association between sarin/cyclosarin and reproductive and developmental effects on the basis of animal data; human data were not available. However, there are chemical similarities between these chemicals and organophosphates. The available animal data centered on the mechanisms and effects of acetylcholinesterase inhibition and neurologic outcomes. No further chemical-specific animal or human data were found to inform conclusions regarding sarin, cyclosarin, or tabun and reproductive and development effects. No data were found on reproductive or developmental endpoints related to sarin/cyclosarin exposure.

The Volume 11 committee concludes that there is inadequate/insufficient evidence to determine whether an association exists between exposure to sarin/cyclosarin and reproductive or developmental effects.

Sulfur Mustard

Sulfur mustard, also known as a mustard gas agent, was used in World War I. This agent can exist in the form of a vapor, liquid, or solid. Military personnel can be exposed to sulfur mustard through inhalation, dermal contact, or drinking contaminated water. Although mustard agents were identified by Congress as a chemical exposure of concern (P.L. 105-368 and P.L. 105-277), the committee found limited information on Gulf War or Post-9/11 veterans exposed to mustard gas during their deployments. However, there is a September 2016 report in the popular press describing a shell containing sulfur-mustard blistering agent landing at a military base in northern Iraq where U.S. military advisers were helping Iraqi forces against the Islamic State militants (Phippen, 2011). There was little reported exposure to mustards during the Gulf War (PAC, 1996, cited in IOM, 2004), and these agents were not reviewed by previous committees. Because it remains unclear to the committee whether exposure to mustard agents occurred after 1991 in the Persian Gulf region or during the Post-9/11 conflicts, the Volume 11 committee reviewed the literature on mustard agents below.

Sulfur mustard was reviewed in 2003 by the Agency for Toxic Substances and Disease Registry (ATSDR). The long-term effects of exposure to sulfur mustard among Iranian survivors of chemical attacks included reduced sperm counts, increased rate of fetal deaths, and altered sex ratios among the offspring. The scarring of genital tissue from direct contact with sulfur mustard was reported to affect reproductive ability. ATSDR noted that the animal data supported the long-term effects observed in humans, including sperm abnormalities, early fetal resorptions, preimplantation losses, and decreases in live embryo implantations associated with male exposure. The limited data available pertaining to developmental outcomes were equivocal, and no conclusions were made (ATSDR, 2003).

Reproductive Effects

Reproductive Effects in Men and Women

The Volume 11 committee examined a study of sulfur mustard effects on Iranian civilians and the Iranian military. Chronic infertility was evaluated in a historical cohort of sulfur-mustard-exposed veterans originally registered in 1990 with mild to severe injuries in the Hamadan province in Iran (Amirzargar et al., 2009). In 2005, semen, fecundity, and follicle-stimulating hormone (FSH) levels were measured in 64 exposed men and 64 veterans with injuries but with no sulfur mustard exposure. At the time of exposure, the mean age was 24.3 years, and a median of 19 years had elapsed since exposure. Male factor infertility was diagnosed in 14 (22.6%) exposed and 3 (4.9%) unexposed subjects ($p=0.007$). Ejaculate volume, sperm concentration, and total sperm count were significantly reduced ($p<0.01$ or 0.001) in the exposed group compared with baseline values obtained in 1990 or to unexposed controls. Out of all semen indices, sperm motility was the only one not affected. FSH was significantly lower ($p<0.05$) in the exposed group than in unexposed controls, but there were no differences between the groups in the levels of luteinizing hormone (LH) or testosterone.

Testicular effects were evaluated in infertile male Iranian service members who had been exposed to mustard gas in the 1985–1988 Iran–Iraq war (Safarinejad, 2001). Injury from exposure was characterized as severe ($n=44$), moderate ($n=20$), or mild ($n=17$) based on the effects on skin, eyes, mouth, respiratory tract, and lungs from the medical record. Semen parameters and hormone levels were evaluated in all participants, and testicular biopsies were taken from 24 individuals. Reference values were used for comparison. FSH was found to be increased in the severely injured group, but no differences were found for LH and testosterone. Of all participants, 42.5% had azoospermia and 57.5% had oligospermia, with all azoospermic men grouped in the severely injured group. Sperm count, motility, and normal morphology were decreased in all groups as compared to reference values, with the most pronounced effects seen in the severely injured group; statistical analyses were not performed. Biopsies showed seminiferous tubules devoid of spermatogonia, intact Sertoli cells, and normal Leydig cells.

The sperm chromatin structure was analyzed in a second study of veterans of the Iraq–Iran war with sulfur mustard exposure (Safarinejad, 2010). Semen and blood samples were collected from groups of 66 to 68 exposed-infertile, exposed-fertile, unexposed-infertile, and unexposed-fertile men. Exposure was categorized as mild, moderate, or severe based on medical records of the injuries. Sperm DNA was evaluated by a sperm chromatin structure assay. Mean serum LH, thyroid stimulating hormone, prolactin, and testosterone levels were similar between the groups, while mean FSH was significantly higher in both exposed groups and in the unexposed-infertile group than in the unexposed-fertile group ($p=0.01$). Ejaculate volume was not different among the groups. Other semen parameters (total sperm/ejaculate, sperm concentration, % motile, and % normal) were significantly lower in both exposed-infertile ($p=0.001$) and exposed-fertile ($p=0.01$) groups and the unexposed-infertile group ($p=0.01$) than in the unexposed-fertile controls. The most marked effects on sperm parameters were seen in the exposed-infertile group. The sperm DNA fragmentation index (DFI) was significantly increased in all groups compared with the unexposed-fertile controls ($p=0.01$), with the greatest difference seen between the exposed-infertile group and the unexposed fertile group (41.6 ± 4.4 versus $21.4\pm2.3\%$, Mann-Whitney U-test, $p=0.001$). Spermatozoa from mustard gas-injured subjects had more ($p=0.001$) abnormal chromatin (increased mean, standard deviation, and DFI) than spermatozoa from their non-mustard-gas-injured counterparts. An evaluation of semen parameters of the exposed groups based on the severity of injury showed more pronounced effects in the moderately and severely injured fertile and infertile individuals than in those of the mildly injured individuals.

Fertility was evaluated in survivors of a 1991 sulfur mustard attack on Sardasht, Iran (Ghanei et al., 2004). Exposure was verified through medical records with follow-up interviews and physical examinations. Participants were divided into those married for at least 1 year prior to exposure (66 males, 34 females) and those married after exposure (30 males, 12 females). Infertility was defined as a failure to conceive after 12 months of unprotected intercourse after marriage. A total of 115 couples were evaluated, 88 of whom reported that only one partner had been exposed and 27 of whom reported that both partners had been exposed. The infertility rate was 7.5% in couples married before exposure and 10.3% in couples married after exposure (p=0.531).

Adverse Pregnancy Outcomes

A cross-sectional study evaluated adverse birth outcomes in Iraqi civilians after the Gulf War (Arnetz et al., 2013). The cohort included 307 individuals living at that time in the metropolitan area of Detroit, Michigan, who had either lived in Iraq during and after the Gulf War (n=185) or who had left before the war (n=122). Data were collected by structured interview, and respondents were asked about environmental chemical exposures, including nerve gas and mustard gas, and stress exposures. Aggregate chemical and stress exposure scores were calculated for each individual. Overall, the results of self-reported data showed that chemical exposures were positively correlated with adverse birth outcomes (OR=2.04, 95% CI 1.12–3.74). Specifically, an exposure to mustard gas was associated with stillbirth (OR=2.54, 95% CI 1.24–5.23, p=0.013) but not congenital anomalies, low birth weight, or preterm delivery. However, the timing between exposure and birth outcome was not specified.

Developmental Effects

A study by Abolghasemi et al. (2010) examined congenital anomalies and childhood illness up to age 16 among 498 children of civilian men with confirmed mustard gas exposure in Sardasht City, Iran. Children whose mothers were also exposed were excluded. The 164 couples with the male exposed were age-matched to 136 controls from a nearby city with no history of chemical attack. Demographic and exposure data were collected by interview, and trained general practitioners evaluated the medical histories of all offspring born at least 9 months after the date of paternal exposure, which ensured that the children themselves were not exposed. The overall frequency of abnormalities and disorders in the exposed group was significantly higher than in the nonexposed group (95 [19%] versus 77 [11%]; OR=1.93, 95% CI 1.37–2.72, p<0.001). Respiratory diseases were found in 20 children (4%), and 21 children (4%) had congenital malformations, as compared with 9 (1%) for both endpoints in the nonexposed group. The frequency of respiratory diseases (OR=3.12, 95% CI 1.43–6.80, p=0.004) and of congenital malformations (OR=3.54, 95% CI 1.58–7.93, p=0.002) were both significantly higher in the offspring from the exposed group than from the nonexposed group, but no significant associations were found for specific respiratory conditions or congenital anomalies. No significant differences were observed for any other disorder as coded by ICD-10 categories. The analyses did not control for potential confounding factors. However, the authors concluded that generational effects can occur from exposure to mustard gas. They also concluded that parental exposure to mustard gas may affect fertility and possibly affect children's health and long-term development.

Animal Studies

One animal study relevant for chemical warfare exposures was identified. Nitrogen mustard, like sulfur mustard, is a blistering agent, and it has similar toxicological effects. He et al. (2007) examined the effects of nitrogen mustard on Sertoli cells in vitro. Sertoli cells were isolated from 20-day-old male Kunming mice and cultured with 0, 50, 100, or 200 μmol/L of nitrogen mustard for up to 24 hours. Treated cells showed smaller cell bodies, a disruption of the cytoplasm, and concentration-related significant decreases in length and area ($p<0.01$ or 0.05). Immunohistochemistry revealed the collapse of vimentin intermediate filaments and a disruption of the network between nuclear and cell membranes. Both messenger ribonucleic acid and protein expression for vimentin were decreased in a concentration- and time-related manner.

Synthesis and Conclusions

Reproductive Effects

Three studies on sulfur mustard found adverse effects on semen parameters in men with exposures sufficient to cause acute effects (Amirzargar et al., 2009; Safarinejad, 2001, 2010). All these studies were conducted on men who had been exposed to sulfur mustard during the Iran–Iraq war in the late 1980s. One study found no association between exposure to sulfur mustard and fertility among Iranian couples where one or both partners were exposed during a chemical attack (Ghanei et al., 2004). Those investigators reported on female fertility following a chemical attack in Iran with sulfur mustard; they found no association.

One study in Iran found a significant association with adverse birth outcomes, specifically for stillbirth but not for congenital anomalies, low birth weight, or preterm delivery (Arnetz et al., 2013). Children born to fathers with prior exposure to sulfur mustard were at a significantly increased risk for respiratory diseases and congenital abnormalities but not for specific diseases or anomalies (Abolghasemi et al., 2010). Although sulfur mustard is a known mutagen, no data were identified to inform conclusions on reproductive or developmental effects.

The Volume 11 committee concludes that there is limited/suggestive evidence of an association between exposure to sulfur mustard and reproductive effects in men.

The Volume 11 committee also concludes that there is inadequate/insufficient evidence of an association between exposure to sulfur mustard and reproductive effects in women, or with adverse pregnancy outcomes.

Developmental Effects

One study in Iran found an increase in congenital anomalies and childhood illness in children born to parents exposed to mustard gas in Iran (Abolghasemi et al., 2010). The authors concluded that parental exposure to mustard gas can affect fertility and possibly have an impact on children's health and long-term development.

The Volume 11 committee concludes that there is inadequate/insufficient of an association between prenatal exposure of women to sulfur mustard and developmental effects.

TABLE 4-1 Summary of Reproductive and Developmental Effects of Chemical Warfare Agents

Study	Population	Exposure	Results
Reproductive Effects			
Reproductive Effects in Men			
Amirzargar et al. (2009)	Historical cohort study. 64 sulfur mustard-exposed and 64 matched unexposed enrolled in the study of the Iraq–Iran conflict. Reproductive status of exposed and unexposed compared 16–22 years after first injury. Mean ages of 24.3±6.3 years (range 17–40 years).	Sulfur mustard	Semen indices lower in exposed men versus baseline values and unexposed men. Male factor infertility increased in exposed (22.6%) versus unexposed (4.9%) ($p=0.007$). FSH higher in infertile men than in exposed men who were fertile ($p<0.0001$). This study provided no ORs for the results.
Ghanei et al. (2004)	115 couples, 88 with 1 partner and 27 with both partners exposed to mustard gas. Study focused on Sardasht, a Kurdish Iranian town. Occurrence of infertility evaluated as failure to conceive after 12 months of unprotected intercourse.	250-kg bombs containing liquid mustard gas released from an aircraft near the city exposing 4,500 civilians to various levels of the toxin.	7.5% rate of infertility was observed among couples who were married at the time of exposure. Infertility rate of 10.3% was noted among individuals single at exposure and subsequently married. Overall infertility rate of 8.3%, compared with a worldwide rate of 10–15%. Using the Fisher exact test, results showed no significant differences among fertility groups 1 and 2 ($p=0.531$). This study provided no ORs for the results.
Safarinejad (2001)	81 Iranian men divided into three groups (44 severely injured men, 20 moderately injured men, and 17 mildly injured men). Ages ranged from 28 to 41, with a mean age of 34.7 years.	Mustard gas exposure during an attack in the 1985–1988 Iran–Iraq War, and some exposed in a contaminated area several hours after the attack.	Azoospermia and severe oligospermia diagnosed in (34) 42.5% and (47) 57.5% of subjects. This study provided no ORs for the results.

continued

TABLE 4-1 Continued

Study	Population	Exposure	Results
Safarinejad (2010)	268 Iranian subjects: Group 1—66 subjects were mustard gas-injured infertile men ages 37 to 55; Group 2—68 subjects were non-mustard-gas-injured fertile men ages 39 to 57; Group 3—68 subjects were non-mustard-gas-injured infertile men who also had oligoastheno-teratozoospermia (ages 35 to 55); and Group 4—66 subjects were non-mustard-gas-injured normozoospermic fertile control men ages 35 to 55.	Mustard gas	The sperm DNA fragmentation index was significantly increased in all groups compared with the unexposed-fertile controls, with the highest value in the exposed-infertile group. Evaluation of semen parameters of the exposed groups based on severity of injury showed more pronounced effects in the moderately and severely injured infertile (41.6±4.4%; p=0.01) and non-mustard-gas-injured infertile individuals (35.8±4.5%; p=0.01) compared with those of the mildly injured individuals. This study provided no ORs for the results.
Adverse Pregnancy Outcomes			
Arnetz et al. (2013)	Random cross-sectional sample of 307 Iraqi families in Detroit, MI. Two groups: those in Iraq during the Gulf War (n=185) and those who left Iraq before (n=122).	Chemicals: depleted uranium, smoke from oil-burning fires, pesticides, nerve gas, contaminated food, prenatal exposure to sulfur/nitrogen dioxide. Aggregate chemical and stress exposure scores calculated for each individual.	Chemical exposures were positively correlated with adverse birth outcome (OR=2.04, 95% CI 1.12–3.74). Exposure to mustard gas was significantly associated with stillbirth (OR=2.55, 95% CI 1.24–5.23, p=0.013). Exposure to burning oil pits and mustard gas increased the risks for specific adverse birth outcomes 2 to 4 times.
Developmental Effects			
Abolghasemi et al. (2010)	Case-control study. 164 couples in Sardasht City, Iran. 164 age-matched controls from a nearby city with no history of chemical attack. Physical abnormalities evaluated in children of fathers who had been exposed.	Sulfur mustard	The overall frequency of abnormalities in the exposed group was significantly higher than in the non-exposed group (95 [19%] versus 77 [11%]; OR=1.93, 1.37–2.72, p<0.001). In offspring from exposed fathers, respiratory diseases were found in 20 (4%) subjects, and 21 (4%) had congenital malformations, compared with 9 (1%) for both endpoints in the nonexposed group. Frequency of respiratory diseases (OR=3.12, 95% CI 1.43–6.80, p=0.004) and congenital malformations (OR=3.54, 95% CI 1.58–7.93, p=0.002) were significantly higher in the offspring of the exposed group vs the nonexposed group.

NOTE: CI=confidence interval; DNA=deoxyribonucleic acid; FSH=follicle-stimulating hormone; OR=odds ratio.

INFECTIOUS DISEASES

Several infectious agents that U.S. service members may have come in contact with during their deployment to the Persian Gulf were identified by P.L. 105-368 and P.L. 105-277, including leishmaniasis. Malaria is also endemic to Afghanistan and was common in Iraq, although it has been eliminated there in recent years (WHO, 2016). The following section discusses these agents because they may exert long-term health effects as described in *Gulf War and Health, Volume 5* (IOM, 2007). That volume characterized the long-term adverse health outcomes associated with infection by the following pathogens: *Brucella* species (spp.), the cause of brucellosis; *Campylobacter* spp., nontyphoidal *Salmonella* spp., and *Shigella* spp., which cause diarrheal disease; *Coxiella burnetii*, the cause of Q fever; *Leishmania* spp., the cause of leishmaniasis; *Mycobacterium tuberculosis*, the cause of tuberculosis; *Plasmodium* spp., the cause of malaria; and West Nile virus, the cause of West Nile fever. The literature search included studies published through January 2005 and included infections relevant to the Post-9/11 population of veterans. The Volume 5 committee noted that orchioepididymitis may occur in up to 20% of men with brucellosis (Ibrahim et al., 1988; Memish and Venkatesh, 2001; Navarro-Martinez et al., 2001; Papatsoris et al., 2002). It is most often unilateral and accompanied by normal urine sediment (Navarro-Martinez et al., 2001). The Volume 5 committee found that there was sufficient evidence of an association between brucellosis and orchioepididymitis.

Among the infectious diseases listed in P.L. 105-277 and P.L. 105-368, *Escherichia coli* and sand fly fever were not included in *Volume 5* for in-depth evaluation because they did not satisfy the criteria for determining the strength of an association between the primary infection and a health outcome in humans. *E. coli*, in particular, is ubiquitous in nature, making it challenging to distinctly identify effects unique to military personnel. Shigellosis, one of the infectious diseases also listed in the legislation, was not exhaustively discussed in *Volume 5* because of the lack of relevant information available on the veteran cohorts of interest.

In the present volume, the committee identified several new studies describing relevant sequela of leishmaniasis. No new data were identified for the other infectious agents of concern. The studies used by the committee to reach its conclusions on infectious agents are summarized in Table 4-2 at the end of this section.

Leishmaniasis

Leishmaniasis is an all-inclusive term for various manifestations of sand-fly-borne parasitic disease, such as cutaneous leishmaniasis, diffuse cutaneous leishmaniasis, mucocutaneous leishmaniasis, visceral leishmaniasis, and viscerotropic leishmaniasis (see IOM, 2007, for a description of the varieties of leishmanisasis). This infectious disease occurs in tropical and temperate climates. Veterans can be exposed to this disease through sand flies, which act as vectors that inject the parasite into humans (IOM, 2007). The infection manifests as skin lesions and damage to internal organs such as the heart, liver, and spleen. Congenital transmission of leishmaniasis from pregnant mother to child has been documented, with transplacental transmission being suspected. In addition to the damage done by direct infection of the child, animal studies suggest that the mother's immune response may also be responsible for adverse birth outcomes (Berger et al., 2017). The Volume 11 committee did not identify any studies of developmental effects in children following prenatal or preconception exposure to leishmaniasis.

Reproductive Effects

Infectious agents such as leishmaniasis plagued U.S. troops deployed to OEF/OIF. Both published reports and presentations available to the public indicate that more than 1,000 U.S. service members received a diagnosis of leishmaniasis contracted during their deployments (IOM, 2007). Three new studies published since the 2007 review were identified: two studies of leishmaniasis in pregnant women and one animal study.

A cross-sectional study of pregnant women diagnosed with visceral leishmaniasis was conducted by Adam et al. (2018). The study was carried out from January 1, 2014, to December 31, 2015, at Gadarif Hospital in Sudan. Demographic and obstetric data were recorded, along with the time span between the onset of visceral leishmaniasis symptoms and hospitalization. Of 45 women, 6 died during pregnancy, and 2 died after delivery. Of the remaining 37 patients who were followed until delivery, 30 (77%) had full-term deliveries with a live neonate who had no observable health issues upon delivery, 6 experienced preterm delivery, 2 had a spontaneous abortion, and 1 had a stillbirth. The authors concluded that visceral leishmaniasis has a very high case fatality rate during pregnancy.

Case reports were described for five women in Brazil who were treated for visceral leishmaniasis during pregnancy (Figueiro-Filho et al., 2008). The women were between 16.5 and 36 weeks of pregnancy at presentation, and the disease was confirmed by positive antibody testing and a demonstration of amastigote forms of leishmania in bone marrow. All patients presented with fever, splenomegaly, and hepatomegaly. One patient died due to hemorrhage after delivery as a result of low platelet count. Treatment with amphotericin B was successful, and no vertical transmission was found. All infants were reported to be healthy at birth. At the 1-year follow-up, the infants and mothers were considered healthy and free of disease.

Animal Studies

A study by Avila-Garcia et al. (2013) discussed the transplacental transmission of cutaneous Leishmania in mice. Transplacental transmission of the parasite from an infected mother to the fetus has been documented in humans with *L. chagasi,* which causes visceral leishmaniasis (Figueiro-Filho et al., 2004), and in mice with *L. Mexicana,* which causes cutaneous leishmaniasis (Avila-Garcia et al., 2013). In the mouse model, infected dams had increased fetal deaths and resorptions. Importantly, both mother and infected infant can be successfully treated (Figueiro-Filho et al., 2004, 2008).

Synthesis and Conclusions

The Volume 5 committee concluded that there is sufficient evidence of an association between leishmaniasis and acute clinical syndrome. That committee did not identify any new data for most agents concerning reproductive and developmental outcomes, with the exception of the study by Adam et al. (2018) showing that Sudanese women who had leishmaniasis during their pregnancy had an elevated risk of having a high fatality rate for their fetuses and infants. Congenital transmission has been documented with leishmaniasis, which can be successfully treated. Results from animal studies provide additional support for a relationship between adverse birth outcomes and maternal immune response to infection (Berger et al., 2017). No data were available on developmental effects.

The Volume 11 committee concludes that there is inadequate/insufficient evidence to determine whether an association exists between exposure to leishmaniasis and reproductive or developmental effects.

The Volume 11 committee also concludes that there is sufficient evidence of an association between leishmaniasis infection during pregnancy and adverse pregnancy outcomes.

TABLE 4-2 Summary of Reproductive Effects of Infectious Diseases

Study	Population	Exposure	Results
Reproductive Effects			
Adam et al. (2018)	Cross-sectional study on 45 pregnant women in Sudan.	VL	Some women had full-term deliveries (77%) of children with no health conditions, and other women had preterm deliveries (15%) and stillbirths (2%). Using univariate analyses, maternal mortality among women with VL among those who had a 1-month time span between their symptoms and onset of hospital presentation: OR=6.2, 95% CI 2.8–13.4; p=0.000.
Figueiro-Filho et al. (2004)	Literature review	VL	VL during pregnancy can be vertically transmitted to the fetus. This is a literature review that provided no ORs.
Figueiro-Filho et al. (2008)	Women admitted to the gynecology–obstetrics service at Federal University of Mato Grosso do Sul, Brazil, from January 2004 to December 2005. 5 cases of pregnant women treated for VL.	VL	VL treatment prevented vertical transmission, even in women who were treated after giving birth. 1 patient with a late diagnosis died.

NOTE: CI=confidence interval; OR=odds ratio; VL=visceral leishmaniasis.

VACCINES

The administration of vaccines to Gulf War military personnel is described and reviewed in *Gulf War and Health, Volume 1* (IOM, 2000). The U.S. military conducts a comprehensive immunization program designed to protect the members of the armed forces against potential disease risks encountered during service. A standard set of vaccinations is required for each military recruit, which varies slightly by branch of service. Additionally, troops assigned to duty stations are given vaccinations that are specifically targeted to protect them from the risks related to their assignment or endemic to their assigned geographic location.

During the Gulf War, a number of different immunobiologics (e.g., cholera, meningitis, rabies, tetanus, and typhoid vaccines) were used to protect against potential exposures to biological threats. An estimated 150,000 U.S. troops received at least one anthrax vaccination, and an estimated 8,000 individuals were vaccinated with botulinum toxoid. However, medical records from the Gulf War contain little or no information about who received which vaccines, how frequently vaccines were administered, or the timing of vaccinations in relation to the other exposures. Furthermore, existing record entries show no consistency in recording the type of vaccine (notations include "A-Vax," "Vacc A," "Vacc B," and "B Vaccination"). A report by the Office of the Special Assistant for Gulf War Illnesses found that documents from the Gulf War indicate uncertainty about where, or whether, the vaccinations were to be used (OSAGWI, 1999).

Vaccinations were used in the Post-9/11 conflicts to aid in preventing communicable or infectious diseases among deployed troops. Vaccinations became so routine that troops would be vaccinated en masse before deployment (IOM, 2000).

Vaccine-related issues of concern to Gulf War veterans, including the safety of anthrax vaccine, botulinum toxoid vaccine, and issues of multiple vaccines, were discussed by the Volume 1 committee (IOM, 2000). Few peer-reviewed, long-term studies focused on the adverse effects of any of these vaccines were available. Even considering other data (not peer-reviewed or published), there was limited information concerning long-term adverse events. Thus, the Volume 1 committee concluded that there was inadequate/insufficient evidence to determine whether an association exists between long-term adverse effects and any of the exposures of interest.

Regarding the anthrax vaccine, the Volume 1 committee noted the lack of human data on adverse events and the lack of long-term monitoring for such effects. No significant adverse events had been reported at that time, leading the Volume 1 committee to conclude that there was inadequate/insufficient evidence to determine whether an association does or does not exist between anthrax vaccine and long-term adverse health effects. The Volume 1 committee encouraged continued investigation and publication of such data.

The Volume 1 committee found that the available data for the anthrax vaccine were sparse and provided no convincing evidence that personnel who received anthrax vaccine had elevated risks of later-onset health events. That committee made many recommendations to DoD and other agencies to support a safe vaccine surveillance program (IOM, 2000). The studies used by the committee to reach its conclusions on vaccines are summarized in Table 4-3 at the end of this section.

Reproductive Effects

Reproductive Effects in Women

The Volume 11 committee identified several studies on anthrax vaccine published after *Volume 1*, including three epidemiologic investigations in military populations, a review of adverse events following the use of the anthrax vaccine, one study in rabbits, and one study of the vaccine in conjunction with smallpox vaccine during pregnancy. No new data on any other vaccines of concern were identified.

Adverse events following anthrax vaccination as reported to the Vaccine Adverse Event Reporting System (VAERS), a national spontaneous reporting system used to monitor the safety of vaccines in the United States from January 1998 through December 2001 were reviewed by Sever et al. (2004). VAERS is a passive surveillance system jointly administered by the Food and Drug Administration (FDA) and the Centers for Disease Control and Prevention. During the study interval, 3,991 adverse events were recorded or 9.4 reports/10,000 doses of anthrax vaccine or 1 event/282 vaccines. Flu-like symptoms, rash, malaise, arthralgia, and headache were the most prevalent adverse events reported. Reproductive system adverse events included two spontaneous abortions and one trisomy 13, which could not be attributed to vaccination.

The effects of anthrax vaccination on semen parameters and pregnancy rates were evaluated in couples seeking assistance at the Walter Reed Army Medical Center Assisted Reproductive Technologies Program (Catherino et al., 2005). Data on 254 vaccinated and 791 unvaccinated men were collected by interview. The mean age of the men in the two groups was similar, and the average ages of the men and the women in the two groups ranged from 34.8 to 35.9. Self-reports of tubal factor infertility were significantly more common among exposed men compared with unexposed men (48% versus 35.2%; $p<0.01$), whereas male factor infertility was significantly lower for exposed men versus unexposed men (19.4% versus 28.2%; $p<0.01$). However, there was no significant difference in 5-day embryo transfers performed on the female partners of the exposed versus unexposed men (20.9% versus 14.5%; $p=0.507$). There were no significant differences in semen parameters—including the mean concentration, total motile concentration per sample, and morphology—between the vaccinated and the unvaccinated men. Fertilization rates and embryo quality were not affected by vaccination. Nor were the pregnancy rates for the vaccinated and unvaccinated groups significantly different (49.6% and 45.9%, respectively).

Wiesen and Littell (2002) evaluated the effect of anthrax vaccination on pregnancy rates, fetal loss, and birth outcome among 3,136 vaccinated and 962 unvaccinated U.S. Army women (ages 17–44). Individual data were obtained from administrative and clinical databases, and the analyses were adjusted for age, marital status, and race. All vaccinated women had received at least one dose of anthrax vaccine, and a majority had been given 2–3 doses. No attempt was made to evaluate a dose–response relationship. In the vaccinated and not-vaccinated groups the annualized pregnancy rates were 159.5 and 160.0 per 1,000 person-years, respectively. No associations were found between anthrax vaccination and pregnancy, birth rate, or adverse birth outcome. Adjusted ORs were 0.94 (95% CI 0.8–1.2) for pregnancy, 0.9 (95% CI 0.5–1.4) for birth rate, and 1.3 (95% CI 0.2–6.4) for low birth weight. No significant increase was found for any structural anomaly in the offspring (OR=0.7, 95% CI 0.2–2.3).

Adverse Pregnancy Outcomes

Pregnancy and infant health outcomes were evaluated in U.S. military women who had received the anthrax vaccine (AVA) during pregnancy (Conlin et al., 2015). The women were registered with the National Smallpox Vaccine in Pregnancy Registry because they had received a smallpox vaccine within the 28 days prior to or during a pregnancy. Analyses included 308 women (312 fetuses) vaccinated for anthrax in pregnancy and 155 women (156 fetuses) not vaccinated for anthrax. Outcomes were compared between the anthrax vaccine-exposed group and expected values determined by a literature review, and additional comparisons were made between the anthrax vaccine-exposed and unexposed groups. Infant health outcomes (preterm birth, low birth weight, major birth defects, and male sex of infant) were similar between the AVA-unexposed group (N=125) and the AVA-exposed group (N=271) for preterm birth (OR=8.8, 95% CI 4.5–15.2 versus OR=10.0, 95% CI 6.7–14.2); low birth weight (OR=9.6, 95% CI 5.1–16.2 versus OR=7.7, 95% CI 4.9–11.6); major birth defects (OR=3.2, 95% CI 0.9–8.0 versus OR=2.6, 95% CI 1.0–5.2); and male sex of infant (OR=52.8, 95% CI 43.7–61.8 versus OR=48.7, 95% CI 42.6–54.8). Adverse fetal outcomes for AVA-unexposed women were higher than or similar to those of AVA-exposed women (ectopic pregnancy: OR=2.6, 95% CI 0.7–6.4 versus OR=0.3, 95% CI 0.0–1.8; elective abortion: OR=7.2, 95% CI 3.7–14.2 versus OR=4.4, 95% CI 2.5–7.9; stillbirth: OR=2.4, 95% CI 0.5–6.8 versus OR=0.7, 95% CI 0.1–2.7). Results were similar when the outcomes among women who received anthrax and smallpox vaccines during pregnancy (not before) were compared with outcomes in women who received the smallpox vaccine during pregnancy and not before.

Conlin et al. (2017) conducted a study to determine if vaccination during pregnancy is associated with the risk of birth defects. Data on 126,839 live infants born in 2003–2010 were obtained from the DoD Birth and Infant Health Registry. Mothers were placed into categories based upon their vaccination exposure and time to pregnancy. The medical records of infants were evaluated for possible birth defect diagnoses that may have occurred within the first year of life. The researchers found that infants born to mothers vaccinated during their first trimester did not have higher risks of birth defects compared with mothers vaccinated at any other time (OR=1.10, 95% CI 0.93–1.29). Infants born to mothers vaccinated before pregnancy had a slightly higher risk of developing a birth defect than infants born to mothers vaccinated after their child's conception (OR=1.11, 95% CI 1.01–1.22). Mothers who were vaccinated after the start of pregnancy had a 10% lower risk of birth defects in their children compared with mothers who never received the vaccination (OR=0.90, 95% CI 0.83–0.99). There was a slight association observed between pre-pregnancy vaccination or never having been vaccinated and birth defects risk when compared with women who were vaccinated after their pregnancy started.

As discussed in Reproductive Effects in Men and Women, Wiesen and Littell (2002) found no association between anthrax vaccination for U.S. Army women and adverse birth outcomes (OR=0.9, 95% CI 0.4–2.4).

Developmental Effects

A retrospective cohort was used to evaluate the association between birth defects and anthrax vaccination in the first trimester among all infants born to U.S. female service members between 1998 and 2004 (Ryan et al., 2008). Data on live-born infants and maternal anthrax vaccination were obtained from DoD databases. A total of 115,169 infants born to 95,595 mothers were studied, including 3,465 infants born to mothers who received a vaccination in the first trimester and 938 who were exposed to more than one dose of a vaccine during the first trimester. After adjusting for preterm birth, male infants, and maternal age more than 35 years, the researchers found that infants with first-trimester exposure did not have a significantly increased risk of having a birth defect (OR=1.18, 95% CI 0.997–1.41) compared with infants born to women vaccinated outside of the first trimester. However, infants exposed in the first trimester had significantly increased odds of birth defects when compared with infants born to mothers who had never been vaccinated (OR=1.20, 95% CI 1.02–1.42). The most common defect, atrial septal defect, was found in 58 infants exposed in the first trimester, which was a statistically significantly higher rate than among women vaccinated outside of the first trimester (OR=1.38, 95% CI 1.04–1.82).

Conlin et al. (2017) conducted an analyses using data from 2003 through 2010 from active-duty Reserve, Army, Air Force, Navy, or Marine mothers. This study included 126,839 infants born to military mothers, categorized by the timing of the anthrax vaccination relative to the pregnancy. Data such as deployment status during pregnancy and the administration of other vaccinations were included in multivariable models. In the study population, 33.3% of mothers were vaccinated for anthrax prior to pregnancy (42,260 women); 3.5% during the first trimester (4,418 women vaccinated during the first trimester); 0.3% during the second or third trimester (423 women vaccinated during the second or third trimester); 19.1% post-pregnancy (24,179 women post-pregnancy); and 43.8% were never vaccinated. Infants born to mothers vaccinated in the first trimester of pregnancy were not at increased odds of a birth defect diagnosis (OR=1.10, 95% CI 0.93–1.29) compared with those whose mothers were vaccinated outside of the first trimester. No increased odds for birth defects were found for vaccination during the first trimester compared with pre-pregnancy, post-pregnancy, or never vaccinated. The infants of mothers who were vaccinated pre-pregnancy had slightly higher odds of birth defects than the infants of women who were vaccinated post-pregnancy (OR=1.11, 95% CI 1.01–1.22), while the infants of those vaccinated post-pregnancy had lower odds than those of never-vaccinated mothers.

Animal Studies

One animal study identified by the committee examined reproductive toxicity in rabbits. Female New Zealand white rabbits were given anthrax vaccination twice before they mated and again on either gestational day (GD) 7 or 17 (Franco et al., 2009). No adverse effects were found on mating and fertility indices, natural delivery observation, clinical signs, gross lesions, in utero growth or survival, morphological development, or kit viability. The data on rabbits support the findings in humans that there is little evidence of an association between vaccinations and reproductive and developmental effects.

Synthesis and Conclusions

The U.S. military implements a comprehensive immunization program that is designed to protect the armed forces from potential disease risks. A standard set of vaccinations is administered to each military recruit, including those specifically targeted to protect against risks related to their assignments or found in their assigned geographic location (e.g., Afghanistan). As was the case in previous reviews, only limited data on the adverse effects of any of these vaccines were available to inform conclusions on potential reproductive or developmental outcomes. New information was found only for the anthrax vaccination.

Studies of military personnel given anthrax vaccination found no effects on male or female fertility (Catherino et al., 2005). One study found that female soldiers who received the anthrax vaccine were not at increased risk for adverse pregnancy outcomes (Wiesen and Littell, 2002).

One large cohort of military women showed a nonsignificant increase in the risk of birth defects following first-trimester vaccination with anthrax (Ryan et al., 2008); however, this was not observed in a second study that compared the timing of vaccination during pregnancy with the occurrence of birth defects (Conlin et al., 2017). Conlin et al. did find a slightly increased significant risk of birth defects for infants born to mothers who were vaccinated prior to pregnancy compared with those vaccinated after their pregnancy. Given that women who are deployed may not be aware that they are pregnant in their first trimester and may receive vaccinations during this time, continued investigation and publication of these data are needed and encouraged.

The Volume 11 committee concludes that there is inadequate/insufficient evidence to determine whether an association exists between anthrax vaccination and reproductive or developmental effects.

TABLE 4-3 Summary of Reproductive and Developmental Effects of Vaccines

Study	Population	Exposure	Results
Reproductive Effects			
Reproductive Effects in Men and Women			
Catherino et al. (2005)	254 men who reported receiving the anthrax vaccination and 791 men who denied vaccination with their partners seeking assisted reproduction services.	Men underwent semen analysis.	Tubal factor infertility was common among the exposed group (48% versus 35.2%; p<0.01); male infertility was less common (19.4% versus 28.2%; p<0.01). Anthrax vaccination did not statistically alter fertility in men who were undergoing assisted reproduction. This study provided no ORs for results.
Wiesen and Littell (2002)	Cohort study from a database of women ages 17–44. Stationed at Fort Stewart, GA/Hunter Army Airfield, GA, from 1999 to 2000.	4,092 women of whom 3,136 received at least one dose of anthrax. 513 pregnancies with 385 following at least one dose of the vaccine. 353 live births and 25 pregnancies lost to follow-up.	Vaccination had no effect on pregnancy, birth rates, or adverse birth outcomes. When comparing the pregnancy ratio for vaccinated women versus unvaccinated women: OR=0.94, 95% CI 0.8–1.2, p=0.60; birth OR=0.9, 95% CI 0.5–1.4, p=0.55; and adverse birth outcomes OR=0.9, 95% CI 0.4–2.4, p=0.88. No associations were found between anthrax vaccination and pregnancy, birth rate, or adverse birth outcome. No significant increase was found for any structural anomaly.
Adverse Pregnancy Outcomes			
Conlin et al. (2015)	Enrollment began in 2003. 517 U.S. military women were chosen who represented 522 pregnancies. 504 eligible women.	Smallpox/anthrax vaccination. 95% of subjects received one or both vaccines before 8 weeks gestational age. 65% of subjects also reported receiving AVA around the time of the smallpox vaccination.	Rates of birth defects and preterm birth remained constant with infants born to military mothers since 2003. Infant health outcomes (preterm birth, low birth weight, major birth defects, etc.) were similar between the AVA-unexposed groups (n=125) and the AVA-exposed group (n=271) for preterm birth (OR=8.8, 95% CI 4.5–15.2 versus OR=10.0, 95% CI 6.7–14.2); low birth weight (OR=9.6, 95% CI 5.1–16.2 versus OR=7.7, 95% CI 4.9–11.6); major birth defects (OR=3.2, 95% CI 0.9–8.0 versus OR=2.6, 95% CI 1.0–5.2); and male sex of infant (OR=52.8, 95% CI 43.7–61.8 versus OR=48.7, 95% CI 42.6–54.8). Adverse fetal outcomes for AVA-unexposed were higher than or similar to those of AVA-exposed women (ectopic pregnancy: OR=2.6, 95% CI 0.7–6.4 versus OR=0.3, 95% CI 0.0–1.8; elective abortion: OR=7.2, 95% CI 3.7–14.2 versus OR=4.4, 95% CI 2.5–7.9; stillbirth: OR=2.4, 95% CI 0.5–6.8 versus OR=0.7, 95% CI 0.1–2.7).

Study	Population	Exposure	Results
Developmental Effects			
Conlin et al. (2017)	126,839 infants born to military mothers during 2003–2010.	AVA	Infants born to mothers vaccinated in the first trimester were not at increased odds of a birth defect diagnosis (OR=1.10, 95% CI 0.93–1.29) compared with those vaccinated outside of the first trimester. No increased odds for birth defects were found for vaccination during the first trimester compared to pre- and post-pregnancy or never vaccinated. Infants born to mothers vaccinated pre-pregnancy had slightly higher odds of birth defects than to mothers vaccinated post-pregnancy (OR=1.11, 95% CI 1.01–1.22).
Ryan et al. (2008)	3,465 infants born to women service members between 1/1/98 and 2/21/04. 115,169 infants born to 95,595 military women.	Anthrax vaccine during first trimester; 938 of infants were exposed to >1 dose during the first trimester. 33,675 infants born to women who received the vaccine outside of their first trimester; 663 of those were exposed in late pregnancy. 14,306 infants' mothers were vaccinated before pregnancy. 18,706 infants' mothers were vaccinated after birth. 78,029 infants were unexposed.	Maternal anthrax vaccination in the first trimester is associated with an increased prevalence of birth defects in infants, mainly atrial septal defects (OR=1.38, 95% CI 1.04–1.82). Women who were vaccinated before pregnancy or in late pregnancy did not have an increased risk of their infants being born with birth defects when compared with women who had not been vaccinated.
Moro et al. (2017)	Birth defects in children from 50 reports.	Vaccinations (some anthrax).	Results showed that infants born to mothers vaccinated in their first trimester experienced a higher rate of deformities than infants born to mothers who were vaccinated in the second or third trimester. This was a review of the VAERS database and did not provide ORs for results.

NOTE: AVA=anthrax vaccine absorbed; CI=confidence interval; OR=odds ratio; VAERS=Vaccine Adverse Effect Reporting System.

DEPLETED URANIUM

DU is a by-product of the enrichment process used to make reactor-grade uranium. It is a weakly radioactive, chemically toxic heavy metal that is derived from natural uranium and used by the U.S. military for munitions and for armor on some tanks. It is well suited as a munition because of its high density and "self-sharpening" nature, both of which help it to penetrate armor. Its high density also makes it an effective shield. DU has been used by all branches of the U.S. military since the 1980s, and it has been used on the battlefield in the Persian Gulf War, the Balkans, and the Iraq War (NRC, 2008).

In the Gulf War, DU was frequently used in an effort to increase the protective layer on heavy-armor tanks to prevent penetration by weaponry. Additionally, the U.S. Army used an estimated 9,500 DU tank rounds during the Gulf War, many of them as training and practice rounds as well as in kinetic energy cartridges and ammunition rounds (IOM, 2000). U.S. service members could be exposed to DU through a variety of pathways, including "friendly fire" incidents, ingestion, inhalation, cleanup operations, and accidents (IOM, 2000). Some military personnel were exposed to DU through contact with contaminated vehicles and inhalation of contaminated dust. Level I exposure, the highest level, occurred in or near combat vehicles when they were struck by DU rounds or when soldiers entered vehicles soon after the impact of such rounds. U.S. military personnel may have experienced Level I exposure as a result of wounds caused by DU fragments, inhalation of airborne DU particles, or ingestion of DU residues. Level II, the intermediate exposure level, occurred when soldiers and civilian employees worked on DU-contaminated vehicles or were involved in cleanup efforts at their installations. More than 700 individuals may have had Level II exposure from the inhalation of dust containing DU particles and residue, ingestion from hand-to-mouth contact, or contamination of clothing. Level III, the lowest level of exposure, occurred when troops entered DU-contaminated Iraqi tanks or when they were downwind from burning DU ammunition, DU-contaminated vehicles, or the Camp Doha fire near Kuwait. Level III exposures could have occurred though inhalation or ingestion. Hundreds of people in both military and civilian cleanup crews are thought to have experienced potential Level III exposure, but there is little additional information on these estimates (OSAGWI, 1998).

In the Post-9/11 conflicts, DU was used to armor tanks and help bullets penetrate enemy armored vehicles. Post-9/11 veterans were exposed to DU via the same routes as Gulf War veterans. Most exposures occurred from DU-containing missiles striking vehicles, producing airborne DU-particles that could be inhaled.

The health effects that may result from DU exposure were reviewed in *Gulf War and Health, Volume 1* (IOM, 2000) and in an updated review in 2008 (IOM, 2008a). The updated review covered literature through 2007. The committees that produced those reviews relied on studies in nonveteran populations and supporting information from animal studies to establish biologic plausibility. Studies on uranium workers were reviewed, but they carried less weight in the committees' final conclusions because radon, which is the primary disease-causing exposure in uranium miners, has different physiochemical properties and deposition patterns in the airways than DU and it also lacks the chemical toxicity (as opposed to radiologic toxicity) of DU. Furthermore, uranium miners have a different array of exposures to other toxic dusts and gases, which makes comparisons with veterans of limited value. Both committees concluded that there was inadequate/insufficient evidence of any association between DU and reproductive or developmental outcomes (IOM, 2000, 2008a).

In 2008, a National Research Council (NRC) committee released a review of the available toxicologic, radiologic, epidemiologic, and toxicokinetic data on DU to help describe the risk of health effects to exposed military personnel. That committee found that long-term surveillance of DU-exposed Gulf War veterans had yielded no evidence of reproductive-system dysfunction in males, abnormalities in sperm, or alterations in neuroendocrine function in the first 14 years after exposure. Nor was there evidence of excess spontaneous abortions, fetal mortality, congenital anomalies, developmental delays, or abnormal infant neurobehavioral difficulties in their offspring. However, animal studies focused on uranium placental transfer. In studies that reported placental uranium transfer, dams were exposed to high doses of uranium (equivalent to about 200 g in a 70-kg person). The NRC committee (2008) recommended that on the basis of available reproductive toxicity and developmental toxicity data, samples of blood, urine, or semen of DU-exposed military personnel should be collected for the measurement of uranium content and signs of abnormal reproductive function in men and women. In addition, the reporting of spontaneous abortions and congenital anomalies should be continued.

In 2013, the ATSDR released *Toxicological Profile for Uranium*, which included information about DU (ATSDR, 2013). The profile reviewed the human and animal literature through 2013 and found that the preponderance of evidence supported renal toxicity, but the data concerning reproductive effects in humans were limited. Reproductive and developmental effects have been studied in mice and rats, but confirmatory studies are needed. The profile did not provide information on depleted uranium specifically.

The studies used by the Volume 11 committee to reach its conclusions on vaccines are summarized in Table 4-4 at the end of this section.

Reproductive and Developmental Effects

Since the uranium update review concluded in 2007, only one new publication has reported on reproductive effects of embedded DU (McDiarmid et al., 2009). The Volume 11 committee did not identify any new studies on the potential developmental effects of preconception or prenatal exposure to DU in humans.

A systematic review by Asghari et al. (2015) focused on multiple studies that were not of sufficient quality or of the necessary focus to be directly relevant to the committee's task. The review found that exposure to DU through in vivo and in vitro procedures caused dysfunction of the gonadal endocrine system leading to hormonal alterations, apoptosis through reactive oxygen species, and musculoskeletal, digestive, and cardiovascular malformations in neonates that resulted from impaired antioxidant enzymes that were related to oxidative stress. Several publications have continued to report on the surveillance of a group of Gulf War veterans with embedded DU shrapnel; of these, one has reported on reproductive outcomes (McDiarmid et al., 2009). Even though DU has been isolated in semen samples from Gulf War veterans with embedded fragments of the material (Todorov et al., 2013), no effects of DU on semen characteristics (data not reported), neuroendocrine parameters (data not reported), or genotoxicity measures (hypoxanthine-guanine phosphoribosyl transferase mutation assay and fluorescent in situ hybridization assay; p-values all greater than 0.08) were observed 16 years after the Gulf War (McDiarmid et al., 2009). In a review of this work, McDiarmid and colleagues noted that even though no health condition has been consistently observed, urinary concentrations of DU continue to be high—and stable—more than 20 years later. Because tissue concentrations will accrue with the continued mobilization of embedded DU, health effects may still be expected to occur, and thus, these veterans will continue to be monitored (McDiarmid et al., 2009; NASEM, 2016).

Animal Studies

The Volume 11 committee identified ATSDR data and seven animal studies that had appeared since the NRC and IOM reviews published in 2008. A two-generation reproductive toxicity study by Arfsten et al. (2009) examined the effects that long-term DU implantation may have on the reproductive system of the F0 generation (249 male and 248 female rats) and on the development and survival of the F1 and F2 generations. F0 rats were implanted with DU pellets and mated 120 days later. The researchers found that the implantation of DU did not have any effect on the survival or well-being of the F0 generation, and they observed no gross abnormalities in the F1 and F2 generations.

Feugier et al. (2008) conducted a study with a total of 101 female mice exposed to DU through contaminated drinking water for 49 days. They found that DU did not influence the intensity of ovulation, but it did affect the quality of the oocyte. The proportion of healthy oocytes was significantly reduced by half in each group ($p<0.001$) from 20 mg/L to 10 mg/L when compared with the control group (healthy proportions=0.537, 0.497, 0.282, and 0.239 in the control, 10 mg/L, 20 mg/L, and 40 mg/L groups, respectively).

Darolles et al. (2010) specifically investigated the effect of DU and enriched uranium on mouse fibroblast cells. After DU treatment (5, 50, or 500 μM), no toxicity or incidence of binucleated cells with one micronucleus (BN-1MN) was detected. However, the study did not have the ability to accurately assess overall uranium genotoxicity. DU had a "low clastogenic effect."[2] Its aneugenic effect was significant and led to a global genotoxic effect equivalent to 12% enriched uranium as assessed by classical cytokinesis-block micronucleus assay (BN-1MN counting).

A study by Hao et al. (2009) investigated 150 male and 150 female 3-week-old hybrid Wistar rats (F0). The rats were exposed to DU through food consumption at doses of 0, 4, or 40 mg/kg/d for 4 months and then mated. F1 rats were exposed to the same doses as their parents for 4 months. Results showed that the uranium content in F1 rats was considerably higher than that in F0 rats in both the kidney and the ovary ($p<0.05$), with significant differences observed by dose and generation in sperm abnormality rate, comet tail length, marrow cell micronuclei rate, and tailed cell percentage. Overall, F1 rats sustained more damage than F0 rats, emphasizing the genotoxic effects of chronic low-dose exposure to DU.

Hao et al. (2012) conducted a follow-up study that tested two generations of Wistar rats. Rats experienced chronic exposure to DU through feed containing DU at doses of 0 (control), 4 (DU4), or 40 (DU40) mg/kg/d for 4 months prior to mating. The FI generation was similarly exposed to DU in feed from postnatal day 21 until death. After 4 months of exposure, the pregnancy rate, normal labor rate, and survival rate of offspring produced by F1 rats were all drastically decreased in comparison with the control group. The DU40 group experienced the largest decrease, with parameters that had fallen by half to two-thirds, while no adverse effects were evident in F0 rats.

Legrand et al. (2016) studied pregnant female Sprague–Dawley rats exposed to DU through drinking water from GD 1 through lactation. Examination of the rats showed that DU decreased cell death in the cortical neuroepithelium of 13 embryos exposed at 40 mg/L and 120 mg/L and in GD18 fetuses exposed at 120 mg/L without altering the number of apoptotic cells. However, postnatal cell death increased in the dentate gyrus in postnatal day (PND) 0 and PND 5 exposed pups at 120 mg/L and was also related to increased apoptotic cell numbers at PND 5. These results showed that DU exposure during the gestational period and during lactation may cause neurogenesis.

A study by Miller et al. (2010) used male transgenic mice (Big Blue strain C57BL/6 hemizygous mice containing 40 copies of a shuttle vector lacI transgene) and non-transgenic female C57BL/6 mice as subjects. These mice were exposed to DU through implantation and drinking water. Within 1 day of DU exposure via implantation or orally through drinking water, male animals (F0) showed significant uranium accumulation in the kidneys, testes, and femur. Final results showed that F0 fathers who

[2] *Clastogenic effects* are visible damage or changes to chromosomes that are virtually microscopic, such as breaks in chromosomes or changes in chromosome numbers.

sustained DU exposure had a significant increase in mutation frequency in their F1 offspring (3.57±0.37 and 4.81±0.43 × 10^{-5}; p<0.001) as compared with controls (2.28±0.31 × 10^{-5}). The mutation frequencies of F1 offspring at low-dose implanted DU (2.71± 0.35 × 10^{-5}) were not notably different from the control levels (2.28±0.31 × 10^{-5}). The results of this study suggest that genomic instability is transmitted from fathers who were exposed to DU to the somatic cells of unexposed offspring.

Synthesis and Conclusions

The effects of DU were reviewed by authoritative bodies (ATSDR, 2013; IOM, 2000, 2008; NRC, 2008), and they concluded that DU was not associated with reproductive or developmental effects. Data published since those reviews show no evidence of reproductive or developmental effects in veterans, although the studies are of male veterans only. Studies in animal models have shown mixed results, with some evidence for male and female reproductive effects and genotoxicity in parents and offspring. The Volume 11 committee did not identify any new studies in humans on the association between exposure to DU and developmental effects.

The Volume 11 committee concludes that there is inadequate/insufficient evidence to determine whether an association exists between exposure to DU and reproductive or developmental effects.

TABLE 4-4 Summary of Reproductive Effects of Depleted Uranium

Study	Design/Population	Exposure	Results
Reproductive Effects			
Reproductive Effects in Men			
McDiarmid et al. (2009)	Subset of 35 members of a larger cohort of 77 Gulf War veterans. Urine uranium concentration and blood uranium concentration tests performed on Gulf War veterans.	DU—exposed during "friendly fire." Length of exposure not specified.	16 years after exposure, veterans showed little to no signs of DU-related health issues. Slight changes in bone formation as a result of DU exposure. Subtle changes in renal proximal tubular function between high and low exposure. Some veterans had embedded DU fragments ($p=0.4$). This review provided no odds ratios for results.

NOTE: DU=depleted uranium.

PYRIDOSTIGMINE BROMIDE

PB is a drug that was used during the Gulf War as a prophylactic agent against potential exposure to nerve agents, such as sarin. PB acts by binding to acetylcholinesterase (IOM, 2000) to act as a reversible cholinesterase inhibitor. It was created in 1945 and approved by FDA in 1955 for the treatment of myasthenia gravis.[3] FDA also approved an injectable form of the drug known for reversing the effects of some anesthetic formulations. The drug is poorly absorbed after oral administration, and peak plasma levels occur 2–3 hours after oral dosing. The drug is eliminated almost exclusively in the urine (IOM, 2000).

PB was first used as an investigational drug during the Gulf War and was not recommended for routine use. FDA, under a then newly-enacted provisional rule, had granted DoD a waiver from the requirement to obtain informed consent from service members taking this drug. Nonetheless, the rule did not address the record keeping that would accompany the use of an investigational drug. DoD reported that 5,328,710 doses were sent into the field and estimated that approximately 250,000 personnel took at least some PB during the Gulf War. It was supplied as a 21-tablet blister pack, and the prescribed dosage was one 30-mg tablet every 8 hours. Variation in use occurred, however, because it was self-administered and supposedly taken only when ordered by the unit commander (IOM, 2000).

The Volume 11 committee found no specific information on exposures of Post-9/11 service members to PB during deployment.

There are ample data pertaining to the use of PB in therapeutic settings, and many studies have examined PB to determine its possible role in causing Gulf War illness. However, few studies have reported on the long-term effects of PB, particularly its reproductive and developmental effects. *Gulf War and Health, Volume 1* concluded that that there is inadequate/insufficient evidence to determine whether an association exists between PB and long-term adverse health effects in military personnel (IOM, 2000).

The Volume 11 committee identified two new publications examining PB's effects on animal reproductive and developmental outcomes that had appeared since the IOM review in 2000. No new studies in humans were identified by the committee.

Animal Studies

One study assessing sperm and testicular changes in animals exposed to a mixture of several toxicants, including PB, that was meant to mirror Gulf War exposures was identified. Male rats were exposed to PB, DEET (N,N-diethyl-meta-toluamide), and permethrin with and without restraint stress for 28 days (Abou-Donia et al., 2003). Stress alone did not influence any of the measured outcomes. The testes of animals exposed to the chemical combination showed histologic abnormalities, including arrested spermatogenesis and seminiferous tubule degeneration, and these effects were enhanced by stress. The authors investigated the causal mechanism and identified it as apoptosis due to an increased expression of two apoptosis-promoting proteins in testicular tissue. This study suggests that exposures such as those experienced by Gulf War veterans may contribute to sperm abnormalities and male infertility; however, the animals in the chemical-plus-stress group gained less weight, suggesting poorer health overall, making interpretation of the findings difficult. Additionally, the results reflect the effects of a mixture, so the effects cannot be attributed to any one component (NASEM, 2016).

Berrios et al. (2015) examined GD 14.5 fetuses removed from pregnant rats. Cultures of rat neural progenitor cells were exposed to up to 300 μM of pyridostigmine over the course of 6 days. Reduced viability was not observed after treatment with 200 μM of pyridostigmine. However, results did show

[3] *Myasthenia gravis* is an autoimmune disorder characterized by antibody blockade of the acetylcholine receptor at the neuromuscular junction.

that PB decreased neurite growth, but it did not affect cell differentiation, and there were changes in protein expression. These results indicated that developmental patterns may have been affected.

Synthesis and Conclusions

PB was previously reviewed by the Volume 1 committee (IOM, 2000). New animal data identified by the Volume 11 committee came from experiments in which the animals were exposed to multiple chemicals and stress, thus making it impossible to identify any single agent as the cause of the observed effects. The combination exposure with PB, DEET, and permethrin did show effects on the testes which were exacerbated by stress. In vitro studies showed possible effects on neurodevelopment. Given the scarcity of data and the complexity of combined exposures, the new data make interpretation difficult and prevent the committee from coming to a definitive conclusion.

The Volume 11 committee concludes that there is inadequate/insufficient evidence to determine whether an association exists between exposure to PB and reproductive or developmental effects.

HEXAVALENT CHROMIUM

In 2003, about 900 U.S. Army personnel and civilian employees were exposed to sodium dichromate at the Qarmat Ali water treatment facility in Iraq, which was being restored by American contractors under the protection of the U.S. Army. Before U.S. control of the site, sodium dichromate was used to filter and treat water from the Tigris River and to prevent the corrosion of pipes and equipment. Vandalism of the facility resulted in sodium dichromate contamination of some parts of the facility (DoD, 2011).

Sodium dichromate contains Cr6, a known carcinogen which causes lung cancer (IARC, 2012). Cr6 is recognized by the European Chemicals Agency as having mutagenic, reproductive, and sensitization effects (ECHA, 2017).

The U.S. Army Center for Health Promotion and Preventative Medicine conducted follow-up medical surveillance and concluded that symptoms such as irritation of eyes, nose, throat, and lungs and the physical findings among exposed personnel were consistent with exposure to the desert environment and that whole blood chromium levels were not elevated (Ciminera et al., 2016). VA enacted a registry and medical surveillance program that began collecting medical data on these individuals in 2009 in collaboration with a parallel DoD program. The health of these service members through January 2012 was recently described by Ciminera et al. (2016), but no information related to reproductive, developmental, or generational outcomes was reported.

An ATSDR profile summarized the literature on Cr6 through 2012, including its reproductive and developmental effects in humans and animals, and it reported that a sensitive endpoint for Cr6 toxicity is the reproductive effects on male reproductive organs, including decreased sperm count and histopathological change to the epididymis (ATSDR, 2012). Because there is a large evidence base regarding the effects of Cr6, the Volume 11 committee focused its review on studies that were not included in the ATSDR review. The committee's literature search identified 11 epidemiologic studies and 8 animal studies on the reproductive or developmental effects of chromium exposure. The studies used by the committee to reach its conclusions on Cr6 are summarized in Table 4-5 at the end of this section.

Several studies reported on molecular changes associated with chromium exposure. Ali et al. (2011) examined a series of lung cancer cases in chromate workers and found that an individual's methylation of DNA *APC*, *hMLH1*, and *MGMT* genes was related to the number of years worked in the industry.

Among a small cohort of steel plant workers exposed to chromium, Bollati et al. (2010) found that two micro RNAs (miRNAs) in peripheral blood leukocytes (miR-21 and miR-146a) were not related to chromium exposure, but that miR-222 expression was associated with chromium (β=0.26, 95% CI 0.0–0.58, p=0.05).

Reproductive Effects

The Volume 11 committee identified two new reviews of epidemiologic studies. No epidemiologic studies examined exposure during the preconception or early pregnancy window or effects in veterans. The committee's search identified several recent studies and one older study that were not considered in the ATSDR profile. Specifically, the committee found three studies of the occupational exposure of men (Ali et al., 2011; Bollati et al., 2010; Yang et al., 2013) and eight studies of environmental exposure: two of which examined Cr6 as a component of air pollution in the United States (Heck et al., 2013; Roberts et al., 2013); three of which studied communities surrounding e-waste recycling operations in China (Guo et al., 2010; Li et al., 2008; Ni et al., 2014); one of which was a study of residents near a factory that used—and emitted—Cr6 (Remy et al., 2017); one of which examined the effects of contaminated drinking water (Aschengrau et al., 1993); and one of which observed Gaza residents exposed to metals, including chromium, as a result of military attacks (Manduca et al., 2014). Many of these studies are confounded by multiple chemical exposures.

Reproductive Effects in Men and Women

An ATSDR (2012) profile summarized the literature on Cr6 through 2012. ATSDR reported reproductive effects in humans associated with occupational exposures, including increased numbers of morphologically abnormal sperm, decreased sperm count and motility, and greater incidences of complications during pregnancy and childbirth (toxicosis and postnatal hemorrhage).

The reproductive impacts of chromium were assessed in one study with a large U.S. population. Residents near a factory in Willits, California, that used Cr6 had greater rates of genitourinary conditions, neoplasms (men and women), and adverse reproductive organ conditions in women (pelvic inflammatory disease, endometriosis, menstrual disorders, ovarian cysts, and reproductive organ surgeries) than compared with the rest of the county and the overall population in California (Remy et al., 2017). Given the large number of subjects and assessments before and after the factory closed, the study authors concluded that chromium was significantly associated with adverse reproductive effects in women. In a meta-analysis of Chinese studies (exact number of studies not given) by Yang et al. (2013), women with occupational Cr6 poisoning were found to have significantly elevated risks of spontaneous abortion (OR=2.31, 95% CI 1.25–4.27) or threatened abortion (OR=20.47, 95% CI 2.60–161.44).

Adverse Pregnancy Outcomes

The Volume 11 committee identified several recent publications and one older one that assessed both pregnancy outcomes and development effects following exposure to chromium. The committee notes that in all cases, pregnant women were exposed to more than one heavy metal or other toxicant. Among pregnant women exposed to contaminated community drinking water in Massachusetts and compared with 1,177 unexposed women, stillbirths (n=77; OR=1.2) and neonatal deaths (n=55; OR not calculated) were not significantly associated with chromium levels in drinking water (Aschengrau et al., 1993). Guo et al. (2010) found no differences in birth length, weight, and gestational age related to placental chromium levels in infants born to mothers residing near e-waste recycling areas in China (all $p>0.7$). There was no significant association ($p=0.53$) between chromium load in the hair of 48 infants born with birth defects and 12 infants born without defects in 2011 whose parents were exposed to metals in Gaza as a result of military weapons in 2009; nor was there a significance difference in chromium load in the hair of 9 infants born prematurely and 12 full-term infants ($p=0.8$) (Manduca et al., 2014). However, children born to mothers residing near a factory in Willits, California, that used Cr6 had significantly higher rates for short gestation (preterm), low birth weight, or small for gestational age (relative risk [RR]=1.14, 95% CI 1.05–1.25); macrosomia (large for gestational age; RR=1.16, 95% CI 1.04–1.29); perinatal jaundice (RR=1.13, 95% CI 1.06–1.20); and conditions affecting the nervous/sensory system (RR=1.17, 95% CI 1.05–1.31) than did children born to women residing elsewhere in the county (Remy et al., 2017). The authors reported that the risk for intrauterine hypoxia/asphyxia and perinatal jaundice dropped significantly after the factory was closed but that the risk of abnormal birth weight and term remained high. Infants born prior to the factory closure were at a significantly elevated risk for congenital anomalies other than genitourinary anomalies (eye, ear, face, neck, cleft, or chromosomal; RR=1.59, $p=0.0489$), but the difference in risk was not significant post-closure (RR=0.93).

Among infants born to women living in an e-waste recycling region in China, the cord blood concentrations of chromium were associated with DNA damage of lymphocytes in the cord blood (cell populations of comet $r=0.95$, $p=0.01$; cell lengths of tail $r=0.89$, $p=0.00$) (Li et al., 2008), and oxidative damage measured by 8-OHdG was associated with Cr ($\beta=0.086$ ng/mL, 95% CI 0.014–0.158 ng/mL) (Ni et al., 2014).

Developmental Effects

ATSDR (2102) reported that there are no studies showing that chromium causes birth defects in humans. In utero exposure to relatively high doses in animals is associated with adverse effects, including decreased numbers of live fetuses/litter, decreased fetal weight, internal and skeletal malformations, and delayed sexual maturation in offspring (ATSDR, 2012).

The Volume 11 committee identified three papers on developmental effects related to Cr6 exposure. One case-control study examined the risk of childhood cancer in California. Using the California Cancer Registry and the California LINE Source Dispersion Model, version 4, to estimate components of air pollution, Heck et al. (2013) reported that prenatal exposure to Cr6 (mean concentration=0.189 ng/m^3) was associated with childhood neuroblastoma in children of mothers who lived within 5 km of an air pollution monitor (OR=1.32, 95% CI 1.00–1.74; 75 cases and 14,602 controls who lived within 5 km of an air pollution monitor), but not for those who lived within 2.5 km of one (OR=1.00, 95% CI 0.25–4.00).

As part of the Nurses' Health Study II, the association between chromium in air pollution and the presence of autism spectrum disorder was examined in 325 cases and 22,101 controls (Roberts et al., 2013). Prenatal exposure to chromium was not significantly associated with autism spectrum disorder for either boys or girls or for both sexes combined among children born between 1987 and 2002, regardless of the quintile of exposure.

McDermott et al. (2015) conducted a systematic review of childhood outcomes associated with in utero exposure to chromium and reported on eight studies, two of which were specific to chromium exposure only (Aschengrau et al., 1993; Li et al., 2008). (Note: Aschengrau et al. [1993] was not included in the ATSDR profile, although the study by Li et al. [2008] of neonates in China was.) The authors reported that one study showed weak associations between chromium exposures and musculoskeletal defects, neuroblastoma, DNA damage, and lymphocyte damage but found no associations with birth weight, gestational age, birth length, autism spectrum disorder, birth defects, or adverse pregnancy outcomes.

Because none of the studies were rated highly for execution and reliability, the authors concluded that there was no association between prenatal chromium exposure and adverse health outcomes in children.

When Aschengrau et al. (1993) compared congenital anomalies in children born to pregnant women (n=1,039) exposed to contaminated community drinking water in Massachusetts with those in children born to 1,177 unexposed women in 1977–1980, they found that congenital anomalies were not significantly associated with chromium levels in drinking water (median concentration=0.5 μg/L) (OR=0.8, 95% CI includes 1).

Animal Studies

ATSDR (2012) found that animal data were robust and that they included primate studies as well as multiple studies in rodents, with most of the studies showing adverse effects on sperm morphology and damage to seminiferous tubules and epididymis in male animals, although some results were not supported in a few studies. Species differences between studies, differences in exposure routes—via water versus via food—and differences in maternal toxicity may have contributed to the variation in animal response. Exposed females showed decreased mating and fertility, increased pre- and postimplantation losses, decreased litter size and number of viable fetuses, and increased resorptions. Conflicting results included reduced implantations and numbers of viable fetuses associated with male chromium exposure (ATSDR, 2012).

The ability of Cr6 to cause testicular damage, including its effects on sperm, by oxidative stress has been demonstrated in several animal studies (Hfaiedh et al., 2014; Marouani et al., 2017) and in vitro studies (Das et al., 2015). An additional in vitro study showed that exposing sperm to Cr6 can lead to detrimental developmental effects on subsequent embryos and blastocysts (Yoisungnern et al., 2016). Testicular toxicity has been observed in the form of histopathological lesions and abnormalities in sperm (Marouani et al., 2012).

Studies of in utero exposures in animals have shown a variety of signs of maternal, embryo, and fetal toxicity. Maternal dosing on GD 6–15 had significant effects on the numbers of viable offspring and was associated with morphological abnormalities (Marouani et al., 2011). Female rats exposed in utero showed age-dependent increases in body and ovary weight, delayed estrous cycle, reduced antioxidant enzyme activity, increased levels of lipid peroxidation and hydrogen peroxide concentration in ovaries, and histopathological changes of the ovaries (Samuel et al., 2014). This reproductive and developmental toxicity in female animals was caused by oxidative stress (Stanley et al., 2014).

Some research has suggested that Cr6 exerts epigenetic effects (Schnekenburger et al., 2007): for example, through Cr6 inhibition of benzo[α]pyrene (BaP)-induced gene methylation. Using an in vitro cell model system, Schnekenburger et al. (2007) showed that the transcriptional repression of Cyp1a1 in response to the procarcinogen BaP is influenced by chromium and that this effect is mediated through an epigenetic mechanism. A chromium–HDAC1–DNMT1–chromatin complex is formed that blocks Cyp1a1 histone promoter acetylation and also the recruitment of RNA polymerase II and inhibits aryl hydrocarbon receptor transactivation of Cyp1a1. Blocking this detoxification pathway increases DNA adduct formation. Schnekenburger et al. (2007) proposed that the repercussions would reflect the timing of the developmental exposure and could include a change in imprinting.

Synthesis and Conclusions

Cr6 has been identified as a reproductive and developmental toxicant by ECHA and ATSDR. ATSDR (2012) reported that human studies showed "a significant increase in the number of morphologically abnormal sperm; significant decreases in sperm count and motility; and greater incidences of complications during pregnancy and childbirth (toxicosis and postnatal hemorrhage)," although these effects were not seen as a result of environmental exposures. The findings in some human epidemiology studies that chromium exposure can lead to increased pregnancy loss and sperm abnormalities in men are supported by a robust animal literature. Animal literature also provides robust support for the effects of Cr6 on semen parameters. Animal studies have exhibited long-term effects on female reproductive organs following in utero and continuous exposure.

Although several studies showed no association between Cr6 exposure and adverse pregnancy outcomes, one study of a community with a plant that used Cr6 showed significant effects of prenatal exposure on both birth weight and duration of gestation (Remy et al. 2017). A strength of this study is that the births were assessed while the plant was in operation and for more than 10 years after the plant had closed. Animal studies also found adverse pregnancy outcomes in rat studies.

On the basis of oral exposure animal studies ATSDR (2012) concluded that Cr6 is a developmental toxicant. In rats and mice, gestational exposure resulted in internal and skeletal malformations and delayed sexual maturation in offspring, although only at relatively high doses (e.g., ≥35mg Cr6/kg/day). Among the studies reviewed by the Volume 11 committee, one study evaluated multiple generations exposed to environmental releases of Cr6, but the exposure was continuous so developmental effects could not be distinguished from transgenerational effects (Roberts et al., 2013). One other study found an association between prenatal chromium exposure, as a component of air pollution, and childhood neuroblastoma (Heck et al. 2013); however, other studies found no association between prenatal Cr6 exposure and birth defects.

None of the available data mimic the potential short-term exposures that veterans often experience.

Epigenetic changes documented in exposed workers are also found in in vitro cell culture studies, but the effects of the epigenetic changes on health are unknown at this time. Cr6 is also recognized as a mutagen (ATSDR, 2012). While teratogenic and epigenetic effects are supported by the data, transgenerational effects have not been clearly established.

The Volume 11 committee concludes that there is sufficient evidence of an association between exposure to Cr6 and reproductive effects in men.

The Volume 11 committee also concludes that there is inadequate/insufficient evidence of an association between exposure to Cr6 and reproductive effects in women.

The Volume 11 committee also concludes that there is limited/suggestive evidence of an association between exposure to Cr6 and adverse pregnancy outcomes.

The Volume 11 committee also concludes that there is sufficient evidence of an association between prenatal exposure to Cr6 and developmental effects.

TABLE 4-5 Summary of Reproductive and Developmental Effects of Hexavalent Chromium

Study	Population	Exposure	Results
Reproductive Effects			
Reproductive Effects in Men			
Ali et al. (2011)	Case series of 36 lung tumor samples in chromate workers, 25 tumor samples from unexposed controls. 1975–1997.	Cr6	DNA methylation of *APC*, *hMLH1*, and *MGMT* genes. Increased methylation associated with time worked (p=0.014). Methylation significantly higher in chromate lung cancers versus non-chromate lung cancers (p=0.0001). This study provided no ORs for results.
Bollati et al. (2010)	Cohort of 63 workers at an electric-furnace steel plant.	Cr6	miRNA in peripheral blood leukocytes miR-21 and miR-146a not related to Cr6 exposure; miR-222 expression associated with Cr6 (β=0.26, 95% CI 0.0–0.58, p=0.05).
Reproductive Effects in Women			
Remy et al. (2017)	Cross-sectional, ecological. Residents near a factory 1983–2014, Willits, CA.	Residence near factory where Cr6 emissions were high in 1963–1995; rest of Mendocino County served as controls.	Based on hospital discharge data, compared to the rest of the county reproductive organ conditions and neoplasms or pregnancy loss, children of residents had higher rates of respiratory conditions (RR=0.99); perinatal jaundice (RR=1.13); birth defects; low birth weight (RR=1.14); and preterm birth (RR=1.14).
Yang et al. (2013)	18 studies of occupational Cr6 poisoning in 14 Chinese cities. 1980–2012. 6,998 workers in China with occupational Cr6 exposures and disease.	Occupational poisoning with Cr6.	Female workers had increased risks of spontaneous abortion (OR=2.31, 95% CI 1.25–4.27) or threatened abortion (OR=20.47, 95% CI 2.60–161.44). Of this group of workers who were pregnant, both spontaneous abortion and threatened abortion were elevated. Minimal ability to ascertain actual Cr6 exposure levels in the plants.
Adverse Pregnancy Outcomes			
Manduca et al. (2014)	Cohort study of babies of parents exposed to weapons in Gaza (48 birth defects, 77 preterm births, 12 healthy babies) in 2011.	Metals in newborn hair samples.	Chromium load in newborn hair not related to birth defects or preterm birth. This study did not provide ORs for results.

continued

TABLE 4-5 Continued

Study	Population	Exposure	Results
Guo et al. (2010)	220 births in Guiyu, China (e-waste recycling region), 119 births from a control area 2008–2009.	Placental concentrations of heavy metals.	Birth length (r=0.002, p=0.977), birth weight (r= –0.029, p=0.675), and gestational age (r=0.002, p=0.971) not related to placental chromium.
Li et al. (2008)	200 newborns from Guiyu, an e-waste recycling region, and 102 newborns from Chaonan, 2006–2007.	Cord blood concentrations of chromium.	DNA damage of lymphocytes in cord blood correlated with cord blood chromium (cell populations of comet r=0.95, p=0.01; cell lengths of tail r=0.89, p=0.00). This study did not provide ORs for results.
Ni et al. (2014)	201 pregnant women living in e-waste recycling region, Guiyu town, China; and 75 living in Shantou city, 2012–2013.	Cord blood concentrations of heavy metals.	Oxidative damage in neonates measured by 8-OHdG associated with Cr (β=0.086 ng/mL, 95% CI 0.014–0.158 ng/mL).
Developmental Effects			
Heck et al. (2013)	Case-control study of 75 cases of neuroblastoma and 14,602 controls from California Cancer Registry, 1990–2007.	Distance of mother's residence to an air monitor (5 km).	Neuroblastoma associated with Cr6 in air pollution, OR=1.32, 95% CI 1.0–1.74.
Roberts et al. (2013)	Nested case-control 325 cases of autism spectrum disorder, 22,101 controls. 1987–2002.	Modeled air pollutants at time and place of birth.	ORs were significant for all metals except for chromium (form unspecified) and arsenic. Autism spectrum disorder not associated with chromium exposure for both sexes in the highest and lowest quintiles. Highest quintile: OR=1.4; 95% CI 0.9–2.0 Lowest quintile: OR=1.0; no CI provided

NOTE: APC=adenomatous polyposis coli; CI=confidence interval; Cr6=hexavalent chromium; DNA=deoxyribonucleic acid; hMLH1=human mutL homolog 1; MGMT=O_6-methylguanine-DNA methyltransferase; miRNA=micro RNA; OR=odds ratio; r=Spearman correlation coefficient; RR=relative risk.

REFERENCES

Abolghasemi, H., M.H. Radfar, M. Rambod, P. Salehi, H. Ghofrani, M.R. Soroush, F. Falahaty, Y. Tavakolifar, A. Sadaghianifar, S.M. Khademolhosseini, Z. Kavehmanesh, M. Joffres, F.M. Burkle, and E.J. Mills. 2010. Childhood physical abnormalities following paternal exposure to sulfur mustard gas in Iran: A case-control study. *Conflict and Health* 4:13–13.

Abou-Donia, M.B., H.B. Suliman, W.A. Khan, and A.A. Abdel-Rahman. 2003. Testicular germ-cell apoptosis in stressed rats following combined exposure to pyridostigmine bromide, n,n-diethyl m-toluamide (DEET), and permethrin. *Journal of Toxicology and Environmental Health Part A* 66(1):57–73.

Adam, G.K., S.M. Omar, M.A. Ahmed, T.M. Abdallah, and A.A. Ali. 2018. Cross-sectional study of the case-fatality rate among patients with visceral leishmaniasis infections during pregnancy in Sudan. *International Journal of Gynecology and Obstetrics* 140(1):119–120.

Alaani, S., M. Tafash, C. Busby, M. Hamdan, and E. Blaurock-Busch. 2011. Uranium and other contaminants in hair from the parents of children with congenital anomalies in Fallujah, Iraq. *Conflict and Health* 5(1):15.

Ali, A.H., K. Kondo, T. Namura, Y. Senba, H. Takizawa, Y. Nakagawa, H. Toba, K. Kenzaki, S. Sakiyama, and A. Tangoku. 2011. Aberrant DNA methylation of some tumor suppressor genes in lung cancers from workers with chromate exposure. *Molecular Carcinogenesis* 50(2):89–99.

Amirzargar, M.A., M. Yavangi, M. Rahnavardi, M. Jafari, and M. Mohseni. 2009. Chronic mustard toxicity on the testis: A historical cohort study two decades after exposure [erratum appears in *International Journal of Andrology* 2012; 35(4):629]. *International Journal of Andrology* 32(4):411–416.

Arfsten, D.P., K.R. Still, E.R. Wilfong, E.W. Johnson, S.M. McInturf, J.S. Eggers, D.J. Schaeffer, and M.Y. Bekkedal. 2009. Two-generation reproductive toxicity study of implanted depleted uranium (DU) in CD rats. *Journal of Toxicology and Environmental Health Part A* 72(6):410–427.

Arnetz, B., A. Drutchas, R. Sokol, M. Kruger, and H. Jamil. 2013. 1991 Gulf War exposures and adverse birth outcomes. *US Army Medical Department Journal* Apr–Jun:58–65.

Aschengrau, A., S. Zierler, and U. Cohen. 1993. Quality of community drinking water and the occurrence of late adverse pregnancy outcomes. *Archives of Environmental Health* 48(2):105–113.

Asghari, M.H., S. Saeidnia, M.A. Rezvanfar, and M. Abdollahi. 2015. A systematic review of the molecular mechanisms of uranium-induced reproductive toxicity. *Inflammation & Allergy—Drug Targets* 14(2):67–76.

ATSDR (Agency for Toxic Substances and Disease Registry). 2003. *Toxicological profile for sulfur mustard (update).* Washington, DC: U.S. Department of Health and Human Services.

ATSDR. 2012. *Toxicological profile for chromium.* Washington, DC: U.S. Department of Health and Human Services.

ATSDR. 2013. *Toxicological profile for uranium.* Washington, DC: U.S. Department of Health and Human Services.

Avila-Garcia, M., J. Mancilla-Ramirez, E. Segura-Cervantes, B. Farfan-Labonne, A. Ramirez-Ramirez, and N. Galindo-Sevilla. 2013. Transplacental transmission of cutaneous leishmania mexicana strain in BALB/c mice. *American Journal of Tropical Medicine and Hygiene* 89(2):354–358.

Berger, A.B., A.H. Bartlett, N.G. Saravia, and N.G. Sevilla. 2017. Pathophysiology of leishmania infection during pregnancy. *Trends in Parasitology* 33(12):935–946.

Berrios, V. O., N.M. Boukli, J.W. Rodriguez, P.D. Negraes, T.T. Schwindt, C.A. Trujillo, S.L.B. Oliveira, L.A. Cubano, P.A. Ferchmin, V.A. Eterovic, H. Ulrich, and A.H. Martins. 2015. Paraoxon and pyridostigmine interfere with neural stem cell differentiation. *Neurochemical Research* 40(10):2091–2101.

Bollati, V., B. Marinelli, P. Apostoli, M. Bonzini, F. Nordio, M. Hoxha, V. Pegoraro, V. Motta, L. Tarantini, L. Cantone, J. Schwartz, P.A. Bertazzi, and A. Baccarelli. 2010. Exposure to metal-rich particulate matter modifies the expression of candidate microRNAs in peripheral blood leukocytes. *Environmental Health Perspectives* 118(6):763–768.

Buller, J., T.S. Albright, A.P. Gehrich, J. Wright, Jr., C.F. Lettieri, and S.G. Dunlow. 2007. Pregnancy during Operation Iraqi Freedom/Operation Enduring Freedom. *Military Medicine* 172(5):511–514.

Catherino, W.H., A. Levi, T.C. Kao, M.P. Leondires, J. McKeeby, and J.H. Segars. 2005. Anthrax vaccine does not affect semen parameters, embryo quality, or pregnancy outcome in couples with a vaccinated male military service member. *Fertility and Sterility* 83(2):480–483.

CIA–DoD (Central Intelligence Agency and Department of Defense). 1997. *Modeling the chemical warfare agent release at the Khamisiyah pit.* Washington, DC: CIA–DoD.

Ciminera, P., M.J. Superior, and T. Bullman. 2016. Findings from the Department of Veterans Affairs Qarmat Ali Medical Surveillance Program. *Military Medicine* 181:307–310.

Conlin, A.M., C. DeScisciolo, C.J. Sevick, A.T. Bukowinski, C.J. Phillpis, and T.C. Smith. 2012. Birth outcomes among military personnel after exposure to documented open air burn pits before and during pregnancy. *Journal of Occupational and Environmental Medicine* 54(6):689–697.

Conlin, A. M. S., A.T. Bukowinski, and G.R. Gumbs. 2015. Analysis of pregnancy and infant health outcomes among women in the National Smallpox Vaccine in Pregnancy Registry who received anthrax vaccine adsorbed. *Vaccine* 33(36):4387–4390.

Conlin, A.M.S., C.J. Sevick, G.R. Gumbs, Z.G. Khodr, and A.T. Bukowinski. 2017. Safety of inadvertent anthrax vaccination during pregnancy: An analysis of birth defects in the U.S. military population, 2003–2010. *Vaccine* 35(34):4414–4420.

Darolles, C., D. Broggio, A. Feugier, S. Frelon, I. Dublineau, M. De Meo, and F. Petitot. 2010. Different genotoxic profiles between depleted and enriched uranium. *Toxicology Letters* 192(3):337–348.

Das, J., M.H. Kang, E. Kim, D. N. Kwon, Y.J. Choi, and J.H. Kim. 2015. Hexavalent chromium induces apoptosis in male somatic and spermatogonial stem cells via redox imbalance. *Scientific Reports* 5:13921.

DoD (Department of Defense). 2011. *Exposure to sodium dichromate at Qarmat Ali, Iraq in 2003*. Arlington, Virginia: Department of Defense.

Dursa, E.K., S.K. Barth, A.I. Schneiderman, and R.M. Bossarte. 2016. Physical and mental health status of Gulf War and Gulf Era veterans: Results from a large population-based epidemiological study. *Journal of Occupational and Environmental Medicine* 58(1):41–46.

ECHA (European Chemicals Agency). 2017. *Sodium dichromate—Substance information*. https://echa.europa.eu/substance-information/-/substanceinfo/100.031.070 (accessed August 9, 2018).

Feugier, A., S. Frelon, P. Gourmelon, and M. Claraz. 2008. Alteration of mouse oocyte quality after a subchronic exposure to depleted uranium. *Reproductive Toxicology* 26(3–4):273–277.

Figueiro-Filho, E.A., G. Duarte, P. El-Beitune, S.M. Quintana, and T.L. Maia. 2004. Visceral leishmaniasis (kala-azar) and pregnancy. *Infectious Diseases in Obstetrics and Gynecology* 12(1):31–40.

Figueiro-Filho, E.A., P. El Beitune, G. T. Queiroz, R.S. Somensi, N.O. Morais, M.E.C. Dorval, S.M. Quintana, and G. Duarte. 2008. Visceral leishmaniasis and pregnancy: Analysis of cases reported in a central-western region of Brazil. *Archives of Gynecology and Obstetrics* 278(1):13–16.

Franco, C., E. Lewis, S. Morseth, L. Simon, and A.T. Waytes. 2009. Reproductive toxicity of biothrax in rabbits. *Birth Defects Research. Part B, Developmental and Reproductive Toxicology* 86(5):370–376.

Ghanei, M., M. Rajaee, S. Khateri, F. Alaeddini, and D. Haines. 2004. Assessment of fertility among mustard-exposed residents of Sardasht, Iran: A historical cohort study. *Reproductive Toxicology* 18(5):635–639.

Guo, Y., X. Huo, Y. Li, K. Wu, J. Liu, J. Huang, G. Zheng, Q. Xiao, H. Yang, Y. Wang, A. Chen, and X. Xu. 2010. Monitoring of lead, cadmium, chromium and nickel in placenta from an e-waste recycling town in China. *Science of the Total Environment* 408(16):3113–3117.

Hao, Y., R. Li, Y. Leng, J. Ren, J. Liu, G. Ai, H. Xu, Y. Su, and T. Cheng. 2009. A study assessing the genotoxicity in rats after chronic oral exposure to a low dose of depleted uranium. *Journal of Radiation Research* 50(6):521–528.

Hao, Y., R. Li, Y. Leng, J. Ren, J. Liu, G.A, H. Xu, Y. Su, and T. Cheng. 2012. The reproductive effects in rats after chronic oral exposure to low-dose depleted uranium. *Journal of Radiation Research* 53(3):377–384.

He, D., D. Zhang, G. Wei, T. Lin, and X. Li. 2007. Cytoskeleton vimentin disruption of mouse sertoli cells injured by nitrogen mustard in vitro. *Journal of Andrology* 28(3):389–396.

Heck, J. E., A. S. Park, J. Qiu, M. Cockburn, and B. Ritz. 2013. An exploratory study of ambient air toxics exposure in pregnancy and the risk of neuroblastoma in offspring. *Environmental Research* 127:1–6.

Hfaiedh, M., D. Brahmi, and L. Zourgui. 2014. Protective role of cactus cladodes extract on sodium dichromate-induced testicular injury and oxidative stress in rats. *Biological Trace Element Research* 159(1–3):304–311.

Hourani, L., and S. Hilton. 2000. Occupational and environmental exposure correlates of adverse live-birth outcomes among 1032 U.S. Navy women. *Journal of Occupational Environmental Medicine* 42(12):1156–1165.

IARC (International Agency for Research on Cancer). 2012. *Chromium (vi) compounds*. https://monographs.iarc.fr/wp-content/uploads/2018/06/mono100C-9.pdf (accessed July 9, 2018).

Ibrahim, A., R. Awad, S. Shetty, M. Saad, and N.E. Bilal. 1988. Genito-urinary complications of brucellosis. *British Journal of Urology* 61(4):294–298.

IOM (Institute of Medicine). 2000. *Gulf War and health, volume 1: Depleted uranium, pyrodostigmine bromide, sarin, vaccines*. Washington, DC: National Academy Press.

IOM. 2004. *Gulf War and health: Updated literature review of sarin*. Washington, DC: The National Academies Press.

IOM. 2005. *Gulf War and health, volume 3: Fuels, combustion products, and propellants*. Washington, DC: The National Academies Press.

IOM. 2006a. *Gulf War and health, volume 4: Health effects of serving in the Gulf War*. Washington, DC: The National Academies Press.

IOM. 2006b. *Posttraumatic stress disorder: Diagnosis and assessment*. Washington, DC: The National Academies Press.

IOM. 2007. *Gulf War and health, volume 5: Infectious diseases*. Washington, DC: The National Academies Press.

IOM. 2008a. *Epidemiologic studies of veterans exposed to depleted uranium: Feasibility and design issues.* Washington, DC: The National Academies Press.

IOM. 2008b. *Gulf War and health, volume 6: Physiologic, psychologic, and psychosocial effects of deployment-related stress.* Washington, DC: The National Academies Press.

IOM. 2010. *Gulf War and health, volume 8: Update of health effects of serving in the Gulf War.* Washington, DC: The National Academies Press.

Ippolito, A.C., A.D. Seelig, T.M. Powell, A.M.S. Conlin, N.F. Crum-Cianflone, H. Lemus, C.J. Sevick, and C.A. LeardMann. 2017. Risk factors associated with miscarriage and impaired fecundity among United States servicewomen during the recent conflicts in Iraq and Afghanistan. *Women's Health Issues* 27(3):356–365.

Katon, J., Y. Cypel, M. Raza, L. Zephyrin, G. Reiber, E.M. Yano, S. Barth, and A. Schneiderman. 2014a. Self-reported infertility among male and female veterans serving during Operation Enduring Freedom/Operation Iraqi Freedom. *Journal of Women's Health* 23(2):175–183.

Katon, J., K. Mattocks, M. Raza, E.M. Yano, L. Callegari., E.B. Schwarz, J. Goulet, J Shaw, C. Brandt, and S. Haskell. 2014b. Gestational diabetes and hypertensive disorders of pregnancy among women veterans deployed in service of operations in Afghanistan and Iraq. *Journal of Women's Health* 23(10):792–800.

Katon, J., Y. Cypel, M. Raza, L. Zephyrin, G. Reiber, E.M. Yano, S. Barth, and A. Schneiderman. 2017. Deployment and adverse pregnancy outcomes: Primary findings and methodological considerations. *Maternal & Child Health Journal* 21:376–386.

Lawrence-Wood, E., S. Kumar, S. Crompvoets, B.G. Fosh, H. Rahmanian, L. Jones, and S. Newhaus. 2016. A systematic review of the impacts of active military service on sexual and reproductive health outcomes among servicewomen and female veterans of armed forces. *Journal of Military and Veterans' Health* 24(3):34–55.

Legrand, M., C. Elie, J. Stefani, N. Flores, C. Culeux, O. Delissen, C. Ibanez, P. Lestaevel, P. Eriksson, and C. Dinocourt. 2016. Cell proliferation and cell death are disturbed during prenatal and postnatal brain development after uranium exposure. *NeuroToxicology* 52:34–45.

Li, Y., X. Xu, J. Liu, K. Wu, C. Gu, G. Shao, S. Chen, G. Chen, and X. Huo. 2008. The hazard of chromium exposure to neonates in Guiyu of China. *Science of the Total Environment* 403(1–3):99–104.

Manduca, P., A. Naim, and S. Signoriello. 2014. Specific association of teratogen and toxicant metals in hair of newborns with congenital birth defects or developmentally premature birth in a cohort of couples with documented parental exposure to military attacks: Observational study at Al Shifa Hospital, Gaza, Palestine. *International Journal of Environmental Research and Public Health* 11(5):5208–5223.

Marouani, N., O. Tebourbi, M. Mokni, M. T. Yacoubi, M. Sakly, M. Benkhalifa, and K.B. Rhouma. 2011. Embryotoxicity and fetotoxicity following intraperitoneal administrations of hexavalent chromium to pregnant rats. *Zygote* 19(3):229–235.

Marouani, N., O. Tebourbi, S. Mahjoub, M.T. Yacoubi, M. Sakly, M. Benkhalifa, and K.B. Rhouma. 2012. Effects of hexavalent chromium on reproductive functions of male adult rats. *Reproductive Biology* 12(2):119–133.

Marouani, N., O. Tebourbi, D. Hallegue, M. Mokni, M.T. Yacoubi, M. Sakly, M. Benkhalifa, and K.B. Rhouma. 2017. Mechanisms of chromium hexavalent-induced apoptosis in rat testes. *Toxicology and Industrial Health* 33(2):97–106.

McDermott, S., D.C. Salzberg, A.P. Anderson, T. Shaw, and J. Lead. 2015. Systematic review of chromium and nickel exposure during pregnancy and impact on child outcomes. *Journal of Toxicology and Environmental Health Part A* 78(21–22):1348–1368.

McDiarmid, M.A., S.M. Engelhardt, C.D. Dorsey, M. Oliver, P. Gucer, P.D. Wilson, R. Kane, A. Cernich, B. Kaup, L. Anderson, D. Hoover, L. Brown, R. Albertini, R. Gudi, and K.S. Squibb. 2009. Surveillance results of depleted uranium-exposed Gulf War I Veterans: Sixteen years of follow-up. *Journal of Toxicology and Environmental Health Part A* 72(1):14–29.

Memish, Z., and S. Venkatesh. 2001. Brucellar epididymo-orchitis in Saudi Arabia: A retrospective study of 26 cases and review of the literature. *Bob Jones University International* 88(1):72–76.

Miller, A.C., M. Stewart, and R. Rivas. 2010. Preconceptional paternal exposure to depleted uranium: Transmission of genetic damage to offspring. *Health Physics* 99(3):371–379.

Moro, P.L., J. Cragan, P. Lewis, and L. Sukumaran. 2017. Major birth defects after vaccination reported to the Vaccine Adverse Event Reporting System (VAERS), 1990 to 2014. *Birth Defects Research* 109(13):1057–1062.

NASEM (National Academies of Sciences, Engineering, and Medicine). 2016. *Gulf War and Health, volume 10: Update of health effects of serving in the Gulf War, 2016.* Washington, DC: The National Academies Press.

Navarro-Martinez, A., J. Solera, J. Corredoira, J. Beato, E. Martinez-Alfaro, M. Atienzar, and J. Ariza. 2001. Epididymoorchitis due to brucella mellitensis: A retrospective study of 59 patients. *Clinical Infectious Diseases* 33(12):2017–2022.

Ni, W., Y. Huang, X. Wang, J. Zhang, and K. Wu. 2014. Associations of neonatal lead, cadmium, chromium and nickel co-exposure with DNA oxidative damage in an electronic waste recycling town. *Science of the Total Environment* 472:354–362.

NRC (National Research Council). 2008. *Review of toxicologic and radiologic risks to military personnel from exposure to depleted uranium during and after combat.* Washington, DC: The National Academies Press.

OSAGWI (Office of the Special Assistant for Gulf War Illnesses). 1998. *Depleted uranium in the Gulf.* Washington, DC: U.S. Department of Defense.

OSAGWI. 1999. *Military medical recordkeeping during and after the Gulf War: Interim report.* Washington, DC: U.S. Department of Defense.

PAC (Presidential Advisory Committee on Gulf War Veterans' Illnesses). 1996. *Presidential Advisory Committee on Gulf War Veterans' Illnesses: Final Report.* Washington, DC: U.S. Government Printing Office.

Papatsoris, A., F. Mpadra, M. Karamouzis, and C. Frangides. 2002. Endemic brucellar epididymo-orchitis: A 10-year experience. *International Journal of Infectious Diseases* 6(4):309–313.

Phippen, J.W. 2016. *A mustard gas attack on U.S. troops.* https://www.theatlantic.com/news/archive/2016/09/mustard-gas-us-troops-iraq/501347/ (accessed October 23, 2017).

Remy, L.L., V. Byers, and T. Clay. 2017. Reproductive outcomes after non-occupational exposure to hexavalent chromium, Willits, California, 1983–2014. *Environmental Health* 16(1):18.

Roberts, A.L., K. Lyall, J.E. Hart, F. Laden, A.C. Just, J.F. Bobb, K. C. Koenen, A. Ascherio, and M.G. Weisskopf. 2013. Perinatal air pollutant exposures and autism spectrum disorder in the children of Nurses' Health Study II participants. *Environmental Health Perspectives* 121(8):978–984.

Ryan, M.A.K., T.C. Smith, C.J. Sevick, W.K. Honner, R.A. Loach, C.A. Moore, and J.D. Erickson. 2008. Birth defects among infants born to women who received anthrax vaccine in pregnancy. *American Journal of Epidemiology* 168(4):434–442.

Ryan, M.A.K., I.G. Jacobson, C.J. Sevick, T.C. Smith, G.R. Gumbs, and A.M.S. Conlin for the U.S. Department of Defense Birth and Infant Health Registry. 2011. Health outcomes among infants born to women deployed to United States military operations during pregnancy. *Birth Defects Research (Part A)* 91(2):117–124.

Safarinejad, M.R. 2001. Testicular effect of mustard gas. *Urology* 58(1):90–94.

Safarinejad, M.R. 2010. Sperm chromatin structure assay analysis of Iranian mustard gas casualties: A long-term outlook. *Current Urology* 4(2):71–80.

Samuel, J.B., J.A. Stanley, P. Sekar, R.A. Princess, M.S. Sebastian, and M.M. Aruldhas. 2014. Persistent hexavalent chromium exposure impaired the pubertal development and ovarian histoarchitecture in Wistar rat offspring. *Environmental Toxicology* 29(7):814–828.

Schnekenburger, M., G. Talaska, and A. Puga. 2007. Chromium cross-links histone deacetylase 1-DNA methyltransferase 1 complexes to chromatin, inhibiting histone-remodeling marks critical for transcriptional activation. *Molecular Cell Biology* 27(20):7089–7101.

Shaw, J.G., D.A. Nelson, K.A. Shaw, K. Woolaway-Bickel, C.S. Phibbs, and L.M. Kurina. 2018. Deployment and preterm birth among United States Army soldiers. *American Journal of Epidemiology* 187(4):687–695.

Sever, J.L., A.I. Brenner, A.D. Gale, J.M. Lyle, L.H. Moulton, B.J. Ward, and D.J. West. 2004. Safety of anthrax vaccine: An expanded review and evaluation of adverse events reported to the Vaccine Adverse Event Reporting System (VAERS). *Pharmacoepidemiology and Drug Safety* 13:825–840.

Stanley, J.A., K.K. Sivakumar, J.A. Arosh, R.C. Burghardt, and S.K. Banu. 2014. Edaravone mitigates hexavalent chromium-induced oxidative stress and depletion of antioxidant enzymes while estrogen restores antioxidant enzymes in the rat ovary in F1 offspring. *Biology of Reproduction* 91(1):12.

Todorov, T.I., J.W. Ejnik, G. Guandalini, H. Xu, D. Hoover, L. Anderson, K. Squibb, M.A. McDiarmid, and J.A. Centeno. 2013. Uranium quantification in semen by inductively coupled plasma mass spectrometry. *Journal of Trace Elements in Medicine and Biology* 27(1):2–6.

WHO (World Health Organization). 2016. *Malaria.* http://www.who.int/malaria/en (accessed April 16, 2018).

Wiesen, A.R., and C.T. Littell. 2002. Relationship between prepregnancy anthrax vaccination and pregnancy and birth outcomes among U.S. Army women. *Journal of the American Medical Association* 287(12):1556–1560.

Winkenwerder, W. 2002. *U.S. demolition operations at Khamisiyah.* Washington, DC: Department of Defense.

Yang, Y., H. Liu, X.H. Xiang, and F.Y. Liu. 2013. Outline of occupational chromium poisoning in China. *Bulletin of Environmental Contamination and Toxicology* 90(6):742–749.

Yoisungnern, T., J. Das, Y.J. Choi, R. Parnpai, and J.H. Kim. 2016. Effect of hexavalent chromium-treated sperm on in vitro fertilization and embryo development. *Toxicology and Industrial Health* 32(9):1700–1710.

5

Pesticides

Pesticides were used in the 1990–1991 Gulf War and Post-9/11 conflicts to combat the endemic insect and rodent populations in Iraq, Afghanistan, and other Persian Gulf areas; one goal was to control insects that were vectors for infectious diseases such as leishmaniasis, malaria, and sand fly fever. More than 35 types of pesticides were used during the Gulf War, while the number of pesticides used in the Post-9/11 conflicts has not been determined by the Volume 11 committee. The U.S. Environmental Protection Agency (EPA) had to approve each insecticide for use in the Gulf War, and the specific types of pesticides and the quantities shipped to military personnel were documented. Military personnel in the Gulf War were exposed to pesticides through both personal and field use. There were specific Department of Defense (DoD) guidelines regarding which pesticides should have been used and for what purposes, but there were reports of both misuse and lack of use. Additionally, reports suggest that pesticide use differed by service, living arrangements, race, rank, and season (Fricker et al., 2000). U.S. Army personnel used pesticides more frequently than members of the other service branches.

DoD indicated that the approximately 700,000 service members deployed to the Persian Gulf had access mainly to two pesticides: permethrin and DEET (IOM, 2003).[1] Service members received spray cans of permethrin to treat their uniforms. It is estimated that 130,894 boxes of 5-oz cans (12/box) and 112,590 boxes of 2-oz tubes (12/box) of permethrin were sent to the Persian Gulf; 44% of service members were estimated to have had some level of exposure. Almost 55,000 boxes of DEET, used as a personal insect repellant, were sent to the Gulf War in the form of a stick or liquid; about 44% of service members were exposed (IOM, 2003). In addition, numerous other pesticides were used. For example, almost 4,000 cases (12 bottles/case) of chlorpyrifos, the most commonly used organophosphate (OP) pesticide, were also shipped to the Persian Gulf region, along with more than 111,000 2-oz cans of

[1] The Volume 2 committee obtained information on the specific pesticides and solvents used during the Gulf War from a variety of sources, including veterans; DoD and, specifically, the Defense Logistics Agency; the Department of Veterans Affairs; the RAND Corporation; the Presidential Advisory Commission (Cecchine et al., 2000; PAC, 1996); and P.L. 105-277 (Gulf War Veterans Act) and P.L. 105-368 (Persian Gulf War Veterans Act) (see Chapter 1). See *Gulf War and Health, Volume 2* (IOM, 2003) for more information on the use of pesticides in the Gulf War.

lindane, an organochlorine pesticide. Furthermore, some service members reportedly used pesticides that were not approved by DoD and were obtained on the local market, such as pet tick-and-flea collars.

Service members deployed to the Post-9/11 conflicts also used pesticides. For example, in Operation Iraqi Freedom in 2003, pesticides were used to repel and control sand flies. U.S. service members serving at Tallil Air Base in Iraq applied DEET to exposed skin, wore permethrin-impregnated uniforms, and slept under permethrin-treated bed nets. In April 2003 a requisition was made for 1,670 boxes of DEET insect repellent (each box contained 12 2-oz tubes), 2,500 boxes of permethrin (each box contained 12 individual dynamic absorption kits for the treatment of uniforms, insect bed nets, or both), and 10,000 insect bed nets. However, service members reported that these pesticides were not very effective against the sand flies. Area spraying of malathion, resmethrin, and pyronyl oil containing 3% permethrin was also conducted in and around the air base for sand fly control. Other pesticides used to treat residential and outdoor areas at the air base included carbaryl, lambda-cyhalothrin, cyfluthrin, bifenthrin, chlorpyrifos, deltamethrin, and cypermethrin (Schleier, 2009). In all, 29,287 oz of pesticides containing 8,258 oz of active ingredient were applied during 2003 at the air base (Coleman et al., 2006). Schleier et al. (2009) reported that these sand fly control efforts were largely unsuccessful. This is just one military installation among many in Iraq and Afghanistan where pesticides were used for insect control.

Although DoD sent rodenticides to the Persian Gulf and to Iraq, the committee did not review the health effects of rodenticide exposure. Inasmuch as those products were sent to the Persian Gulf in pellet form (Cecchine et al., 2000), exposure would have probably required ingestion. The use of rodenticides was also reported by Coleman et al. (2006) at Tallil Air Base in Iraq in 2003. Attempts to eliminate the mouse population on the base were made using Maki rodent pellets (whose active ingredient is 3-[3-(4'-bromo[1,1'- biphenyl]-4-yl)-3-hydroxy-1-phenylpropyl]-4-hydroxy- 2H-1-benzopyran-2-one) (Coleman et al., 2006). Because there were no accounts of military personnel consuming rodenticides or coming in direct contact, neither the Volume 2 committee nor the Volume 11 committee reviewed the adverse health effects of rodenticides. The Volume 11 committee was unable to identify further specific information in the literature on the exposure of Post-9/11 service members to pesticides, although it had no reason to conclude that any reproductive or developmental effects from exposure to the pesticides would be different for Post-9/11 veterans than for Gulf War veterans.

This chapter focuses on the active ingredients of pesticides (the mechanisms of action for these chemicals were discussed in *Gulf War and Health, Volume 2*); however, it is important to remember that the toxicity of a pesticide can be altered by its formulation. Agents contributing to formulation of a pesticide are often listed as "inert ingredients" (for example, petroleum products, xylenes, oils, and surfactants), but they can alter the toxicokinetics of a pesticide, potentially increasing the absorption of active ingredients, or can be toxic themselves (Petrelli et al., 1993; Ware, 1989). Many of these "inert ingredients" are considered elsewhere in this report because they act as solvents or fuels, and they may also be found in combustion products from oil-well fires and burn pits.

There are several overarching concerns when considering the possible reproductive, developmental, and generational health effects that may occur in Gulf War and Post-9/11 veterans and their descendants. First, there were several routes by which service members may have been exposed to pesticides, such as dermal contact, which could have occurred through the use of repellant or the wearing of contaminated clothing; inhalation from breathing polluted air or being downwind of spraying activities; and oral ingestion as a result of hand-to-mouth contact. The route of exposure can have significant implications for the toxicity of the pesticide. For example, the oral LD_{50} of carbofuran is 5 mg/kg in the rat, while the dermal LD_{50} is 120 mg/kg, indicating that oral exposure can be 24 times more toxic than dermal exposure (Roberts and Reigart, 2013). Second, as is evident from the description of the leishmaniasis control program used at Tallil Air Base, service members were often exposed to more than one pesticide at a time or within a short time span. Exposures to mixtures of pesticides and to pesticides mixed with other chemicals are a common occurrence not only for service members but also for individuals who are occupationally exposed to toxicants, and even the general public. Nevertheless, many studies assessing adverse effects resulting from possible exposures to pesticides have focused on the effects of a single pesticide or group of pesticides (e.g., OPs), rather than on mixtures of pesticides or the combined exposure with other chemicals.

Most of the information on the exposure of service members to pesticides is based on information for the 1990–1991 Gulf War and described in detail in *Volume 2*. That committee concluded that there was inadequate/insufficient evidence to determine whether an association exists between exposure to pesticides and "male or female infertility after cessation of exposure," "parental preconception exposure to pesticides and spontaneous abortion or other adverse pregnancy outcomes," and "parental preconception exposure to pesticides and congenital malformations" (IOM, 2003). These conclusions were applicable to all the Gulf War pesticides considered in *Volume 2* and were the only reproductive or developmental endpoints identified.

The Volume 11 committee notes that pesticides, unlike many other commonly used chemicals, must be registered for use by EPA, and those registrations are periodically renewed. Some of the pesticides sent to the 1990–1991 Gulf War were no longer registered for use by the time that the Post-9/11 conflicts began or else have had their registrations terminated since 2001.

In the sections below, the committee considers the reproductive and developmental effects that may result from exposure to the following pesticides: OPs, carbamates, pyrethroids, lindane, and DEET (N,N-diethyl m-toluamide).

ORGANOPHOSPHATES

The class of OP pesticides is large and includes a number of pesticides that are in wide use, primarily in agriculture. P.L. 105-277, the Persian Gulf War Veterans Act, lists four specific OP pesticides—chlorpyrifos, diazinon, dichlorvos, and malathion—that were used in the 1990–1991 Gulf War. Since that war, three of the OP pesticides—chlorpyrifos, diazinon, and dichlorvos—have had their use as residential pesticides restricted and therefore are unlikely to have been sent to the Post-9/11 conflicts. Beginning in 2000, most registered household use of diazinon and chlorpyrifos was to be phased out and eventually cancelled; most household use of dichlorvos was cancelled in 1995 (ATSDR, 1997b). Malathion continues to be used in public health pest control programs for controlling mosquito-borne illnesses. It is available to the general public for residential use, and it was sprayed on military installations in Iraq (Schleier, 2009). As all four OPs were used in the Gulf War and malathion was used in Post-9/11 conflicts, the Volume 11 committee considered the possible reproductive and developmental effects for all four OPs.

OPs are alkylating agents that can lead to deoxyribonucleic acid (DNA) damage (Ojha and Gupta, 2015). These agents were developed for their ability to inhibit the enzyme acetylcholinesterase (AChE). AChE is responsible for the breakdown of the neurotransmitter acetylcholine. When acetylcholine does not break down in the presence of OPs, the neuromuscular synapses become overstimulated, which can lead to nervousness, delirium, hallucinations, and psychoses (Ecobichon, 2001).

Exposure to OP pesticides may be assessed by AChE activity in erythrocytes as a proxy to indicate the enzyme status in the nervous system. Exposure to OPs may also be determined by detecting OP metabolites in urine or blood (IOM, 2003). OP metabolites, usually dialkylphosphates (DAPs), may be measured as individual metabolites or as a sum of several DAPs (ΣDAPs). Among the commonly measured urinary DAPs of OPs are dimethylphosphate (DMP), dimethylthiophosphate (DMTP), dimethyldithiophosphate (DMDTP), diethylphosphate (DEP), diethylthiophosphate (DETP), and diethyldithiophosphate (DEDTP). Most of the OPs considered in this report may be metabolized to one or more DAPs, so the detection of a specific DAP does not necessarily indicate which OP an individual may have been exposed to. However, some other metabolites are specific for a given OP; for example, the detection of 3,5,6-trichloro-2-pyridinol (TCPy) in the urine is indicative of an exposure to chlorpyrifos (Bicker et al., 2005). These pesticides have a short half-life on the order of hours or days, and therefore a single measure may not adequately reflect exposure over a critical window of development. In addition, the nonspecific metabolites may reflect exposure to the metabolites themselves, not just the parent compound (Bradman et al., 2015; Eskenazi et al. 2014; Quirós-Alcalá et al., 2012), and excretion may differ from individual to individual according to their metabolism (Wessels et al., 2003).

Reproductive Effects

In 1997, ATSDR published toxicological profiles of chlorpyrifos and dichlorvos. The profile for chlorpyrifos contained no information on reproductive effects in humans by any route of exposure. Similarly, the profile for dichlorvos also had no information on reproductive effects in humans by any exposure route. The 2003 ATSDR *Toxicological Profile for Malathion* included one study in which women had been exposed to malathion as a result of spraying for insect control in an urban area. There was a "moderate association" of malathion exposure with stillbirths, but not with spontaneous abortions. In a study that compared birth outcomes in 1,016 couples in which the men applied malathion as well as other pesticides with 1,020 couples in which the men were not exposed to pesticides, the exposed couples had more stillbirths (8.73% versus 2.65%) and more abortions (26.0% versus 15.0%) than the unexposed couples. The study also found a significantly lower percentage of fertile males (80.8% in the exposed males versus 94.9% in controls) and a decreased percentage of live births (53.0% versus 80.1%) (ATSDR, 2003a; Rupa et al., 1991). Finally, the 2008 ATSDR *Toxicological Profile for Diazinon* contained no studies of the effects of diazinon exposure on human reproduction.

Gulf War and Health, Volume 2 (IOM, 2003) reported on one study of time to pregnancy (TTP) in Ontario farm couples exposed to OPs (Curtis et al., 1999). Neither men nor women had a significantly altered time to pregnancy with OP exposure. *Volume 2* reported no other reproductive effects in human or animals that may have occurred from exposure to the four OPs listed in the Persian Gulf War Veterans Act.

Reproductive Effects in Men and Women

The Volume 11 committee identified several new studies on reproductive effects and exposure to the OPs of interest. The new studies assessing OP exposure and reproductive effects in men and women are listed in Table 5-2. The effects of OPs on male fertility have been studied by several researchers, including a recent systematic review by Martenies and Perry (2013). In general, human studies have focused on sperm quality associated with either environmental or occupational exposures.

Meeker et al. (2004a) assessed TCPy, a urinary marker of chlorpyrifos exposure, in 272 men who were not occupationally exposed to pesticides and who were attending an infertility clinic in Massachusetts. They reported that increasing urinary TCPy levels were associated, although not significantly, with increased risk of having sperm concentrations below 20 million/mL, less than 50% motile sperm, and less than 4% of sperm with normal morphology. Meeker et al. (2004b) further studied sperm DNA integrity, which they assessed by neutral comet assay and reported as comet extent, percentage DNA in comet tail (Tail%), and tail distributed moment (TDM). Statistically significant increases in Tail% for an interquartile range (IQR) increase in TCPy (β=2.8, 95% confidence interval [CI] 0.9–4.6) were reported, while a decrease in TDM was associated with IQR changes in TCPy (β= –2.5, 95% CI –4.7– –0.2).

Using the same population as Meeker et al. (2004b), Figueroa et al. (2015) examined whether exposure to OPs was associated with sperm chromosomal abnormalities—specifically XX18, YY18, XY18, and total disomy in sperm nuclei. Increasing levels of urinary metabolites, both individual and total sum of DAPs, were significantly associated with increased levels of disomy, particularly XX18 and XY18, although the increases were not monotonic. The highest significant association was observed between the third exposure quartile of DMTP (2.21–6.47 ng/mL) and XX18, with a 52% increase in the incidence rate ratio (95% CI 1.36–1.69).

Sperm integrity, specifically the sperm chromatin structure, was also evaluated in 33 men occupationally exposed to OPs in Mexico (Sánchez-Peña et al., 2004). About 75% of the men had semen with altered sperm chromatin structure (>30% of DNA fragmentation index [DFI]) that would classify them as having poor fertility potential, compared with only 4% of the unexposed men. Only the DAP concentrations for DETP were significantly associated with mean DFI (p=0.026) and standard deviation-DFI (p=0.022) and marginally associated with DFI% (p=0.079) after adjustment for potential confounders, such as the presence of immature germ cells (IGCs). No other DAPs had any associations with measured outcomes. No significant associations were found between semen quality parameters, including IGCs, and DETP or any other DAP, although IGC values were above the reference value for 82% of the samples versus only 9% of unexposed men. There was a negative correlation between mean DFI and sperm viability (r=0.254; p<0.027) and also seminal volume (r=0.333; p<0.004).

A further assessment of the effect of exposure to environmental OPs on sperm parameters and male reproductive hormones was conducted by Melgarejo et al. (2015). This was a study of 116 men attending an infertility clinic in southern Spain, all of whom had detectable concentrations of at least one urinary OP metabolite (the possible sources of exposure were not discussed). The serum levels of reproductive hormones were within the normal range, and only DEDTP showed a positive association with luteinizing hormone (LH) levels (β=11.4, 95% CI 0.81–22.1) and follicle-stimulating hormone (FSH) levels (β=3.2, 95% CI 0.08–6.2) and a negative association with the testosterone/LH ratio (β= –9.6, 95% CI –18.7– –0.50). However, the semen quality parameters were inversely correlated with the urinary OP metabolites. The sperm concentration and total sperm count were both significantly inversely associated with urinary concentrations of the DMP, DMDP, and DMDTP as well as ΣDAP. There was a significant inverse association between the percentage of motile sperm and DMTP, DMDTP, and DEP, and the total motile count was significantly inversely associated with urinary DMP and DMDTP concentrations (all significant at the ≤0.05 level). The seminal volume and percentage of sperm with normal morphology were not affected by DAP levels.

Although their study was not specific for any particular OP or carbamate pesticide (the latter are discussed in the next section), Miranda-Contreras et al. (2013) measured erythrocyte AChE and plasma butyrylcholinesterase (BuChE) levels in 64 male agricultural workers in Venezuela with exposure to these and other pesticides and also in 35 unexposed men. A total of 87.5% of the exposed workers showed exposure to OP and carbamate pesticides, and 82.8% had mild inhibition of BuChE activity. The levels of reproductive hormones and sperm quality were assessed in the workers. In the exposed group, there were significant adverse effects observed in semen pH, sperm motility, abnormal sperm, the number of live sperm, and the DNA fragmentation index versus those values in the unexposed group. Reproductive and thyroid hormones (testosterone, prolactin, free T4, and thyroid stimulating hormone) were normal in most of the exposed workers, although 44% had levels of LH and 21% had levels of FSH above reference values.

In a systematic review that assessed exposure to OPs and semen parameters, Martenies and Perry (2013) found that all six studies published between 2007 and 2012 reported significant adverse associations between OP exposure and at least one semen parameter (Hossain et al., 2010; Perez-Herrera et al., 2008; Perry et al., 2007, 2011; Recio-Vega et al., 2008; Yucra et al., 2008). The Volume 11 committee notes that exposures in most of the studies cited in this review were generally to more than one class of pesticide, e.g., OPs and carbamates, and to more than one pesticide within a class.

In a small biomonitoring study in China, Perry et al. (2007) examined sperm concentration in 18 men who did not work directly with pesticides but who had visited an agricultural area. Urine samples were analyzed for 13 parent OPs or their metabolites. Only the crude difference in sperm concentration for low versus high concentrations of DETP in urine was statistically significant (absolute sperm concentration difference= –1.0, 95% CI –1.8– –0.2). In a larger study of 94 exposed men and 95 controls in eastern China, Perry et al. (2011) confirmed that men with lower sperm concentration and motility were more likely to have higher urinary levels of DMP (odds ratio [OR]=1.30, 95% CI 1.02–1.65) than men with higher sperm concentrations; there was no association with five other urinary OP metabolites.

Recio-Vega et al. (2008) found similar effects on sperm quality in a study of 52 male agricultural workers in Mexico who were exposed to a number of pesticides, including diazinon. OP metabolites were found in the urine of 83% of the occupationally exposed participants. Of the seven semen parameters evaluated, only semen volume and total sperm count were significantly lower (p=0.004 and p=0.01, respectively) in the most exposed subjects compared with unexposed controls, and in the highly exposed group there was a negative correlation between semen volume and sperm count; there were no other significant associations. There were seasonal variations in the application of pesticides, with a corresponding variation in the levels of urinary metabolites and semen quality. Yucra et al. (2008) also found that exposure to OPs as reflected in the levels of urinary metabolites, particularly DETP and DEDTP, was associated with semen quality among 31 pesticide workers in Peru who were compared with 31 unexposed workers. Men with the highest levels of these two metabolites had lower volumes of semen and higher seminal pH than men with lower levels of DEDTP and DETP; there were no other significant associations. The reported use of the pesticides paraquat and/or malathion was correlated with semen quality in a group of 62 farmers in Malaysia who were compared with nonexposed controls (Hossain et al., 2010). The risk of having impaired semen parameters (lower semen volume, lower sperm concentration, a smaller percentage of motile sperm, and more abnormal sperm) was significantly increased (ORs 4.5–8.7) in exposed workers; seminal pH was not significantly changed. The committee notes that in the Hossain et al. study, exposure to the pesticides was not confirmed nor were the various pesticides distinguished by metabolite analysis.

Finally, Pérez-Herrera et al. (2008) evaluated the role of the $PON1_{Q192R}$[2] polymorphism on the susceptibility to OP toxicity in 54 male agricultural workers in Mexico. All participants had abnormal sperm morphology, 46% had low ejaculate volume, 30% had low sperm motility, and 13% had low sperm viability. OP exposure, either at the month of sample collection or during the preceding 3 months before sampling, was not associated with any parameters of semen quality or with DNA integrity. However, for men with the 192RR but not QQ genotype, there was a significant negative association between OP exposure during the 3 months before sampling (representing one spermatogenic cycle) and decreased sperm viability (p=0.086).

[2] OP deactivation occurs primarily by serum paraoxonase (PON1), which is encoded by a single gene on chromosome 7q21–22. PON1 activity in serum shows a wide variation among individuals, which may be attributed to the presence of polymorphisms in the PON1 gene at positions 55 and 192; the latter has two isoforms (Q and R). The 192R alloenzyme hydrolyzes paraoxon (the parathion oxon metabolite) faster than the 192Q isoform, while diazoxon (the oxon of diazinon) is hydrolyzed faster by the 192Q isoform (Pérez-Herrera et al., 2008).

The Volume 11 committee identified two studies on female reproductive effects from exposure to OPs (Al-Hussaini et al., 2018; Hu et al., 2018). In the first study, Al-Hussaini and colleagues reported on 94 couples at an infertility clinic in Egypt. Follicular fluid from each woman was collected during in vitro fertilization/embryo transfer and analyzed for the presence of chlorpyrifos (mean=146.9±43 [s.d.] μg/L), diazinon (mean=284.7±108.2 μg/L), and malathion (mean=38.5±9.5 μg/L), among other pesticides and polychlorinated biphenyls. There were negative correlations between the follicular fluid concentrations of all three pesticides and endometrial thickness ($p<0.05$ for diazinon and malathion and $p<0.01$ for chlorpyrifos). The concentrations of diazinon and chlorpyrifos, but not of malathion, were negatively associated with the number of oocytes retrieved ($p<0.01$ for both pesticides) and with the implantation rate (that is, the number of sacs; $p<0.01$ for both pesticides). None of the OPs were associated with reduced fertilization or early embryo cleavage rates.

Hu et al. (2018) conducted a TTP study with 569 women recruited from two preconception care clinics in Shanghai, China, from August 2013 and April 2015. The subjects were enrolled in the study before conceiving a child and were followed for approximately 1 year. Exposure to organophosphates (and pyrethroids) was determined through the measurement of urinary metabolites. After adjustments were made for age, body mass index (BMI) before pregnancy, smoking, and education, women in the highest quartile for urinary levels of DETP were found to have significantly longer TTP (fecundability OR=0.68, 95% CI 0.51–0.92) and increased infertility (OR=2.17, 95% CI 1.19–3.93) than women in the lowest quartile.

Adverse Pregnancy Outcomes

Numerous researchers have examined the effects of exposure to OPs on a variety of pregnancy outcomes, such as infant body weight and length and head circumference, preterm birth, and duration of gestation. Some studies have included large cohorts of mother–child pairs and have followed the children for several years after birth. The postnatal developmental effects observed in these children are discussed in the section on developmental effects. In this section the committee focuses on fetal growth and birth outcomes, including spontaneous abortion, as important reproductive effects.

The committee notes that none of the studies considered in this section provide information on maternal or paternal exposures during the preconception period or the first trimester of pregnancy. Rather, the studies usually assess maternal and fetal exposure by measuring OP metabolites in maternal or cord blood or maternal urine samples during pregnancy. In addition, for the Columbia Center for Children's Environmental Health (CCCEH) study the mothers wore personal air monitors during pregnancy to measure ambient exposures, and the researchers measured the parent compounds chlorpyrifos and diazinon in maternal blood within one day of delivery.

There are four major longitudinal U.S. birth cohort studies of pesticide exposure and child health that have examined the effects of prenatal exposure to OPs and other pesticides on fetal growth: the CCCEH study in New York City; the Center for the Health Assessment of Mothers and Children of Salinas (CHAMACOS) study in California; the Health Outcomes and Measures of the Environment (HOME) study in Cincinnati, Ohio; and the Children's Environmental Cohort Study at Mount Sinai Hospital in New York City. Each of these studies has combined an assessment of maternal pesticide exposure with some measure of birth outcomes. Harley et al. (2016) evaluated birth outcomes across all four U.S. cohorts.

The CCCEH study followed a cohort of 263 inner-city African American or Dominican women enrolled between 1998 and 2002 (Perera et al., 2003). Women wore personal air monitors for 48 hours in the second or third trimester to determine their exposure to airborne toxicants. Blood and urine were also sampled. Chlorpyrifos was detected in 98% of maternal blood samples and 94% of cord blood samples at birth. Prenatal chlorpyrifos exposure (pg/g blood) was associated with a significant decrease in birth weight (grams) overall (β= –0.04, p=0.01) and among African Americans (β= –0.05, p=0.04), but not among Dominican infants (β= –0.03, p=0.11). It was also associated with reduced birth length overall (β = –0.01, p=0.003) and in Dominicans (β= –0.02, p<0.001); chlorpyrifos exposure was not significantly associated with reduced head circumference in any group.

The CHAMACOS study investigated a group of 488 low-income Latina women and their infants in an agricultural area of Salinas Valley, California, in 1999–2000 (Eskenazi et al., 2004). DAPs were measured in maternal urine at about 13 weeks of gestation and again at 26 weeks of gestation, and cholinesterase (ChE) and BuChE were measured in maternal and umbilical cord blood at delivery. Increased DAP concentrations were associated with increased infant body length (p=0.06) and were significantly associated with an increased head circumference (p=0.03). A 10-fold increase in DMP, but not DEP, metabolites was associated with a 3-day decrease in gestational duration (β= –0.41 weeks/log10 unit increase; 95% CI –0.75– –0.02; p=0.02), but only after 22 weeks of gestation. DAP metabolites were not associated with birth weight, infant ponderal index (a weight–height index used to measure fetal growth), the risk of preterm delivery, low birth weight, or small-for-gestational-age births. Lower levels of ChE in umbilical cord blood were associated with a significantly shorter length of gestation (β=0.34 weeks/unit increase; 95% CI, 0.13–0.55; p=0.001), increased risk of preterm delivery (OR=2.3, 95% CI 1.1–4.8; p=0.02), and lower birth weight (OR=4.3, 95% CI 1.1–17.5; p=0.04). However, 6 of the 11 low-birth-weight infants were also preterm. BuChE levels in maternal and umbilical cord blood were not associated with any birth outcome.

A further analysis of the CHAMACOS cohort by Harley et al. (2011) examined whether *PON1* would modify the effect of OPs on adverse fetal outcomes. Maternal and cord blood samples were analyzed for the *PON1* genotype and enzyme activity. Associations of *PON1* with decreased gestational age were found only in those infants who had susceptible *PON1* genotypes ($PON1_{-108TT}$); the presence of susceptible *PON1* genotypes in mothers was not associated with decreased gestational age. No associations were found between any marker of *PON1* genotype or activity as measured in maternal blood and the gestational age or infant birth weight, length, or head circumference. There was some evidence of effect modification with DAPs: maternal DAP concentrations were associated with shorter gestational age only among infants with the susceptible $PON1_{-108TT}$ genotype (p-value interaction=0.09). However, maternal DAP concentrations were associated with larger birth weight (p-value interaction=0.06) and head circumference (p-value interaction 0.01) in infants with a nonsusceptible genotype ($PON1_{192QQ}$).

In the Cincinnati HOME study, 344 women less than 19 weeks pregnant were assessed for residential exposure to toxicants between 2003 and 2006 (Rauch et al., 2012). Urine samples collected at 16 and 26 weeks of gestation were analyzed for six DAPs; all mothers had detectable levels of at least one DAP. A 10-fold increase in total DAP concentration was significantly associated with a decrease in gestational age (β= –0.5 weeks, 95% CI –0.8– –0.1) and with a lower birth weight (β= –151 g, 95% CI –287– –16), and the association with decreases in gestation age was stronger for white mothers than for black mothers, but the reverse was true for birth weight. Decrements in birth weight and gestational age associated with ΣDAP concentrations were greatest among infants with the $PON1_{192QR}$ and PON_{-108CT} genotypes.

Berkowitz et al. (2004) reported on the Children's Environmental Cohort Study at Mount Sinai Hospital in New York City, a cohort of 404 multiethnic mother–infant pairs with babies born between 1998 and 2002. TCPy (a metabolite of chlorpyrifos) and 3-phenoxybenzoic acid (PBA; a pyrethroid metabolite) were each detected in more than 40% of prenatal maternal urines. There were no associations between maternal pesticide exposures or urinary levels of TCPy, PBA, or pentachlorophenol and adjusted birth weight, adjusted length, adjusted head circumference, or adjusted gestational age. A positive trend was found between maternal blood PON1 activity and head circumference, but the trend was only significant for mothers whose TCPy levels were above the level of detection. No trends were seen for birth weight or birth length for TCPy or for the other metabolite levels when maternal *PON1* genotype level was taken into account. Infant PON1 activity had no association with any of the fetal growth measures.

Harley et al. (2016) pooled data from the four U.S. cohort studies and found that there were no significant associations between DAP metabolites and birth weight, length, or head circumference. However, when the mothers were stratified by ethnicity, there was an association between increasing urinary DAP concentrations and decreased birth weight for non-Hispanic black women. Infants with the $PON1_{192RR}$ genotype were at greater risk for decreased birth length with increasing prenatal exposure to DAP metabolites. Gestational duration was not examined in the pooled analysis.

The committee identified one study in Shanghai, China, that also sought to determine whether prenatal exposure to pesticides resulted in any adverse fetal growth outcomes (Wang et al., 2012). Women (n=187) were recruited into the study between 2006 and 2007, and they provided urine samples at the onset of labor for DAP analysis. There were no significant associations between prenatal OP exposure and infant body weight or length or length of gestation, with the exception of DEP, which showed a significant inverse relationship with duration of gestation for infant girls but not boys ($\beta = -1.79$; $p=0.001$ versus $\beta=0.17$; $p=0.164$, respectively).

In an in vitro study with human villous cytotrophoblast cells isolated from human placentas, exposure to chlorpyrifos was found to cause marked changes in placental tissues including chorionic villi, suggesting the placenta may be a target of chlorpyrifos toxicity (Ridano et al., 2017).

Animal Studies

Although the Volume 2 committee (IOM, 2003) did not report on human or animal studies of reproductive effects and OP exposure, information from animal studies was available at the time. In 1997, ATSDR had published toxicological profiles of dichlorvos and of chlorpyrifos that included the results of animal studies on the reproductive effects of those pesticides. Dermal exposure to chlorpyrifos had resulted in transient adverse effects on semen volume and quality in bulls. Oral exposure to chlorpyrifos had no effect on female reproduction in mice, rats or dogs; however, the doses of chlorpyrifos needed to cause death in pregnant mice were approximately six times lower than those needed to cause death in nonpregnant mice. Chlorpyrifos administered via inhalation had no effect on rat testes (ATSDR, 1997a). ATSDR concluded that in several animal species oral and inhalation exposures to dichlorvos did not have reproductive effects in either males or females (ATSDR, 1997b). The ATSDR *Toxicological Profile for Malathion* (2003a) indicated that malathion was not a reproductive toxicant in animals; however, several animal studies had found that the oral administration of malathion did produce transient testicular effects. Finally, ATSDR concluded that animal studies had provided no evidence that diazinon was a reproductive toxicant. The studies on which that conclusion was based had involved oral exposures in mice, rats, and dogs (ATSDR, 2008).

In the past 10 years, rodent research has focused on characterizing the testicular toxicity of OPs. As discussed below, these studies have treated rodents with OPs, usually over at least one sperm cycle, and found effects on sperm quality, serum hormones, testes and epididymis histopathology, biochemistry, and gene expression.

DNA damage in sperm, which has been associated with OP exposure in humans (Meeker et al., 2004b), has also been observed in animal studies after in vivo treatment with diazinon (Pina Guzman et al., 2005; Sarabia et al., 2009) and malathion (Giri et al., 2002) as well as in vitro with human sperm after exposure to chlorpyrifos (Salazar-Arredondo et al., 2008). These findings in sperm agree with the in vitro genotoxicity that has been observed relating to chromosomal disruption in lymphocytes (Ohja and Gupta, 2015).

As in human studies such as Meeker et al. (2008a), rodent experiments in male animals have found decreased levels of serum testosterone as well as of the gonadotropins FSH and LH after short-term exposure to chlorpyrifos (Alaa-Eldin et al., 2017; Mandal and Das, 2012; Sai et al., 2014), dichlorvos (Dirican and Kalender, 2012), diazinon (Leong et al., 2013), and malathion (Bustos-Obregón and González-Hormazabal, 2003; Geng et al., 2015; Uzun et al., 2009). These hormone effects were seen in connection with sperm abnormalities and testicular histopathology. Hormone effects were observed consistently, as was testicular toxicity, when measured, with the exception of the two dichlorvos studies (Okamura et al., 2005, 2009).

Two mechanisms for OP reproductive toxicity have been studied. The suggestion that OPs generate reactive oxygen species (ROS) is supported by the presence of tissue oxidative damage markers in male reproductive organs after treatment with chlorpyrifos (Mandal and Das, 2011, 2012; Mosbah et al., 2016; Sai et al., 2014; Umosen et al., 2012). ROS-mediated genotoxicity has been established for in vitro chlorpyrifos exposures (Chauhan et al., 2016). Other studies have supported this hypothesis by showing that antioxidants provide protection against testicular toxicity (Alaa-Eldin et al., 2017; Dirican and Kalender, 2012; Dutta and Sahu, 2013; Elmazoudy et al., 2011; Elsharkawy et al., 2014; Mosbah et al., 2016; Umosen et al., 2012; Uzun et al., 2009). A second line of mechanistic work demonstrated a failure in the final steps of sperm maturation in the epidydimis after treatment with malathion and dichlorvos (Akbarsha et al., 2000). ROS are known to be involved in sperm capacitation (Aitken, 2017).

OP animal studies that included a mating trial after the males had been treated found that preconception exposure to chlorpyrifos reduced fertility (85% negative fertility using mating exposure test; Joshi et al., 2007) and decreased the number of live fetuses, increased the number of dead fetuses, and increased the number of early resorptions (Farag et al., 2010). The treatment of male rats with malathion prior to mating caused an 80% decrease in fertility (Choudhary et al., 2008).

As with humans, there is little information on female animal reproductive toxicity resulting from exposures prior to pregnancy. Chebab et al. (2017) found that 6.75 mg/kg chlorpyrifos administered to female rats for 30 days significantly decreased the serum concentrations of sex hormones and thyroid hormones.

A study with dichlorvos did not find any effects on pregnancy when female mice were treated before mating (Dean and Blair, 1976). Gomes and Lloyd (2009) and Gomes et al. (2008) found effects on both pregnancy outcome and the incidence of malformation when a mixture of OPs was given to female mice before mating. The mixture included chlorpyrifos and dichlorvos (both OPs used in the Gulf War) as well as other pesticides at LD_{50} levels. Such high doses coupled with the use of commercial formulations and the large number of agents make these findings difficult to interpret. Malathion has also been shown to affect the maturation of porcine cumulus–oocyte complexes in vitro by inducing oxidative stress (Flores et al., 2017).

The Volume 11 committee found a lack of relevant information in the animal literature on adverse birth outcomes associated with preconception or prenatal exposure to any of the relevant OPs considered in this chapter.

Developmental Effects

Numerous studies have examined developmental effects in children following prenatal exposures to OPs. The research for the most part has focused on potential neurodevelopmental effects that may occur in infants and children exposed in utero. Several longitudinal studies have examined neurodevelopmental deficits in children as they grow. Respiratory effects, childhood cancers, birth defects, and ear infections in children have also been studied in the context of prenatal OP exposure. The Volume 11 committee identified only a few studies that related preconception exposure to OPs to health outcomes in children (e.g., Monge et al., 2007).

In the sections below and in Table 5-3, the Volume 11 committee reviews the literature on postnatal effects in children following prenatal exposures to OPs, with subsections devoted to each developmental effect. As noted in the introduction to this chapter, the Volume 2 committee (IOM, 2003) concluded that there was inadequate/insufficient evidence to determine whether an association exists between "parental preconception exposure to insecticides and childhood leukemia, brain and other central nervous system cancers, and non-Hodgkin's lymphoma" or between "parental preconception exposure to insecticides and congenital malformations" in children, but that committee made no conclusions for OPs specifically.

Neurodevelopmental Effects

The *Gulf War and Health, Volume 2* committee did not discuss any studies on developmental effects that may result in children whose parents were exposed to OPs. On the other hand, that committee did consider a number of animal studies, which are discussed later in this section.

In November 2016, EPA released *Chlorpyrifos: Revised Human Health Risk Assessment for Registration Review* as part of the Federal Insecticide, Fungicide, and Rodenticide Act Section 3(g) Registration Review program. The review gave special consideration to chlorpyrifos' neurodevelopmental effects on children. The risk assessment document (EPA, 2016) stated:

> In the 2015 updated literature review (USEPA, D331251, 09/15/2015), the agency conducted a systematic review expanding the 2012/2014 review which was focused only on US cohort studies with particular emphasis on chlorpyrifos. The expanded 2015 review includes consideration of the epidemiological data on any OP pesticide, study designs beyond prospective cohort studies, and non-U.S. based studies. The updated literature review identified seven studies which were relevant (Bouchard et al. 2010; Fortenberry et al. 2014; Furlong et al. 2014; Guodong et al. 2012; Oulhote and Bouchard, 2013; Zhang et al. 2014; Shelton et al. 2014). These seven studies have been evaluated in context with studies from the 2012/2014 review (D. Drew et al. D424485, 12/29/2014). In addition, the agency has also reviewed more recent studies from CCCEH (Rauh et al. 2015) and a pooled analysis of U.S. cohort studies (Engel et al. 2015) (E. Holman, D432184, 03/25/2016). As discussed below, Rauh et al. (2015) provides further evidence of neurodevelopmental outcomes in the CCCEH study. The Engel et al. (2015) study shows relatively consistent results compared to previous studies conducted at 24 months (Engel et al. 2011; Rauh et al. 2006). . . . The agency continues to conclude that the 3 U.S. cohort studies (CCCEH, CHAMACOS, and Mt. Sinai) provide the most robust available epidemiological evidence.
>
> The agency acknowledges the lack of established MOA/AOP pathway [mode of action/adverse outcome pathway], the inability to make strong causal linkages, and the unknown window(s) of susceptibility. These uncertainties do not undermine or reduce the confidence in the findings of the epidemiology studies. The epidemiology studies reviewed in the 2012/2014 and 2015 literature reviews represent different investigators, locations, points in time, exposure assessment procedures, and outcome measurements. Despite differences in study design, with the exception of two negative studies in the 2015 literature review (Guodong et al. 2012; Oulhote and Bouchard, 2013) and the results from the more recent Engel et al. (2015) study, all other study authors have identified associations with neurodevelopmental outcomes associated with OP exposure; these conclusions were across four cohorts and twelve study citations. Specifically, there is evidence of delays in mental development in infants (24-36 months), attention problems and autism spectrum disorder in early childhood, and intelligence decrements in school age children who

> were exposed to OPs during gestation. Investigators reported strong measures of statistical association across several of these evaluations (odds ratios 2-4 fold increased in some instances), and observed evidence of exposures-response trends in some instances, e.g., intelligence measures. . . .
>
> In summary, the EPA's assessment is that the CCCEH study, with supporting results from the other 2 U.S. cohort studies and the seven additional epidemiological studies reviewed in 2015, provides sufficient evidence that there are neurodevelopmental effects occurring at chlorpyrifos exposure levels below that required for AChE inhibition.

On December 15, 2017, the California Environmental Protection Agency, Office of Environmental Health Hazard Assessment, Developmental and Reproductive Toxicant Identification Committee determined that chlorpyrifos was "clearly shown through scientifically valid testing according to generally accepted principles to cause reproductive toxicity," based on the developmental endpoint (OEHHA, 2017).

The Volume 11 committee considered a number of studies on the developmental effects, particularly neurological outcomes, in children whose mothers or fathers had been exposed to organophosphate pesticides, primarily chlorpyrifos. In addition to studies conducted in Spain, Mexico, and China, researchers have also used four U.S. cohort studies to look at the effects of prenatal OP exposure on a variety of neurodevelopmental outcomes in children. Only studies not cited in *Chlorpyrifos: Revised Human Health Risk Assessment for Registration Review* (EPA, 2016) and considered by the committee to be relevant to its assessment are included in Table 5-3.

The CCCEH study assessed children born between February 1998 and May 2002 for psychomotor and cognitive development at 12, 24, and 36 months (Rauh et al., 2006), and at 7 years of age (Rauh et al., 2012). Younger children were administered the Bayley Scales of Infant Development II (BSID-II), and their mothers completed the Child Behavior Checklist (CBCL); the 7-year-olds were administered the Wechsler Intelligence Scale for Children, 4th edition (WISC-IV). Prenatal exposure of chlorpyrifos levels was measured in maternal blood or cord blood samples obtained at delivery, and the results were categorized as high exposure (>6.17 pg chlorpyrifos/g plasma) or low exposure (≤6.17 pg/g). At 12 and 24 months of age, there were no differences in mental or motor function between high- and low-exposure children. However, at 36 months of age, children with high prenatal exposure to chlorpyrifos scored significantly lower on the psychomotor development index (PDI; $p=0.01$) than children with low exposure; were in the clinical problems range for all five CBCL scales, particularly the attention problems and attention deficit–hyperactivity disorder (ADHD) scales ($p=0.03$ each); and were more likely than the low-exposure children to have mental delays (OR=2.4, 95% CI 1.12–5.08) and motor delays (OR=4.5, 95% CI 1.61–12.70) (Rauh et al., 2006). At 7 years of age, there were significant inverse associations between chlorpyrifos exposure and two of the WISC-IV scales: working memory ($r= -0.21$, $p <0.0001$) and full-scale intelligence quotient ($r= -0.13$, $p=0.02$) (Rauh et al., 2011). Horton et al. (2012) found a significant interaction between exposure and the child's sex, suggesting that boys had a greater decrement in working memory than girls ($\beta= -1.714$, 95% CI –3.753–0.326). At 11 years of age, there was a significant association of prenatal chlorpyrifos exposure with tremor (Rauh et al., 2015). A subgroup of 40 CCCEH 7-year-old children (20 from the upper tertile and 20 from the lowest tertile) also underwent magnetic resonance imaging of the brain. Children in the high-exposure group had a significant enlargement of several brain areas (e.g., superior temporal, posterior middle temporal, and inferior postcentral gyri bilaterally; gyrus rectus) as well as frontal and parietal cortical thinning and an inverse dose–response relationship between chlorpyrifos and cortical thickness (Rauh et al., 2012).

A second New York City study, the Mount Sinai Children's Environmental Health Cohort, recruited 404 mother–infant pairs during pregnancy in 1998–2001 (Engel et al., 2007, 2011). Prenatal exposure to OPs (including malathion) was determined by an analysis of maternal blood and urine samples taken at about pregnancy week 31. The Brazelton Neonatal Behavioral Assessment Scale (BNBAS) was administered to 311 neonates before they left the hospital (Engel et al., 2007). BNBAS scores showed that neonates born to women with elevated urinary malathion dicarboxylic acid (MDA) levels had a greater number of abnormal reflexes (OR=2.24, 95% CI 1.55–3.24) than children born with elevated total DEP metabolites (OR=1.49, 95% CI 1.12–1.98). Increasing levels of total DAP and DMP metabolites were also associated with an increase in abnormal reflexes. In a further study of this cohort (n=169 children or more, depending on which assessment), neurodevelopment was assessed within 5 days of birth, at 12 and 24 months, and at 6–9 years of age (Engel et al., 2011). At 12 and 24 months, in black and Hispanic infants decreased mental development (as measured with the BSID-II) was associated with higher exposure to prenatal total DAP metabolites, whereas among whites, increasing exposure was associated with improved mental development index (MDI) scores. Furthermore, prenatal maternal DAP levels were inversely associated with children's 24-month MDI but not their PDI. At 7–9 years of age, there were only modest effects of any prenatal OP metabolites on any psychometric measure in the children (Engel et al., 2011). A further evaluation of the 7- to 9-year-old children was done using the Social Responsiveness Scale (SRS) to assess for characteristics of autism spectrum and related disorders. No associations overall were found between any of the total DAP, DEP, or DMP metabolites and total SRS scores. However, increasing total DEP levels were associated with poorer SRS scores among blacks (β=5.1 points, 95% CI 0.8–9.4) and boys (β=3.5 points, 95% CI 0.2–6.8), although not among whites and Hispanics (β=0.2 points, 95% CI –2.8–3.2), or among girls (β= –0.4 points, 95% CI –4.1–3.3) (Furlong et al., 2014). Further analysis of the children found that DMP metabolites were negatively associated with internalizing factor scores (β= –0.13, 95% CI –0.26–0.00), but positively associated with executive functioning factor scores (β=0.18, 95% CI 0.04–0.31). However, DEP metabolites were negatively associated with the working memory index (β= –0.17, 95% CI –0.33– –0.03) (Furlong et al., 2017a).

The longitudinal CHAMACOS cohort study has tracked children born between October 1999 and October 2000 to mothers residing in an agricultural area of the Salinas Valley in California. The mothers were generally young, of Mexican origin, and from farm-working families, and most had not completed high school. Urine samples were collected from the mothers (n=381) during the first and the second half of pregnancy, and each sample was analyzed for DAP metabolites of OP pesticides. Children (n=327) were assessed for developmental parameters at 6, 12, and 24 months, 3.5 years, 5 years, and 7 years of age (Eskenazi et al., 2014). Newborn infants showed a significant increase in the number of abnormal reflexes on the BNBAS which was correlated with increasing levels of maternal total DAP, DMP, and DEP levels measured in urine (β=0.23, 95% CI 0.05–0.41; β=0.18, 95% CI 0.02–0.34; β=0.22, 95% CI 0.04–0.40, respectively); however, none of the maternal metabolite levels were correlated with any of the other BNBAS scores (Young et al., 2005). Eskenazi et al. (2007) found that maternal prenatal DAP levels were negatively associated with the child's MDI on the BSID-II and that this association reached statistical significance at 24 months of age (per 10-fold increase in prenatal DAPs: β= –3.5 points; 95% CI –6.6– –0.5). Prenatal DAPs were also associated with pervasive developmental disorder (per 10-fold increase in prenatal DAPs: OR=2.3, p=0.05). Prenatal DAPs were not significantly associated with attention problems or ADHD when the children were 3.5 years of age, but they were associated with both outcomes by the time the children were 5 years of age (CBCL attention problems: β=0.7 points; 95% CI 0.2–1.2; ADHD: β=1.3, 95% CI 0.4–2.1), and some associations were found only among boys (Marks et al., 2010). Finally, at 7 years of age, a 10-fold increase in maternal DAP concentrations was associated with lower cognitive scores on all four cognitive subtests of the WISC-IV. The most significant associations were for verbal comprehension (β= –5.3, 95% CI –8.6– –2.0) and a decrease of 5.6 full-scale IQ points (95% CI –9.0– –2.2). Higher DAP levels later in pregnancy were associated with greater deficits in the children than were levels in the first half of pregnancy (Bouchard et al., 2011). The association between DAPs and full-scale IQ was strongest for the children of mothers with the lowest-tertile levels of arylesterase, a measure of the enzyme activity of PON1. This relationship held for both diethyl and dimethyl DAPs and for all subscales of the WISC (Eskenazi et al., 2014). Further assessment of neurobehavior in 238 of the 7-year-old children in the CHAMACOS cohort found consistent but not significant negative associations between DNA methylation at several CpG sites close to the PON1 transcription start site in the children's cord blood and full-scale IQ and other composite measures of cognition as measured with the WISC-IV. Nonsignificant associations were also found between cord blood methylation at cg15887283 and the children's working memory scores (Huen et al., 2018). Studies using Pesticide Use Reporting data from California reported an association between the use of OPs in fields near the maternal residence during pregnancy and WISC Full Scale and Verbal Comprehension IQ scores in children at age 7 (Gunier et al., 2017).

A further study by Sagiv et al. (2018) of the CHAMACOS cohort examined whether there is an association between prenatal exposure to OP pesticides and autism spectrum disorder (ASD) traits in children and adolescents. Women were interviewed twice during pregnancy, once after delivery and then when the children reached the ages of 6 months, 1, 2, 3.5, 5, 7, 9, 10.5, 12, and 14 years. Exposure was assessed by measuring DAPs in urine and by collecting information on the mother's residential proximity to OP application while pregnant, using California's Pesticide Use Reporting data. The authors measured traits in 247 children based on the parents' and teachers' reporting on the child's performance at ages 7, 10.5, 12, and 14 years on tests specifically aimed at evaluating a child's ability to use facial expressions and to recognize the mental state of others. Results showed that prenatal exposure to DAPs was associated with unfavorable social behavior reported by parents and teachers. DAP levels were also associated with a 2.7-fold increase in social responsiveness among children at 14 years of age (β=2.7, 95% CI 0.9–4.5). The SRS subscales are social awareness, social cognition, social communication, social motivation, and restricted interests and repetitive behavior. Normal scores are below 59, and scores above 75 are interpreted as indicating severe deficiencies in reciprocal social behaviors. No association was found between proximity to an area where OPs were used during pregnancy and ASD traits in children. In short, this study presented inconsistent results on the association between OP pesticides and ASD-related traits.

The committee considered two studies that examined pregnant women recruited into the HOME study (Donauer et al., 2016; Millenson et al., 2017). Urine from 327 women was collected at about gestation week 16 and again around gestation week 26 and analyzed for metabolites of OPs. Children were administered the BSID-II at 1, 2, and 3 years of age; the Clinical Evaluation of Language Fundamentals at age 4; and the Weschsler Preschool and Primary Scale of Intelligence at age 5 (Donauer et al., 2016). No association was found between prenatal exposure and cognition at any age from 1 through 5 after adjustment for relevant covariates. Millenson et al. (2017) further examined the children for PON1 polymorphisms from cord blood. Children were assessed with the SRS. Total DAP levels were not associated with changes in SRS scores (β= –1.2, 95% CI –4.0–1.6), nor were the associations modified by the child's PON1 genotype.

Engel et al. (2016) attempted to pool data from the CHAMACOS study, the HOME study in Cincinnati, and the CCCEH and Mount Sinai cohort studies in New York City. Those researchers found significant heterogeneity for estimates of the association between DAPs and MDI (p=0.09) and also found that PON1 genotypes, ethnicity, and the center performing the study all influenced the results. Despite the limitations, the authors concluded that some population subgroups were at risk of neurodevelopment problems as shown by changes in the MDI.

The Childhood Autism Risk from Genetics and Environment (CHARGE) study in California also attempted to link pesticide use near the mother's residence to children having ASD (n=486) or developmental disorder (n=168) (Shelton et al., 2014). Each pregnancy was given an exposure profile based on the pesticide applications made near the mother's home and the days of her pregnancy on which those applications occurred. Children were eligible for the study if they were 2–5 years of age (mean 36–38 months). Any prenatal proximity (within 1.25 km) to OPs was associated with an increased risk for ASD (OR=1.6, 95% CI 1.02–2.51); the risks were higher the later in the pregnancy the exposure occurred, but except for third-trimester exposures, those risks were not significant (OR=1.37, 95% CI 0.76–2.50 for preconception exposure; OR=1.53, 95% CI 0.87–2.68 for first trimester; OR=1.57, 95% CI 0.87–2.83 for second trimester; and OR=1.99, 95% CI 1.11–3.56 for third trimester). For developmental disorder and residential proximity to agricultural pesticide application the ORs were 1.23 (95% CI 0.65–2.31) for all pregnancies, 1.20 (95% CI 0.54–2.65) for preconception exposure, 1.29 (95% CI 0.60–2.79) for the first trimester, 1.62 (95% CI 0.75–3.48) for the second trimester, and 1.10 (95% CI 0.46–2.67) for the third trimester. The authors concluded that prenatal exposure to OPs could be linked with neurodevelopmental disorders.

Several studies in China assessed the effect of prenatal exposure to OPs on child neurodevelopment. Zhang et al. (2014a) administered the Neonatal Behavioral Neurological Assessment (NBNA) to 3-day-old infants in Shenyang, China. Urine samples of 249 pregnant women were analyzed for five nonspecific OP metabolites. Higher prenatal DAP concentrations were associated with lower scores in all NBNA scales, especially the Behavior Scale (β for a 10-fold increase in concentration= –0.65, 95% CI –0.84– –0.45, p=0.01). In a further assessment of the effects of prenatal exposure to over 30 OPs on child neurodevelopment, Silver et al. (2017) analyzed cord blood from 237 Chinese infants born in Fuyang Maternal and Children's Hospital between 2008 and 2011. Exposure to chlorpyrifos, as determined by gas chromatography, was associated with significant motor function deficits in 199 infants assessed at 6 weeks and 9 months of age using the Peabody Developmental Motor Scales, 2nd edition. In another study, Wang et al. (2017) measured six DAP metabolites in urine specimens from 436 women taken at delivery. Women were part of the Laizhou Wan Birth Cohort study in Shandong, China. Children were assessed for neurodevelopment at 12 months (n=297) and 24 months (n=262). Prenatal OP concentrations were not correlated with any neurodevelopmental deficits, as measured with the Gesell Developmental Schedules, at 12 months. At 24 months, however, prenatal, but not postnatal, OP exposure was associated with a reduced developmental quotient, especially among boys.

González-Alzaga et al. (2015) used the WISC-IV to study the effects of high and low exposure to OP applications on cognitive functioning in 305 6- to 11-year-old children in Spain. Maternal prenatal residential exposure to OPs was associated with a poorer score on the processing speed subtest for boys (β= –5.7; 95% CI –9.6– –1.8), but not for girls (β= –1.6, 95% CI –6.4– –3.3). No other associations were significant for either high or low exposures or any of the WISC-IV subtests. The authors concluded that there was a weak association between prenatal OP exposure and neurological deficits.

The Early Life Exposures in Mexico to Environmental Toxicants (ELEMENT) study measured metabolites in maternal urine to assess prenatal exposure to chlorpyrifos and ADHD in children ages 6–11 years old in Mexico City (Fortenberry et al., 2014). There were no significant associations between chlorpyrifos metabolite concentrations in maternal urine and ADHD outcomes in the children.

A recent integrative review by Burke et al. (2017) examined the developmental neurotoxicity of OPs with an emphasis on chlorpyrifos and summarized the extensive epidemiologic studies of chlorpyrifos (most of which are discussed earlier in this section). The authors concluded that a "disruption of the structural integrity of the brain can be an important determinant of the cognitive deficits" associated with prenatal exposure to the pesticide. The authors also considered eight studies of cognitive and locomotor phenotypes following prenatal exposure to chlorpyrifos in rats and mice. The authors argued that "it is unclear to what extent, if any, AChE inhibition contributes to the developmental neurotoxicity of chlorpyrifos" and concluded that this made it difficult to extrapolate from animal models to humans.

Respiratory Effects

Respiratory effects in children following prenatal exposures were not reported in *Gulf War and Health, Volume 2*, nor were they discussed in EPA's 2016 *Chlorpyrifos: Revised Human Health Risk Assessment for Registration Review*, ATSDR's 2008 *Toxicological Profile for Diazinon*, or ATSDR's 1997 *Toxicological Profile for Dichlorvos*.

The Volume 11 committee identified two recent publications by Raanan et al. (2015, 2016) that assessed respiratory effects in young children after prenatal exposure to OPs and other pesticides in the CHAMACOS cohort. The assessments of maternal exposures to OPs were based on an analysis of DAPs in maternal urine at gestation weeks 13 and 26. Mothers reported their children's respiratory symptoms at 5 and 7 years of age, with 359 children assessed. Children's respiratory symptoms were not associated with any maternal DAP concentrations in the first half of pregnancy. However, there were significantly increased risks of respiratory symptoms in children whose mothers had elevated prenatal total DAPs and diethyl metabolite levels during the second half of pregnancy (ΣDAPs OR for a 10-fold increase in concentration=1.77, 95% CI 1.06–2.95; DEPs OR=1.61, 95% CI 1.08–2.39); there was no increased risk observed for elevated dimethyl metabolites (Raanan et al., 2015). A spirometric assessment of lung function in the 7-year-old children found that the mothers' DAP urinary concentrations, whether in the first half or second half of pregnancy, were not significantly associated with lung function measurements (FEV_1, FVC, FEV_1/FVC ratio, and FEF_{25-75}) in their children (Raanan et al., 2016).

Childhood Cancer

Genotoxicity studies of OPs reveal primarily chromosomal abnormalities and DNA fragmentation. IARC has classified two of the Gulf War OPs—diazinon and malathion—as probable human carcinogens (IARC, 2016a,b). IARC has also classified dichlorvos as a possible human carcinogen (IARC, 1991). No transplacental cancer studies were reviewed for any of the three OPs.

The committee found only one new study that assessed the risk of childhood cancers and exposure to OPs before birth. Monge et al. (2007) examined the effects of maternal exposures (n=876) and paternal exposures (n=762) to pesticides on the risk of childhood leukemia (n=334) in Costa Rica in 1995–2000. Parents were interviewed about risk factors for childhood leukemia, and their exposures were rated as to hazard value at the time of occurrence. The mothers' exposure to OPs in the first trimester of pregnancy was significantly associated with total leukemia (OR=3.5, 95% CI 1.0–12.2) and acute lymphoblastic leukemia (ALL) (OR=3.7, 95% CI 1.0–13.1). Although the risk of any leukemia and ALL was elevated in children whose mothers were exposed in the year before conception (leukemia OR=2.3, 95% CI 0.9–6.0; ALL OR=2.5, 95% CI 0.9–6.7) and during the second trimester (leukemia OR=2.5, 95% CI 0.7–9.5; ALL OR=3.0, 95% CI 0.8–11.5), the increases were not significant. In the fathers, exposure to OPs was associated with a increased risk of leukemia at all time points: the year before conception (OR=1.5, 95% CI 1.0–2.2), the first trimester (OR=1.6, 95% CI 1.0–2.6), and the second trimester (OR=1.4, 95% CI 0.8–2.3). Further analysis of the fathers' exposures to specific pesticides showed that exposure to malathion in the year before conception was associated with an increased risk of leukemia and of ALL for boys (OR=8.5, 95% CI 1.1–74.1 and OR=10.4, 95% CI 1.2–91.1, respectively), but not for girls (OR=0.9, 95% CI 0.2–4.9 and OR=0.5, 95% CI 0.1–4.8, respectively).

Other Developmental Effects

Carmichael et al. (2014) examined the association between exposure to pesticides during pregnancy and the prevalence of eight types of congenital heart defects in a population-based case-control study. Pesticide exposure within a 500-meter radius of each mother's residence was estimated for the 3 months prior to conception to delivery using geospatial coding for eight San Joaquin counties. The California Pesticide Use Reporting records were used to identify any pesticides applied at more than 100 lbs per year in any of the eight counties. Using data from the California Birth Defects Monitoring Program from 1997 to 2006, the exposures of the mothers of 569 case infants was compared with 785 mothers who had an infant without a birth defect. Prenatal exposure to chlorpyrifos was significantly associated with pulmonary valve stenosis (OR=2.4, 95% CI 1.0–6.3) and atrial septal defects, secundum (OR=1.9, 95% CI 1.1–3.4). A further assessment for five types of other birth defects was conducted (Carmichael et al., 2016), based on the exposure of 367 mothers of case infants compared with the same 785 control mothers. Prenatal exposure to OPs as a group (based on mechanism of action) was associated with a reduced risk of anorectal atresia/stenosis (OR=0.4, 95% CI 0.2–0.9) but was significantly associated with an increased risk of craniosynostosis (OR=1.9, 95% CI 1.1–3.2). Chlorpyrifos specifically was significantly associated with anotia (OR=2.0, 95% CI 1.1–3.8) and craniosynostosis (OR=2.4, 95% CI 1.2–4.6). The ORs for all other OPs or birth defects were not significant and ranged from 0.5 to 2.0.

Buscail et al. (2015) used the French PELAGIE mother–child cohort to examine the prevalence of otitis media in children at 2 years of age. They found that the children of 246 mothers who had exposure to OPs, determined by an analysis of DAP, DMP, and DEP metabolites in the mother's urine taken before the 19th week of pregnancy, were not at an increased risk of having one or more occurrences of otitis media before age 2 years.

The Volume 11 committee identified one small study on epigenetic effects associated with prenatal exposure to pesticides. Declerck et al. (2017) examined 25 children born in Denmark between 1996 and 2001 to mothers who had occupational exposures to a variety of pesticides during the first trimester of pregnancy and 23 unexposed control children. Blood samples taken from the children at 6–11 years of age were analyzed for the *PON1* Q192R genotype and genome-wide DNA methylation patterns related to prenatal pesticide exposure was determined. The majority of mothers (91%) were exposed to organophosphate pesticides, including chlorpyrifos, dichlorvos, and dimethoate, as well as pyrethroid pesticides (e.g., deltamethrin) and carbamate pesticides (e.g., methomyl). Prenatal pesticide exposure was found to be associated with changes in DNA methylation patterns in children with the *PON1* 192R-allele compared with the 192Q-genotype and the control children, and the hypermethylation changes were significantly associated with higher body fat content ($p<0.001$) and serum leptin concentrations ($p=0.02$).

Animal Studies

In studies of pregnant women exposed to toxicants, including OPs, there are three confounding issues: exposures are seldom limited to one insecticide (i.e., exposures are typically to mixtures of toxicants); exposures are rarely limited to one period of time (i.e., preconception, pregnancy or trimester of pregnancy, or postnatal); and outcome assessments are typically made in early childhood and not at later stages of development, such as adolescence. These issues can be addressed in animal models. Socioeconomic status can also be a confounder in human studies, but it is not in animal studies.

The ATSDR *Toxicological Profile for Malathion* (2003a) indicated that malathion was not a developmental toxicant in animals at doses that did not induce maternal toxicity.

Animal models have been used extensively to study sensitive periods for chlorpyrifos exposure in pregnancy. This is important for female veterans whose deployments are terminated shortly after pregnancy is identified. Researchers using rodent models to compare the effects of chlorpyrifos exposure in early and late pregnancy found that early pregnancy exposure had various long-lasting effects on brain development in rats, including altered behavior (Icenogle et al., 2004), brain morphology (Chen et al., 2017; Qiao et al., 2004), modified brain chemistry (Aldridge et al., 2003, 2004, 2005; Meyer et al., 2004a,b; Qiao et al., 2002), and altered brain development (Qiao et al., 2003). For example, adult rats that had been exposed to chlorpyrifos on gestational days (GDs) 9–12 or 17–20 showed significant changes in the adenylyl cyclase signaling cascade, which mediates the cellular responses to numerous neurotransmitters, in a wide variety of brain regions in adulthood (Meyer et al., 2004a). However, exposure during GD 9–12 was less sensitive and required doses that resulted in decreased maternal weight gain. In another study, early pregnancy exposure resulted in cardiac and hepatic effects in offspring (Meyer et al., 2004b).

Exposure to chlorpyrifos later in pregnancy (GDs 14–20) also produced anxiety-like symptoms in rats assessed on postnatal day (PND) 21, but the anxious behavior was reversed by PND 70 (Silva et al., 2017). There were no depressive symptoms.

Studies of mid- to late-pregnancy exposure (GDs 14–17) of CD-1 mice to chlorpyrifos at a dose of 6 mg/kg resulted in early effects on pup vocalizations (Venerosi et al., 2009) and, later, alterations in social vocalizations and social investigation in female offspring (Venerosi et al., 2006, 2015). There was "specific and sex-dependent vulnerability of affective/emotional domains" and a disruption of serotoninergic transmission in both male and female animals (Venerosi et al., 2010). Lan et al. (2017) also treated pregnant mice in mid-gestation and found a delayed development of neonatal reflexes; by PND 90 the mice at the high dose had reduced social behavior, while the low-dose mice showed increased restricted interest behaviors. Thus, these animal studies demonstrate that chlorpyrifos exposure during sensitive brain development periods may affect various behavioral domains, including cognition, motor behavior, anxiety, and social behavior, and these detrimental neurodevelopmental effects may persist to adulthood.

While chlorpyrifos has been the most extensively studied OP with regard to neurodevelopmental effects, one study did demonstrate long-term effects on behavior in rodents following early pregnancy exposure to dichlorvos (Lazarini et al., 2004).

The associations between early pregnancy exposure to OPs and malformations and transplacental cancer have also been studied. All registered pesticides are assessed for teratogenicity before EPA approval. For malathion, diazinon, and dichlorvos there are published studies that reported finding no teratogenesis (ATSDR 1997b, 2003a, 2008). Recently, studies using chlorpyrifos doses with high systemic toxicity during embryogenesis did produce malformations (Akhtar et al., 2006), and studies testing mixtures of OPs, or mixtures including OPs with other pesticides, were also positive (Gomes and Lloyd, 2009; Yu et al., 2017). At doses that produce high systemic toxicity, pregnancy outcome measures (resorption, fetal loss, neonatal death, growth retardation) were also affected by OPs. However, it is important to note that the studies that identified neurodevelopmental toxicity of OPs used doses below the threshold for systemic maternal toxicity.

Oxidative damage has been implicated as a possible mechanism of action for the developmental effects of OPs (Qiao et al., 2004). While it has been demonstrated that antioxidants protect against the reproductive effects of OPs in males (Mosbah et al., 2016), this has not been studied for neurodevelopmental effects in offspring.

Synthesis and Conclusions

Reproductive Effects

Chlorpyrifos exposure has been shown to result in significant effects on sperm quality and lead to significantly increased levels of disomy in sperm chromosomes (Figueroa et al., 2015; Martenies and Perry, 2013; Meeker et al., 2004a,b; Melgarejo et al., 2015; Miranda-Contreras et al., 2013; Sánchez-Peña et al., 2004). Occupational exposure to OPs has been associated with altered sperm integrity, specifically the sperm chromatin structure, although the association was only with the presence of the OP metabolite DETP (Sánchez-Peña et al., 2004). Adverse effects on sperm parameters and some reproductive hormones were also seen in agricultural workers with OP exposure, although the men were also exposed to other pesticides (Miranda-Contreras et al., 2013). Similar adverse effects on sperm parameters were seen in men with environmental exposures to OPs, although reproductive hormones were largely unaffected (Melgarejo et al., 2015). A systematic review of six studies assessing the effects of exposure to OPs on male reproduction concluded that all six studies reported significant negative associations between OP exposure, whether occupational or otherwise, and at least one semen parameter. However, the Volume 11 committee noted that in many of these studies exposure was assessed using a single nonspecific urinary measure of the metabolites to which most OPs devolve, and, as indicated above, these biomarkers have some inherent limitations (e.g., they reflect only recent exposure, they may reflect exposure to preformed metabolites, etc.). Meeker et al. (2004a,b) examined six sperm parameters and reported no significant associations between urinary levels of TCPy, a metabolite of chlorpyrifos, and sperm concentration, motility, morphology, or percentage DNA tail or comet extent in sperm; only a decrease in tail distributed moment reached significance.

Recent rodent studies also focused on the testicular toxicity of OPs. These studies treated rodents with a pesticide, usually over at least one sperm cycle, and found effects on sperm quality, serum hormones, testes and epididymis histopathology, biochemistry, and gene expression. Such rodent studies have been conducted for all the OPs recognized for Gulf War toxicants: chlorpyrifos (Mandal and Das, 2012; Sai et al., 2014), dichlorvos (Dirican and Kalender, 2012), diazinon (Leong et al., 2013; Zidan, 2009), and malathion (Bustos-Obregón and González-Hormazabal, 2003; Geng et al., 2015; Uzun et al., 2009). The Volume 11 committee found that these animal studies described findings that were supportive of male reproductive effects being associated with OPs. These studies used measures similar to those used in human studies (serum hormones, sperm quality, sperm DNA damage) and were able to add testes histopathologic and biochemical measures. Although sperm production is affected by chlorpyrifos exposure in both animal and human studies, the effects on spermatogenesis and male fertility after the discontinuation of exposure have not been elucidated in humans. The Volume 11 committee concludes that these animal studies are supportive of male reproductive effects associated with OPs in human studies, as both human and animal studies assess the same sperm parameters. Additionally, animal studies of ROS generation as the mechanism of testicular toxicity provide biological plausibility for the associations reported in human studies.

The Volume 11 committee identified two studies that assessed the effects of OP exposure on female reproduction. Although the study in China (Hu et al., 2018) showed increased TTP and reduced fertility, the second study did not show decreased fertility. OP effects on ovarian function either during or after exposure have not been examined in any human studies and have been examined in only a few animal studies.

The Volume 11 committee considered several major longitudinal U.S. birth cohorts—the CCCEH study in New York City, the CHAMACOS study in California, the Children's Environmental Cohort Study at Mt. Sinai Hospital in New York City, and the HOME study in Cincinnati, Ohio—that examined the association between prenatal exposure to one or more pesticides, including OPs, and birth outcomes.

The effects of prenatal exposure to chlorpyrifos specifically, or OPs in general, on birth outcomes were not consistent across the studies. In particular, the Volume 11 committee notes that there were ethnic and sex differences for several of the outcomes related to specific DAPs. The Harley et al. (2016) pooled analysis found no significant associations between increases in maternal DAP concentrations and decreases in birth weight, birth length, or infant head circumference for white and Hispanic women, but it did find among black women that increased prenatal OP exposure was associated with decreased infant birth weight, length, and head circumference. However, gestational duration could not be examined in this pooled analysis, and an association between OP exposure and shortened gestational duration was noted in two of the studies (CHAMACOS and HOME) that examined length of gestation (Eskenazi et al., 2004; Rauch et al., 2012). The Volume 11 committee also emphasizes that it was not possible in any of these cohort studies to say which particular OP the subjects were exposed to. Furthermore, maternal OP exposure may not be restricted to preconception, to the first trimester of pregnancy, or to pregnancy.

The Volume 11 committee found a lack of relevant information in the animal literature on adverse birth outcomes associated with preconception or prenatal exposure to any of the relevant OPs considered in this chapter.

The Volume 11 committee concludes that there is limited/suggestive evidence of an association between exposure to OPs and reproductive effects in men.

The Volume 11 committee also concludes that there is inadequate/insufficient evidence to determine whether an association exists between exposure to OPs and reproductive effects in women, or with adverse pregnancy outcomes.

Developmental Effects

Research into the developmental effects in infants or children following prenatal exposure to OPs has focused primarily on neurodevelopmental effects, although effects on the respiratory system and the presence of childhood cancers have also been assessed (see Table 5-1).

The potential neurodevelopmental effects associated with prenatal exposure to OPs—and to chlorpyrifos in particular—have been the subject of several comprehensive reviews. In 2016 EPA concluded that the CCCEH study in New York City, along with other epidemiologic studies, provided "sufficient evidence that there are neurodevelopmental effects occurring at chlorpyrifos exposure levels below those required for AChE inhibition." The Volume 11 committee reviewed a number of studies of child neurodevelopment and prenatal OP exposure conducted in Spain, Mexico, and China, as well as the CCCEH, CHAMACOS, and Mount Sinai, and HOME cohort studies. Results of many, but not all, of these studies indicate that prenatal exposure to OPs can result in lower scores on developmental indices such as IQ and other assessment scales and that these deficits may persist up to at least the 9th year of life. In addition, associations have been found with attention deficits and tremor. The CHARGE study in California found that close prenatal proximity to OP application was associated with an increased risk for ASD (Shelton et al., 2014), and Burke et al. (2017) stated that "the association between cord blood levels of chlorpyrifos and neurodevelopmental outcomes cannot be ignored."

Assessment of the CHAMACOS cohort found increased respiratory symptoms, but no impairment of lung function, in children at 5 and 7 years of age as reported by mothers, although the increase was not associated with maternal DAP measures in the first half of pregnancy. Studies on the effects of prenatal OP exposure and the risks of childhood leukemia were inconsistent, although the one positive study examined both the father's and the mother's exposure prior to conception and in the first trimester. There was little information on the effects of prenatal OP exposure on the risk of birth defects or on other adverse childhood health effects.

In addition to the numerous epidemiologic studies discussed above, the Volume 11 committee considered more than 50 new animal studies, many of which discussed a variety of reproductive and developmental endpoints. Because of the large number of studies that assessed developmental effects from prenatal exposure to OPs, the committee described only those that specifically showed effects in early pregnancy compared with effects seen later in pregnancy. Animal studies indicate that early pregnancy exposures produce developmental toxicity, but it is unclear whether these effects would be expected for human pregnancies initiated after deployment ends since organ systems in animals and humans develop at different times during gestation.

The Volume 11 committee concludes that there is sufficient evidence of an association between prenatal exposure to OPs and neurodevelopmental effects.

The Volume 11 committee also concludes that there is inadequate/insufficient evidence to determine whether an association exists between prenatal exposure to OPs and other developmental effects.

TABLE 5-1 Summary of Neurodevelopmental Effects of Organophosphate Pesticides

Cohort	OP Exposure Measurements	Child's Age at Time of Assessment	Neurodevelopmental Effects
CCCEH Rauh et al. (2006, 2012, 2015)	Cord blood at delivery	12, 24, 36 months	At 36 months, decrease in PDI scores and motor skills with increase in ADHD and pervasive development disorder.
		7 years	Decrease in IQ and working memory; decrease greater in boys than girls. Adverse brain morphology.
Mt. Sinai Engel et al. (2007, 2011); Furlong et al. (2014)	Blood/urine in third trimester	<5 days	Increase in abnormal reflexes.
		12, 24 months, 6–9 years	Decrease MDI in nonwhites at 12, 24 months; whites had increased MDI; all effects more modest by 7–9 years old.
		7-9 years	No association of DAPs with Social Responsiveness Scale scores in whites and Hispanics; association with blacks; boys scored poorly compared with girls.
CHAMACOS Eskenazi et al. (2007, 2014); Young, et al. (2005); Marks et al. (2010); Bouchard et al. (2011); Eskenazi et al. (2014); Sagiv et al. (2018)	Urine in the third trimester	3 days	Increased DAPs associated with increase abnormal reflexes.
		6, 12, 24 months	Increased DAPs associated with decreased MDI at 24 months; increased risk of pervasive development disorder, but no effect on ADHD.
		3.5 and 5 years	ADHD not increased at 3.5 years but increased at 5 years; some effects associated only in boys.
		7 years	Increased DAP associated with decreased cognitive and IQ scores.
		6 months–14 years	DAPs showed association with poor social behavior and test performance. No association between proximity and ASD-related traits.
		7, 9, 10.5, 12, and 14 years	Increased DAPs associated with poor social skills but no other consistent associations with ASD symptoms.
HOME Donauer et al. (2016); Millenson et al. (2017)	Urine at 16 wks pregnancy	1, 2, 3, 4, 5 years	No association of DAPs with cognition at 1–5 years; at 5 years increased DAPs associated with increased verbal IQ, but attenuated after adjustment for covariates.
		8 years	No association of DAPs with child's social behavior.

Cohort	OP Exposure Measurements	Child's Age at Time of Assessment	Neurodevelopmental Effects
CHARGE study (Shelton et al., 2014)	Residential proximity to OP application	2–5 years	OPs in first trimester not associated with ASD, but increased risk for ASD with any OP exposure during pregnancy, highest for third-trimester exposures.
González-Alzaga et al. (2015) Spain	Urine sample prenatal	6–11 years	Increased prenatal OP exposure associated with decreased processing speed performance for boys but not girls.
Zhang et al. (2014a) China	Urine samples during pregnancy	3 days	Increased DAPs associated with decreased scores on neonatal behavioral neurological assessment test for both boys and girls.
Fortenberry et al. (2014) Mexico	Urine samples	6–11 years	No association of TCPy with ADHD.

NOTE: ADHD=attention deficit–hyperactivity disorder; ASD=autism spectrum disorder; CCCEH=Columbia Center for Children's Environmental Health study; CHAMACOS=Center for the Health Assessment of Mothers and Children of Salinas study; CHARGE=Childhood Autism Risk from Genetics and Environment; DAP=dialkylphosphates; DEP=diethylphosphate; HOME=Health Outcomes and Measures of the Environment study; IQ=intelligence quotient; MDI=mental development index; Mt. Sinai=Mount Sinai Children's Environmental Health Cohort; OP=organophosphate; PDI=psychomotor development index; TCPy=3,5,6-trichloro-2-pyridinol.

TABLE 5-2 Summary of Reproductive Effects of Organophosphate Pesticides

Study	Population	Exposure Assessment	Results
Reproductive Effects			
Reproductive Effects in Men			
Meeker et al. (2004a)	330 men in subfertile couples seeking infertility diagnosis at Massachusetts General Hospital (Boston) between January 2000 and April 2003.	No men reported occupational exposure to pesticides. A single spot urine sample was collected from each subject on the same day as the semen sample and analyzed for TCPy.	Suggestive but not statistically significant associations between TCPy levels with sperm concentration (medium level OR=2.1, 95% CI 0.8–5.6; high level OR=2.4, 95% CI 0.9–6.3; p-value for trend=0.09), sperm motility (medium OR=1.6, 95% CI 0.8–3.0; high OR=1.7, 95% CI 0.9–3.2; p-value for trend=0.09), and sperm morphology (medium OR=1.2, 95% CI 0.5–2.7; high OR=1.9, 95% CI 0.9–4.0; p-value for trend=0.10) compared to those with low TCPy levels.
Meeker et al. (2004b)	See Meeker et al. (2004a); semen samples available for 260 men; 46 samples excluded with specific gravity >1.03 or <1.01.	See Meeker et al. (2004a). TCPy measured in urine (geometric mean of 2.59 μg/L). Semen analyzed for DNA damage by the neutral comet assay and reported as comet extent, percentage DNA in comet tail (Tail%), and tail distributed moment (TDM).	A statistically significant increase in Tail% was found for an IQR increase in TCPy (β=2.76, 95% CI 0.89–4.62), while a decrease in TDM was associated with IQR changes in TCPy (β= –2.5, 95% CI –4.71– –0.22), the change in comet extent was not significant. A negative correlation between Tail% and TDM was present only when stratified by comet extent, suggesting that Tail% and TDM may measure different types of DNA damage within comet extent strata.
Figueroa et al. (2015)	Same population as Meeker et al. (2004a,b). 159 male subjects.	See Meeker et al. (2004a).	Of the 159 men, 10% (n=16) had sperm concentrations <15 million/mL, 21% (n=33) had <32% motile sperm, and 18% (n=28) had <4% normally shaped sperm based on the most recent WHO reference values for sperm concentration and the Tygerberg Strict Criteria for morphology. A significant inverse association was observed between DMP and total disomy.
Sánchez-Peña et al. (2004)	33 male agricultural workers in Durango, Mexico, ages 18–50.	Men provided semen and urine samples. Urine samples were analyzed for 6 DAPs: DMDTP, DMTP, DEDTP, DETP, DMP, and DEP. 87% of workers had at least one OP metabolite in their urine.	Most sperm samples had altered chromatin structure. About 75% of semen samples were classified as having poor fertility potential (>30% of DFI%) and 12% were classified as potentially fertile (<15% of DFI%), whereas only 4% of unexposed urban men were classified as having poor fertility potential. There were significant associations between urinary DETP concentrations and mean DFI (p=0.026), and standard deviation-DFI (p=0.022); no associations with any other DAP were found. 82% of exposed men versus 9% of unexposed men had immature germ cell values above the reference value. There were no significant associations found between DAP and semen quality parameters, although there was a negative correlation between mean DFI and sperm viability (r=0.254, p<0.027) and seminal volume (r=0.333; p<0.004).

Study	Population	Exposure Assessment	Results
Melgarejo et al. (2015)	Cross-sectional study in Murcia Region, Spain. Subjects recruited between December 2012 and July 2013. 162 men 25–38 years old (median age 35); 116 returned for semen analysis, had blood drawn, gave urine sample, and completed questionnaires.	Length of exposure not specified. Men attending infertility clinic. Urine analyzed for 6 DAPs.	At least one urinary OP metabolite detected for all men. Urinary DMP concentrations were signficiantly inversely correlated with percentage of motile sperm ($r = -0.23$, 95% CI –0.34– –0.05) and sperm with normal morphology ($r = -0.20$, 95% CI –0.36– –0.02); no other associations. Reproductive hormone levels within normal range for all men, but positive associations between DEDTP concentrations and LH ($\beta=11.4$, 95% CI 0.81–22.1) and FSH levels ($\beta=3.2$, 95% CI 0.08–6.2) and a negative correlation with the testosterone/LH ratio. Significant inverse association between concentrations of DMP, DMTP, and DMDTP, and ΣDAP and sperm concentration and total sperm count; between DMTP, DMDTP, and DEP concentrations and motile sperm; and between DMP and DMDTP concentrations and total motile sperm count.
Miranda-Contreras et al. (2013)	64 male farm workers (ages 18–52 years), 35 control males from city 90 km away.	Agricultural community in Venezuela; mixed exposure to OPs, carbamates, pyrethroids, and triazines. Exposed lived in area ≥2 years prior to the study, 53.5% of exposed males had worked in agriculture for >5 years; 75% sprayed pesticides 1–3 times/wk.	Levels of BuChE activity indicated that 87.5% of the pesticide sprayers had been exposed to OP and carbamate pesticides; 82.8% had mild BuChE inhibition. Significant differences in 3 of 9 semen parameters for exposed group: higher seminal pH ($p<0.004$), lower percent live sperm ($p<0.0001$), and rapid and progressive sperm motility ($p < 0.04$); the levels of testosterone, prolactin, FT4, and TSH appeared to be normal; a tendency for increased LH and FSH levels in the exposed group.
Perry et al. (2007)	Pilot biomonitoring study in 2004. 18 men living in Anhui, China; men were young and newly married.	Men lived in city and visited family in rural area where OPs and pyrethroids used. Urine samples analyzed for 24 pesticide metabolites, including 6 DAPs, TCPy, malathion dicarboxylic acid, 2-isopropyl-4-methyl-6-hydroxypyrimidinol (a diazinon metabolite); baseline sperm collected.	Significant difference in sperm concentration between men with high and low urine concentrations of DETP, but not DMTP (the only metabolites reported), with absolute sperm concentration difference for DETP= –1.0 (95% CI –1.8– –0.2).

continued

TABLE 5-2 Continued

Study	Population	Exposure Assessment	Results
Perry et al. (2011)	Continuation of Perry et al. (2007); 94 men and 95 controls living in Anqing City, China, who returned to rural area in winter.	Baseline urine analyzed for 6 DAPs. Cases (those with sperm concentrations and motility below population median) and controls were based on their median residual value of sperm concentration and motility adjusted for covariates.	Lower sperm concentration and motility in men with higher urinary concentration of DMP in cases compared with men with lower urinary concentrations (OR=1.30, 95% CI 1.02–1.65). No significant differences were seen between cases and controls for the other DAPs.
Recio-Vega et al. (2008)	Longitudinal follow-up study. 52 men living in Durango, Mexico, who provided 2 or more semen samples (total 139 samples).	Men lived in agricultural area, 17 non-occupationally exposed, 16 occupationally exposed but not OP sprayers, and 19 OP sprayers (highly exposed). Semen collected at times of low, median, and high OP use. Urine collected morning of day semen collected and analyzed for 6 DAPs.	DAPs were found in urine of 83% of participants, and levels were highest during heavy spraying season. Only semen volume and total sperm count were significantly lower in the highly exposed group (p=0.004 and p=0.01, respectively), the other semen parameters (sperm concentration, viability, motility, dead sperm, and rapid progressive motility) were not significantly different.
Yucra et al. (2008)	Cross-sectional study of 31 male OP pesticide applicators in Peru (ages 20–60) and 31 unexposed controls.	Urine, blood, and semen samples collected day after last pesticide application; urine analyzed for 6 DAPs.	Nine semen parameters were analyzed. DEDTP (p=0.04) and DETP (p=0.02) were more related to occupational exposure than other OP metabolites. Seminal pH was the only parameter significantly associated with urinary concentrations of ethylated (p=0.02) or methylated (p=0.002) DAPs; methylated DAPs were also associated with lower seminal vesicle function (p=0.04, seminal fructose levels). Holm's test used to correct for multiple comparisons.
Hossain et al. (2010)	Cross-sectional study of 62 male farmers in 3 communities in Malaysia with exposure to malathion (15 men) or paraquat (39 men) or both (8 men); 90 unexposed.	Pesticide exposure based on interviews with farmers; semen samples analyzed for volume, pH, sperm concentration, motility, morphology, and white blood count.	Results presented for exposed versus unexposed. The committee notes that grouping of all pesticide types together makes assessment impossible for malathion specifically. Exposed workers had a greater risk of abnormal sperm volume (OR=6.5, 95% CI 2.7–15.2), sperm concentration (OR=8.7, 95% CI 4–19), lower sperm motility (OR=5.1, 95% CI 2.5–10.5), sperm morphology (OR=4.9, 95% CI 1.6–14.6), and white blood cell count (OR=4.5, 95% CI 1.5–13.4).

Study	Population	Exposure Assessment	Results
Perez-Herrera et al. (2008)	Cross-sectional study; 54 agricultural workers (18–55 years old) in Yucatan, Mexico.	Men had chronic, year-round exposure to pesticides, mostly OPs (including CPF, malathion, and diazinon). Semen and blood samples collected.	Abnormal sperm morphology was seen in all 54 participants; 46% had low ejaculate volume, 30% had low sperm motility, and 13% had low sperm viability; however, sperm parameters were not associated with OP exposure during the month of semen collection or the 3 months prior to collection. For men with 192RR phenotype, there were significant associations between OP exposure at the month of sampling and NT-positive cells and sperm viability and a dose–effect relationship between OP exposure during 3 months before sampling and sperm quality parameters and NT-positive cells.
Al-Hussaini et al. (2018)	94 women in Egypt undergoing in vitro fertilization.	Follicular fluid collected from each woman at time of embryo transfer and analyzed for CPF, diazinon, and malation among other pesticides.	All three pesticide concentrations in follicular fluid were negatively correlated with endometrial thickness ($p<0.05$ for diazinon, $p<0.024$ for malathion, and $p<0.098$ for CPF). Diazinon and CPF, but not malation, were negatively associated with the number of oocytes retrieved and with a lower implantation rate (number of sacs) ($p<0.01$ for both pesticides and endpoints); none of the three were associated with reduced fertilization or early embryo cleavage rates.
Hu et al. (2018)	615 women (≥20 years of age) in Shanghai, China, recruited from two preconception care clinics during 2013–2015. 569 women were nulliparous. Women followed for 1 year prior to pregnancy.	4 DAPs measured in urine. Pyrethroid exposure also measured. Women asked about pesticide exposure and perceived stress and lifestyle.	Women in the highest quartile for DETP had longer TTP (fecundability OR=0.68, 95% CI 0.51–0.92) and increased infertility (OR=2.17, 95% CI 1.19–3.93) compared with women in lowest quartile. For nulliparous women only, the fecundability OR for TTP was 0.67 (95% CI 0.50–0.91), and the fertility OR was 2.30 (95% CI 1.23–4.30). There were no significant associations with the other 3 DAPs.
Adverse Pregnancy Outcomes			
Perera et al. (2003)	CCCEH cohort of 269 African American and Dominican women, 18–35 years old, enrolled into the cohort between 1998 and 2002.	Women wore personal monitor during the daytime hours for 2 consecutive days and placed the monitor near the bed at night. Maternal blood (30–35 mL) was collected within 1 day postpartum, and umbilical cord blood (30–60 mL) was collected at delivery.	CPF was detected in 98% of the maternal and 94% of the cord samples. CPF was significantly associated with decreased birth weight overall ($\beta= -0.04$, $p=0.01$) and among African Americans ($\beta= -0.05$, $p=0.04$), but not among Dominicans ($\beta= -0.03$, $p=0.11$). CPF was also associated with reduced birth length overall ($\beta= -0.01$, $p=0.003$) and in Dominicans ($\beta= -0.02$, $p<0.001$), but it was not significantly associated with head circumference.

continued

TABLE 5-2 Continued

Study	Population	Exposure Assessment	Results
Eskenazi et al. (2004)	CHAMACOS cohort of women living in agricultural area of Salinas Valley, CA; children born October 1999–October 2000; eligible n=488) women were ≥18 years of age, <20 weeks gestation at enrollment; DAP metabolites were measured in urine from mothers twice during pregnancy (mean=13 and 26 weeks gestation).	Gestational and preconception exposure, half of the women resided in United States for <5 years; approximately 28% had worked in the fields during pregnancy, another 14% worked at other agriculture jobs (e.g., packing shed, nursery, and greenhouse work). 85% of the women had agricultural workers living in their homes during their pregnancy. Exposure to OPs was measured in 3 ways: (1) DAP metabolites in maternal urine during pregnancy; (2) 7 different pesticide-specific metabolites in maternal urine during pregnancy; and (3) ChE in whole blood and BuChE in plasma collected from mothers during pregnancy and at delivery, and from the umbilical cord.	A 10-fold increase in average DAP metabolite concentration was associated with an increase in infant's body length of 0.52 cm (p=0.06) and in head circumference of 0.32 cm (p=0.03); similar increases in body length and head circumference were seen when DMP and DEP were examined separately, although these increases were not statistically significant. A 10-fold increase in average DMP but not DEP was associated with a 3-day decrease in gestational duration (p=0.02). After 22 weeks gestation, increasing levels of DMP had significant adverse association with gestational duration. DMP, DEP, and total DAP levels were not associated with birth weight, infant ponderal index, risk of preterm delivery, low birth weight, or small for gestational age births. Lower ChE levels in cord blood were associated with significantly shorter length of gestation, averaging 0.34 weeks (p=0.001) for each unit decrease in ChE (in moles/m/mL; range of ChE in cord blood is 4.4 units), with an increased risk of preterm delivery (OR=2.3, 95% CI 1.1–4.8, p=0.02), and with low birth weight (OR=4.3, 95% CI 1.1–17.5, p=0.04); however, 6 of the 11 low-birth-weight infants were also preterm. BuChE levels in maternal and cord blood were not associated with any birth outcome.
Harley et al. (2011)	CHAMACOS cohort; see Eskenazi et al. (2004).	See Eskenazi et al. (2004).	All women had detectable levels of OP pesticide metabolites in their urine during pregnancy; average DAP concentration during pregnancy was 146 nmol/L (95% CI 133–160); associations of PON1 with birth outcome were found only with PON1 measured in infants, not in mothers. No associations were found between any marker of *PON1* genotype or activity measured in maternal blood and gestational age or infant birth weight, length, and head circumference. Each 10-fold increase in maternal DAPs during pregnancy was associated with decrease in gestational age among $PON1_{-108TT}$ infants (β= –0.5, 95% CI –0.9–0.0) compared with $PON1_{192QQ}$ infants.

Study	Population	Exposure Assessment	Results
Rauch et al. (2012)	HOME Study, prospective birth cohort in Cincinnati area between March 2003 and January 2006. 344 women who met eligibility criteria.	Continuous residential exposure. Mothers gave blood and spot urine samples at 16 and 26 weeks gestation, and within 24 hours of delivery. Measured 6 urinary DAPs.	All mothers had detectable levels of at least one DAP metabolite. A 10-fold increase in ΣDAP concentrations was associated with a 0.5-week decrease in gestational age (95% CI –0.8– –0.1]); birth weight was also inversely associated with ΣDAP concentrations (–151 g, 95% CI –287– –16); no evidence for main effects of *PON1* genotype on either birth weight or length of gestation.
Berkowitz et al. (2004)	Mount Sinai Children's Environmental Cohort Study of ethnically diverse mother–infant pairs in New York City. Babies born between May 1998 and July 2002 (n=404); maternal blood and urine samples taken at 26 weeks gestation.	Mothers in third trimester answered questionnaire about pesticide and other environmental exposures. 46.2% of women reported that they or a household member had used indoor pesticides during the pregnancy. Cord blood samples used to determine maternal and infant PON1 activity and polymorphisms.	No significant associations between adjusted birth outcomes and TCPy, PBA, or PCP levels above and below the LOD. A significant positive trend was found between maternal PON1 activity and head circumference among the offspring of mothers whose TCPy levels were above the LOD. A similar trend was seen for mothers with TCPy levels below the LOD, but this was not significant. The test for interaction among TCPy level, PON1 activity, and head circumference was not statistically significant ($p>0.05$). PON1 activity had no association with any of the fetal growth measures.
Harley et al. (2016)	See Engel et al. (2016); (1) CHAMACOS, (2) HOME, (3) CCCEH, and (4) Mt. Sinai birth cohorts.	See Engel et al. (2016).	No significant associations of ΣDEP, ΣDMP, or ΣDAPs with birth weight, length, or head circumference overall. Among non-Hispanic black women, increasing urinary ΣDAP and ΣDMP concentrations were associated with decreased birth length (β= –0.4 cm; 95% CI –0.9–0.0 and β= –0.4 cm; 95% CI –0.8–0.0, respectively, for each 10-fold increase in metabolite concentration). Among infants with the $PON1_{192RR}$ genotype, ΣDAP and ΣDMP were negatively associated with length (β= –0.4 cm; 95% CI –0.9–0.0 and β= –0.5 cm; 95% CI –0.9– –0.1).

continued

TABLE 5-2 Continued

Study	Population	Exposure Assessment	Results
Wang et al. (2012)	187 healthy pregnant women from Shanghai, China, were recruited to participate in this study from September 1, 2006 to January 31, 2007.	Information about pesticide use for a woman herself or other household members during pregnancy and, if so, the types of pesticides and frequency of use; paternal OP exposure and occupation were also collected through personal interview. Urine samples collected at onset of labor; urine analyzed for 5 DAPs.	No significant associations between fetal growth (assessed as birth weight and body length) or length of gestation and any measure of in utero OP exposure. However, a significant inverse association was found between DEP level and duration of gestation ($\beta = -1.79$; $p=0.001$) for infant girls after stratification by gender; this association was not seen for boys ($\beta=0.17$; $p=0.164$).

NOTE: BuChE=butyryl cholinesterase; CCCEH=Columbia Center for Children's Environmental Health study; CHAMACOS=Center for the Health Assessment of Mothers and Children of Salinas study; ChE=cholinesterase; CI=confidence interval; CPF=chlorpyrifos; DAP=dialkyl phosphate; DEDTP=diethyldithiophosphate; DEP=diethylphosphate; DETP=diethylthiophosphate; DFI=DNA fragmentation index; DMDTP=dimethyldithiophosphate; DMP=dimethylphosphate; DMTP=dimethyl thiophosphate; DNA=deoxyribonucleic acid; FT4=free thyroxine; FSH=follicle-stimulating hormone; HOME=Health Outcomes and Measures of the Environment study; IQR=interquartile range; LH=luteinizing hormone; LOD=level of detection; NT=nick translation; OP=organophosphate; OR=odds ratio; PBA=3-phenoxybenzoic acid; PCP=pentachlorophenol; PON1=paraoxonase; TCPy=3,5,6-trichloro-2-pyridinol; TDM=tail distributed moment; TTP=time to pregnancy; TSH=thyroid-stimulating hormone; WHO=World Health Organization.

TABLE 5-3 Summary of Developmental Effects of Organophosphate Pesticides

Study	Population	Exposure	Outcomes
Neurodevelopmental Effects			
Rauh et al. (2012)	CCCEH cohort, 40 children.	Subgroup of 20 children who had CPF exposure levels in the upper tertile of distribution and 20 children from the lowest tertile. All children had no/very low prenatal ETS exposure and low prenatal PAH exposure levels measured by third-trimester personal monitoring of mothers; children had usable MRI imaging data and 7-year cognitive testing using the WISC-IV.	Overall brain size did not differ significantly across exposure groups, adjusted for age, sex, and height; high-CPF group had significant enlargement of several brain areas: superior temporal, posterior middle temporal, and inferior postcentral gyri bilaterally, and enlarged superior frontal gyrus, gyrus rectus, cuneus, and precuneus along the medial wall of the right hemisphere. Group differences were derived from exposure effects on underlying white matter. Significant exposure × IQ interaction was derived from CPF disruption of normal IQ associations with surface measures in low-exposure children. High-exposure children did not show expected sex differences in the right inferior parietal lobule and superior marginal gyrus, and they displayed reversal of sex differences in the right medial superior frontal gyrus; they also showed frontal and parietal cortical thinning and an inverse dose–response relationship between CPF and cortical thickness.
Horton et al. (2012)	CCCEH cohort study. Subjects included 335 mother–child pairs selected from an ongoing prospective cohort study. Pregnant women ages 18–35 years who self-identified as either African American or Dominican.	Children assessed at age 7 with WISC-IV. Children's home environments were evaluated at 3 years of age; maternal prenatal urine samples from third trimester.	Significant interaction between prenatal exposure to CPF and child sex (β= –1.714, 95% CI –3.753–0.326), suggesting males experience a greater decrement in working memory than females following prenatal CPF exposure.

continued

TABLE 5-3 Continued

Study	Population	Exposure	Outcomes
Engel et al. (2007)	Mount Sinai Children's Environmental Health Cohort is a prospective multiethnic cohort study; 404 mother–infant pairs were recruited during pregnancy between May 1998 and July 2001.	Mothers answered exposure questionnaire and gave blood and urine samples about gestational week 31.2; neonatal behavior and/or primitive reflexes measured with BNBAS w/in 5 days of birth; mother's urine analyzed for MDA and 6 DAPs: DMDTP, DMTP, DEDTP, DETP, DMP, and DEP.	Urine MDA levels above the LOD and ΣDEP metabolites were associated with RRs of 2.24 (95% CI 1.55–3.24) and 1.49 (95% CI 1.1–1.98), respectively, for the number of abnormal reflexes. Mothers with elevated MDA levels delivered infants who were 3.6 times more likely to have at least 2 abnormal reflexes (95% CI 1.5–8.8), and babies born to mothers with elevated ΣDEP were 2.3 times more likely to have at least 2 abnormal reflexes (95% CI 1.1–5.0). Higher levels of ΣDEP and ΣDAPs were associated with increase in abnormal reflexes. Strong interaction between PON1 expression levels and ΣDMP on risk of abnormal reflexes: infants born to women in the first (interaction p=0.002) and second (interaction p=0.01) tertiles (slower metabolizers) had a greater risk of abnormal reflexes than infants in the highest tertile (fast metabolizers). For women in the highest tertile of PON1 expression, no increased risk of abnormal reflexes with increasing exposure was found. There was no interaction between ΣDEP and PON1.
Furlong et al. (2017a)	Mt. Sinai cohort study; see Engel et al. (2007).	Children assessed at 6–9 years using WPPSI-III at age 6 and WISC-IV between the ages of 7 and 9 years. Parents completed the BRIEF questionnaire and BASC at child's age 6 and 7–9 years.	Factor analysis used to derive 7 neurodevelopment phenotypes. Maternal DMP metabolites in urine were negatively associated with one phenotype internalizing factor (β= –0.13, 95% CI –0.26–0.00) but positively associated with the executive functioning factor (β=0.18, 95% CI 0.04–0.31). However, DEP metabolites were negatively associated with the working memory index of the WISC-IV (β= –0.17, 95% CI –0.33– –0.03).

Study	Population	Exposure	Outcomes
Marks et al. (2010)	CHAMACOS cohort, see Eskenazi et al. (2004). Children were assessed at ages 3.5 years (n=331) and 5 years (n=323).	Mothers completed the CBCL. NEPSY-II visual attention subtest administered to children at 3.5 years and K-CPT at 5 years. The K-CPT yielded a standardized ADHD confidence index score. Psychometricians scored behavior of the 5-year-olds during testing using the Hillside Behavior Rating Scale. Total DAPs were measured in maternal urine collected at two time points during pregnancy and in child urine collected at the 3.5-year and 5-year visits.	Prenatal DAPs were not associated with maternal reports of attention problems and ADHD at age 3.5 years but were significantly related at age 5 years (CBCL attention problems: β=0.7 points, 95% CI 0.2–1.2; ADHD: β=1.3, 95% CI 0.4–2.1). Prenatal DAPs were associated with scores on the K-CPT ADHD confidence index >70th percentile (OR=5.1, 95% CI 1.7–15.7) and with a composite ADHD indicator of the various measures (OR=3.5, 95% CI 1.1–10.7). Some outcomes exhibited evidence of effect modification by sex, with associations found only among boys.
Bouchard et al. (2011)	CHAMACOS cohort; mothers of 329 7-year-old children were slightly older and breast-fed longer than those from the initial cohort.	Most commonly used OP pesticides in the Salinas Valley are CPF and diazinon (which devolve to DE) and malathion and oxydemeton-methyl (which devolve to DM). Maternal urine samples from first (median, 13th week of gestation) and second half (median, 26th week of gestation) of pregnancy analyzed for 3 DAPs. Administered WISC-IV at the 7-year study visit.	DAP levels were associated with lower cognitive scores on all subtests in children at 7 years old, but were most significant for verbal comprehension (13-wk β= –2.6, 95% CI –5.1– –0.1; 26-wk β= –3.1, 95% CI –6.4–0.2) and full-scale IQ (13-wk β= –2.4, 95% CI –4.9–0.2; 26-wk β= –3.5, 95% CI –6.9– –0.1). Higher prenatal DAP concentrations were associated with lower scores on all four cognitive domains, the strongest associations being for verbal comprehension (β for a 10-fold increase in concentration= –5.3; 95% CI –8.6– –2.0). A 10-fold increase in DAP concentrations was associated with 5.6-point decrease in full-scale IQ (95% CI –9.0– –2.2).
Eskenazi et al. 2014	CHAMACOS cohort; 296 children assessed at 5 years of age and 327 assessed at 7 years of age.	Children administered the K-CPT at 5 years and the WISC-IV at 7 years; DAPs measured in maternal and child urine samples, and analyzed $PON1_{192}$ and $PON1_{-108}$ genotypes and enzyme activity [arylesterase (ARYase), paraoxonase (POase)] in maternal and child blood.	Maternal and child *PON1* genotype was not related to performance on K-CPT or WISC. Pregnancy ARYase levels were positively associated with all WISC subscales (e.g., 4.0 point increase in full-scale IQ per ARYase increase, 95% CI 1.6–6.4). Pregnancy POase levels were positively associated with WISC processing speed only. The association between DAPs and full-scale IQ was strongest for children of mothers with lowest-tertile ARYase levels (p interaction=0.27).

continued

TABLE 5-3 Continued

Study	Population	Exposure	Outcomes
Huen et al. 2018	CHAMACOS cohort; 238 children assessed at 7 years of age	Cord blood and blood samples from children collected at 7 years old assessed for *PON1* DNA methylation using Illumina 450K and EPIC BeadChip arrays; administered WISC-IV full-scale IQ and 4 composite measures (verbal comprehension, perceptual reasoning, working memory, and processing) at the 7-year study visit.	Cord blood *PON1* DNA methylation CpG sites were not significantly associated with any decrements in the 5 neurobehavioral scores after adjustment for false discovery rate (p-values all >0.05).
Gunier et al. (2017)	CHAMACOS cohort, see Eskenazi et al. (2004) 283 mother–child pairs.	Children assessed for neurodevelopment at 7 years old using WISC-IV. Agricultural pesticide use within 1 km of mother's residence during pregnancy estimated using California Pesticide Use Reporting data from 1999–2001. Maternal urine analyzed for 6 DAPs.	Increased exposure to OPs during pregnancy was significantly associated with an estimated 2.2-point decrease in full-scale IQ (95% CI –3.9 – –0.5) and a 2.9-point decrease in verbal comprehension (95% CI –4.4– –1.3). Only increases in CPF and diazinon use were significantly associated with a decrease in verbal comprehension, malathion was not. There were no significant changes in other WISC domains.
Sagiv et al. (2018)	CHAMACOS cohort, see Eskenazi et al. (2004) 246 mother–child pairs.	Children assessed at 7, 10.5, and 14 years old. Parents reported child's social behavior with SRS-2 at age 14 years and BASC-2 at 7, 10.5, and 14 years. Teachers also used BASC-2 for 7-year-olds. At 9 years old, children tested with Evaluación Neuropsicológica Infantil Facial Expression Recognition Test and at age 12 years, the NEPSY-II Affect Recognition subtest.	In 14-year-olds, a 10-fold increase in prenatal DAPs was associated with 2.7-point increase (95% CI 0.9–4.5) in parent-reported SRS-2 T-scores (a measure of ASD behaviors). Scores on the social communication and interaction test and the restricted and repetitive behaviors tests were not significantly associated with DAP concentrations. Increased DAPs were associated with parent and teacher reports of BASC-2 social skills T-scores, which indicate poorer social skills. In 9-year- and 12-year-olds, DAPs were not associated with affect recognition measured with the Evaluación Neuropsicológica Infantil or the NEPSY-II, respectively. There were no consistent associations across sex for any of the outcomes.

Study	Population	Exposure	Outcomes
Donauer et al. (2016)	HOME study. Prospective pregnancy and birth cohort study. Subjects were 327 mother–infant pairs in Cincinnati, Ohio, between February 2003 and January 2006.	Spot urine samples were collected from the mothers at 2 time points about 16 and 26 weeks' gestation. BSID-II MDI and PDI administered at ages 1, 2, and 3 years, the Clinical Evaluation of Language Fundamentals-Preschool, Second Edition, at age 4, and the WPPSI-III at age 5.	No associations between prenatal exposure to OPs and cognition at 1–5 years of age. At 2-year visit, total DMP and total DEP were associated with BSID-II MDI at the $p<0.20$ level after controlling for relevant covariates ($\beta=0.002$ and $\beta=0.002$). At 5 years, total DAP and total DM were positively associated with full-scale IQ at the $p<0.20$ level after controlling for relevant covariates ($\beta=0.001$ and $\beta=0.002$, respectively). Finally, total DAP, total DM, and total DE were positively associated with verbal IQ at the $p<0.20$ level after controlling for relevant covariates ($\beta=0.003$, $\beta=0.003$, and $\beta=-0.027$, respectively). No associations between prenatal exposure to OPs and cognition at 1–5 years of age.
Millenson et al. (2017)	Prospective cohort study. 224 pregnant women in the Cincinnati HOME study. Child PON1 polymorphisms determined from cord blood. Children 8 years old.	6 OP insecticide metabolite concentrations from two urine samples collected at ~16 and ~26 weeks gestation; analyzed for 6 DAPs. Children administered SRS.	ΣDAP concentrations were not associated with SRS scores ($\beta=-1.2$, 95% CI –4.0–1.6). Among 8-year-old children with the $PON1_{-108TT}$ genotype, ΣDAP concentrations were associated with 2.5-point higher (95% CI –4.9–9.8) SRS scores; however, the association was not different from the 1.8-point decrease (95% CI –5.8–2.2) among children with $PON1_{-108CT/CC}$ genotypes (ΣDAP × $PON1_{-108}$ p-value=0.54). The association between ΣDAP concentrations and SRS scores was not modified by $PON1_{192}$ (ΣDAP × $PON1_{192}$ p value=0.89). Urinary DAP concentrations were not associated with children's social behaviors; these associations were not modified by child PON1 genotype.

continued

TABLE 5-3 Continued

Study	Population	Exposure	Outcomes
Engel et al. (2016) (Analysis of 4 cohort studies)	Pooled data from (1) CHAMACOS; (2) HOME in Ohio; (3) Columbia Center for Childrens' Environmental Health study of urban population residing in South Bronx or Northern Manhattan in New York City; (4) urban population consisting of women receiving antenatal care at the Mount Sinai Hospital or two private obstetric practices in New York City.	Variable, maternal residential exposures preconception, during pregnancy and postnatal. (1) 2 urine samples at 13 and 26 weeks gestation averaged on a creatinine corrected basis; (2) 2 urine samples at 16 and 26 weeks gestation averaged on a creatinine-corrected basis; (3) 1 urine sample at 32 weeks gestation; (4) 1 urine sample at 31 weeks gestation.	10-fold increase in prenatal exposure to ΣDAPs is associated with an approximate 1-point decrease in the 24-month MDI, whether pooled across four cohorts without adjustment for race/ethnicity (β= –1.28, 95% CI –2.58–0.03) or pooled across race/ethnicities without adjustment for cohort (β= –1.48, 95% CI –2.77– –0.19). Evidence of heterogeneity in associations of ΣDAPs with the MDI according to $PON1_{-108C/T}$ genotype among whites, heterogeneity with ΣDEPs and MDI according to $PON1_{Q192R}$ in the whole population, and with ΣDAPs and $PON1_{Q192R}$ among both whites and blacks. There was no evidence of an association with the psychomotor development index.
Silver et al. (2017)	Zhejiang province, China. 237 infants born in Fuyang Maternal and Children's Hospital between 2008 and 2011.	30 OPs analyzed for in cord blood. Motor function assessed at 6 weeks and 9 months with PDMS.	CPF detected in 36.7% of samples. At 6 weeks, no significant associations between CPF and PDMS outcomes. At 9 months, chlorpyrifos-exposed infants had significantly lower PDMS scores than unexposed infants for reflexes (p=0.04), locomotion (p=0.02), grasping (p=0.05), visuomotor integration (p<0.001), gross motor (p=0.007), fine motor (p=0.002), and total motor (p<0.001) scores.
Wang et al. (2017)	Laizhou Wan Birth Cohort study in Shandong, China. 436 mothers recruited from March 2011 to December 2013, 297 12-month-old infants and 262 24-month-old children.	Urine samples collected from mothers at delivery and from 12- and 24-month-old children. Analyzed for 6 DAP metabolites. Gesell Developmental Schedules (motor, adaptive, language, and social domains) used to assess neurodevelopment.	Prenatal OP exposure was negatively associated with 24-month-old children's development quotients, especially among boys. A 10-fold increase in prenatal diethyl and total DAPs was associated with a 2.59- and 2.49-point decrease in social domain development quotient scores in 24-month-old children (n=262), respectively. Prenatal exposure to OPs was not related to 12-month-old infants' development quotients.

Study	Population	Exposure	Outcomes
González-Alzaga et al. (2015)	This was an ambispective study. Subjects included 305 (156 boys and 149 girls) children ages 6–11 years old who were randomly selected from public schools in southeastern Spain. Average age was 8.1 years for boys and 8.4 for girls. 291 (149 boys and 142 girls) children provided a urine sample in the period of low exposure and 270 (137 boys and 133 girls) in the period of high exposure.	OP exposure assessed by biomonitoring of maternal urinary levels of metabolites of these compounds at two time points of the same crop season, representing low and high pesticide use (January–February and October 2010). Both prenatal and postnatal residential exposure to pesticides estimated by developing a GIS-technology-based index that integrated distance-weighted measure of agricultural surface, time-series of crop areas per municipality and year, and land-use maps. Cognitive performance measured with WISC-IV.	Prenatal exposure index was significantly associated with a poorer score in processing speed subtest in boys (β= –5.7, 95% CI –9.6 – –1.8) but not in girls (β= –1.6, 95% CI –6.4–3.3). There was a non-significant inverse association with performance in the remaining subtests of the WISC-IV scale for full-scale IQ, verbal comprehension, and perceptual reasoning, but not for working memory.
Respiratory Effects			
Raanan et al. (2015)	CHAMACOS cohort; see Eskenazi et al. (2004); examined relationship between early-life exposure to OPs and respiratory outcomes.	See Eskenazi et al. (2004). (Note: Only data on prenatal exposure in first half of pregnancy is given as closest to Gulf War exposures; postnatal exposures are not relevant for this report.)	Higher prenatal DAP concentrations in the first half of pregnancy were nonsignificantly associated with respiratory symptoms in the previous 12 months at 5 or 7 years of age (OR per 10-fold increase=1.11, 95% CI 0.72–1.72) and with exercise-induced coughing (OR=1.24, 95% CI 0.58–2.66).
Raanan et al. (2016)	See Raanan et al. (2015).	Spirometry was performed at age 7 years.	Mothers' DAP urinary concentrations in either half of pregnancy were not significantly associated with lung function measurements (FEV_1, FVC, FEV_1/FVC ratio and $FEF_{25–75}$) in their children.

continued

TABLE 5-3 Continued

Study	Population	Exposure	Outcomes
		Childhood Cancer	
Monge et al. (2007)	N=334 subjects with cases of leukemia ages 0–14 years old. Diagnosed in Costa Rica during 1995–2000. Population controls (N=579).	22 pesticides were identified as high priority on the basis of historical data on use and toxicity data. OPs included malathion and dichlorvos.	Mothers' exposures to any pesticides during the year before conception and during the first and second trimesters were associated with risk of leukemia (OR=2.4, 95% CI 1.0–5.9; OR=22, 95% CI 2.8–171.5; OR=4.5, 95% CI 1.4–14.7, respectively) and during anytime (OR=2.2, 95% CI 1.0–4.8). Association with fathers' exposures to any pesticides during the second trimester (OR=1.5, 95% CI 1.0–2.3). Increased risk with mother's exposure to OPs during the first trimester (OR=3.5, 95% CI 1.0–12.2) and for fathers during the year before conception and the first trimester (OR=1.5, 95% CI 1.0–2.2 and OR=0.6, 95% CI 1.0–2.6, respectively).
Other Developmental Effects			
Carmichael et al. (2014)	569 cases of children born 1997–2006 with 1 of 7 congential heart defects in 1 of 8 counties in San Joaquin Valley, CA, and 785 infants born without birth defects. Birth defects (heterotaxia; tetralogy of Fallot; hypoplastic left heart syndrome; coarctation of the aorta; pulmonary valve stenosis; ventricular spetal defect, perimembranous; and atrial septal defect, secundum) based on California Birth Defects Monitoring Program.	Pesticide exposure was estimated for each mother on the basis of her residence from 3 months prior to conception to delivery using geospatial coding for eight San Joaquin counties and the Pesticide Use Reporting records for pesticides applied at greater than 100 lbs in any of the eight counties.	Prenatal exposure to CPF was significantly associated with pulmonary valve stenosis (OR=2.4, 95% CI 1.0–6.3) and with atrial septal defects, secundum (OR=1.9, 95% CI 1.1–3.4). Prenatal exposure to OPs as a group was associated with an increase in pulmonary valve stenosis as well (OR=2.5, 95% CI 1.2–5.0).

Study	Population	Exposure	Outcomes
Carmichael et al. (2016)	367 cases of children born with 1 of 5 birth defects. See Carmichael et al. (2014). Birth defects (anotia/microtia; anorectal atresia/stenosis; transverse limb deficiency; craniosynostosis; and diaphragmatic hernia) based on California Birth Defects Monitoring Program.	See Carmichael et al. (2014).	Prenatal exposure to OPs as a group (based on mechanism of action) was not significantly associated with anorectal atresia/stenosis (OR=0.4, 95% CI 0.2–0.9), but was significantly associated with craniosynostosis (OR=1.9, 95% CI 1.1–3.2); CPF specifically was significantly associated with anotia (OR=2.0, 95% CI 1.1–3.8) and craniosynostosis (OR=2.4, 95% CI 1.2–4.6). The ORs for all other OPs or birth defects were ≥0.5 or ≤2.0 or the CI included 1.0.
Buscail et al. (2015)	PELAGIE cohort of subsample of 248 pregnant women from Brittany, France, from January 2002 to February 2006, recuited before the 19th week of gestation; women provided urine sample, cord blood sample, and umbilical cord sample.	Urine analyzed for 6 DAPs; maternal exposure during pregnancy reported via questionnaire.	No association between any outcome and residential proximity to crops. Positive association between the highest tertile of DMPs and recurrent otitis media occurrence was found in the complete-case analysis (OR=2.90, 95% CI 1.12–7.48, p-value for trend=0.02), but it was no longer statistically significant after multiple imputations (OR=1.76, 95% CI 0.82–3.77, p-value for trend=0.13). No statistically significant association was found between urinary concentrations of other OP insecticide metabolites and either otitis media or recurrent otitis media.

NOTE: ADHD=attention deficit–hyperactivity disorder; ASD=autism spectrum disorder; BASC=Behavior Assessment System for Children; BNBAS=Brazelton Neonatal Behavioral Assessment Scale; BRIEF=Behavior Rating Inventory of Executive Functioning; BSID-II=Bayley Scales of Infant Development II; CBCL= Child Behavior Checklist; CCCEH=Columbia Center for Children's Environmental Health study; CHAMACOS=Center for the Health Assessment of Mothers and Children of Salinas study; CI=confidence interval; CPF=chlorpyrifos; CpG=cytosine-adjacent-to-guanine; DAP=dialkyl phosphate; DE=diethyl alkyl metabolites; DEDTP=diethyldithiophosphate; DEP=diethylphosphate; DETP=diethylthiophosphate; DM=dimethyl alkyl metabolites; DMDTP=dimethyldithiophosphate; DMP=dimethylphosphate; DMTP=dimethylthiophosphate; ETS=environmental tobacco smoke; FEF_{25-75}=forced expiratory flow at 25–75%; FEV_1=forced expiratory volume in 1 second; FVC=forced vital capacity; GIS=geospatial information system; HOME=Health Outcomes and Measures of the Environment study; IQ=intelligence quotient; K-CPT=Conners' Kiddie Continuous Performance Test; LOD=level of detection; MDA=malathion dicarboxylic acid; MDI=mental development index; MRI=magnetic resonance imaging; Mt. Sinai=Mount Sinai Children's Environmental Health Cohort; NEPSY-II=Developmental NEuroPSYchological Assessment; OP=organophosphate; OR=odds ratio; PAH=polyaromatic hydrocarbons; PDI=psychomotor development index; PDMS=Peabody Developmental Motor Scales; PON1=paraoxonase; SRS=Social Responsiveness Scale; WISC-IV=Wechsler Intelligence Scale for Children, 4th edition; WPPSI-III=Wechsler Preschool and Primary Scales of Intelligence-III.

CARBAMATES

Three carbamate pesticides—propoxur, carbaryl, and methomyl—are among the agents listed in Gulf War legislation P.L. 105-277 and P.L. 105-368[3] and therefore were considered by the Volume 2 and Volume 11 committees. Carbamates have a similar mechanism of toxicity to that of OPs—that is, they both inhibit acetylcholinesterases. Not all carbamates are pesticides; some, such as pyridostigmine bromide (discussed as a distinct deployment-related exposure in Chapter 4), have medicinal uses. Unlike OPs, the effects of carbamate poisoning tend to be of shorter duration because their inhibition of nervous tissue acetylcholinesterase is reversible, and carbamates are more rapidly metabolized (Roberts and Reigart, 2013).

Indoor residential uses of propoxur were cancelled in 2007, and as of 2016, it is no longer used in pet flea collars. However, it continues to be sold for commercial and residential control of cockroaches and other insect infestations. Methomyl is used as fly bait and in agricultural applications, but it has no residential uses. Carbaryl has both agricultural and residential uses and is widely sold under the brand name Sevin®.

As with the OP pesticides, metabolites of carbamate pesticides detected in the urine and blood can be used to indicate exposure. Urinary metabolites of carbaryl include 1- and 2-naphthol, and 2-isopropoxyphenol is a propoxur metabolite that has been detected in human blood. The elimination half-life in humans of 1-naphthol in urine is about 3.6 hours for an oral carbaryl dose of 0.008 mg/kg (Sams, 2017).

There are no ATSDR toxicological profiles available for any of the carbamates. The California Office of Environmental Health Hazard Assessment lists carbaryl as a male and female toxicant as well as a developmental toxicant (OEHHA, 2018).

Table 5-4 at the end of this section summarizes the studies used by the Volume 11 committee to draw its conclusions.

Reproductive Effects

Reproductive Effects in Men and Women

The Volume 2 committee found little relevant information on the reproductive and developmental effects of human or animal exposure to propoxur and methomyl. The committee did review several epidemiologic studies that assessed reproductive effects associated with exposure to either carbamates in general or to carbaryl specifically. The Volume 11 committee found a similar dearth of epidemiologic information on propoxur and methomyl and only one set of studies on carbaryl published since *Volume 2*.

In *Volume 2*, two studies on sperm effects in the same cohort of male carbaryl production workers were assessed (Whorton et al., 1979; Wyrobek et al., 1981); they reported that compared with unexposed controls there was an exposure-dependent increase in the number of oligospermic men among the male carbaryl production workers (p=0.07). There was also an increase in teratospermic men (having more than 60% abnormal sperm), but the increase was not dose-dependent. The latter study also found that men who were younger or who had more years of exposure had a greater proportion of abnormal sperm. The Volume 2 committee concluded that both of these cross-sectional studies had flaws in their methodology, including the choice of chemical workers as controls and crude measures of exposure.

The Volume 11 committee identified two new studies that examined reproductive effects in men (see Table 5-4). Meeker and colleagues (2004a,b, 2006, 2008a) completed a series of reports on the effects of low-level environmental exposure on human sperm and male reproductive hormones. Men (n=330) who were recruited from an infertility clinic provided semen and urine samples; the latter were analyzed for

[3] Persian Gulf War Veterans Act of 1998—P.L. 105-277; Veterans Program Enhancement Act of 1998—P.L. 105-368.

1-naphthol, a urinary metabolite of carbaryl. None of the subjects reported being occupationally exposed to carbaryl or other pesticides. Compared with the lowest-exposure tertile, ORs for the medium and high tertiles of 1-naphthol and below-reference sperm concentration were 4.2 (95% CI 1.4–13.0), and 4.2 (95% CI 1.4–12.6; p-value for trend=0.01); for 1-naphthol exposures and sperm motility, the ORs were 2.5 (95% CI 1.3–4.7) and 2.4 (95% CI 1.2–4.5; p-value for trend=0.01). There was no association between 1-naphthol and abnormal sperm morphology. However, increasing carbaryl exposure was associated with increasing DNA damage as determined by the neutral comet assay. Reduced testosterone and estradiol levels were associated with carbaryl exposures but were not dose-dependent.

In a study of 16 production workers in China who had occupational exposure to carbaryl for at least 1 year, no significant differences in semen volume, sperm concentration, sperm number per ejaculum, or sperm motility were seen between the carbaryl-exposed workers and members of two control groups (12 unexposed workers in the same plant and 18 workers outside the plant) (Xia et al., 2005). However, morphological defects such as sperm abnormalities were significantly higher in the exposed workers than in the external control group ($p=0.008$), as were the frequencies of disomic sex-chromosome-bearing (highest the XY-bearing) and disomic chromosome 18 spermatozoa ($p<0.05$ and/or $p<0.01$, respectively).

The Volume 2 committee also considered several studies on fertility and carbamate exposure. Several researchers reported on the large Ontario Farm Family Health Study, which assessed both male and female exposures to pesticides during the month of attempted conception or at any time during the previous 2 months. Neither maternal-only nor paternal-only exposure to carbaryl was associated with significant effects on TTP; the close correlation of exposures between members of a couple made it difficult to determine whether any effects were specifically maternally or paternally mediated (Curtis et al., 1999).

Adverse Pregnancy Outcomes

In the Ontario Farm Family Health Study reviewed by the Volume 2 committee, both male and female exposures to pesticides were assessed during the month of attempted conception or at any time during the previous 2 months (Curtis et al., 1999). For men who reported working with carbaryl, there was a significant increase in spontaneous abortions, although there was no association with altered sex ratios, small for gestational-age deliveries, or preterm births (Savitz et al., 1997). A further analysis of preconception exposure for the couple as a unit showed no increased risk for overall, early, or late spontaneous abortions (Arbuckle et al., 2001).

Bell et al. (2001) studied the relationship between fetal death and maternal residential proximity to agricultural areas in California with pesticide applications. They found that exposure to carbamates from the third to eighth week of pregnancy was not significantly associated with an increased risk of fetal death due to congenital abnormalities. Wives of pesticide applicators were at increased risk of spontaneous abortion, although the Volume 2 committee noted that the study had few details on its methodology.

The Volume 11 committee reviewed one study (see Table 5-4) and one EPA summary on the effects of exposure to carbamate pesticides on fetal growth and birth outcomes.

Whyatt et al. (2004, 2005) assessed birth outcomes in women enrolled in the CCCEH study between 1998 and 2002. All women had detectable levels of chlorpyrifos, diazinon, and propoxur in personal air samples collected at their homes over a 48-hour period during their third trimester. The insecticides were detected in 45–74% of blood samples collected from the mothers and newborns at delivery. Among the birth outcomes measured in newborns (birth weight, birth length, and head circumference), for those born before 2001 only the association between 2-isopropoxyphenol (a propoxur metabolite) and decreased birth length was statistically significant ($\beta=-0.73$ cm/unit, $p=0.01$); for those born after January 1, 2001, the association remained inverse, but the magnitude of the effect was less and no longer significant ($\beta=-0.30$ cm/unit, $p=0.56$).

Animal Studies

Volume 2 reported on two animal studies on the effects of carbaryl on sperm. When 50 mg or 100 mg carbaryl/kg was fed to rats 5 days per week for 60 or 90 days, dose- and age-dependent decreases in sperm count and motility and increased abnormal sperm structure were observed, particularly in young animals (Pant et al., 1995, 1996). In a sperm-abnormality assay, rats fed carbaryl for 3, 6, 9, 12, 15, and 18 months at 12.5, 25, and 250 mg/kg per day had genotoxic effects (Luca and Balan, 1987).

The Volume 2 committee further reported that the reproductive toxicity of carbaryl has been examined in rats, gerbils, dogs, and primates following a variety of protocols, including multigeneration studies and studies to determine whether carbamate pesticides act as endocrine modulators. The oral administration of carbaryl to rats for 1 year resulted in a decreased sperm count, decreased motility, and abnormalities (Kitagawa et al., 1977). In a three-generation reproductive study in rats, even the lowest dose (100 mg/kg per day) decreased weaning weights (Collins et al., 1971). In a three-generation study of gerbils, a dose of 150 mg/kg per day was found to be the no-observed-effect level; higher doses were associated with decreases in fertility, litter size, viability, and survival (Collins et al., 1971). In two dog studies, teratogenesis was seen at doses similar to those that did not result in fetotoxicity (Imming et al., 1969; Smalley et al., 1968).

The EPA *Integrated Risk Information System (IRIS) Chemical Assessment Summary* (EPA, 1987) reported on one dog study in which doses of methomyl up to 1,000 ppm had no effect on reproductive organs. A 2016 EPA fact sheet for propoxur reported that no information was available on the reproductive or developmental effects of propoxur in humans and that no adverse reproductive or developmental effects had been observed in an oral study of rabbits; however, a few studies of rats orally exposed to propoxur found fetotoxic effects, decreased numbers of pups, and depressed fetal weight (EPA, 2000). No studies on adverse effects on maternal reproduction or fetal outcomes were identified.

The Volume 11 committee identified no additional studies of carbaryl exposure in animals, but it did identify one on propoxur and one on methomyl. Male rats exposed to propoxur at a dose of 5.2 mg/kg body weight had significant ($p<0.05$) decreases in body weight gain, sperm density, serum and intratesticular total cholesterol concentration, and intratesticular total protein. However, there were no significant effects on gestation, fertility and parturition indices, average birth weight, litter size, and pups' sex ratio for untreated females mated with treated males (Ngoula et al., 2007).

Male rats that were administered methomyl orally (17 mg/kg in saline) daily for 2 months had a significant decrease in their levels of testosterone, while their levels of FSH, LH, and prolactin were significantly increased. The testes had degenerative changes in the seminiferous tubules up to total cellular destruction (Mahgoub and El-Medany, 2001).

The 1992 EPA *IRIS Chemical Assessment for Baygon* (a brand name for propoxur) briefly summarized three animal studies conducted by the chemical industry: a three-generation reproduction study in rats that found decreased pup numbers at 37.5 mg/kg/day (the generation in which the effects were seen was not stated); a no-observed-effect level of 500 mg/kg/day in a teratogenicity study in rabbits; and a fetotoxicity study in rats that showed a significantly lower average fetal weight, at 150 mg/kg/day (EPA, 1992).

Developmental Effects

Volume 2 identified several studies that reported an increased risk of childhood leukemia and brain cancers in children born to mothers who reported exposure to pesticides, including carbamates, during pregnancy. However, none of the studies examined preconception exposure, and the exposure to carbamates specifically was based on the researchers' assessment of likely uses around the house; none of the studies actually confirmed the use of carbamate pesticides.

The Volume 11 committee identified several studies of developmental effects and carbamate exposure (see Table 5-4). One case-control study found no significant association between the prevalence of hypospadias in children born to parents living in agricultural areas where carbaryl was used and in children from areas where carbaryl was not used (OR=0.80, 95% CI 0.20–3.18) (Meyer et al., 2006). Exposure was based on agricultural pesticide application records and geographic information system modeling.

In a second case-control study of the association between exposure to agricultural pesticides in the San Joaquin Valley in California and the presence of any of five birth defects, Carmichael et al. (2016) found that prenatal exposure to methomyl was significantly associated only with craniosynostosis (OR=3.0, 95% CI 1.1–7.8).

Lafiura et al. (2007) analyzed umbilical cord blood samples obtained from 49 infants, 39 of whom had prenatal exposure to propoxur, as determined by meconium analysis and maternal blood samples. The mothers lived in an agricultural area of the Philippines. Cord blood was analyzed for the presence of t(8;21)(q22;q22), a common cytogenetic abnormality in childhood acute myeloid leukemia (AML). Propoxur-exposed infants had a nonsignificant twofold increase in the incidence of t(8;21) compared with unexposed infants (20.5% versus 10%). A follow-up analysis of this cohort found that at 24 months of age, prenatal exposure to propoxur was negatively related to motor development ($\beta = -0.14$, $p < 0.001$) but was unrelated to social and performance development in the children (Ostrea et al., 2012). The committee notes that this was a small number of infants, which made it difficult to extrapolate the results to the general population.

In a further follow-up of the CHAMACOS study in California described in the section on OPs, Gunier et al. (2017) analyzed the Pesticide Use Reporting data from California to determine the use of OPs and carbamate pesticides in fields near the maternal residence during pregnancy. Greater application of carbamates was associated with a significant decrease at age 7 in children's WISC verbal comprehension scores ($\beta = -2.4$, 95% CI –3.9– –1.0) but not in scores on the other scales. Greater application of OPs and carbamates combined also was associated with significantly lower WISC full-scale IQ ($\beta = -2.1$, 95% CI –3.7– –0.4) and verbal comprehension scores ($\beta = -2.9$, 95% CI –4.5– –1.4) at age 7; however, by age 10 there were no significant differences for any WISC score and maternal residential exposure to OPs and carbamates combined (Rowe et al., 2016).

Monge et al. (2007), discussed in the OP section, also examined the effects of maternal (n=876) and paternal (n=762) exposures to pesticides on the risk of childhood leukemia (n=334) in Costa Rica in 1995–2000. Parents were interviewed about risk factors for childhood leukemia and their exposures were rated by hazard value and time of occurrence. The fathers' exposure to carbamates in the year prior to conception or at any time during the mother's pregnancy was not significantly associated with an increased risk of total leukemia in their children. Specific information on the mother's exposures to carbamates and any increased risk of leukemia in their children was not reported.

Animal Studies

No animal data on developmental effects from exposure to carbamate pesticides was reported in *Volume 2*, nor did the Volume 11 committee identify any new animal studies on the relevant carbamates.

Synthesis and Conclusions

Reproductive Effects

Information on the reproductive and developmental toxicity of the carbamate pesticides is limited almost exclusively to carbaryl, with little information on propoxur or methomyl. With the exception of occupational studies in carbaryl workers—the CCCEH study and the studies by Meeker et al.—virtually all other epidemiologic studies on male or female reproductive effects relied on self-reports of exposure to carbamates, often in conjunction with other potential pesticide exposures. This poses considerable challenges for the interpretation of the findings. The Volume 2 committee found adverse effects on sperm in the two occupational studies it reviewed, but it concluded that the studies were flawed. The Volume 11 committee identified one new occupational study in China that found an increase in sperm abnormalities (Xia et al., 2005) and a second study of men with no occupational exposure to carbaryl who attended an infertility clinic in the United States (Meeker et al., 2004a,b). The latter study also found sperm damage and decreased sperm concentrations to be associated with carbaryl exposure. Animal studies with carbaryl, propoxur, or methomyl supported the adverse effects on sperm seen in humans; other studies had inconsistent results for other reproductive effects in male animals, and there were no studies on female reproduction. Additional animal evidence indicates that carbamates, specifically carbaryl, act as an endocrine-disrupting compound, providing biological plausibility and mechanistic support for the reproductive effects in humans. There were no relevant animal studies on female reproductive effects.

Studies on adverse pregnancy outcomes associated with carbamate exposure reviewed by the Volume 2 committee showed that paternal occupational exposure to carbaryl increased the risk of spontaneous abortion, but when couples were analyzed as a unit, there was no increased risk (Curtis et al., 1999). Maternal exposure had no significant effects on birth outcomes. The Volume 11 committee identified only one new study that examined birth outcomes for women with exposure to chlorpyrifos, diazinon, and propoxur during pregnancy. Only propoxur was significantly associated with birth length, and it was not associated with birth length or head circumference at birth. The animal data provide inconsistent evidence of an association between exposure to carbamates and adverse reproductive effects in male and female animals. Adverse pregnancy outcomes were reported in two multigeneration studies of carbaryl.

The Volume 11 committee concludes that there is sufficient evidence of an association between exposure to carbamates and reproductive effects in men.

The Volume 11 committee also concludes that there is inadequate/insufficient evidence to determine whether an association exists between exposure to carbamates and reproductive effects in women, or with adverse pregnancy outcomes.

Developmental Effects

The epidemiologic studies on developmental effects in children exposed prenatally to carbamates, particularly the prevalence of childhood cancers, are of concern. While the CHAMACOS study (Gunier et al., 2017) indicated that there are some early neurocognitive deficits associated with maternal residential proximity to carbamate application, these deficits resolved with age (Rowe et al., 2016). The small study by Lafiura (2007) also showed neurodevelopmental effects with maternal carbamate exposure. Other studies were not restricted to carbamates alone. There is a lack of animal data on developmental effects in offspring following parental exposure to carbamates reported in *Volume 2*, and the Volume 11 committee did not identify any new animal studies.

The Volume 11 committee concludes that there is inadequate/insufficient evidence to determine whether an association exists between prenatal exposure to carbamates and developmental effects.

TABLE 5-4 Summary of Reproductive and Developmental Effects of Carbamate Pesticides

Study	Population	Exposure	Results
Reproductive Effects			
Reproductive Effects in Men			
Meeker et al. (2004a)	330 men who were partners in subfertile couples seeking infertility diagnosis at Massachusetts General Hospital (Boston) between January 2000 and April 2003.	1-N, a metabolite of carbaryl, was detected in 99.7% of men's urine.	Compared with men in the lowest 1-N concentration tertile, men in both the medium and high 1-N tertiles were more likely to have below-reference sperm concentration (ORs low exposure=1.0; medium exposure=4.2, 95% CI 1.4–13.0; high exposure=4.2, 95% CI 1.4–12.6) and sperm motility (low=1.0, medium=2.5, 95% CI 1.3–4.7; high=2.4, 95% CI 1.2–4.5). Sperm morphology was not significantly associated with 1-N.
Meeker et al. (2004b)	See Meeker et al. (2004a); semen samples available for 260 men; 46 samples excluded with specific gravity >1.03 or <1.01.	See Meeker et al. (2004a).	For an IQR increase in 1-N, Tail% significantly increased by 4.13% (95% CI 1.92–6.32). An IQR increase in 1-N resulted in a nonsignificant reduction in TDM (–2.18 mm, 95% CI –4.88–0.50) and a nonsignificant decrease in comet extent (–0.92 mm, 95% CI –7.39–5.55).
Meeker et al. (2006)	See Meeker et al. (2004a); 330 men with semen, urine, and nonfasting blood samples taken on same day.	See Meeker et al. (2004a).	Regression model results show an inverse association between 1-N and testosterone. An IQR range increase in 1-N was associated with a 6.0% (–11% to –1%) decrease in median testosterone level.
Meeker et al. (2008a)	See Meeker et al. (2004a).	See Meeker et al. (2004a).	No significant association between increased 1-N levels and decreased estradiol (p=0.09). Highest four quintiles of 1-N were associated with declined estradiol but not in a dose-related manner. No statistically significant associations between 1-N and prolactin.

continued

TABLE 5-4 Continued

Study	Population	Exposure	Results
Xia et al. (2005)	46 sperm donors ages 21–48 years in Changzhou, China; 16 were carbaryl-exposed workers; 12 internal controls were clerical or official workers in the same pesticide factory but far away from the pesticide workshop; 18 external control group were selected from professions other than pesticide workers.	Exposed workers worked in the plant for >1 year and had been working continuously for 6 months before biological sampling.	No significant differences in semen volume, sperm concentration, sperm number per ejaculum, and sperm motility between carbaryl-exposed and two control groups. Carbaryl group had significantly more morphological defects (e.g., sperm abnormalities) than external control group (p=0.008), significantly higher mean percentage of spermatozoa with fragmented DNA than internal (p=0.035) or external controls (p=0.030), and significant differences in the frequencies of disomic sex-chromosome-bearing (highest the XY-bearing) and disomic chromosome 18 spermatozoa (p<0.05 and p<0.01, respectively). Nullisomies of sex chromosomes and chromosome 18 were significantly higher than those in the external (p<0.01) but not internal controls. No significant differences in percentage of normal spermatozoa with X- or Y-chromosome or diploidy rates between any two groups.
Adverse Pregnancy Outcomes			
Whyatt et al. (2004)	CCCEH cohort; 314 African American and Dominican women, 18–35 years old, enrolled into the cohort between 1998 and 2002. Umbilical cord blood collected at birth; and maternal blood collected within 2 days postpartum.	85% reported using some form of pest control measures during pregnancy, and 35% reported using an exterminator; 56.5% of users reported using one or more of the more highly toxic pest control methods (can sprays, pest bombs, or sprays by exterminator). Measured 2-isopropoxyphenol, a metabolite of propoxur.	2-isopropoxyphenol in cord plasma was inversely associated with birth length (p=0.05). Among newborns born before 2001, the association between (ln)2-isopropoxyphenol and birth length was statistically significant (β= –0.73 cm/unit, p=0.01). Among newborns born after January 1, 2001, the association remained inverse, but the magnitude of effect was less and not significant (β= –0.30 cm/unit, p=0.56). No association was seen between infant head circumference and levels of propoxur or its metabolite in maternal personal air and cord blood samples.
Whyatt et al. (2005)	CCCEH cohort; see Whyatt et al. (2004).	See Whyatt et al. (2004)	No significant associations between 2-isopropoxyphenol levels in cord plasma and birth weight for infants born before or after 2001 (p=0.12 and p=0.27, respectively). For infants born before 2001, statistically significant inverse relationship between 2-isopropoxyphenol in cord blood and birth length (β= –0.73, p=0.01), but not for infants born after 2001 (p=0.56).

Study	Population	Exposure	Results
Developmental Effects			
Meyer et al. (2006)	354 cases of hypospadias in male children born between 1998 and 2002 in eastern Arkansas; 727 controls were selected from birth certificates.	Classified exposure based on pounds of pesticides (estimated by crop type) applied or persisting within 500 m of each child's home during gestational weeks 6–16.	Hypospadias were not significantly associated with increases in carbaryl application (OR=0.80, 95% CI 0.20–3.18).
Carmichael et al. (2016)	367 cases of children born 1997–2006 with 1 of 5 birth defects in any one of 8 counties in San Joaquin Valley, CA, and 785 infants born without birth defects. Birth defects (anotia/microtia; anorectal atresia/stenosis; transverse limb deficiency; craniosynostosis; and diaphragmatic hernia) based on California Birth Defects Monitoring Program.	Pesticide exposure within 500-m radius was estimated for each mother's residence from 1 month before to 2 months after her reported date of conception using geospatial coding for San Joaquin Valley counties and the Pesticide Use Reporting records for pesticides applied at >100 lbs in any of the counties.	Prenatal exposure to methomyl was significantly associated with craniosynostosis (OR=3.0, 95% CI 1.1–7.8) but not with other birth defects.
Lafiura et al. (2007)	Pregnant women prospectively enrolled into the study at mid-gestation, living in Bulacan, an agroindustrial province of the Philippines.	49 meconium and umbilical cord blood samples were obtained of which 39 were exposed prenatally to propoxur and 10 were unexposed.	Incidence of t(8;21)(q22;q22), a common cytogenetic abnormality seen in AML, was twofold higher in the exposed children than in the unexposed children. Levels of AML1-ETO fusion transcripts resulting from t(8;21) abnormality were positively associated with propoxur concentrations in meconium.

continued

TABLE 5-4 Continued

Study	Population	Exposure	Results
Ostrea et al. (2012)	Same population as Lafiura et al. (2007). 696 mother–infant pairs assessed.	Cyfluthrin/propoxur major pesticide used in 73% of homes/farms. Neuro-development at 24 months assessed with Griffith Mental Development Scales: (1) locomotor subscale (gross motor development, including balance and coordination of movements), (2) social development (personal–social [daily activities and child interaction] and language subscales [receptive and expressive language]), and (3) performance subscale (visuospatial skills and reaction time).	Exposure to propoxur negatively associated with motor development ($\beta = -0.14$, $p<0.001$), but not with social and performance development.
Gunier et al. (2017)	CHAMACOS cohort of women living in agricultural area of Salinas Valley, CA; children born October 1999–October 2000; eligible n=488) women were ≥18 years of age, <20 weeks gestation at enrollment.	Gestational and preconception exposure, half of the women resided in United States for <5 years; approximately 28% had worked in the fields during pregnancy, another 14% worked at other agriculture jobs (e.g., packing shed, nursery, and greenhouse work). 85% of the women had agricultural workers living in their homes during their pregnancy. Exposure to OPs was measured as DAP metabolites in maternal urine during pregnancy (mean=13 and 26 weeks gestation) and ChE in whole blood and BuChE in plasma collected	Increased exposure to carbamates during pregnancy was significantly associated with an estimated 2.4-point decrease in verbal comprehension (95% CI –3.9– –1.0), but not with the other WISC subscales of full-scale IQ, working memory, processing speed, and perceptual reasoning.

Study	Population	Exposure	Results
		from mothers during pregnancy and at delivery, and from the umbilical cord. Children assessed for neurodevelopment at 7 years using WISC-IV. Pesticide use within 1 km of mother's residence during pregnancy estimated using California Pesticide Use Reporting data from 1999–2001.	
Rowe et al. (2016)	CHAMACOS cohort, see Grunier et al. (2007). 501 10-year-old children.	Exposure based on kgs of OPs and carbamates used near the residence where each woman lived the longest during pregnancy. WISC-IV used to test neuro-development at 10 years of age.	WISC scores were significantly decreased only at the fourth quintile of combined OP and carbamate use (highest usage) during pregnancy (full-scale IQ $\beta = -3.0$, 95% CI –5.6– –0.3; verbal comprehension $\beta = -1.3$, 95% CI –4.1–1.4; perceptual reasoning $\beta = -4.0$, 95% CI –7.6– –0.4; working memory $\beta = -2.8$, 95% CI –5.6– –0.1; and processing speed $\beta = -0.7$, 95% CI –3.8–2.4).
Monge et al. (2007)	334 cases of leukemia and 579 population controls. Children ages 0–14 years diagnosed in Costa Rica in 1995–2000.	Childhood leukemia identified from Cancer Registry and the Children's Hospital of Costa Rica. Parents interviewed in 2001–2003 about occupational, environmental, and home pesticide exposures of both parents from 12 months prior to conception to diagnosis of cancer.	No increased risk of childhood leukemia associated with paternal exposure to carbamates at any time prior to birth (ORs=1.3, 95% CI 0.6–2.5) or for year before conception (OR=1.2, 95% CI 0.4–3.3 for first trimester; OR=1.6, 95% CI 0.6–4.1 for second trimester; and OR=2.0, 95% CI 0.7–5.8 for third trimester).

NOTE: 1-N=1-naphthol; AML=acute myloid leukemia; BuChE=butyryl cholinesterase; CCCEH=Columbia Center for Children's Environmental Health study; CHAMACOS=Center for the Health Assessment of Mothers and Children of Salinas study; ChE=cholinesterase; CI=confidence interval; DAP=dialkyl phosphate; DNA=deoxyribonucleic acid; IQR=interquartile range; OP=organophosphate; OR=odds ratio; TDM=tail distributed moment; WISC-IV=Wechsler Intelligence Scale for Children, 4th edition.

PYRETHROIDS

Pyrethrins are naturally occurring pesticides found in chrysanthemum flowers. They degrade rapidly in the environment, particularly in the presence of sunlight. Pyrethroids are commercially manufactured pesticides with a chemical structure similar to pyrethrins, which have been in use for more than 40 years. They are more toxic to insects and mammals than pyrethrins, and they persist longer in the environment (ATSDR, 2003b). Pyrethroids were used extensively during the 1990–1991 Gulf War, with estimates that each service member deployed to the Persian Gulf received 2.2 cans of permethrin (as 6-oz aerosol cans) to treat their uniforms (PAC, 1996). Service members in the Post-9/11 conflicts also used permethrin-treated uniforms and bed nets to help prevent sand fly bites.

The acute neurotoxicity of pyrethroids to human adults is well established (Shafer et al., 2005). Permethrin is metabolized by the cytochrome P450 enzyme and esterases to at least 80 metabolites (Casida et al., 1983), but most of them are inactive. Half-lives vary among the different pyrethroid compounds, but they range from 6.4 to 16.5 hours in humans, with elimination mostly completed within 5 days (ATSDR, 2003b). Among the pyrethroid metabolites found in urine and blood and discussed in this section are PBA, cis- and trans-3-(2,2-dichlorovinyl)-2,2-dimethylcyclopropane carboxylic acid (CDCCA and TDCCA, respectively), and cis-2,2-dibromovinyl-2,2-dimethylcyclopropane-carboxylic acid (DBCA).

Based on the Defense Logistics Agency list of pesticides sent to the Gulf War (IOM, 2003) and the reported use of pyrethroids in Iraq in 2003 (Schleier et al., 2009), the Volume 11 committee paid particular attention to the pyrethroids permethrin, cypermethrin, deltamethrin, and resmethrin.

Reproductive Effects

The Volume 2 committee did not consider specific reproductive effects that may result from the exposure of men or women to pyrethroid insecticides. The ATSDR publication *Toxicological Profile on Pyrethrins and Pyrethroids* (2003b) reported that standard reproductive toxicity studies, including some that were performed for three successive generations, did not indicate that pyrethrins or pyrethroids are of particular concern to reproductive success.

Reproductive Effects in Men and Women

The Volume 11 committee considered several papers that explored the association between environmental exposure of men to pyrethroids and the impacts on their reproductive systems, particularly sperm quality (see Table 5-5). The majority of the studies assessed exposure to pyrethroids by analyzing for urinary metabolites, including PBA, CDCCA, TDCCA, and DBCA. In general, the men in the studies were recruited from infertility clinics.

Xia et al. (2008) reported a dose–response relationship between increasing urinary PBA quartiles and decreased sperm concentration in 376 Chinese men. ORs for the first, second, third, and fourth concentration quartiles were 1.00, 1.31 (95% CI 0.65–2.64), 1.73 (95% CI 0.87–3.45), and 2.04 (95% CI 1.02–4.09), respectively (p-value for trend=0.027), whereas sperm volume, sperm number per ejaculum, and sperm motility showed no significant associations with PBA quartiles. In another study of Chinese men, Ji et al. (2011) found a significant inverse correlation between urinary PBA levels and sperm concentration ($\beta = -0.27$, 95% CI –0.41– –0.12, $p<0.001$) and a significant positive correlation between PBA levels and sperm DNA fragmentation ($\beta=0.27$, 95% CI 0.15–0.39, $p<0.001$).

Imai et al. (2014) found in a sample of 323 Japanese men (university students) that environmental exposure to pyrethroid insecticides as determined by urinary PBA did not affect semen volume, sperm concentration, motility, the total number of sperm, or the total number of motile sperm. Furthermore, the researchers did not find any association between PBA and the levels of FSH, LH, testosterone, sex hormone-binding globulin, inhibin B, or calculated free testosterone. More than 91% of the men had detectable levels of PBA in their urine (Yoshinaga et al., 2014).

In a study of 195 men in Poland conducted to evaluate sperm DNA damage (Jurewicz et al., 2015) and aneuploidy (Radwan et al., 2015), there was a positive association between CDCCA greater than the 50th percentage concentration distribution in urine and the percentage of medium DFI, the percentage of immature sperm, and disomy of chromosome 18 ($p=0.04$, $p=0.04$, and $p=0.05$, respectively). A level of PBA was positively related to the percentage of high DFI ($p=0.03$). The TDCCA, DBCA levels, and the sum of pyrethroid metabolites were not associated with any sperm DNA damage measures. PBA concentrations in the urine that were both below and above the 50th percentile were associated with disomy of sex chromosomes, although to different degrees—XY disomy ($p=0.05$ and $p=0.02$, respectively), Y disomy ($p=0.04$ and 0.02, respectively), disomy of chromosome 21 ($p=0.04$ and $p=0.04$, respectively), and total disomy ($p=0.03$ and $p=0.04$, respectively); while PBA levels that were above the 50th percentile were associated with disomy of chromosome 18 ($p=0.03$). Urinary levels of TDCCA above the 50th percentile were related to XY disomy ($p=0.04$) and disomy of chromosome 21 ($p=0.05$) but not with any sperm DNA damage. The levels of DBCA and the sum of pyrethroid metabolites also were not associated with any sperm DNA damage measures. The three metabolites were also significantly associated with an increase in the number of sperm having abnormal morphology and a decrease in sperm concentration and levels of testosterone (Radwan et al., 2014).

One study of U.S. men also found environmental exposure to pyrethroids to be associated with semen quality. In a study of 207 men attending an infertility clinic in Massachusetts, Meeker et al. (2008b) found that increasing levels of urinary PBA and CDCCA were associated with increased sperm DNA damage. TDCCA levels showed a dose-dependent increase in the risk of having sperm concentration, motility and morphology below the reference values. Further assessment of these men showed that all three metabolites were associated with an increased incidence of disomy of chromosomes X, Y, and 18. Specifically, disomy was increased in YY18 for PBA, CDCCA, and TDCCA (incidence ratio rates [IRRs]=1.28, 95% CI 1.15–1.42; 1.18, 95% CI 1.05–1.31; and 1.19, 95% CI 1.06–1.34, respectively). Both CDCCA and TDCCA were significantly associated with increased disomy for XY18 and total disomy, but PBA was not. None of the metabolites were associated with disomy for XX18 or 1818 (Young et al., 2013).

Meeker et al. (2009) assessed the effects of pyrethroids on serum hormone levels in men and found that PBA, TDCCA, and CDCCA were all positively associated with FSH levels (all p-values for trend <0.05). CDCCA was also significantly associated with luteinizing hormone; however, CDCCA and TDCCA were inversely associated with inhibin B (p-values for trend=0.03 and 0.02, respectively).

In a systematic review of three papers—Ji et al. (2011); Meeker et al. (2008b); Xia et al. (2008)—published between 2007 and 2012 on the effects of exposure to pyrethroid insecticides on sperm parameters, Martenies and Perry (2013) concluded that although all three studies reported inverse associations between pyrethroid metabolites in urine and decreased sperm concentrations, the results were suggestive but not definitive.

The Volume 11 committee identified only one study on the effects of pyrethroids on female reproduction. Hu et al. (2018) conducted a TTP study of 615 women in Shanghai, China, who were recruited from two preconception care clinics between August 2013 and April 2015. Women were enrolled in the study before conceiving a child and were followed for approximately 1 year after they had stopped using a contraceptive. Exposures to pyrethroids were determined by measuring PBA, TDCCA, and CDCCA in urine. After adjustments were made for age, BMI before pregnancy, smoking, and education, women who had never been pregnant and were in the highest quartile for PBA concentrations had significantly longer TTP (fecundability OR=0.72, 95% CI 0.53–0.98) and increased infertility (OR=2.03, 95% CI 1.10–3.74) than women in the lowest quartile.

Adverse Pregnancy Outcomes

The ATSDR review *Toxicological Profile for Pyrethrins and Pyrethroids* (2003b) reported that no studies had been identified on the reproductive effects, including birth outcomes, of pyrethroid pesticides following inhalation, oral, or dermal exposures in humans. Several studies in Poland, China, and Japan have been published since the ATSDR profile. The studies examine the impact of prenatal exposure to pyrethroid pesticides on fetal outcomes.

In a 2003 study of the effect of first- and second-trimester exposures to pesticides on birth outcomes in Poland, women (n=95) who reported residential or occupational exposure to pesticides, including pyrethroids, were found to be at an increased risk (p=0.01) of delivering a low-birth-weight infant, but the risk was not significant for pyrethoid exposure specifically (p=0.286), and there was no effect on pregnancy duration (Dabrowski et al., 2003). The study is limited in that exposures were to mixtures of pesticides and based on the mother's recall of pesticide use at the time of delivery. As such, pesticide-specific effects cannot be evaluated.

The Volume 11 committee considered one study of birth outcomes in babies born to women in rural China who had prenatal exposure to pyrethroids (Ding et al., 2015). Maternal urine samples were analyzed for CDCCA, TDCCA, and PBA. The authors found that $\log_{10}$ unit increases in the total concentration of the metabolites, but not individual metabolite levels, were associated with a decrease in birth weight (β= –96.76, 95% CI= –173.15– –20.37). No associations were found between individual or total metabolite levels and birth length, head circumference, or gestational duration.

Zhang et al. (2014b) analyzed the urine of 147 Japanese women in their first trimester of pregnancy for PBA metabolites. Thyroid hormone levels—free thyroxine (FT4) and thyroid-stimulating hormone (TSH)—were determined in neonatal and maternal blood at birth. The levels of both thyroid hormones were within the normal range for all infants except one. There was no significant correlation between PBA concentrations in maternal urine and neonatal thyroid hormone concentration or with body size at birth (p=0.05), nor was there a significant correlation between the levels of maternal PBA and other neonatal outcomes of body weight, body length, head circumference, or chest circumference. However, in a multiple-regression analysis the authors found that PBA concentrations in maternal urine sampled in the first trimester were significantly associated with reduced birth weight (β=0.183, p=0.017) and head circumference (β=0.243, p=0.010).

The Baltimore THREE (Tracking Health Related to Environmental Exposures) study collected cord blood from 300 singleton live births delivered between November 2004 and March 2005 at Johns Hopkins Hospital. The cord blood was analyzed for the cis- and trans-isomers of permethrin, for the permethrin synergist piperonyl butoxide, and for nine cytokines. Infants were evaluated for birth weight, length, head circumference, ponderal index, and gestational age. Permethrin was negatively associated with the anti-inflammatory cytokine IL-10 (β= –0.14, 95% CI –0.22– –0.05). The permethrin concentrations measured in the cord blood had no significant associations with gestational age, birth weight, length, head circumference, or ponderal index (Neta et al., 2011).

Animal Studies

The Volume 2 committee considered several studies on the reproductive effects of pyrethroids in animal models. Pyrethroids at 100–10,000 nM were found not to be estrogenic or antiestrogenic, nor did they alter human estrogen-receptor α-mediated mechanisms in vitro (Saito et al., 2000; Sumida et al., 2001). The Volume 2 committee cited numerous studies that indicated that pyrethroids are not gonadotoxic, embryotoxic, or teratogenic (EPA, 1983; Hallenbeck and Cunningham-Burns, 1985; Kaloianova and El Batawi, 1991; Kidd and James, 1991; Litchfield, 1985; Miyamoto, 1976; Polakova and Vargova, 1983; Ray, 1991), although high oral doses (250 mg/kg per day) of permethrin during GDs 6–15 were found to reduce the number of offspring (Wauchope et al., 1992). A three-generation study of resmethrin reported slight increases in premature stillbirths and a decrease in pup weight (Ray, 1991). The Volume 2 committee concluded that pyrethroids are unlikely to cause reproductive and teratogenic effects (IOM, 2003).

The ATSDR review *Toxicological Profile on Pyrethrins and Pyrethroids* (2003b) reported that a few studies have indicated that relatively low-level, intermediate-duration oral exposure of adult male rats to some pyrethroids may result in damage to reproductive organs, abnormal sperm characteristics, reduced plasma testosterone levels, and reduced fertility. Relative to controls, male rats administered oral doses of deltamethrin had significantly reduced sperm cell concentrations, live cell percentage, and motility index; had a significantly higher percentage of total sperm abnormalities; and had significantly reduced plasma testosterone levels. Male fertility, determined by successful matings to untreated female rats, was 50% that of controls (Abd El-Aziz et al., 1994).

ATSDR also reported on an EPA study that showed decreased pup survival in rats following parental oral exposure to resmethrin at 70.8 mg/kg/day prior to mating and throughout gestation and lactation; rats receiving 80 mg/kg/day during GDs 6–15 had slight increases in skeletal variations and delayed ossification (EPA, 1994).

The Volume 11 committee identified several animal studies that assessed the reproductive toxicology of all three pyrethroids of interest. One study examined the effect of 20 or 40 mg/kg/day permethrin on rat ovaries (Kotil and Yon, 2015). After treatment for 14 days via gavage, dose-dependent degenerative changes were seen in the follicular and corpus luteum cell morphology, with evidence of apoptotic cell death. All the other studies assessed the reproductive toxicity of pyrethroids in male animals.

In studies of male reproductive effects, Zhang et al. (2007, 2008) dosed male ICR mice with cis-permethrin at 0, 35, or 70 mg/kg/day for 6 weeks. Caudal epididymal sperm count and sperm motility, testicular testosterone production, and plasma testosterone concentrations were all significantly and dose-dependently decreased, with an increase in LH. Testicular mitochondrial mRNA expression was also reduced, with mitochondrial membrane damage in the Leydig cells. Cis-permethrin administered at 90 μmol/kg/day for 6 weeks did not affect plasma testosterone levels, although the co-exposure of animals with 10 μmol/kg/day diazinon reduced plasma testosterone levels to 45% of those in the control animals. Cis-permethrin alone also reduced translocator protein mRNA levels by 46% compared with controls but did not reduce P450scc mRNA levels. Administration of permethrin to adult male rats at 35 mg/kg/day for 60 days resulted in reductions in reproductive organ weights, the number of live sperm and Leydig cells, sperm motility, and serum testosterone levels and in increased abnormal sperm morphology (Khaki et al., 2017).

Deltamethrin was also found to have adverse effects on male reproduction in animal studies, including reduced sperm quality, sex hormones, and libido and increased testicular damage (Ben Slima et al., 2017). Issam et al. (2009) treated male rats with deltamethrin at 2 ppm for 30 days, 20 ppm for 45 days, and 200 ppm for 60 days and reported a significant decrease in FSH, LH, and testosterone at the highest dose. The deltamethrin treatment of rats also arrested spermatogenesis and produced a significant increase in malondialdehyde levels that was related to dose, the length of treatment, and lipid peroxidation. Abdallah et al. (2010) studied the effect of deltamethrin at doses of 0, 10, 50, 100 and 200 μmol on the oxidative stress response in rat spermatozoa after 3 hours of incubation. This in vitro exposure caused a significant decline in sperm motility and viability and increased abnormal sperm morphology as well as levels of malondialdehyde, superoxide dismutase, and catalase. The administration of deltamethrin at 5 mg/kg/day to male rats for 4 weeks resulted in decreased serum testosterone, LH, and FSH levels and significantly increased testicular total oxidant capacity, poly(ADP-ribose) polymerase, lactate dehydrogenase, and DNA damage (Ismail and Mohamed, 2012). A dose of 1 mg/kg deltramethrin administered intraperitoneally for 5 days/week for 1 month increased the weight of rat testes and produced adverse histopathologic changes. There was also a significant reduction in the number of seminiferous tubules per unit area and adverse morphologic changes in the tubules (Kumar and Nagar, 2014).

Cypermethrin was found to have similar effects to deltamethrin on male rodents. Elbetieha et al. (2001) studied the effects of cypermethrin on reproductive and fertility parameters in male mice receiving 0, 13.15, 18.93, and 39.66 mg cypermethrin in drinking water for 12 weeks. All doses resulted in a significant reduction in the number of viable fetuses in females mated to the treated males, lower body weight gain in the treated males, a significant increase in preputial gland weights, and a significant decrease in epididymal and testicular sperm counts and daily sperm production. At the two higher doses, there was a significant increase in the weight of the testes and seminal vesicles and a significant reduction in the perimeter and number of cell layers of the seminiferous tubules, along with hemorrhage in the testes and a large number of immature spermatids in the tubules. The two lower doses (13.15 and 18.93 mg) produced significantly reduced fertility, as indicated by fewer females being impregnated by the treated males, while 39.66 mg cypermethrin caused a significant reduction in the number of implantation sites. On the other hand, Al-Hamdani and Yajurvedi (2010) did not see a decrease in fertility in mice administered cypermethrin by gavage at 1.38, 2.76, and 5.52 mg/kg/day for 6 or 12 weeks. All doses and both durations caused a significant reduction in epididymal spermatozoa count and an increase in abnormal spermatozoa, but 6 weeks after dosing ceased, the counts returned to normal in mice administered the two lower doses but not the highest dose. All mice had normal fertility, although the weight of the litters was significantly lower than for controls; the gestation period and the litter size were unaffected. Dahamna et al. (2010) also found that cypermethrin administered to male mice at 20% and 5% of the LD_{50} (485 mg/kg) for 2 weeks and 4 weeks, respectively, and at 20% of the LD_{50} for 12 weeks, resulted in a 20% decrease in sperm count and an increase in abnormal sperm and in testicular and epididymal morphology. Similar results were seen by Hu et al. (2013) who treated rats with cypermethrin at 0, 6.25, 12.5, 25 and 50 mg/kg/day by gavage for 15 days. At 25 and 50 mg/kg there was a significant reduction in sperm production and changes in the seminiferous tubules, including reduced and deformed spermatogonia. Furthermore, at 50 mg/kg cypermethrin, androgen receptor levels were significantly reduced, as were serum testosterone levels. Rodriguez et al. (2017) also found adverse effects on Sertoli cells in mice administered 20% of the LD_{50} intraperitoneally.

Sharma et al. (2018) found that the administration of cypermethrin, deltamethrin, or a combination of the two pesticides significantly reduced sperm count and motility and concentrations of some steroidogenic enzymes and increased the number of abnormal sperm; the combination of the two pesticides had a greater effect on all sperm parameters and enzyme levels. Both pesticides and their combination also significantly reduced testosterone and LH concentrations, but only the combination of the two pesticides significantly reduced concentrations of FSH.

The mechanism by which pyrethroids act on male fertility was explored by Taylor et al. (2010) using an in vitro mouse Sertoli cell assay. Pyrethroids, at both low and high serum concentrations, affected the expression of the two estrogen receptors; however, the influence on estrogen receptor gene expression was different from the effect of exposure to 17beta-estradiol.

Developmental Effects

The ATSDR review *Toxicological Profile on Pyrethrins and Pyrethroids* (2003b) did not report any studies of developmental effects in humans following maternal or paternal exposure to pyrethroids by any route of exposure. The majority of the studies published since the ATSDR profile examined neurodevelopmental outcomes in children following prenatal exposures to pyrethroids, although the committee did consider a few other studies that examined other developmental outcomes in children.

The Volume 11 committee considered several studies of the developmental effects of pyrethroids. The studies are summarized in Table 5-5 and discussed in the following section.

Neurodevelopmental Effects

The CCCEH study assessed 348 children born between February 1998 and May 2002 for psychomotor and cognitive development at several times during their childhoods (Horton et al., 2011). In this study, the children were administered the BSID-II to generate MDI and PDI scores. Prenatal exposure to permethrin was measured in maternal and umbilical cord plasma collected on delivery, and permethrin and piperonyl butoxide levels were measured in personal air collected during pregnancy. When the children were assessed at 36 months of age, the authors found no significant associations between their MDI or PDI scores and permethrin concentrations in either the personal air samples or the maternal or umbilical cord plasma samples. However, the highest prenatal piperonyl butoxide exposure was associated with a 3.9-point mean decrement in MDI scores (95% CI –0.25– –7.49), and the most highly exposed children had the greatest risk (OR=3.11, 95% CI 1.38–6.98) of delayed mental development.

In a further follow-up of the CHAMACOS study in California described in the section on OPs, Gunier et al. (2017) used the Pesticide Use Reporting data from California to determine the use of pyrethroids in fields near the maternal residence during pregnancy. Neurodevelopment in children at age 7 was assessed using WISC-IV. Pyrethroid use was associated with lower scores on the full-scale IQ (β= –2, 95% CI –3.7– –0.3), verbal comprehension (β= –1.8, 95% CI –3.4– –0.3), and perceptual reasoning (β= –2.1, 95% CI –4.0– –0.2) subscales, but not on the working memory or processing speed scores.

The Mt. Sinai Children's Environmental Health Cohort, described in the section on OPs, assessed 162 mother–infant pairs during pregnancy in 1998–2001. Prenatal exposure to pyrethroids was determined by an analysis of maternal urine samples taken in the third trimester of pregnancy; the samples were analyzed for PBA, TDCCA, and CDCCA. Children were assessed for neurodevelopment at 4, 6, and 7–9 years of age. Parents reported on their children's development using the Behavioral Assessment System for Children and the Behavior Rating Inventory of Executive Function. Detectable levels of PBA during pregnancy were associated with lower scores for the indices of internalizing (β= –4.50, 95% CI –8.05– –0.95), depression (β= –3.21, 95% CI –6.38– –0.05), somatization (β= –3.22, 95% CI –6.38– –0.06), behavioral regulation (β= –3.59, 95% CI –6.97– –0.21), emotional control (β= –3.35, 95% CI –6.58– –0.12), shifting (β= –3.42, 95% CI –6.73– –0.11), and monitoring (β= –4.08, 95% CI –7.07– –1.08). Detectable levels of CDCCA were associated with worse externalizing (β= –4.74, 95% CI –9.37– –0.10), conduct problems (β= –5.35, 95% CI –9.90– –0.81), behavioral regulation (β= –6.42, 95% CI –11.39– –1.45), and inhibitory control (β= –7.20, 95% CI –12.00– –2.39) (Furlong et al., 2017b).

The impact of maternal exposure to pyrethroids on the development of 102 18-month old Japanese infants was examined by Hisada et al. (2017) using the Kinder Infant Development Scale, which is based on a questionnaire completed by the caretaker. Infants whose mothers had higher levels of PBA in their urine at 10–12 weeks of gestation had higher development quotient scores than infants whose mothers had lower PBA concentrations (p=0.017), which the authors considered to be unexpected.

Other studies have found in utero pyrethroid exposure to be associated with adverse effects on neurodevelopment. Xue et al. (2013) found that among 497 mother–infant pairs in China, increasing levels of pyrethroid metabolites in maternal urine during pregnancy were inversely correlated with the development quotient of the infants at 1 year of age (β= –0.1527, p=0.05), although there was no such correlation for the MDI. The Development Screen Test scale was used to assess the intellectual development of infants. Children born to mothers residing in rural areas had greater impairment than children born to mothers living in cities. The impairment was correlated with higher levels of pyrethroid metabolites in the urine of mothers residing in rural areas.

The impact of maternal exposure to pyrethroids on child neurodevelopment was also assessed by Watkins et al. (2016) in the ELEMENT longitudinal study of a mother–child cohort in Mexico City recruited from 1997 to 2001. PBA was measured in the urine of 187 mothers during their third trimester, and children were administered the BSID-II Spanish version (BSID-IIS) to assess the developmental functioning of infants and children at 24 and 36 months of age using the MDI and PDI. Children whose mothers had medium and high urinary PBA levels had nonsignificantly lower MDI scores (β= –3.54, 95% CI –7.86–0.78 and β= –3.80, 95% CI –8.44–0.84, respectively) at 24 months than those with mothers in the low (reference) PBA category (p-value for trend=0.07), and the effect was lower at 36 months (p-value for trend=0.14). At 24 months the associations were significantly stronger for female children (β= –6.20, 95% CI –12.3– –0.14) than for males (β= –2.58, 95% CI –9.10–3.94) of mothers with medium PBA levels, but the differences were not significant at 36 months. The third-trimester prenatal level of maternal PBA was not associated with PDI scores at either time point.

Eskenazi et al. (2018) assessed the effects of prenatal exposure to multiple pesticides on neurodevelopment, as measured by the BSID-II, in 752 children in South Africa participating in the Venda Health Examination of Mothers, Babies and Their Environment (VHEMBE) birth cohort study. Maternal exposure to pyrethroids during pregnancy was determined through the identification of four urinary pyrethroid metabolites—DBCA, CDCCA, TDCCA, and PBA. Maternal urine samples were collected around the time of delivery. When the children were 1 year of age, each 10-fold increase in CDCCA, TDCCA, and PBA was significantly associated with a decrement in social–emotional scores (β= –0.63, 95% CI –1.14– –0.12; β= –0.48, 95% CI –0.92– –0.05; and β= –0.58, 95% CI –1.11– –0.06, respectively). At 2 years of age, each 10-fold increase in maternal CDBCA levels was associated with significant decrements in language composite scores (β= –1.74, 95% CI –3.34– –0.13) and expressive communication scores (β= –0.40, 95% CI –0.77– –0.04). The authors noted that "significant differences by sex were estimated for pyrethroid metabolites and motor function scores at 2 years of age, with higher scores for boys and lower scores for girls."

The PELAGIE study in Brittany, France, is a large mother–child cohort that has assessed child development since the children were born between 2002 and 2006 (Viel et al., 2015). Maternal exposure to pyrethroids was determined on the basis of urine samples collected between 6 and 19 weeks of pregnancy and adjusted for exposure to OPs. At a child's sixth birthday, the mother and child participated in a neuropsychological follow-up using the WISC-IV; a total of 287 mother–child pairs took part. None of the WISC scores were associated with maternal pyrethroid metabolite concentrations (PBA, TDCCA, or CDCCA). The children's behavior was further evaluated for three subscales of the Strengths and Difficulties Questionnaire: prosocial behavior, internalizing disorders, and externalizing disorders (Viel et al., 2017). Maternal prenatal CDCCA was associated with internalizing difficulties, while maternal prenatal PBA was associated with externalizing difficulties and higher odds of abnormal or borderline social behavior per the maternal report on the Strengths and Difficulties Questionnaire (Viel et al., 2017).

The CHARGE study in California attempted to link pesticide use near the mother's residence with children having ASD (n=486) or developmental disorder (n=168) (Shelton et al., 2014). Prenatal residence proximity (within 1.5 km) to areas sprayed with pyrethroids was associated with an increased risk for ASD if the exposure was prior to conception (OR=1.82, 95% CI 1.00–3.31) or in the third trimester (OR=1.87, 95% CI 1.02–3.43). Exposure at 1.75 km was associated with an increased risk for ASD only in the third trimester (OR=1.83, 95% CI 1.04–3.23). For developmental disorders and residential proximity to agricultural pesticide application, there was a significant risk only for a distance of 1.75 km during the third trimester (OR=2.34, 95% CI 1.18–4.67), indicating that the timing of exposure during pregnancy had a significant effect on the risk of ASD and developmental disorder.

Other Developmental Effects

Researchers have linked other developmental endpoints to prenatal exposure to pyrethroids. Carmichael et al. (2014), discussed in the section on OPs, compared the exposure of mothers of 569 infants with any of eight congenital heart defects with 785 mothers who had an infant without a birth defect. Prenatal exposure to permethrin was nonsignificantly associated with ventricular septal defect, perimembranous (OR=2.2, 95% CI 0.8–5.7), but not with any of the heart defects. Monge et al. (2007) examined the effect of maternal (n=876) and paternal (n=762) exposures to pesticides on the risk of childhood leukemia (n=334) in Costa Rica in 1995–2000. Parents were interviewed about risk factors for childhood leukemia, and their exposures were rated by hazard value and by time of occurrence. Neither maternal nor paternal exposure to pyrethroid insecticides, primarily deltamethrin, at any time prior to birth was significantly associated with childhood leukemia for either boys or girls.

The association between prenatal exposure to permethrins and piperonyl butoxide, a synergist for residential pyrethroid pesticides, and the presence of childhood cough at 5–6 years of age was examined by Liu et al. (2012) as part of the CCCEH birth cohort. Prenatal exposure to cis- and trans-permethrin was not significantly associated with a noninfectious cough at age 5–6 years, but there was a positive association between a noninfectious cough and prenatal piperonyl butoxide in children ages 5–6 years (OR=1.27 for unit change in log piperonyl butoxide, 95% CI 1.09–1.48). Exposure to piperonyl butoxide or permethrins at ages 5–6 years was not associated with an increase in childhood cough.

Coker et al. (2018) assessed the effects of prenatal exposure to multiple pesticides on child body weight and body composition in 708 children in South Africa's VHEMBE birth cohort. Maternal exposure was determined by the identification of four urinary pyrethroid metabolites—DBCA, CDCCA, TDCCA, and PBA. Maternal urine samples were collected around the time of delivery. The length or height and the weight of the children were measured at 1 and 2 years of age; maternal exposure to dichlorodiphenyltrichloroethane (i.e., DDT) was also assessed. Using a single-pollutant linear mixed-effects model, BMI-for-age and weight-for-height were inversely related to DBCA and TDCCA levels; the effects were more pronounced for boys than for girls for both measures and metabolites. Weight-for-age was also inversely related to TDCCA for boys only, but not overall. None of the four metabolites significantly affected any of the measures for girls.

Animal Studies

The Volume 2 committee reported that pyrethroids administered to female rats during pregnancy did not affect the development of their offspring (Extoxnet, 1994). No other animal studies on the developmental effects of pyrethroids were cited in *Volume 2*.

The ATSDR review *Toxicological Profile on Pyrethrins and Pyrethroids* (2003b) did not find the typical signs of developmental toxicity in animals exposed to pyrethrins or pyrethroids, particularly deltamethrin. There were no studies of reproductive or developmental effects following inhalation.

ATSDR reported that numerous studies of pyrethorids administered orally in rats and mice did not indicate any developmental toxicity at doses below those which cause maternal toxicity. In utero exposure of rats resulted in cellular changes indicative of compromised immunological function. Santoni et al. (1997, 1998, 1999) reported treatment-related increases in natural killer (NK) cell and antibody-dependent cytotoxic activity, impaired thymocyte function, increased levels of T cells in peripheral blood, and decreased levels of T cells in the spleen in rats after their mothers were given 50 mg/kg/day cypermethrin orally during gestation—a dose schedule that did not result in clinical signs of maternal toxicity. Malaviya et al. (1993) observed significant increases in the levels of dopamine and muscarinic receptors of striatal membrane in rat pups that had been exposed to 15 mg cypermethrin/kg on GDs 5–21.

The Volume 11 committee identified three new studies and a systematic review that assessed the effects of preconception and prenatal exposure to permethrin on the development of offspring. In a two-generation study with mice, males and females were given 0, 4.9, 9.8, and 19.6 mg/kg/d permethrin by gavage for 4 weeks before mating (Farag et al., 2006). The highest dose produced signs of toxicity in the F0 mice, with body weight loss in the females during gestation and lactation. There was a significant ($p<0.05$) reduction in fetal weight and in the number of live pups born to females receiving the two highest doses. Postnatal assessment of the F1 offspring showed that at 9.8 and 19.6 mg/kg there was a significant reduction in righting reflexes, swimming ability, and open field activity and a slowed development of cliff avoidance; these effects were not seen in pups whose dams received 4.9 mg/kg permethrin. Imanishi et al. (2013) found other effects of prenatal permethrin exposure on neurodevelopment. Pregnant mice received a single dose of 0, 2, 10, 50, or 75 mg/kg permethrin on GD 10.5. On GD 17.5, exposure to 10 mg/kg resulted in significant increases in abnormalities of the anterior communicating arteries in the brain of male fetuses but not of female fetuses. Fetal brains obtained on GD 17.5 had anatomical abnormalities, including altered vascular formation, and on PND 7 rat brains had alterations in the thickness of the neocortex and hippocampus and significantly increased norepinephrine and dopamine levels. Even the lowest dose of 2 mg/kg showed significant influences on vascular development in fetuses and on adult offspring behaviors. At 8 and 12 weeks of age, male mice had a significant reduction in standing ability and locomotor activity at the 2 mg/kg dose; these effects were not observed in female offspring.

One new study on the effects of deltamethrin on adult male offspring of treated dams was identified (Ben Slima et al., 2012). Pregnant mice received 5 mg/kg/day deltamethrin by gavage from GD 3 to GD 21. Male offspring were assessed for fertility when the animals achieved sexual maturity. Although the body weights of the dams were significantly reduced, there were no significant differences in absolute and relative epididymides weights in offspring. However, there were significant differences in absolute and relative testes weights (reduced to approximately half of the control value, $p\leq0.05$); reduced spermatozoa counts and percent of motile and viable sperm; increased abnormal sperm; and increases in testicular histopathology.

Saillenfait et al. (2017) assessed the effects of prenatal exposure to cypermethrin on fetal testicular steroidogenesis. Cypermethrin (0.1, 1, 5, or 10 mg/kg/day) administered on GDs 13–19 had no effect on anogenital distance of the male fetuses assessed on GD 19, but the two highest doses reduced testosterone production. Testicular mRNA expressions of HMG-CoA synthase and reductase, and the genes *SRB1*, *StAR*, *P450scc*, *3βHSD*, *P450 17A1*, and *17βHSD*, were not affected at any dose.

A systematic review of inherited transgenerational effects was conducted by the National Institute of Environmental Health and Sciences (Walker et al., 2018). The researchers found that there was no evidence of transgenerational effects of pesticide exposure in humans. However, there were three rodent studies—all from the same group of investigators—that examined whether transgenerational effects might occur following gestational exposure to a mixture of permethrin and DEET. The studies assessed the effects of the pesticide mixture on growth and development, reproductive effects in offspring, and renal effects in offspring. Two studies evaluated the body weight of F3 offspring and reported no impact of exposure on post-weaning weight at PND 21, but an increased weight at 12 months of age (Manikkam et al., 2012a,b). Two studies reported on male reproductive effects with no associations for most endpoints (Manikkam et al., 2012a,b). Three studies (Manikkam et al., 2012a,b; Nilsson et al., 2012) reported decreased ovarian follicle counts and increased ovarian cysts in female rats of the F3 generation of F0 gestating females exposed to 190 mg/kg/day permethrin and DEET, but inconsistent effects on puberty and no effects on fertility and ovarian weight were reported. Confidence in these findings is limited by inconsistencies across the studies (heterogeneity of endpoints, differences in the measurement of endpoints), a lack of studies from other research groups, and a lack of analysis using the litter as the unit of analysis.

Synthesis and Conclusions

Pyrethroid insecticides have been used for many years and were widely used in both the 1990–1991 Gulf War and the Post-9/11 conflicts. In particular, permethrin was used to treat uniforms and bed nets to control sand flies, which were vectors for infectious diseases such as leishmanisis.

Reproductive Effects

Several studies have assessed the effects of exposure to pyrethroids on human male reproductive parameters. Most of the studies assessed pyrethroid exposure by measuring the levels of the metabolite PBA in urine. With the exception of one study in Japanese men (Imai et al., 2014), which found no association between PBA levels and semen parameters or male reproductive hormones, the other five studies considered by the committee found that increasing levels of pyrethroid metabolites in urine were associated with decreased sperm concentrations and motility and increased sperm abnormal morphology and DNA damage and disomy. Numerous animal studies in rats and mice also indicate that exposure to permethrin, cypermethrin, and deltamethrin has adverse effects on male reproduction, especially sperm parameters and reproductive hormones. One limitation of these studies is that the PBA reflects only recent exposure, given the short half-life of pyrethroids, and in most cases only a single measurement of pyrethroid metabolites was made.

The Volume 11 committee identified one study of the effects of pyrethroid exposure on female reproduction and it showed increased TTP and reduced fertility (Hu et al., 2018).

Several epidemiologic studies on the effects of prenatal exposure to pyrethroids on birth outcomes were considered. When the assessed exposure to pyrethroids was based on the concentration of metabolites in urine, there was a negative association between exposure and birth weight, although this was not seen in a study where permethrin exposure was based on its concentration in cord blood. There were no animal studies that added to the evidence base for effects on female reproduction or birth outcomes.

The Volume 11 committee concludes that there is limited/suggestive evidence of an association between exposure to pyrethroid pesticides and reproductive effects in men.

The Volume 11 committee also concludes that there is inadequate/insufficient evidence to determine whether an association exists between exposure to pyrethroid pesticides and reproductive effects in women, or with adverse pregnancy outcomes.

Developmental Effects

The effects of prenatal pyrethroid exposure on the neurodevelopment of children were assessed in several studies with mixed results. Hisada et al. (2017) found that mothers' exposure to pyrethroids during the first trimester of pregnancy was positively associated with their children's development scores at 18 months of age—that is, greater exposure in the mothers was associated with better performance in the children. This conclusion was contradicted by several other studies, including that of Watkins et al. (2016), who found that children born to mothers with higher PBA concentrations during any trimester of pregnancy had lower scores on developmental tests at 24 months of age; a study by Xue et al. (2013) in China that reported an association between pyrethroid metabolite concentrations in the mother's urine and the developmental quotient in their children at 1 year of age; a study by Gunier et al. (2017) that used geospatial data to estimate prenatal exposure and found negative associations with child IQ at age 7 years; a study by Furlong et al. (2017b) that found increased PBA and CDCCA were both associated with decrements in children's neurodevelopment at 4, 6, and 7–9 years of age; and a study by Shelton et al. (2014) that found that preconception or third-trimester exposure (but not first- or second-trimester exposure) to pyrethroids (as determined by proximity to areas of agricultural pesticide application) was associated with an increased risk of ASD. However, the PELAGIE study in France found no significant association between a mother's urinary pyrethroid metabolite concentrations during early pregnancy and cognitive outcomes in their children at age 6 years, with the exception of one developmental subscale (Viel et al., 2015, 2017), and a study from Japan (Hisada et al., 2017) found better developmental quotients associated with prenatal exposure.

Prenatal exposure to pyrethroids was not associated with childhood leukemia. Studies of the effects of prenatal exposure to permethrin and piperonyl butoxide on noninfectious cough at ages 5–6 years were inconclusive. Although exposure to pyrethroids was associated with reduced child growth at 1 and 2 years of age, the effect was limited to boys only and for only two of the four metabolites measured (Coker et al., 2018).

Animal studies reviewed by the Volume 2 committee and ATSDR did not indicate that prenatal exposure of animals to pyrethroids causes postnatal developmental effects, although one research group did find effects on immune function that deserve further study. The Volume 11 committee considered two additional animal studies of pyrethroids that indicated that prenatal exposure at levels that do not cause maternal toxicity may result in neurodevelopmental effects (structural brain abnormalities, poor performance on neurodevelopmental tests) in offspring. Although there is evidence in rodent models that transgenerational effects are possible (Walker et al., 2018), their relevance to human health is not yet clear.

The Volume 11 committee concludes that there is limited/suggestive evidence of an association between prenatal exposure to pyrethroid pesticides and developmental effects.

TABLE 5-5 Summary of Reproductive and Developmental Effects of Pyrethroid Pesticides

Study	Population	Exposure	Results
Reproductive Effects			
Reproductive Effects in Men			
Xia et al. (2008)	376 eligible men provided semen and urine samples at infertility clinic in Nanjing, China; recruited between March 2004 and March 2006.	Urinary concentrations of PBA were assessed.	Compared with men in the lower PBA quartiles, men in higher quartiles were more likely to have below-reference sperm concentration (ORs for increasing exposure quartiles, 1.00, 1.31 [95% CI 0.65–2.64]; 1.73 [95% CI 0.87–3.45]; 2.04 [95% CI 1.02–4.09]; p-value for trend=0.027). No statistical significance was found between the three higher 3 PBA quartiles and the lowest PBA quartile in terms of below-reference sperm number per ejaculum and sperm motility. For semen volume, although the OR of quartile 3 was significantly higher than that of quartile 1, the exposure–response trends were not monotonic.
Ji et al. (2011)	240 men recruited from an infertility clinic in China between April 2005 and March 2007.	Urinary concentrations of PBA were assessed.	Significant inverse correlation was observed between the urinary PBA level and the sperm concentration ($\beta = -0.27$, 95% CI –0.41– –0.12, $p<0.001$). A significant positive correlation between urinary PBA level and sperm DNA fragmentation ($\beta=0.27$, 95% CI 0.15–0.39, $p<0.001$) was found.
Imai et al. (2014)	323 men from a larger cross-sectional, multi-center study. Inclusion criteria were (1) university student, (2) 18–24 years old, and (3) he and his mother were born in Japan. Recruitment in Tokyo May 1999–May 2000 and April 2002–May 2003.	Urine and semen collection. Urine analyzed for PBA; PBA was detected in 294 of 322 samples of urine (91.3%).	No significant difference in PBA levels between men with a semen parameter below the 2010 WHO lower reference limit (n=23–52, depending on the parameter) and those with a value greater than the lower reference limit (t-test, $p>0.05$).
Yoshinaga et al. (2014)	See Imai et al. (2014) above.	Urine, blood, and semen samples collected. Concentrations of LH, FSH, SHBG, testosterone, and inhibin B in serum.	There was no significant difference between the four quartiles of urinary PBA excretion for any of the hormones except for testosterone/LH). Mean testosterone/LH was significantly higher in the 3rd quartile than in the 4th quartile ($p<0.05$); however, no linear trend was found.

continued

TABLE 5-5 Continued

Study	Population	Exposure	Results
Jurewicz et al. (2015)	See Radwan et al. (2014); 286 men participated.	See Radwan et al. (2014). Comet assay procedure used to assess sperm DNA damage.	A positive association was observed between CDCCA >50th percentage distribution of concentration and the percentage of medium DFI and the percentage of immature sperm ($p=0.04$, $p=0.04$, respectively). The level of PBA >50th percentage distribution in urine was positively related to the percentage of high DFI ($p=0.03$). TDCCA and DBCA levels and the sum of pyrethroid metabolites were not associated with any sperm DNA damage measures.
Radwan et al. (2015)	See Radwan et al. (2014); 195 men participated.	Semen and urine analysis as in Radwan et al. (2014). Sperm aneuploidy was measured by multicolor fluorescence in situ hybridization (FISH) test.	Association between CDCCA >50th percentile and disomy of chromosome 18 ($p=0.05$), but TDCCA in urine >50th percentile was related to XY disomy ($p=0.04$) and disomy of chromosome 21 ($p=0.05$). PBA level ≤50th and >50th percentile was related to disomy of sex chromosomes: XY disomy ($p=0.05$ and $p=0.02$, respectively), Y disomy ($p=0.04$ and 0.02, respectively), disomy of chromosome 21 ($p=0.04$ and $p=0.04$, respectively), and total disomy ($p=0.03$ and $p=0.04$, respectively). Disomy of chromosome 18 was positively associated with PBA >50th percentile ($p=0.03$). No association was found between DBCA level in urine and any of analyzed chromosome disomy.
Radwan et al. (2014)	334 men who attended infertility clinics in Lodz, Poland, for diagnostic purposes. The mean age of men was 32.2 years. Semen and urine samples were collected.	A spot urine sample was collected from each subject and analyzed for PBA, CDCCA, TDCCA, and DBCC.	Positive association was observed between CDCCA levels in urine >50th percentile and the percentage of sperm with abnormal morphology ($p=0.05$). The level of TDCCA in urine >50th percentile was negatively related to sperm concentration and the level of testosterone ($p=0.04$ and $p=0.04$, respectively). In addition, the level of TDCCA in urine <50th percentile and >50th percentile increases the percentage of sperm with abnormal morphology ($p=0.01$ and $p=0.02$, respectively). The concentrations of PBA and DBCC >50th percentile were negatively associated with one of the computer-aided semen analysis parameters, LIN ($p=0.05$ and $p=0.01$, respectively). The sum of pyrethroids >50th percentile was positively associated with the percentage of sperm with abnormal morphology ($p =0.04$).

Study	Population	Exposure	Results
Meeker et al. (2008b)	207 men between 18 and 54 years of age were recruited between January 2000 and April 2003 from Massachusetts General Hospital.	Comet assay procedure used to assess sperm DNA damage. A spot urine sample was collected from each subject and analyzed for PBA, CDCCA, and TDCCA.	Men in the highest PBA category had declines in sperm concentration and sperm motility. TDCCA concentration >75th percentile was also associated with a suggestive 20.3 million sperm/ml decline in sperm concentration (95% CI 235.3– +2.6) and a statistically significant 10% (95% CI –19% – –21%) reduction in sperm motility. In the comet assay, PBA and CDCCA were associated with increased sperm DNA damage measured as Tail%, but not comet extent or TDM. Association of PBA categories and Tail% was monotonic (p-value for trend=0.02). Regression coefficients for medium and high PBA groups were equivalent to increases in Tail% of 7.5% (95% CI –10–25%) and 20% (3–37%), respectively, relative to the study population median of 32.3% of DNA in comet tail.
Young et al. (2013)	75 men who were selected from a parent study of 341 patients at Massachusetts infertility clinic (see Meeker et al., 2008b). 90% of the men were white and non-Hispanic (96%), average age 35 years.	Three pyrethroid metabolites—PBA, CDCCA, and TDCCA—measured in urine. Multiprobe fluorescence in situ hybridization for chromosomes X, Y, and 18 was used to determine XX, YY, XY, 1818, and total sex chromosome disomy in sperm nuclei.	Disomy rates were increased by 7% to 30% across the aneuploidy outcomes, with the highest risk seen for TDCCA and XX18 (IRR=1.30, 95% CI 1.17–1.46), the lowest risk seen for TDCCA and XY18 (IRR=1.07, 95% CI 1.00–1.14), and no association with 1818. In men with PBA concentrations >LOD versus those <LOD, rates of YY18 disomy were 1.28 times higher (95% CI 1.15–1.42), whereas a lower rate (IRR=0.82, 95% CI 0.77–0.87) was seen for XY18 and total disomy (IRR=0.93, 95% CI 0.87–0.97). No association was observed between PBA and XX18 or 1818 disomy.

continued

TABLE 5-5 Continued

Study	Population	Exposure	Results
Meeker et al. (2009)	161 men from an infertility clinic recruited during 2000–2003 from Massachusetts General Hospital; 18–54 years of age; measured serum reproductive and thyroid hormone levels.	Measured pyrethroid metabolites PBA, CDCCA, and TDCCA in spot urine samples.	Compared with men who had values below the median, men in the highest PBA category had significantly higher FSH levels ($p=0.001$; p-value for trend among low, medium, and high categories=0.002) but not higher levels of LH ($p=0.054$). When adjusting for potential confounders, categories for all three metabolites, as well as their summed values, were positively associated with FSH (all p-values for trend <0.05). Statistically significant relationships with LH were also found. CDCCA and TDCCA were inversely associated with inhibin B (p for trend=0.03 and 0.02, respectively). Finally, there was evidence that TDCCA was inversely associated with testosterone and the free androgen index (the ratio of testosterone to sex hormone binding globulin; p-value for trend=0.09 and 0.05, respectively).
Reproductive Effects in Women			
Hu et al. (2018)	615 women in Shanghai, China, recruited from two preconception care clinics between August 2013 and April 2015. 496 women left for study analysis.	PBA, TDCCA, and CDCCA measured in urine. OP exposure also measured. Women asked about pesticides exposure and perceived stress and lifestyle.	Women in the highest quartile for PBA had longer TTP (fecundability OR=0.72, 95% CI 0.53–0.98) and increased infertility (OR=2.03, 95% CI 1.10–3.74). Concentrations of TDCCA and CDCCA were below the level of detection and were not further examined.
Adverse Pregnancy Outcomes			
Dabrowski et al. (2003)	Women who delivered their children in 25 maternity hospitals in the region of Lodz, central Poland. 389 women and 377 infants with birth weight ≥2,500 g. Infants delivered randomly on 70 selected days between January 31, 1998, and June 30, 2001.	Questionnaire on pesticide use and involvement in heavy physical work on the farm in each pregnancy trimesters was administered by a physician 1-2 days after delivery. 95 women (19.3%) reported pesticide exposure in first or second trimester of pregnancy.	Infants born to women exposed to pesticides in first or second trimester had birth weight lower by 189 g than that of infants of the nonexposed women. When adjusted for pregnancy duration, the women exposed to pesticides delivered infants with birth weight lower by about 100 g ($p=0.067$) compared with nonexposed women. Mothers exposed to pesticides on average delivered half a week earlier than those nonexposed ($p=0.05$).

Study	Population	Exposure	Results
Ding et al. (2015)	Prospective cohort in rural northern China. 454 mother–infant pairs recruited between September 2010 and 2012.	Pyrethroid metabolites in maternal urine at delivery analyzed. Assessed birth outcomes, including birth weight, length, head circumference, and gestational duration. Creatinine-adjusted medians of pyrethroid metabolites in urine were 0.51 μg/g for CDCCA, 0.65 μg/g for TDCCA, and 0.68 μg/g for PBA.	Increase in total metabolites, but not any individual metabolite, was associated with a decrease in birth weight (adjusted β= −96.76 g per log_{10} unit increase, 95% CI −173.15– −20.37).
Zhang et al. (2014b)	147 mother–infant pairs recruited during early pregnancy at a Tokyo hospital in Japan 2009–2011. Blood and urine samples obtained in the first trimester; infant blood collected 5 days postpartum.	Concentrations of FT4, TSH, and TBG in maternal serum; PBA and iodine concentrations in maternal urine; and of FT4 and TSH in neonatal blood were determined.	No significant correlation of PBA concentration in maternal urine of the first trimester of gestation with neonatal thyroid hormone concentration (FT4, p=0.09; and TSH, p=0.69) or with body size at birth (p>0.05). No nonlinear relationship between prenatal pyrethroid exposure and neonatal outcomes.
Neta et al. (2011)	Baltimore Tracking Health Related to Environmental Exposures study; cord blood was collected from 341 births between November 26, 2004, and March 16, 2005.	185 (62%) cord blood samples were analyzed for cis- and trans-permethrin isomers and PBO.	Permethrin levels were (p-value <0.05) negatively associated with anti-inflammatory response (cytokine component 3) and positively associated with an IL-1β response (cytokine component 5). Associations were significant only for most highly exposed group versus lowest exposure group. A one-unit change in permethrin levels was associated with a nonsignificant 1-day decrease in gestational age (95% CI −2–0.2 days); most highly exposed group was significantly associated with a 2-day decrease versus lowest-exposure group.
Developmental Effects			
Neurodevelopmental Effects			
Horton et al. (2011)	CCCEH cohort study. Subjects included 230 mother–child pairs selected from an ongoing prospective cohort study. Pregnant women ages 18–35 years who self-identified as either African American or Dominican.	Children assessed at age 36 months with BSID-II. Children's home environments were evaluated at 3 years of age; maternal prenatal urine samples from third trimester and maternal personal air samples (48 hrs) were collected during the third trimester of pregnancy.	No significant association between permethrin concentration in air and 36-month MDI. However, there was a significant risk of lower MDI scores associated with the highest quartile PBO concentrations versus controls (OR= −4.57, 95% CI −0.30– −8.84). The highest category of PBO exposure was associated with a 3.9-point mean decrement in MDI score (95% CI −0.25– −7.49).

continued

TABLE 5-5 Continued

Study	Population	Exposure	Results
Gunier et al. (2017)	CHAMACOS cohort, see Eskenazi et al. (2004) 283 mother–child pairs.	Children assessed at 7 yrs old for neurodevelopment using WISC-IV. Agricultural pesticide use within 1 km of mother's residence during pregnancy estimated using California Pesticide Use Reporting data from 1999–2001.	Pyrethroid use was associated with lower scores on the full-scale IQ (β= –2, 95% CI –3.7– –0.3) and the verbal comprehension (β= –1.8, 95% CI –3.4– –0.3) and perceptual reasoning (β= –2.1, 95% CI –4.0– –0.2) subscales, but not working memory or processing speed scores. There were no significant changes in other WISC-IV domains.
Furlong et al. (2017b)	Mount Sinai Children's Environmental Health Cohort assessed 162 mother–infant pairs during pregnancy in 1998–2001 in New York City.	Maternal urine samples in third trimester of pregnancy analyzed for PBA, TDCCA, and CDCCA. Children were assessed for neurodevelopment at 4, 6, and 7–9 years of age using parent reports on the BASC and BRIEF.	Detectable levels of PBA during pregnancy were associated with worse scores on internalizing (β= –4.50, 95% CI –8.05– –0.95), depression (β= –3.21, 95% CI –6.38– –0.05), somatization (β= –3.22, 95% CI –6.38– –0.06), behavioral regulation (β= –3.59, 95% CI –6.97– –0.21), emotional control (β= –3.35, 95% CI –6.58– –0.12), shifting (β= –3.42, 95% CI –6.73– –0.11), and monitoring (β= –4.08, 95% CI –7.07– –1.08) scales. Detectable levels of CDCCA were associated with worse scores on externalizing (β= –4.74, 95% CI –9.37– –0.10), conduct problems (β= –5.35, 95% CI –9.90– –0.81), behavioral regulation (β= –6.42, 95% CI –11.39– –1.45), and inhibitory control (β= –7.20, 95% CI –12.00– –2.39). TDCCA was not associated with adverse performance for any composite or subscale except for better performance on the BASC anxiety subscale (β=4.61, 95% CI 0.05–9.16). No effects of sex or race at 0.10 level.
Hisada et al. (2017)	See Zhang et al. (2014b) above.	Maternal urine analyzed for PBA; infant blood for TSH. Mothers completed Kinder Infant Development Scale, Index of Child Care Environment.	Infants whose mother had higher pyrethroid exposure during pregnancy had a higher development quotient score, and infants whose Index of Child Care Environment scores were higher had a higher development quotient. A positive canonical correlation coefficient (0.216, p=0.03) was found, indicating that a higher subscale score on "social relationships with children" was obtained for children whose mother had higher pyrethroid exposure during pregnancy.

Study	Population	Exposure	Results
Xue et al. (2013)	Prenatal urine of 497 pregnant women from Henan province, China, was collected in July–December 2010. Infants assessed at 1 year of age.	Mother answered questions about chemical exposure during pregnancy.	Increasing levels of pyrethroid metabolites in the urine of mothers was associated with a gradual downward trend ($p=0.47$) in the development quotient of the 1-year infants.
Watkins et al. (2016)	187 pregnant women enrolled between 1997 and 2001 into the Early Life Exposures in Mexico to Environmental Toxicants study, a longitudinal cohort study in Mexico City; subset of 21 women. Children assessed for developmental functioning at 24 and 36 months of age.	Measured maternal urinary PBA concentrations during each trimester of pregnancy. Used BSID-IIS to assess developmental functioning of infants and children using the MDI and PDI.	Lower MDI scores at 24 months were seen in the medium and high PBA categories compared with those with non-detectable urinary PBA (–3.5 and –3.8, respectively); p-value for trend=0.07). Findings were slightly stronger among girls, with MDI-24 scores among those in the medium and high PBA groups 6 points below scores of girls in the nondetectable category (95% CI= –12.3– –0.14 and –12.4–1.3, respectively; p-value for trend=0.08). At 36 months there was no statistical difference in scores among children in the high PBA category versus children with undetectable levels of PBA (p-value for trend=0.14). No associations between maternal PBA levels during the third trimester of pregnancy and PDI scores at 24 or 36 months of age among all participants or in sex-stratified analyses.
Eskenazi et al. (2018)	708 mother–child pairs living in Venda district of South Africa as part of the Venda Health Examination of Mothers, Babies and Their Environment (VHEMBE) longitudinal birth cohort assessed in 2012–2013.	Maternal urine and blood samples collected just before or after delivery and analyzed for PBA, CDCCA, DBCA, and TDCCA. Neurodevelopment assessed in children at 1 and/or 2 years of age using 7 or 8 scales of BSID-III.	At 1 year of age, each 10-fold increase in CDCCA, TDCCA, and PBA was significantly associated with a decrement in Social-Emotional scores (β= –0.63, 95% CI –1.14– –0.12; β= –0.48, 95% CI –0.92– –0.05; and β= –0.58, 95% CI –1.11– –0.06, respectively). At 2 years of age, each 10-fold increase in maternal DBCA levels was associated with significant decrements in Language Composite scores (β= –1.74, 95% CI –3.34– –0.13) and Expressive Communication scores (β= –0.40, 95% CI –0.77– –0.04). Significant differences by sex were estimated for pyrethroid metabolites and motor function scores at 2 years of age, with higher scores for boys and lower scores for girls.

continued

TABLE 5-5 Continued

Study	Population	Exposure	Results
Viel et al. (2015)	PELAGIE cohort in France. 3,421 pregnant women from Brittany, France, were recruited January 2002 to February 2006 before the 19th week of gestation.	Urine samples were collected during early pregnancy (6–19 gestational weeks) for mothers and at the visit at 6 years of age for children. 287 children received cognitive assessments with the WISC at age 6 as did mothers. Urine analyzed for pyrethroid metabolites PBA, 4-F-PBA, CDCCA, TDCCA and DBCA.	Assessed association between maternal prenatal pyrethroid metabolite concentrations and neurocognitive scores, adjusting for potential confounders of the associations, urinary creatinine levels, DMP and DEP prenatal concentrations, and the corresponding childhood pyrethroid metabolite concentrations. No consistent association was found, although some evidence suggested a potentially negative trend between TDCCA concentrations and WISC-Working memory index (p-value for trend=0.18).
Viel et al. (2017)	See Viel et al. (2015), PELAGIE cohort.	The children's behavior was further evaluated for three subscales of the Strengths and Difficulties Questionnaire: prosocial behavior, internalizing disorders, and externalizing disorders.	Only increasing concentrations of CDCCA in prenatal urine were associated with any abnormal or borderline scores on the Strengths and Difficulties Questionnaire and only for internalizing disorders (p=0.05).
Shelton et al. (2014)	Childhood Autism Risks from Genetics and Environment study is a population-based case-control study of 970 participants with ASD (n=486) or developmental disorder (n=168) with typically developing referents (n=316).	Commercial pesticide application data from the California Pesticide Use Report (1997–2008) were linked to the addresses during pregnancy. One-third of mothers lived within 1.5 km of an agricultural pesticide application.	Prenatal proximity (within 1.5 km) to pyrethroids was associated with an increased risk for ASD if the exposure was prior to conception (OR=1.82, 95% CI 1.00–3.31) or in the third trimester (OR=1.87, 95% CI 1.02–3.43). Exposure at 1.75 km was associated with an increased risk for ASD only in the third trimester (OR=1.83, 95% CI 1.04–3.23). For developmental disorder and residential proximity to agricultural pesticide application, there was a significant risk only for a distance of 1.75 km during the third trimester (OR=2.34, 95% CI 1.18–4.67).

Study	Population	Exposure	Results
Other Developmental Effects			
Carmichael et al. (2014)	569 cases of children born during 1997–2006 with 1 of 8 congenital heart defects in 8 counties in San Joaquin Valley, CA, and 785 infants born without birth defects. Heart defects (heterotaxia; tetralogy of Fallot; hypoplastic left heart syndrome; coarctation of the aorta; pulmonary valve stenosis; ventricular septal defect, perimembranous; and atrial septal defect, secundum) based on California Birth Defects Monitoring Program.	Pesticide exposure was estimated for each mother on the basis of her residence from 3 months prior to conception to delivery using geospatial coding for eight San Joaquin counties and the Pesticide Use Reporting records for pesticides applied at greater than 100 lbs in any of the eight counties.	Prenatal exposure to permethrin was not significantly associated with any heart defect and only the ventricular septal defect, perimembranous showed a nonsignificant increase (OR=2.2, 95% CI 0.8–5.7).
Monge et al. (2007)	N=334 subjects with cases of leukemia ages 0–14 years old. Diagnosed in Costa Rica during 1995–2000. Population controls (N=579).	Parents were interviewed about risk factors for childhood leukemia, and their exposures were rated as to hazard value and by time of occurrence. 22 pesticides were identified, including deltamethrin.	Neither maternal nor paternal exposure to deltamethrin at any time prior to birth was significantly associated with childhood leukemia for either boys or girls.
Liu et al. (2012)	CCCEH birth cohort. Children 5–6 years of age.	PBO and permethrins were measured in personal air during the third trimester of pregnancy. Air samples collected for 2 consecutive days. Mothers reported on their children's coughs.	Prenatal exposure to cis- and trans-permethrin was not significantly associated with noninfectious cough at age 5–6 years; however, there was a positive association between noninfectious cough and prenatal PBO and non-infectious cough in children ages 5–6 years (OR=1.27 for unit change in log PBO, 95% CI 1.09–1.48, $p<0.01$). Exposure to PBO or permethrins at ages 5–6 years was not associated with an increase in childhood cough.

continued

TABLE 5-5 Continued

Study	Population	Exposure	Results
Coker et al. (2018)	708 mother–child pairs in VHEMBE longitudinal birth cohort.	Maternal urine and blood samples collected just before or after delivery and analyzed for PBA, DCCA, DBCA, and TDCCA. Anthropometric measures of children taken at least at one or both follow-up visits around age 1 or 2 years old.	DBCA and TDCCA were inversely related to BMI-for-age and weight-for-height overall; however, results suggested that weight-for-age and weight-for-height associations for TDCCA (sex interaction p-value weight-for-age=0.02; p-value weight-for-height=0.13) and CDCCA (sex interaction p-value weight for-age=0.02; p-value weight-for-height=0.08) were strongest and most consistent in boys relative to girls. Only boys had significant decreases in BMI-for-age (p=0.05) and weight-for-height (p=0.05) for DBCA exposure, and for weight-for-age (p=0.05), BMI-for-age (p=0.04), and weight-for-height (p=0.03) for exposure to TDCCA. None of the other exposures or measures were significantly related.

NOTE: ASD=autism spectrum disorder; BASC=Behavior Assessment System for Children; BMI=body mass index; BSID=Bayley Scales of Infant Development II; BRIEF=Behavior Rating Inventory of Executive Functioning; CCCEH=Columbia Center for Children's Environmental Health study; CDCCA=cis-3-2,2-dichlorovinyl)-2,2-dimethylcyclopropane carboxylic acid; CHAMACOS=Center for the Health Assessment of Mothers and Children of Salinas study; CI=confidence interval; DBCA=cis-2,2-dibromovinyl-2,2-dimethylcyclopropane-1-carboxylic acid; DEP=diethyl phosphate; DFI=DNA fragmentation index; DMP=dimethyl phosphate; DNA=deoxyribonucleic acid; FSH=follicle-stimulating hormone; FT4=free thyroxine; IQ=intelligence quotient; IRR=incidence rate ratio; LH=luteinizing hormone; LOD=level of detection; MDI=mental development index; OP=organophosphate; OR=odds ratio; PBA=3-phenoxybenzoic acid; PBO=piperonyl butoxide; PDI=psychomotor development index; SHBG=sex hormone binding globulin; TBG=thyroxin-binding globulin; TDCCA=trans-3-2,2-dichlorovinyl)-2,2-dimethylcyclopropane carboxylic acid; TSH=thyroid-stimulating hormone; TTP=time to pregnancy; VHEMBE=Venda Health Examination of Mothers, Babies and Their Environment; WHO=World Health Organization; WISC-IV=Wechsler Intelligence Scale for Children, 4th edition.

LINDANE

Lindane is the only organochlorine pesticide considered by the committee in this report. It is the γ-isomer of 1,2,3,4,5,6-hexachlorocyclohexane (HCH), a persistent organochlorine pesticide commonly used to treat ectoparasites (e.g., scabies and lice). It is available as a 1% shampoo and lotion to topically treat lice infestations on humans. The Food and Drug Administration recommends that lindane be used only when other treatments have not worked or if the person cannot use other treatments (FDA, 2018). Service members are most likely to be exposed to lindane during deployment as a result of its use as an ectoparasiticide and ovicide. Fricker et al. (2000) reported that lindane was used to delouse prisoners of war in the 1990–1991 Gulf War, but U.S. service members were also issued small containers of lindane as a powder for personal use, and several soldiers indicated they used the powder more frequently than directed. Lindane was also reported to be used to treat uniforms (VA, 2017). The Volume 11 committee was unable to identify any information on the extent of lindane use in the Post-9/11 conflicts.

Lindane is a central nervous system stimulant and may cause neurologic effects, including seizures, even when used correctly. Chlorophenols are the primary urinary metabolites of lindane, with 2,3,5-, 2,4,6-, and 2,4,5-trichlorophenol accounting for more than 50% of the metabolites (ATSDR, 2005). Chlorophenols have also been detected in blood in animal studies following lindane exposure (ATSDR, 2005).

The reproductive and developmental effects of lindane are summarized in Table 5-6 at the end of this section and in the following section.

Reproductive Effects

Reproductive Effects in Men and Women

The Volume 2 committee (IOM, 2003) and ATSDR (2005) both identified only one study that assessed lindane's reproductive effects in men—an examination of workers at a lindane production facility for 8 years (Tomczak et al., 1981). Blood samples from the exposed workers showed elevated serum LH concentrations, somewhat elevated levels of FSH, and somewhat depressed testosterone levels.

The Volume 11 committee identified three studies on female reproductive effects from exposure to lindane. In a study of 94 couples at a fertility clinic in Egypt, follicular fluid from each woman was collected during in vitro fertilization–embryo transfer and analyzed for the presence of lindane (mean=418.6±171.4 [sd] µg/L) among other pesticides and polychlorinated biphenyls (Al-Hussaini et al., 2018). There were negative correlations between the follicular fluid concentration of lindane and endometrial thickness (p=0.0001), and a high concentration of lindane was associated with a lower implantation rate (p=0.006). Lindane did not reduce fertilization or early embryo cleavage rates.

In an earlier study of the association between exposure to lindane and endometriosis, Buck Louis et al. (2012) assessed 473 women 18–44 years of age scheduled for a laparoscopy or laparotomy (operative cohort) and an age and residence matched population cohort of 127 women in San Francisco, California, between 2007 and 2009. Serum and fat samples were analyzed for HCH and its β and γ isomers along with other persistent organic pollutants. Lindane in the fat of the operative cohort was significantly associated with endometriosis (OR=1.27, 95% CI 1.01–1.59). Serum β-HCH was significantly associated with endometriosis in the population cohort (OR=1.72, 95% CI 1.09–2.72), but not the operative cohort; fat samples were not analyzed for the population cohort, only sera. In another study in western Washington State, conducted from 1996 to 2001, Upson et al. (2013) compared levels of several endocrine-disrupting chemicals in the sera of 248 women with endometriosis and 538 population-based women. β-HCH—but not γ-HCH (lindane)—was associated with endometriosis (third versus lowest quartile OR=1.7, 95% CI 1.0–2.8; highest versus lowest quartile OR=1.3, 95% CI 0.8–2.4), and the risk was even greater for ovarian endometriosis specifically (highest versus lowest quartile OR=2.5, 95% CI 1.1–5.3). A third study of 55 women in France with endometriosis (24 with deep infiltrating endometriosis only and 25 with deep infiltrating endometriosis and ovarian endometriosis) and 44 controls was conducted between 2013 and 2015 (Ploteau et al., 2017). Concentrations of β-HCH in adipose tissue collected during surgery were not associated with an increased risk of deep infiltrating endometriosis (OR=1.58, 95% CI 0.94–2.80), but there was a significant association with deep infiltrating endometriosis combined with ovarian endometriosis (OR=3.64, 95% CI 1.52–11.15). The researchers analyzed for γ-HCH in the fat tissue, but the detection rate was so low that further analysis was not performed (Ploteau et al., 2016).

Adverse Pregnancy Outcomes

Volume 2 discussed two studies that examined the effects of lindane on fetal outcomes; however, lindane was not a unique exposure in either study. Willis et al. (1993) found that among 535 pregnant women who resided in an agricultural area in San Diego, California, only those who were not exposed to pesticides—which included carbaryl and lindane—had spontaneous abortion or preterm delivery; furthermore, the unexposed women also had a greater incidence of low-birth-weight infants. The Volume 2 committee found this study hard to interpret because critical information such as the number of exposed women in the cohort was not presented.

The second study assessed paternal insecticide exposure and pregnancy outcomes among 32 Italian pesticide applicators and their wives (Petrelli et al., 2000). Although there was an increased risk of spontaneous abortion among the exposed wives (OR=3.8, 95% CI 1.2–12.0), there was little information on the selection and recruitment of study subjects, and a crude exposure measurement was used.

The 2005 ATSDR review *Toxicological Profile for Alpha-, Beta-, Gamma-, and Delta-Hexachlorocyclohexane* had no reports on fetal outcomes following inhalation exposure in humans. One study found that babies born to pregnant Indian women with higher blood levels of HCH isomers, including the gamma isomer, also had higher levels of lindane and were more likely to have intrauterine fetal growth retardation (Siddiqui et al., 2003); however, mothers also had exposure to other organochlorine pesticides.

The Volume 11 committee identified one new study that examined the effects of prenatal exposure to organochlorine pesticides in infants born in an urban area of Northern India (Tyagi et al., 2015). The levels of γ-HCH in maternal blood and placental tissue were measured in 50 women who were at less than 37 weeks of gestation and 50 women who were at 37 weeks or more; γ-HCH residues were detected in the blood of all the women. There was a negative correlation between the blood levels of γ-HCH and placental weight (r= –0.401, p=0.006) but no correlation with the weight of the infant or length of gestation.

Animal Studies

The Volume 2 committee found mixed results from studies of the reproductive effects of lindane in animals. Lindane was found to produce reversible decreases in the total number of sperm in mice (Smith, 1991), testicular degeneration in rats (Chowdhury et al., 1987), and reduced "reproductive behavior" in young rams (Beard et al., 1999). Lindane also had adverse effects on reproduction in female animals. Low doses (10 mg/kg/day for 138 days) of lindane reduced fecundity and litter size in rats (Trifonova et al., 1970); increased the number of resorbed fetuses in hamsters, rabbits, and rats (Dzierzawski, 1977);

and increased the duration of diestrus, shortened the duration of estrus, lengthened the gestation period, decreased the number of fetuses, increased the number of dead fetuses, and decreased the growth of the young in rats (Nayshteyn and Leybovich, 1971). However, another study found lindane to have no effect on the numbers of pregnancies, abortions, and dead or resorbed fetuses when given to rats on GDs 6-15 (Khera et al., 1979).

The 2005 ATSDR review *Toxicological Profile for Alpha-, Beta-, Gamma-, and Delta-Hexachlorocyclohexane* found no studies on reproductive effects in animals following inhalation exposure to any HCH isomer. Anti-estrogenic properties were found in female rats given γ-HCH by the oral route (Chadwick et al., 1988), and female rabbits treated orally with γ-HCH had a reduced ovulation rate (Lindenau et al., 1994). The results of single and multigeneration reproduction studies in rats and mink indicate that exposure to γ-HCH reduces receptivity to mating and reduces whelping rate, decreases numbers of offspring at birth, reduces neonatal viability, and delays the maturation of pups. Those effects were primarily the result of prenatal or postnatal developmental toxicity (Beard and Rawlings, 1998; Beard et al., 1997; King, 1991).

The Volume 11 committee identified five new animal studies on the reproductive effects of lindane. In a two-generation study in rats, lindane administered in the diet to male and females for 10 weeks through mating was found to have no reproductive effects in males; in females, a lack of maternal behavior was seen in the F0 and F1 generations, but no effects were observed on mating, fertility, pregnancy, or parturition in F1 females (Matsuura et al., 2005).

Oral administration of lindane to male rats at 5 mg/kg for 30 days resulted in significantly reduced weights of the reproductive organs and in reductions of testicular DNA, RNA, protein, and enzymes (Sujatha et al., 2001). Damage to Leydig cells was seen in rats treated dermally with a single 1% dose of lindane (the medical dose for scabies) (Suwalsky et al., 2000).

Two in vitro animal studies were considered by the committee. Walsh and Stocco (2000) found that alpha-, delta-, and gamma-HCH inhibited steroidogenesis by reducing StAR protein expression, an action that may contribute to the pathogenesis of lindane-induced reproductive dysfunction. Ronco et al. (2001) also found that lindane produced a dose-dependent inhibition of testosterone production in hCG-stimulated Leydig cells.

Developmental Effects

The Volume 2 committee found no studies of developmental effects in humans following either maternal or paternal exposure. Furthermore, the 2005 ATSDR review *Toxicological Profile for Alpha-, Beta-, Gamma-, and Delta-Hexachlorocyclohexane* also found no studies of developmental effects of lindane in humans following either maternal or paternal exposure by any route of exposure.

The Volume 11 committee identified only one new study of developmental effects in infants following maternal exposure to lindane. Lindane levels in placentas were analyzed in infants with and without neural tube defects who had been born to 130 women in an agricultural area of China. Higher levels of γ-HCH in the placenta were associated with an increased risk for any neural tube defects (OR=3.36, 95% CI 1.10–6.44) (Ren et al., 2011).

Animal Studies

In *Volume 2*, a number of studies indicated that lindane is not teratogenic. A three-generation study of rats (Palmer et al., 1978) and experiments with mice (Chernoff and Kavlock, 1983; Gray and Kavlock, 1984) did not demonstrate any teratogenic effects.

The 2005 ATSDR review *Toxicological Profile for Alpha-, Beta-, Gamma-, and Delta-Hexachlorocyclohexane* reported that there were no inhalation data on the developmental effects of lindane in animals. Adverse effects on testicular histology and sperm numbers occurred in the adult male offspring of mice that were exposed to γ-HCH during gestation (Traina et al., 2003).

No adverse prenatal developmental effects of γ-HCH from oral exposure have been found in rats or rabbits (Khera et al., 1979; Palmer et al., 1978; Seiler et al., 1994). Decreases in fetal weight, fetal thymic weight, and placental weight were reported in mice exposed to a single oral dose of γ-HCH on day 12 of gestation (Hassoun and Stohs, 1996). No effects on embryonic development were seen in rabbits treated orally with γ-HCH (Seiler et al., 1994). Due to the lack of developmental toxicity studies in humans as well as the lack of inhalation and dermal data in animals, insufficient information is available to indicate whether HCH affects development via all three routes of exposure. Pharmacokinetic data suggest that HCH isomers might have the potential to affect development across all routes of exposure.

The Volume 11 committee identified three studies of oral exposure to lindane in animals. In a series of experiments, pregnant mice were treated on GDs 9 to 16 with 15 or 25 mg/kg lindane, and male and female offspring were assessed for developmental effects. There were no significant effects on gross malformations in pups, the average number of live pups per litter, the incidence of stillbirths or runts, sex ratio, survival to weaning, or developmental landmarks. Adult F1 males had changes in testicular enzyme activity, germ cell distribution, and chromatic abnormalities of the sperm at PND 60 (i.e., sexual maturity) that were not significant by PND 100 (Di Consiglio et al., 2009; Traina et al., 2003). Female F1 mice showed early increases in uterus weight that were not evident at PND 100; only the diameter of follicular oocytes was significantly reduced in treated females (Maranghi et al., 2007). Preimplantation embryotoxicity with degenerating two-cell embryos was induced by exposure of preovulatory oocytes in mice at the highest lindane dose tested (25 mg/kg); no other signs of embryotoxicity were observed (e.g., apoptosis or micronucleus induction). In one of the few studies to assess preconception exposure only, female mice were given up to 64.4 mg/kg/day lindane in drinking water for 2 weeks prior to mating. There were no cytopathological effects on the male offspring germ cells (Lopez-Casas et al., 2012).

Synthesis and Conclusions

Reproductive Effects

There is little epidemiologic information available on lindane. Both the Volume 2 committee and ATSDR found little information on the effects of lindane exposure on male reproduction in humans and none for lindane's effects on female reproduction. Three studies of endometriosis found that serum levels of β-HCH were associated with an increased risk of endometriosis, but only one of the studies found an increased risk specifically with lindane exposure (Buck Louis et al., 2012). Lindane was also associated with reduced endometrial thickness but not embryo implantation in one study of in vitro fertilization (Al-Hussaini et al., 2018). Thus, all three studies suggest that hexachlorocyclohexane may affect endometrial tissue but the association is stronger for the β-isomer and not the γ-isomer (lindane). Thus, the committee finds that more research on the association between the γ-isomer and female reproductive effects is warranted as lindane is still available to the general public.

The studies of the effects of lindane on birth outcomes are difficult to interpret because lindane was not the only pesticide to which the mothers were exposed. The single new study identified by the Volume 11 committee, Tyagi et al. (2015), found only a negative correlation with lindane and placental weight and no other adverse effects.

In general, the animal studies examined by ATSDR and the Volume 2 and Volume 11 committees found that oral exposure to lindane was associated with numerous reproductive outcomes in both male and female animals, including reduced mating behavior in both sexes and poor fetal outcomes. This body of animal evidence suggests that additional studies of the effects of lindane in humans is warranted to ascertain whether effects seen in animals may be occurring in humans. Furthermore, animals studies with gestational exposures that are equivalent to human organogenesis would be helpful.

The Volume 11 committee concludes that there is inadequate/insufficient evidence to determine whether an association exists between exposure to lindane and reproductive effects in men, or with adverse pregnancy outcomes.

The Volume 11 committee also concludes that there is limited/suggestive evidence of an association between exposure to lindane and reproductive effects in women.

Developmental Effects

There is a lack of information on developmental effects in humans following prenatal exposures to lindane; only one study of women in China found an association—in this case, between the women's lindane exposure and neural tube defects in their children (Ren et al., 2011).

Lindane has not been shown to be teratogenic in animals, and the results of studies to ascertain adverse developmental outcomes following oral exposure prenatally are mixed. Developmental effects were seen in two-generation studies of mice; adult offspring of both sexes displayed altered reproductive parameters at sexual maturity, although the effects appeared to resolve with age. ATSDR (2005) indicated that there was insufficient information to determine if lindane affects development in animals or humans. Although the animal studies indicate that lindane may be both a reproductive and a developmental toxicant, confirmation of the effects in humans is lacking. The available human studies are generally small and may be confounded by exposure to other pesticides or organochlorines; and exposure may have occurred at any point prior to or during pregnancy.

The Volume 11 committee concludes that there is inadequate/insufficient evidence to determine whether an association exists between prenatal exposure to lindane and developmental effects.

TABLE 5-6 Summary of Reproductive and Developmental Effects of Lindane

Study	Population	Exposure Assessment	Results
Reproductive Effects			
Reproductive Effects in Men and Women			
Al-Hussaini et al. (2018)	94 couples (women ages 20 to 38 years) at a university-affiliated fertility center in Assiut, Egypt; cross-sectional observation study.	Follicular fluid samples collected during in vitro fertilization–embryo transfer and analyzed for pesticides, including lindane.	Higher lindane concentrations were significantly associated with lower implantation rate ($p=0.006$) and reduced endometrial thickness ($p<0.01$) but there was no effect on the number of eggs retrieved, number of fertilized oocytes, or number of cleaved embryos.
Buck Louis et al. (2012)	473 menstruating women 18–44 years of age scheduled for a laparoscopy or laparotomy (190 with a diagnosis of endometriosis and 293 without) and an age and residence matched population cohort of 127 women (14 with endometriosis and 113 without).	Blood and urine collected from all participants and omental (abdominal) fat collected from operative cohort only.	Lindane levels in the fat of women in the operative cohort were significantly associated with endometriosis (OR=1.27, 95% CI 1.01–1.59). β-HCH in the sera of women in the population cohort was significantly associated with endometriosis (OR=1.72, 95% CI 1.09–2.72) but not in the operative cohort (OR=0.77, 95% CI 0.54–1.14).
Upson et al. (2013)	248 women ages 18–49 years with surgically confirmed endometriosis and 538 population based controls enrolled in a large health care system in western Washington State in 1996–2001.	Organochlorine pesticides were determine in serum of all participants, including β- and γ-HCH (lindane).	Serum concentrations of β-HCH were significantly associated with an increased risk of endometriosis (third versus lowest quartile OR=1.7, 95% CI 1.0–2.8; highest versus lowest quartile OR=1.3, 95% CI 0.8–2.4); the association was stronger when analysis restricted to cases of ovarian endometriosis (third versus lowest quartile OR=2.5, 95% CI 1.5–5.2; highest versus lowest quartile OR=2.5, 95% CI 1.1–5.3). γ-HCH was not significantly associated with any endometriosis or ovarian endometriosis.

Study	Population	Exposure Assessment	Results
Ploteau et al. (2017)	55 women, ages 18–45, in France with endometriosis (24 with deep infiltrating endometriosis only and 25 with deep infiltrating endometriosis and ovarian endometriosis) and 44 controls; assessed between 2013 and 2015.	Subcutaneous or abdominal adipose tissue taken during surgery was analyzed for 76 persistent organic pollutants, including the α-, β-, and γ-isomers of HCH.	Concentrations of β-HCH in adipose tissue were not associated with an increased risk of deep infiltrating endometriosis (OR=1.58, 95% CI 0.94–2.80), but there was a significant association with deep infiltrating endometriosis combined with ovarian endometriosis (OR=3.64, 95% CI 1.52–11.15). Low detection of γ-HCH in the adipose tissue precluded further analysis.
Adverse Pregnancy Outcomes			
Tyagi et al. (2015)	50 women who had below 37 weeks of gestation and 50 women who had a gestation period of 37 weeks or above term labor in Delhi, India, between November 2011 and April 2013.	Maternal blood collected at time of labor and placenta at delivery. Analyzed for residues of organochlorine pesticides, including lindane.	All samples contained lindane residue. Increased levels of γ-HCH were associated with reduced placental weight ($r= -0.401$, $p=0.006$). Lindane was not significantly associated with reduced birth weight or length of gestation.
Developmental Effects			
Ren et al. (2011)	130 women in a rural area of China; 80 women who had pregnancies with neural tube defects (cases) and 50 women who delivered healthy infants (controls).	Placental samples of cases and controls analyzed for persistent organic pollutants; concentrations of lindane were significantly higher in case than in control placentas.	Higher levels of γ-HCH were associated with increased risk for any NTDs (OR=3.36, 95% CI 1.10–6.44). Median concentration γ-HCH was higher in the placental samples of cases with anencephaly and spina bifida than those of controls, although differences in the concentration of γ-HCH for the two subtypes of NTDs were not statistically significant, and there was no apparent dose–response relationship between levels of γ-HCH and the risk of any subtype of NTDs.

NOTE: β-HCH=beta-hexachlorocyclohexane; γ-HCH=gamma-hexachlorocyclohexane; CI=confidence interval; NTD=neural tube defects; OR=odds ratio.

DEET (N,N-DIETHYL-3-METHYLBENZAMIDE)

DEET is a widely used liquid insect repellant. It is the active ingredient in a number of commercially available products such as Off® and Cutter® insect repellants. DEET may be present in these repellants at a concentration of up to 30% and, according to the label, may be used on children as young as 2 years old (ATSDR, 2017).

During the 1990–1991 Gulf War, DoD shipped approximately two 2-oz tubes of 33% DEET per service member (PAC, 1996). It was unclear to the committee if this allotment per service members was the only supply of DEET they received for the duration of their deployment.

There were no epidemiologic or other human studies of the possible reproductive or developmental effects of DEET considered by the Volume 2 committee. One animal study found an increased permeability of the blood–brain barrier and the blood–testis barrier for male rats exposed dermally to DEET and permethrin for 60 days (Abou-Donia et al., 2001). Milder effects were reported for DEET alone, but not for permethrin alone. There were no other reports on any animal reproductive or developmental effects of DEET.

The 2017 ATSDR review *Toxicological Profile for DEET (N,N-diethyl-meta-toluamide)* reported that there were no reproductive studies of DEET in humans and that there were no developmental effects of DEET found in two epidemiological studies of women and their children. In animal studies, DEET was not observed to affect fertility in male or female rats in a two-generation continuous feeding study, nor did it affect reproductive organs in intermediate- or chronic-duration oral studies in animals. One 90-day study found that the dermal application of a high dose of DEET (≥624 mg/kg/day) increased the incidence of tubular degeneration in hamster testes. One relevant animal inhalation study of male and female Sprague-Dawley rats given up to 1,511 mg/m^3 of aerosolized DEET for 13 weeks found no gross or microscopic alterations in the reproductive organs.

The Volume 11 committee found little new information on possible reproductive or developmental effects from exposure to DEET. Because there are only two new studies to be considered, there is no table of reproductive or developmental effects provided here.

In one study of the effect of DEET on human fertility, Segal et al. (2017) evaluated urine and semen samples from 90 men participating in a prospective cohort study at the Massachusetts General Hospital Fertility Center. Urinary concentrations of the DEET metabolite 3-(diethylcarbamoyl)benzoic acid were not associated with any semen parameters, and there were no differences in the parameters between the highest and lowest metabolite concentrations.

A review by Koren et al. (2003) examined the potential for increased risks to children and pregnant women from DEET use. The researchers found that the available evidence did not support an increased risk for adverse reproductive or developmental outcomes in mothers who used DEET during their second and third trimesters or in their children. There were no studies on first-trimester exposures. In the era of Zika virus, Wylie et al. (2016) also summarized available reproductive and developmental toxicity literature on DEET and concluded that DEET did not pose a health risk when used as directed.

Only one study was identified that assessed the level of DEET in cord blood and birth outcomes in Fuyang, China (Wickerham et al., 2012). Of the 112 women recruited at 36 weeks gestation who reported a healthy, uncomplicated singleton pregnancy, 73% had detectable levels of DEET in cord blood collected at delivery, the most of any pesticide. However, there was no association between DEET levels and a change in birth weights (β=110, 95% CI –49.2–269).

Synthesis and Conclusions

DEET has been used for more than 50 years as an effective insect repellant around the world. Unlike most pesticides, however, there is a dearth of information on its long-term toxicity, including its possible reproductive or developmental effects, in both humans or animals. Nonetheless, the few available data indicate that, when used as directed, DEET appears to pose no risks for reproductive or developmental effects in humans, although there do not appear to be any long-term studies of any potential reproductive or developmental effects in humans or animals to confirm this. Given the widespread use of this pesticide by men, women, and children, studies on its long-term reproductive and developmental effects in animals are warranted.

The Volume 11 committee concludes that there is inadequate/insufficient evidence to determine whether an association exists between exposure to DEET and reproductive or developmental effects.

REFERENCES

Abd El-Aziz, M.I., A.M. Sahlab, and M. Abd El-Khalik. 1994. Influence of diazinon and deltamethrine on reproductive organs and fertility of male rats. *Deutsche Tieräerztliche Wochenshrift* 101:213–248.

Abdallah, F.B., K. Hamden, I. Galeraud-Denis, A. El Feki, and L. Keskes-Ammar. 2010. An in vitro study on reproductive toxicology of deltamethrin on rat spermatozoa. *Andrologia* 42(4):254–259.

Abou-Donia, M. B., L.B. Goldstein, A. Dechovskaia, S. Bullman, K.H. Jones, E.A. Herrick, A.A. Abdel-Rahman, and W.A. Khan. 2001. Effects of daily dermal application of DEET and epermethrin, alone and in combination, on sensorimotor performance, blood-brain barrier, and blood-testis barrier in rats. *Journal of Toxicology and Environmental Health Part A* 62(7):523–541.

Aitken, R.J. 2017. DNA damage in human spermatozoa; Important contributor to mutagenesis in the offspring. *Translational Andrology and Urology* 6(Suppl 4):S761–S764.

Akbarsha, M. A., P.N. Latha, and P. Murugaian. 2000. Retention of cytoplasmic droplet by rat cauda epididymal spermatozoa after treatment with cytotoxic and xenobiotic agents. *Journal of Reproduction & Fertility* 120(2):385–390.

Akhtar, N., M.K. Srivastava, and R.B. Raizada. 2006. Transplacental disposition and teratogenic effects of chlorpyrifos in rats. *Journal of Toxicological Science* 31(5):521–527.

Alaa-Eldin, E.A., D.A. El-Shafei, and N.S. Abouhashem. 2017. Individual and combined effect of chlorpyrifos and cypermethrin on reproductive system of adult male albino rats. *Environmental Science and Pollution Research International* 24(2):1532–1543.

Aldridge, J.E., F.J. Seidler, A. Meyer, I. Thillai, and T.A. Slotkin. 2003. Serotonergic systems targeted by developmental exposure to chlorpyrifos: Effects during different critical periods. *Environmental Health Perspectives* 111(14):1736–1743.

Aldridge, J.E., F.J. Seidler, and T.A. Slotkin. 2004. Developmental exposure to chlorpyrifos elicits sex-selective alterations of serotonergic synaptic function in adulthood: Critical periods and regional selectivity for effects on the serotonin transporter, receptor subtypes, and cell signaling. *Environmental Health Perspectives* 112(2):148–155.

Aldridge, J.E., A. Meyer, F.J. Seidler, and T.A. Slotkin. 2005. Alterations in central nervous system serotonergic and dopaminergic synaptic activity in adulthood after prenatal or neonatal chlorpyrifos exposure. *Environmental Health Perspectives* 113(8):1027–1031.

Al-Hamdani, N.M., and H.N. Yajurvedi. 2010. Cypermethrin reversibly alters sperm count without altering fertility in mice. *Ecotoxicology and Environmental Safety* 73(5):1092–1097.

Al-Hussaini, T.K., A.A. Abdelaleem, I. Elnashar, O.M. Shabaan, R. Mostafa, M.A.H. El-Baz, S.E.M. El-Deek, and T.A. Farghaly. 2018. The effect of follicullar fluid pesticides and polychlorinated biphenyls concentrations on intracytoplasmic sperm injection (ICSI) embryological and clinical outcome. *European Journal of Obstetrics & Gynecology and Reproductive Biology* 220:39–43.

Arbuckle, T.E., Z. Lin, and L.S. Mery. 2001. An exploratory analysis of the effect of pesticide exposure on the risk of spontaneous abortion in an Ontario farm population. *Environmental Health Perspectives* 109(8):851–857.

ATSDR (Agency for Toxic Substances and Disease Registry). 1997a. *Toxicological profile for chlorpyrifos*. Atlanta, GA: U.S. Department of Health and Human Services.

ATSDR. 1997b. *Toxicological profile for dichlorvos*. Atlanta, GA: U.S. Department of Health and Human Services.

ATSDR. 2003a. *Toxicological profile for malathion*. Atlanta, GA: U.S. Department of Health and Human Services.

ATSDR. 2003b. *Toxicological profile for pyrethrins and pyrethroids*. Atlanta, GA: U.S. Department of Health and Human Services.

ATSDR. 2005. *Toxicological profile for alpha-, beta-, gamma-, and delta-hexachlorocyclohexane*. Atlanta, GA: U.S. Department of Health and Human Services.

ATSDR. 2008. *Toxicological profile for diazinon*. Atlanta, GA: U.S. Department of Health and Human Services.

ATSDR. 2017. *Toxicological profile for DEET (N,N-diethyl-meta-toluamide)*. Atlanta, GA: U.S. Department of Health and Human Services.

Beard, A.P., and N.C. Rawlings. 1998. Reproductive effects in mink (*Mustela vison*) exposed to the pesticides lindane, carbofuran and pentachlorophenol in a multigenerational study. *Journal of Reproduction & Fertility* 113:93–104.

Beard, A.P., A.C. McRae, and N.C. Rawlings. 1997. Reproductive efficiency in mink (*Mustela vison*) treated with the pesticides lindane, carbofuran and pentachlorophenol. *Journal of Reproduction & Fertility* 111:21–28.

Beard, A.P., P.M. Bartlewski, R.K. Chandolia, A. Honaramooz, and N.C. Rawlings. 1999. Reproductive and endocrine function in rams exposed to the organochlorine pesticides lindane and pentachlorophenol from conception. *Journal of Reproduction & Fertility* 115(2):303–314.

Bell, E., I. Hertz-Picciotto, and J.J. Beaumont. 2001. Case-cohort analysis of agricultural pesticide applications near maternal residence and selected causes of fetal death. *American Journal of Epidemiology* 154:702–710.

Ben Slima, A., F. Ben Abdallah, L. Keskes-Ammar, Z. Mallek, A. El Feki, and R. Gdoura. 2012. Embryonic exposure to dimethoate and/or deltamethrin impairs sexual development and programs reproductive success in adult male offspring mice. *Andrologia* 44(Suppl 1):661–666.

Ben Slima, A., Y. Chtourou, M. Barkallah, H. Fetoui, T. Boudawara, and R. Gdoura. 2017. Endocrine disrupting potential and reproductive dysfunction in male mice exposed to deltamethrin. *Human & Experimental Toxicology* 36(3):218–226.

Berkowitz, G.S., J.G. Wetmur, E. Birman-Deych, J. Obel, R.H. Lapinski, J.H. Godbold, I.R. Holzman, and M.S. Wolff. 2004. In utero pesticide exposure, maternal paraoxonase activity, and head circumference. *Environmental Health Perspectives* 112(3):388–391.

Bicker, W., M. Lämmerhofer, and W. Lindner. 2005. Determination of chlorpyrifos metabolites in human urine by reversed-phase/weak anion exchange liquid chromatography-electrospray ionisation-tandem mass spectrometry. *Journal of Chromatography B: Analytical Technologies in the Biomedical and Life Sciences* 822(1–2):160–169.

Bouchard, M.F., J. Chevrier, K.G. Harley, K. Kogut, M. Vedar, N. Calderon, C. Trujillo, C. Johnson, A. Bradman, D.B. Barr, and B. Eskenazi. 2011. Prenatal exposure to organophosphate pesticides and IQ in 7-year-old children. *Environmental Health Perspectives* 119(8):1189–1195.

Bradman, A., L. Quirós-Alcalá, R. Castorina, R. Aguilar Schall, J. Camacho, N.T. Holland, D.B. Barr, and B. Eskenazi. 2015. Effect of organic diet intervention on pesticide exposures in young children living in low-income urban and agricultural communities. *Environmental Health Perspectives* 123(10):1086–1093.

Buck Louis, G.M., Z. Chen, C.M. Peterson, M.L. Hediger, M.S. Croughan, R. Sundaram, J.B. Stanford, M.W. Varner, V.Y. Fujimoto, L.C. Giudice, A. Trumble, P.J. Parsons, and K. Kannan. 2012. Persistent lipophilic environmental chemicals and endometriosis: The ENDO Study. *Environmental Health Perspectives* 120:811–816.

Burke, R.D., S.W. Todd, E. Lumsden, R.J. Mullins, J. Mamczarz, W.P. Fawcett, R.P. Gullapalli, W.R. Randall, E.F.R. Pereira, and E.X. Albuquerque. 2017. Developmental neurotoxicity of the organophosphorus insecticide chlorpyrifos: From clinical findings to preclinical models and potential mechanisms. *Journal of Neurochemistry* 142(Suppl 2):162–177.

Buscail, C., C. Chevrier, T. Serrano, P. Fabienne, C. Monfort, S. Cordier, and J. Viel. 2015. Prenatal pesticide exposure and otitis media during early childhood in the PELAGIE mother–child cohort. *Occupational and Environmental Medicine* 72:837–844.

Bustos-Obregón, E., and P. González-Hormazabal. 2003. Effect of a single dose of malathion on spermatogenesis in mice. *Asian Journal of Andrology* 5(2):105–107.

Carmichael, S.L., W. Yang, E. Roberts, S.E. Kegley, A.M. Padula, P.B. English, E.J. Lammer, and G.M. Shaw. 2014. Residential agricultural pesticide exposures and risk of selected congenital heart defects among offspring in the San Joaquin Valley of California. *Environmental Research* 135:133–138.

Carmichael, S.L., W. Yang, E. Roberts, S.E. Kegley, T.J. Brown, P.B. English, E.J. Lammer, and G.M. Shaw. 2016. Residential agricultural pesticide exposures and risks of selected birth defects among offspring in the San Joaquin Valley of California. *Birth Defects Research (Part A)* 106:27–35.

Casida, J.E., D.W. Gammon, A.H. Glickman, and L.J. Lawrence. 1983. Mechanisms of selective action of pyrethroid insecticides. *Annual Review of Pharmacology and Toxicology* 23:413–438.

Cecchine, G., B.A. Golomb, L.H. Hilborne, D. Spektor, and C.R. Anthony. 2000. *A review of the scientific literature as it pertains to Gulf War illnesses: Pesticides. Volume 8.* Arlington, VA: National Defense Research Institute (RAND).
Chadwick, R.W., R.L. Cooper, J. Chang, G.L. Rehnberg, and W.K. McElroy. 1988. Possible antiestrogenic activity of lindane in female rats. *Journal of Biochemistry and Toxicology* 3:147–158.
Chauhan, L.K., M. Varshney, V. Pandey, P. Sharma, V.K. Verma, P. Kumar, and S.K. Goel. 2016. ROS-dependent genotoxicity, cell cycle perturbations and apoptosis in mouse bone marrow cells exposed to formulated mixture of cypermethrin and chlorpyrifos. *Mutagenesis*. 31(6):635–642.
Chebab, S., F. Mekircha, and E. Leghouchi. 2017. Potential protective effect of pistacia lentiscus oil against chlorpyrifos-induced hormonal changes and oxidative damage in ovaries and thyroid of female rats. *Biomedicine & Pharmacotherapy* 96:1310–1316.
Chen, X.P., Y.S. Chao, W.Z. Chen, and J.Y. Dong. 2017. Mother gestational exposure to organophosphorus pesticide induces neuron and glia loss in daughter adult brain. *Journal of Environmental Science and Health, Part B* 52(2):77–83.
Chernoff, N., and R.J. Kavlock. 1983. A teratology test system which utilizes postnatal growth and viability in the mouse. *Environmental Science Research* 27:417–427.
Choudhary, N., R. Goyal, and S.C. Joshi. 2008. Effect of malathion on reproductive system of male rats. *Journal of Environmental Biology* 29(2):259–262.
Chowdhury, A.R., H. Venkatakrishna-Bhatt, and A.K. Guatam. 1987. Testicular changes of rats under lindane treatment. *Bulletin of Environmental Contamination and Toxicology* 38:154–156.
Coker, E., J. Chevrier, S. Rauch, A. Bradman, M. Obida, M. Crause, R. Bornman, and B. Eskenazi. 2018. Association between prenatal exposure to multiple insecticides and child body weight and body composition in the VHEMBE South African birth cohort. *Environment International* 113C:122–132.
Coleman, R. E., D.A. Burkett, J.L. Putnam, V. Sherwood, J.B. Caci, B.T. Jennings, L.P. Hochberg, S.L. Spradling, E.D. Rowton, K. Blount, J. Ploch, G. Hopkins, J.W. Raymond, M.L. O'Guinn, J.S. Lee, and P.J. Weina. 2006. Impact of phlebotomine sand flies on U.S. Military operations at Tallil Air Base, Iraq: 1. Background, military situation, and development of a "leishmaniasis control program." *Journal of Medical Entomology* 43(4):647–662.
Collins, T.F.X., W.H. Hansen, and H.V. Keeler. 1971. The effect of carbaryl (Sevin) on reproduction of the rat and gerbil. *Toxicology and Applied Pharmacology* 19(2):202–216.
Curtis, K.M., D.A, Savitz, C.R. Weinberg, and T.E. Arbuckle. 1999. The effect of pesticide exposure on time to pregnancy. *Epidemiology* 10(2):112–117.
Dabrowski, S., W. Hanke, K. Polanska, T. Makowiec-Dabrowska, and W. Sobala. 2003. Pesticide exposure and birthweight: An epidemiological study in Central Poland. *International Journal of Occupational Medicine and Environmental Health* 16(1):31–39.
Dahamna, S., F. Bencheikh, D. Harzallah, S. Boussahel, A. Belgeit, M. Merghem, and H. Bouriche. 2010. Cypermetherin toxic effects on spermatogenesis and male mouse reproductive organs. *Communications in Agricultural and Applied Biological Sciences* 75(2):209–216.
Dean, J.B., and D. Blair. 1976. Dominant lethal assay in female mice after oral dosing with dichlorvos or exposure to atmospheres containing dichlorovos. *Mutation Research* 40(1):67–72.
Declerck, K., S. Remy, C. Wohlfahrt-Veje, K.M. Main, G. Van Camp, G. Schoeters, W. Vanden Berghe, and H.R. Andersen. 2017. Interaction between prenatal pesticide exposure and a common polymorphism in the *PON1* gene on DNA methylation in genes associated with cardio-metabolic disease risk—an exploratory study. *Clinical Epigenetics* 9:35.
Di Consiglio, E., G. De Angelis, M.E. Traina, E. Urbani, and E. Testai. 2009. Effect of lindane on CYP-mediated steroid hormone metabolism in male mice following in utero exposure. *Journal of Applied Toxicology* 29(8):648–655.
Ding, G., C. Cui, L. Chen, Y. Gao, Y. Zhou, R. Shi, and Y. Tian. 2015. Prenatal exposure to pyrethroid insecticides and birth outcomes in rural northern China. *Journal of Exposure Science and Environmental Epidemiology* 25:264–270.
Dirican, E. K., and Y. Kalender. 2012. Dichlorvos-induced testicular toxicity in male rats and the protective role of vitamins C and E. *Experimental and Toxicologic Pathology* 64(7–8):821–830.
Donauer, S., M. Altaye, Y. Xu, H. Sucharew, P. Succop, A.M. Calafat, J.C. Khoury, B. Lanphear, and K. Yolton. 2016. An observational study to evaluate associations between low-level gestational exposure to organophosphate pesticides and cognition during early childhood. *American Journal of Epidemiology* 184(5):410–418.
Dutta, A.L., and C.R. Sahu. 2013. Protective effect of emblica officinalis on chlorpyrifos (an organophosphate insecticide) induced male reproductive system in rats. *International Journal of Pharma and Bio Sciences* 4(1):B49–B58.
Dzierzawski, A. 1977. Embryotoxicity studies of lindane in the golden hamster, rat and rabbit. *Bulletin of the Veterinary Institute in Pulawy* 21:85–93.
Ecobichon, D.J. 2001. Pesticide use in developing countries. *Toxicology* 160(1–3):27–33.

Elbetieha, A., S. I. Da'as, W. Khamas, and H. Darmani. 2001. Evaluation of the toxic potentials of cypermethrin pesticide on some reproductive and fertility parameters in the male rats. *Archives of Environmental Contamination and Toxicology* 41(4):522–528.

Elmazoudy, R.H., A.A. Attia, and H.S. Abdelgawad. 2011. Evaluation of developmental toxicity induced by anticholinesterase insecticide, diazinon in female rats. *Birth Defects Research. Part B, Developmental and Reproductive Toxicology* 92(6):534–542.

Elsharkawy, E.E., D. Yahia, and N.A. El-Nisr. 2014. Chlorpyrifos induced testicular damage in rats: Ameliorative effect of glutathione antioxidant. *Environmental Toxicology* 29(9):1011–1019.

Engel, S.M., G.S. Berkowitz, D.B. Barr, S.L. Teitelbaum, J. Siskind, S.J. Meisel, J.G. Wetmur, and M.S. Wolff. 2007. Prenatal organophosphate metabolite and organochlorine levels and performance on the Brazelton Neonatal Behavioral Assessment Scale in a multiethnic pregnancy cohort. *American Journal of Epidemiology* 165(12):1397–1404.

Engel, S.M., J. Wetmur, J. Chen, C. Zhu, D.B. Barr, R. L. Canfield, and M.S. Wolff. 2011. Prenatal exposure to organophosphates, paraoxonase 1, and cognitive development in childhood. *Environmental Health Perspectives* 119(8):1182–1188.

Engel, S.M., A. Bradman, M.S. Wolff, V.A. Rauh, K.G. Harley, J.H. Yang, L.A. Hoepner, D.B. Barr, K. Yolton, M.G. Vedar, Y. Xu, R.W. Hornung, J.G. Wetmur, J. Chen, N.T. Holland, F.P. Perera, R.M. Whyatt, B.P. Lanphear, and B. Eskenazi. 2016. Prenatal organophosphorus pesticide exposure and child neurodevelopment at 24 months: An analysis of four birth cohorts. *Environmental Health Perspectives* 124(6):822–830.

EPA (U.S. Environmental Protection Agency). 1983. Tolerances in food administered by EPA: Pemethrin. *Federal Register* 48:36246–36247.

EPA. 1987. *Integrated Risk Information System (IRIS) Chemical Assessment Summary: Methomyl; CASRN 16752-77-5.* https://cfpub.epa.gov/ncea/iris/iris_documents/documents/subst/0069_ summary.pdf (accessed June 15, 2018).

EPA 1992. *Baygon; CASRN 114-26-1. Integrated Risk Information System (IRIS) Chemical Assessment Summary.* National Center for Environmental Assessment.

EPA. 1994. Memorandum: Resmethrin: Evaluation of 2-generation reproduction study in rat and reevaluation of the following previously submitted studies: 3-generation reproduction study in rat, six month dog, rat. Toxicological Review 011329. Washington, DC: EPA, Office of Pesticides and Toxic Substances.

EPA. 2000. *Propoxur (Baygon).* https://www.epa.gov/sites/production/files/2016-09/documents/propoxur.pdf (accessed August 16, 2018).

EPA. 2016. Chlorpyrifos: Revised human health risk assessment for registration review. Memorandum. Washington, DC: EPA Office of Chemical Safety and Pollution Prevention. November 3, 2016.

Eskenazi, B., K. Harley, A. Bradman, E. Weltzien, N.P. Jewell, D.B. Barr, C.E. Furlong, and N.T. Holland. 2004. Association of in utero organophosphate pesticide exposure and fetal growth and length of gestation in an agricultural population. *Environmental Health Perspectives* 112(10):1116–1124.

Eskenazi, B., A.R. Marks, A. Bradman, K. Harley, D.B. Barr, C. Johnson, N. Morga, and N.P. Jewell. 2007. Organophosphate pesticide exposure and neurodevelopment in young Mexican-American children. *Environmental Health Perspectives* 115(5):792–798.

Eskenazi, B., K. Kogut, K. Huen, K.G. Harley, M. Bouchard, A. Bradman, D. Boyd-Barr, C. Johnson, and N. Holland. 2014. Organophosphate pesticide exposure, PON1, and neurodevelopment in school-age children from the CHAMACOS study. *Environmental Research* 134:149–157.

Eskenazi, B., A. Sookee, S.A. Rauch, E.S.Coker, A. Maphula, M. Obida, M. Crause, K.R. Kogut, R. Bornman, and J. Chevrier. 2018. Prenatal exposure to DDT and pyrethroids for malaria control and child neurodevelopment: The VHEMBE cohort, South Africa. *Environmental Health Perspectives* 126(4):047004.

Extoxnet. 1994. *Pyrethrins and pyrethroids.* http://ace.orst.edu/info/extoxnet/pips/pyrethri.htm (accessed August 12, 2018).

Farag, A.T., N.F. Goda, A.H. Mansee, and N.A. Shaaban. 2006. Effects of permethrin given before mating on the behavior of F1-generation in mice. *NeuroToxicology* 27(3):421–428.

Farag, A.T., A. Radwan, F. Sorour, A. El Okazy, E.-S. El-Agamy, and A. El-Khaliek El-Sebae. 2010. Chlorpyrifos induced reproductive toxicity in male mice. *Reproductive Toxicology* 29:80–85.

FDA (U.S. Food and Drug Administration). 2018. *Lindane shampoo.* https://www.accessdata.fda.gov/drugsatfda_docs/label/2003/006309shampoolbl.pdf (accessed June 26, 2018).

Figueroa, Z.I., H.A. Young, J.D. Meeker, S.E. Martenies, D. Boyd Barr, G. Gray, and M.J. Perry. 2015. Dialkyl phosphate urinary metabolites and chromosomal abnormalities in human sperm. *Environmental Research* 143(0):256–265.

Flores, D., V. Souza, M. Betancourt, M. Teteltitla, H. Gonzalez-Marquez, E. Casas, E. Bonilla, P. Ramírez-Noguera, M.C. Gutierrez-Ruíz, and Y. Ducolomb. 2017. Oxidative stress as a damage mechanism in porcine cumulus–oocyte complexes exposed to malathion during in vitro maturation. *Environmental Toxicology* 32:1669–1678.

Fortenberry, G., J.D. Meeker, B.N. Sánchez, D. Boyd Barr, P. Panuwet, D. Bellinger, L. Schnaas, M. Solano-González, A.S. Ettinger, M. Hernandez-Avila, H. Hu, and M.M. Tellez-Rojo. 2014. Urinary 3,5,6-trichloro-2-pyridinol (TCPy) in pregnant women from Mexico City: Distribution, temporal variability, and relationship with child attention and hyperactivity. *International Journal of Hygiene and Environmental Health* 217(0):405–412.

Fricker, R.D., E. Reardon, D.M. Spektor, S.K. Cotton, J. Hawes-Dawson, J.E. Pace, and S.D. Hosek. 2000. *Pesticide use during the Gulf War: A survey of Gulf War veterans*. Santa Monica, CA: RAND; National Defense Research Institute.

Furlong, M.A., S.M. Engel, D.B. Barr, and M.S. Wolff. 2014. Prenatal exposure to organophosphate pesticides and reciprocal social behavior in childhood. *Environment International* 70:125–131.

Furlong, M.A., A. Herring, J.P. Buckley, B.D. Goldman, J.L. Daniels, L.S. Engel, M.S. Wolff, J. Chen, J. Wetmur, D. B. Barr, S.M. Engel. 2017a. Prenatal exposure to organophosphorus pesticides and childhood neurodevelopmental phenotypes. *Environmental Research* 158:737–747.

Furlong, M.A., D.B. Barr, M.S. Wolff, and S.M. Engel. 2017b. Prenatal exposure to pyrethroid pesticides and childhood behavior and executive functioning. *Neurotoxicology* 62:231–238.

Geng, X., H. Shao, Z. Zhang, J.C. Ng, and C. Peng. 2015. Malathion-induced testicular toxicity is associated with spermatogenic apoptosis and alterations in testicular enzymes and hormone levels in male Wistar rats. *Environmental Toxicology and Pharmacology* 39(2):659–667.

Giri, S., S.B. Prasad, A. Giri, and G.D. Sharma. 2002. Genotoxic effects of malathion: An organophosphorus insecticide, using three mammalian bioassays in vivo. *Mutation Research* 514(1–2):223–231.

Gomes, J., and O.L. Lloyd. 2009. Oral exposure of mice to formulations of organophosphorous pesticides: Gestational and litter outcomes. *International Journal of Environmental Health Research* 19(2):125–137.

Gomes, J., O.L. Lloyd, and Z. Hong. 2008. Oral exposure of male and female mice to formulations of organophosphorous pesticides: Congenital malformations. *Human & Experimental Toxicology* 27(3):231–240.

González-Alzaga, B., A.F. Hernandez, M. Rodríguez-Barranco, I. Gómez, C. Aguilar-Garduño, I. López-Flores, T. Parrón, and M. Lacasaña. 2015. Pre- and postnatal exposures to pesticides and neurodevelopmental effects in children living in agricultural communities from South-Eastern Spain. *Environment International* 85:229–237.

Gray, L.E., Jr., and R.J. Kavlock. 1984. An extended evaluation of an in vivo teratology screen utilizing postnatal growth and viability in the mouse. *Teratogenesis, Carcinogenesis, and Mutagenesis* 4(5):403–426.

Gunier, R., A. Bradman, K.G. Harley, K. Kogut, and B. Eskenazi. 2017. Prenatal residential proximity to agricultural pesticide use and IQ in 7-year-old children. *Environmental Health Perspectives* 125(5):057002.

Hallenbeck, W.H., and K.M. Cunningham-Burns. 1985. *Pesticides and human health*. New York: Springer-Verlag.

Harley, K.G., K. Huen, R.A. Schall, N.T. Holland, A. Bradman, D.B. Barr, and B. Eskenazi. 2011. Association of organophosphate pesticide exposure and paraoxonase with birth outcome in Mexican-American women. *PLOS ONE* 6(8):e23923.

Harley, K.G., S.M. Engel, M.G. Vedar, B. Eskenazi, R.M. Whyatt, B.P. Lanphear, A. Bradman, V.A. Rauh, K. Yolton, R.W. Hornung, J.G. Wetmur, J. Chen, N.T. Holland, D.B. Barr, F.P. Perera, and M.S. Wolff. 2016. Prenatal exposure to organophosphorous pesticides and fetal growth: Pooled results from four longitudinal birth cohort studies. *Environmental Health Perspectives* 124(7):1084–1092.

Hassoun, E.A., and S.J. Stohs. 1996. Comparative teratological studies on TCDD, endrin, and lindane in C57BL/6J and DBA/2J mice. *Comparative Biochemistry and Physiology* 113C(3):393–398.

Hisada, A., J. Yoshinaga, J. Zhang, T. Kato, H. Shiraishi, K. Shimodaira, T. Okai, N. Ariki, Y. Komine, M. Shirakawa, Y. Noda, and N. Kato. 2017. Maternal exposure to pyrethroid insecticides during pregnancy and infant development at 18 months of age. *International Journal of Environmental Research and Public Health* 14(1):E52.

Horton, M.K., A. Rundle, D.E. Camann, D. Boyd Barr, V.A. Rauh, and R.M. Whyatt. 2011. Impact of prenatal exposure to piperonyl butoxide and permethrin on 36-month neurodevelopment. *Pediatrics* 127(3):e699–e706.

Horton, M.K., L.G. Kahn, F. Perera, D.B. Barr, and V. Rauh. 2012. Does the home environment and the sex of the child modify the adverse effects of prenatal exposure to chlorpyrifos on child working memory? *Neurotoxicology and Teratology* 34(5):534–541.

Hossain, F., O. Ali, U.J.A. D'Souza, and D.K. Saw Naing. 2010. Effects of pesticide use on semen quality among farmers in rural areas of Sabah, Malaysia. *Journal of Occupational Health* 52(6):353–360.

Hu, J.X., Y.F. Li, J. Li, C. Pan, Z. He, H.Y. Dong, and L.C. Xu. 2013. Toxic effects of cypermethrin on the male reproductive system: With emphasis on the androgen receptor. *Journal of Applied Toxicology* 33(7):576–585.

Hu, Y., L. Ji, Y. Zhang, R. Shi, W. Han, L. A. Tse, R. Pan, Y. Wang, G. Ding, J. Xu, Q. Zhang, Y. Gao, and Y. Tian. 2018. Organophosphate and pyrethroid pesticide exposures measured before conception and associations with time to pregnancy in Chinese couples enrolled in the Shanghai Birth Cohort. *Environmental Health Perspectives* 126(7):077001.

Huen, K., O. Solomon, K. Kogut, B. Eskenazi, and N. Holland. 2018. *PON1* DNA methylation and neurobehavior in Mexican-American children with prenatal organophosphate exposure. *Environment International* 121:312–340.

IARC (International Agency for Research on Cancer). 1991. *Deltamethrin*. IARC Monographs on the Evaluation of Carcinogenic Risks to Humans 53. Lyon, France: IARC Press.

IARC. 2016a. *Malathion*. IARC Monographs on the Evaluation of Carcinogenic Risks to Humans 112. Lyon, France: IARC Press.

IARC. 2016b. *Diazinon*. IARC Monographs on the Evaluation of Carcinogenic Risks to Humans 112. Lyon, France: IARC Press.

Icenogle, L.M., N.C. Christopher, W.P. Blackwelder, D.P. Caldwell, D. Qiao, F.J. Seidler, T.A. Slotkin, and E.D. Levin. 2004. Behavioral alterations in adolescent and adult rats caused by a brief subtoxic exposure to chlorpyrifos during neurulation. *Neurotoxicology and Teratology* 26(1):95–101.

Imai, K., J. Yoshinaga, M. Yoshikane, H. Shiraishi, M.N. Mieno, M. Yoshiike, S. Nozawa, and T. Iwamoto. 2014. Pyrethroid insecticide exposure and semen quality of young Japanese men. *Reproductive Toxicology* 43:38–44.

Imanishi, S., M. Okura, H. Zaha, T. Yamamoto, H. Akanuma, R. Nagano, H. Shiraishi, H. Fujimaki, and H. Sone. 2013. Prenatal exposure to permethrin influences vascular development of fetal brain and adult behavior in mice offspring. *Environmental Toxicology* 28(11):617–629.

Imming R.J., B.C. Shaffer, and G. Woodward. 1969. Sevin®. Safety evaluation by feeding to female beagles from day one of gestation through weaning of the offspring. Report from Woodward Research Corporation to Union Carbide Agricultural Products Company, Inc. Research Triangle Park, NC (as cited in R. L. Baron. 1991. Carbamate insecticides. In: W.J. Hayes, Jr., and E.R. Laws, Jr. (eds.). *Handbook of pesticide toxicology. Vol. 3. Classes of pesticides*. San Diego: Academic Press Inc. Pp. 1125–1189).

IOM (Institute of Medicine). 2003. *Gulf War and health, volume 2: Insecticides and solvents*. Washington, DC: The National Academies Press.

Ismail, M.F., and H.M. Mohamed. 2012. Deltamethrin-induced genotoxicity and testicular injury in rats: Comparison with biopesticide. *Food and Chemical Toxicology* 50(10):3421–3425.

Issam, C., H. Samir, H. Zohra, Z. Monia, and B.C. Hassen. 2009. Toxic responses to deltamethrin (DM) low doses on gonads, sex hormones and lipoperoxidation in male rats following subcutaneous treatments. *Journal of Toxicological Sciences* 34(6):663–670.

Ji, G., Y. Xia, A. Gu, X. Shi, Y. Long., L. Song, S. Wang, and X. Wang. 2011. Effects of non-occupational environmental exposure to pyrethroids on semen quality and sperm DNA integrity in Chinese men. *Reproductive Toxicology* 31:171–176.

Joshi, S.C., R. Mathur, and N. Gulati. 2007. Testicular toxicity of chlorpyrifos (an organophosphate pesticide) in albino rat. *Toxicology and Industrial Health* 23:439–444.

Jurewicz, J., M. Radwan, B. Wielgomas, W. Sobala, M. Piskunowicz, P. Radwan, M. Bochenek, and W. Hanke. 2015. The effect of environmental exposure to pyrethroids and DNA damage in human sperm. *Systems Biology in Reproductive Medicine* 61(1):37–43.

Kaloianova, F.P., and M.A. El Batawi. 1991. *Human toxicology of pesticides*. Boca Raton, FL: CRC Press.

Khaki, A., A.A. Khaki, and A. Rajabzadeh. 2017. The effects of permethrin and antioxidant properties of Allium cepa (onion) on testicles parameters of male rats. *Toxin Reviews* 36(1):1–6.

Khera, K.S., C. Whalen, G. Trivett, and G. Angers. 1979. Teratogenicity studies on pesticidal formulations of dimethoate, diuron, and lindane in rats. *Bulletin of Environmental Contamination and Toxicology* 22(4–5):522–529.

Kidd, H., and D.R. James (eds.). 1991. *The agrochemicals handbook*. 3rd ed. Cambridge, UK: Royal Society of Chemistry Information Services.

King, V. 1991. Lindane: Reproductive performance study in rats treated continuously through two successive generations: Final Report. (Addendum to MRID 422210). Lab Project Number 91/0948: 91CIL004-0948. CIL-004-LIND. Unpublished study prepared by Life Science Research, Ltd. MRID Number 42246101.

Kitagawa, K., M. Wakakura, and S. Ishikawa. 1977. Light microscopic study of endocrine organs of rats treated by carbamate pesticide. *Journal of Toxicological Sciences* 2:53–60.

Koren, G., D. Matsui, and B. Bailey. 2003. DEET-based insect repellents: Safety implications for children and pregnant and lactating women. *CMAJ* 169(3):209–212.

Kotil, T., and N.D. Yon. 2015. The effects of permethrin on rat ovarian tissue morphology. *Experimental and Toxicologic Pathology* 67(3):279–285.

Kumar, A., and M. Nagar. 2014. Histomorphometric study of testis in deltamethrin treated albino rats. *Toxicology Reports* 1:401–410.

Lafiura, K.M., D.M. Bielawski, N.C. Posecion, Jr., E.M. Ostrea, Jr., L.H. Matherly, J.W. Taub, and Y. Ge. 2007. Association between prenatal pesticide exposures and the generation of leukemia-associated T(8;21). *Pediatric Blood & Cancer* 49(5):624–628.

Lan, A., M. Kalimian, B. Amram, and O. Kofman. 2017. Prenatal chlorpyrifos leads to autism-like deficits in C57Bl6/J mice. *Environmental Health* 16(43):1–10.

Lazarini, C.A., R.Y. Lima, A.P. Guedes, and M.M. Bernardi. 2004. Prenatal exposure to dichlorvos: Physical and behavioral effects on rat offspring. *Neurotoxicology and Teratology* 26(4):607–614.

Leong, C. T., U.J.A. D'Souza, M. Iqbal, and Z.A. Mustapha. 2013. Lipid peroxidation and decline in antioxidant status as one of the toxicity measures of diazinon in the testis. *Redox Report* 18(4):155–164.

Lindenau, A., B. Fischer, P. Seiler, and H.M. Beier. 1994. Effects of persistent chlorinated hydrocarbons on reproductive tissues in female rabbits. *Human Reproduction* 9:772–780.

Litchfield, M.H. 1985. Toxicity to mammals. In J.P. Leahey (ed.). *The pyrethroid insecticides*. London: Taylor & Francis. Pp. 99–150.

Liu, B., K.H. Jung, M.K. Horton, D.E. Camann, X. Liu, A.M. Reardon, M.S. Perzanowski, H. Zhang, F.P. Perera, R.M. Whyatt, and R.L. Miller. 2012. Prenatal exposure to pesticide ingredient piperonyl butoxide and childhood cough in an urban cohort. *Environment International* 48:156–161.

Lopez-Casas, P.P., S.C. Mizrak, L.A. Lopez-Fernandez, M. Paz, D.G. de Rooij, and J. del Mazo. 2012. The effects of different endocrine disruptors defining compound-specific alterations of gene expression profiles in the developing testis. *Reproductive Toxicology* 33(1):106–115.

Luca, D., and M. Balan. 1987. Sperm abnormality assay in the evaluation of the genotoxic potential of carbaryl in rats. *Morphologie et Embryologie* 33(1):19–22.

Mahgoub, A.A., and A.H. El-Medany. 2001. Evaluation of chronic exposure of the male rat reproductive system to the insecticide methomyl. *Pharmacological Research* 44(2):73–80.

Malaviya, M., R. Husain, and P.K. Seth. 1993. Perinatal effect of two pyrethroid insecticides on brain neurotransmitter function in the neonatal rat. *Veterinary and Human Toxicology* 35(2):119–122.

Mandal, T.K., and N.S. Das. 2011. Correlation of testicular toxicity and oxidative stress induced by chlorpyrifos in rats. *Human and Experimental Toxicology* 30(10):1529–1539.

Mandal, T.K., and N.S. Das. 2012. Testicular gametogenic and steroidogenic activities in chlorpyrifos insecticide-treated rats: A correlation study with testicular oxidative stress and role of antioxidant enzyme defence systems in Sprague-Dawley rats. *Andrologia* 44(2):102–115.

Manikkam, M., C. Guerrero-Bosagna, R. Tracey, M.M. Haque, and M.K. Skinner. 2012a. Transgenerational actions of environmental compounds on reproductive disease and identification of epigenetic biomarkers of ancestral exposures. *PLOS ONE* 7(2):e31901.

Manikkam, M., R. Tracey, C. Guerrero-Bosagna, and M.K. Skinner. 2012b. Pesticide and insect repellent mixture (permethrin and DEET) induces epigenetic transgenerational inheritance of disease and sperm epimutations. *Reproductive Toxicology* 34(4):708–719.

Maranghi, F., M. Rescia, C. Macri, E. Di Consiglio, G. De Angelis, E. Testai, D. Farini, M. De Felici, S. Lorenzetti, and A. Mantovani. 2007. Lindane may modulate the female reproductive development through the interaction with ER-beta: An in vivo–in vitro approach. *Chemico-Biological Interactions* 169(1):1–14.

Marks, A.R., K. Harley, A. Bradman, K. Kogut, D.B. Barr, C. Johnson, N. Calderon, and B. Eskenazi. 2010. Organophosphate pesticide exposure and attention in young Mexican-American children: The CHAMACOS study. *Environmental Health Perspectives* 118(12):1768–1774.

Martenies, S.E., and M.J. Perry. 2013. Environmental and occupational pesticide exposure and human sperm parameters: A systematic review. *Toxicology* 307:66–73.

Matsuura, I., T. Saitoh, E. Tani, Y. Wako, H. Iwata, N. Toyota, Y. Ishizuka, M. Namiki, N. Hoshino, M. Tsuchitani, and Y. Ikeda. 2005. Evaluation of a two-generation reproduction toxicity study adding endpoints to detect endocrine disrupting activity using lindane. *Journal of Toxicological Sciences* 30(Spec Iss.):135–161.

Meeker, J.D., L. Ryan, D.B. Barr, R.F. Herrick, D.H. Bennett, R. Bravo, and R. Hauser. 2004a. The relationship of urinary metabolites of carbaryl/naphthalene and chlorpyrifos with human semen quality. *Environmental Health Perspectives* 112(17):1665–1670.

Meeker, J.D., N.P. Singh, L. Ryan, S.M. Duty, D.B. Barr, R.F. Herrick, D.H. Bennett, and R. Hauser. 2004b. Urinary levels of insecticide metabolites and DNA damage in human sperm. *Human Reproduction* 19(11):2573–2580.

Meeker, J.D., L. Ryan, D.B. Barr, and R. Hauser. 2006. Exposure to nonpersistent insecticides and male reproductive hormones. *Epidemiology* 17(1):61–68.

Meeker, J. D., S.R. Ravi, D.B. Barr, and R. Hauser. 2008a. Circulating estradiol in men is inversely related to urinary metabolites of nonpersistent insecticides. *Reproductive Toxicology* 25(2):184–191.

Meeker, J.D., D.B. Barr, and R. Hauser. 2008b. Human semen quality and sperm DNA damage in relation to urinary metabolites of pyrethroid insecticides. *Human Reproduction* 23(8):1932–1940.

Meeker, J.D., D.B. Barr, and R. Hauser. 2009. Pyrethroid insecticide metabolites are associated with serum hormone levels in adult men. *Reproductive Toxicology* 27(2):155–160.

Melgarejo, M., J. Mendiola, H.M. Koch, M. Moñino-García, J.A. Noguera-Velasco, and A. Torres-Cantero. 2015. Associations between urinary organophosphate pesticide metabolite levels and reproductive parameters in men from an infertility clinic. *Environmental Research* 137:292–298.

Meyer, A., F.J. Seidler, and T.A. Slotkin. 2004a. Developmental effects of chlorpyrifos extend beyond neurotoxicity: critical periods for immediate and delayed-onset effects on cardiac and hepatic cell signaling. *Environmental Health Perspectives* 112(2):170–178.

Meyer, A., F.J. Seidler, J.E. Aldridge, C.A. Tate, M.M. Cousins, and T.A. Slotkin. 2004b. Critical periods for chlorpyrifos-induced developmental neurotoxicity: Alterations in adenylyl cyclase signaling in adult rat brain regions after gestational or neonatal exposure. *Environmental Health Perspectives* 112(3):295–301.

Meyer, K.J., J.S. Reif, D.N. Rao Veeramachaneni, T.J. Luben, B.S. Mosley, and J.R. Nuckols. 2006. Agricultural pesticide use and hypospadias in Eastern Arkansas. *Environmental Health Perspectives* 114(10):1589–1595.

Millenson, M.E., J.M. Braun, A.M. Calafat, D.B. Barr, Y.T. Huang, A. Chen, B.P. Lanphear, and K. Yolton. 2017. Urinary organophosphate insecticide metabolite concentrations during pregnancy and children's interpersonal, communication, repetitive, and stereotypic behaviors at 8 years of age: The HOME study. *Environmental Research* 157:9–16.

Miranda-Contreras, L., R. Gomez-Perez, G. Rojas, I. Cruz, L. Berrueta, S. Salmen, M. Colmenares, S. Barreto, A. Balza, L. Zavala, Y. Morales, Y. Molina, L. Valeri, C. A. Contreras, and J. A. Osuna. 2013. Occupational exposure to organophosphate and carbamate pesticides affects sperm chromatin integrity and reproductive hormone levels among Venezuelan farm workers. *Journal of Occupational Health* 55(3):195–203.

Miyamoto J. 1976. Degradation, metabolism and toxicity of synthetic pyrethroids. *Environmental Health Perspectives* 14:15–28.

Monge, P., C. Wesseling, J. Guardado, I. Lundberg, A. Ahlbom, K.P. Cantor, E. Weiderpass, and T. Partanen. 2007. Parental occupational exposure to pesticides and the risk of childhood leukemia in Costa Rica. *Scandinavian Journal of Work, Environment & Health* 33(4):293–303.

Mosbah, R., M.I. Yousef, F. Maranghi, and A. Mantovani. 2016. Protective role of Nigella sativa oil against reproductive toxicity, hormonal alterations, and oxidative damage induced by chlorpyrifos in male rats. *Toxicology and Industrial Health* 32(7):1266–1277.

Nayshteyn, S.Y., and D.L. Leybovich. 1971. Low doses of DDT, γ-HCCH and mixtures of these: Effect on sexual function and embryogenesis in rats. *Gigiena i Sanitariia* 36(5):19–22 [In Russian]. As cited in: W.J. Hayes, Jr., and E.J. Laws, Jr. (eds.). 1991. *Handbook of pesticide toxicology. Vol. 2, Classes of pesticides.* San Diego: Academic Press, Inc.

Neta, G., L.R. Goldman, D. Barr, B.J. Apelberg, F.R. Witter, and R.U. Halden. 2011. Fetal exposure to chlordane and permethrin mixtures in relation to inflammatory cytokines and birth outcomes. *Environmental Science and Technology* 45(4):1680–1687.

Ngoula, F., P. Watcho, T.S. Bouseko, A. Kenfack, J. Tchoumboue, and P. Kamtchouing. 2007. Effects of propoxur on the reproductive system of male rats. *African Journal of Reproductive Health* 11(1):125–132.

Nilsson, E., G. Larsen, M. Manikkam, C. Guerrero-Bosagna, M.I. Savenkova, M.K. Skinner. 2012. Environmentally induced epigenetic transgenerational inheritance of ovarian disease. *PLOS ONE* 7:e36129.

OEHHA (California Office of Environmental Health Hazard Assessment). 2017. Meeting synopsis and slide presentations from the Developmental and Reproductive Toxicant Identification Committee Meeting held on November 29, 2017. Sacramento, CA: California Environmental Protection Agency.

OEHHA. 2018. *OEHHA chemical database*. https://oehha.ca.gov/chemicals/carbaryl (accessed July 2, 2018).

Ojha, A., and Y.K. Gupta. 2015. Evaluation of genotoxic potential of commonly used organophosphate pesticides in peripheral blood lymphocytes of rats. *Human and Experimental Toxicology* 34(4):390–400.

Okamura, A., M. Kamijima, E. Shibata, K. Ohtani, K. Takagi, J. Ueyama, Y. Watanabe, M. Omura, H. Wang, G. Ichihara, T. Kondo, and T. Nakajima. 2005. A comprehensive evaluation of the testicular toxicity of dichlorvos in Wistar rats. *Toxicology* 213(1–2):129–137.

Okamura, A., M. Kamijima, K. Ohtani, O. Yamanoshita, D. Nakamura, Y. Ito, M. Miyata, J. Ueyama, T. Suzuki, R. Imai, K. Takagi, and T. Nakajima. 2009. Broken sperm, cytoplasmic droplets and reduced sperm motility are principal markers of decreased sperm quality due to organophosphorus pesticides in rats. *Journal of Occupational Health* 51(6):478–487.

Ostrea, Jr., E.M., A. Reyes, E. Villanueva-Uy, R. Pacifico, B. Benitez, E. Ramos, R.C. Bernardo, D.M. Bielawski, V. Delaney-Black, L. Chiodo, J.J. Janisse, and J.W. Ager. 2012. Fetal exposure to propoxur and abnormal child neurodevelopment at 2 years of age. *NeuroToxicology* 33(4):669–675.

PAC (Presidential Advisory Committee on Gulf War Veterans' Illnesses). 1996. *Presidential Advisory Committee on Gulf War Veterans' Illnesses: Final report*. Washington, DC: US Government Printing Office.

Palmer, A.K., D.D. Cozens, E.J.F. Spicer, and A.N. Worden. 1978. Effects of lindane upon reproductive function in a 3-generation study in rats. *Toxicology* 10(1):45–54.

Pant, N., S.C. Srivastava, A.K. Prasad, R. Shankar, and S.P. Srivastava. 1995. Effects of carbaryl on the rat's male reproductive system. *Veterinary and Human Toxicology* 37(5):421–425.

Pant. N., R. Shankar, and S.P. Srivastava. 1996. Spermatotoxic effects of carbaryl in rats. *Human and Experimental Toxicology* 15(9):736–738.

Perera, F.P., V. Rauh, W.Y. Tsai, P. Kinney, D. Camann, D. Barr, T. Bernert, R. Garfinkel, Y.H. Tu, D. Diaz, J. Dietrich, and R.M. Whyatt. 2003. Effects of transplacental exposure to environmental pollutants on birth outcomes in a multiethnic population. *Environmental Health Perspectives* 111(2):201–205.

Pérez-Herrera, N., H. Polanco-Minaya, E. Salazar-Arredondo, M.J. Solis-Heredia, I. Hernandez-Ochoa, E. Rojas-Garcia, J. Alvarado-Mejia, V.H. Borja-Aburto, and B. Quintanilla-Vega. 2008. PON1Q192R genetic polymorphism modifies organophosphorous pesticide effects on semen quality and DNA integrity in agricultural workers from southern Mexico. *Toxicology and Applied Pharmacology* 230(2):261–268.

Perry, M.J., S.A. Venners, D. Barr, and X. Xu. 2007. Environmental pyrethroid and organophosphorus insecticide exposures and sperm concentration. *Reproductive Toxicology* 23:113–118.

Perry, M.J., S.A. Venners, X. Chen, and X. Liu. 2011. Organophosphorous pesticide exposures and sperm quality. *Reproductive Toxicology* 31:75–79.

Petrelli, G., G. Siepi, L. Miligi, and P. Vineis. 1993. Solvents in pesticides. *Scandanavian Journal of Work, Environment & Health* 19(1):64–65.

Petrelli, G., I. Figa-Talamanca, R. Tropeano, M. Tangucci, C. Cini, S. Aquilani, L. Gasperini, and P. Meli. 2000. Reproductive male-mediated risk: Spontaneous abortion among wives of pesticide applicators. *European Journal of Epidemiology* 16(4):391–393.

Pina-Guzman, B., M.J. Solis-Heredia, and B. Quintanilla-Vega. 2005. Diazinon alters sperm chromatin structure in mice by phosphorylating nuclear protamines. *Toxicology and Applied Pharmacology* 202(2):189–198.

Ploteau, S., J.-P. Antignac, C. Volteau, P. Marchand, A. Vénisseau, V. Vacher, and B. Le Bizec. 2016. Distribution of persistent organic pollutants in serum, omental, and parietal adipose tissue of French women with deep infiltrating endometriosis and circulating versus stored ratio as new marker of exposure. *Environment International* 97:125–136.

Ploteau, S., G. Cano-Sancho, C. Volteau, A. Legrand, A. Vénisseau, V. Vacher, P. Marchand, B. Le Bizec, and J.-P. Antignac. 2017. Associations between internal exposure levels of persistent organic pollutants in adipose tissue and deep infiltrating endometriosis with or without concurrent ovarian endometrioma. *Environment International* 108:195–203.

Polakova, H., and M. Vargova. 1983. Evaluation of the mutagenic effects of decamethrin: Cytogenetic analysis of bone marrow. *Mutation Research* 120(2–3):167–171.

Qiao, D., F.J. Seidler, S. Padilla, and T.A. Slotkin. 2002. Developmental neurotoxicity of chlorpyrifos: What is the vulnerable period? *Environmental Health Perspectives* 110(11):1097–1103.

Qiao, D., F.J. Seidler, C.A. Tate, M.M. Cousins, and T.A. Slotkin. 2003. Fetal chlorpyrifos exposure: Adverse effects on brain cell development and cholinergic biomarkers emerge postnatally and continue into adolescence and adulthood. *Environmental Health Perspectives* 111(4):536–544.

Qiao, D., F.J. Seidler, Y. Abreu-Villaça, C.A. Tate, M.M. Cousins, and T.A. Slotkin. 2004. Chlorpyrifos exposure during neurulation: Cholinergic synaptic dysfunction and cellular alterations in brain regions at adolescence and adulthood. *Brain Research Developmental Brain Research* 148(1):43–52.

Quirós-Alcalá, L., A. Bradman, K. Smith, G. Weerasekera, M. Odetokun, D.B. Barr, M. Nishioka, R. Castorina, A.E. Hubbard, M. Nicas, S.K. Hammond, T.E. McKone, and B. Eskenazi. 2012. Organophosphorous pesticide breakdown products in house dust and children's urine. *Journal of Exposure Science and Environmental Epidemiology* 22(6):559–568.

Raanan, R., K.G. Harley, J.R. Balmes, A. Bradman, M. Lipsett, and B. Eskenazi. 2015. Early-life exposure to organophosphate pesticides and pediatric respiratory symptoms in the CHAMACOS cohort. *Environmental Health Perspectives* 123(2):179–185.

Raanan, R., J.R. Balmes, K.G. Harley, R.B. Gunier, S. Magzamen, A. Bradman, and B. Eskenazi. 2016. Decreased lung function in 7-year-old children with early-life organophosphate exposure. *Thorax* 71:148–153.

Radwan, M., J. Jurewicz, B. Wielgomas, W. Sobala, M. Piskunowicz, P. Radwan, and W. Hanke. 2014. Semen quality and the level of reproductive hormones after environmental exposure to pyrethroids. *Journal of Occupational and Environmental Medicine* 56(11):1113–1119.

Radwan, M., J. Jurewicz, B. Wielgomas, M. Piskunowicz, W. Sobala, P. Radwan, L. Jakubowski, W. Hawula, and W. Hanke. 2015. The association between environmental exposure to pyrethroids and sperm aneuploidy. *Chemosphere* 128:42–48.

Rauch, S.A., J.M. Braun, D.B. Barr, A.M. Calafat, J. Khoury, M.A. Montesano, K. Yolton, and B.P. Lanphear. 2012. Associations of prenatal exposure to organophosphate pesticide metabolites with gestational age and birth weight. *Environmental Health Perspectives* 120(7):1055–1060.

Rauh, V.A., R. Garfinkel, F.P. Perera, H.F. Andrews, L. Hoepner, D.B. Barr, R. Whitehead, D. Tang, and R.W. Whyatt. 2006. Impact of prenatal chlorpyrifos exposure on neurodevelopment in the first 3 years of life among inner-city children. *Pediatrics* 118(6):e1845–e1859.

Rauh, V., S. Arunajadai, M. Horton, F. Perera, L. Hoepner, D.B. Barr, and R. Whyatt. 2011. Seven-year neurodevelopmental scores and prenatal exposure to chlorpyrifos, a common agricultural pesticide. *Environmental Health Perspectives* 119(8):1196–1201.

Rauh, V.A., F.P. Perera, M.K. Horton, R.M. Whyatt, R. Bansal, X. Hao, J. Liu, D.B. Barr, T.A. Slotkin, and B.S. Peterson. 2012. Brain anomalies in children exposed prenatally to a common organophosphate pesticide. *Proceedings of the National Academy of Sciences* 109(20):7871–7876.

Rauh, V.A., W.E. Garcia, R.M. Whyatt, M.K. Horton, D.B. Barr, and E.D. Louis. 2015. Prenatal exposure to the organophosphate pesticide chlorpyrifos and childhood tremor. *NeuroToxicology* 51:80–86.

Ray, D. E.1991. Pesticides derived from plants and other organisms. In W.J. Hayes, Jr., and E. R. Laws, Jr. (eds.). *Handbook of pesticide toxicology*. San Diego: Academic Press. Pp. 585–636.

Recio-Vega, R., G. Ocampo-Gomez, V.H. Borja-Aburto, J. Moran-Martinez, and M.E. Cebrian-Garcia. 2008. Organophosphorus pesticide exposure decreases sperm quality: Association between sperm parameters and urinary pesticide levels. *Journal of Applied Toxicology* 28(5):674–680.

Ren, A., X. Qiu, L. Jin, J. Ma, Z. Li, L. Zhang, H. Zhu, R.H. Finnell, and T. Zhu. 2011. Association of selected persistent organic pollutants in the placenta with the risk of neural tube defects. *Proceedings of the National Academy of Sciences* 108(31):12770–12775.

Ridano, M.E., A.C. Racca, J.B. Flores-Martin, R. Fretes, C.L. Bandeira, L. Reyna, E. Bevilacqua, and S. Genti-Raimondi. 2017. Impact of chlorpyrifos on human villous trophoblasts and chorionic villi. *Toxicology and Applied Pharmacology* 329:26–39.

Roberts, J.R., and J.R. Reigart. 2013. *Recognition and management of pesticide poisonings, sixth edition*. EPA/735/R-98/003. Washington, DC: U.S. Environmental Protection Agency, Office of Pesticide Programs.

Rodriguez, H., H. Jara, S. Legua, D. Campos, J. Morales, and O. Espinoza-Navarro. 2017. Effects of cypermethrin on cytokeratin 8/18 and androgen receptor expression in the adult mouse Sertoli cell. *Revista Internacional de Andrologia* 15(2):51–57.

Ronco, A.M., K. Valdes, D. Marcus, and M. Llanos. 2001. The mechanism for lindane-induced inhibition of steroidogenesis in cultured rat Leydig cells. *Toxicology* 159(1–2):99–106.

Rowe, C., R. Gunier, A. Bradman, K.G. Harley, K. Kogut, K. Parra, and B. Eskenazi. 2016. Residential proximity to organophosphate and carbamate pesticide use during pregnancy, poverty during childhood, and cognitive functioning in 10-year-old children. *Environmental Research* 150:128–137.

Rupa, D.S., P.P Reddy, and O.S. Reddi. 1991. Reproductive performance in population exposed to pesticides in cotton fields in India. *Environmental Research* 55:123-128.

Sagiv, S.K., M.H. Harris, R.B. Gunier, K.R. Kogut, K.G. Harley, J. Deardorff, A. Bradman, N. Holland, and B. Eskenazi. 2018. Prenatal organophosphate pesticide exposure and traits related to autism spectrum disorders in a population living in proximity to agriculture. *Environmental Health Perspectives* 126(4):047012.

Sai, L., X. Li, Y. Liu, Q. Guo, L. Xie, G. Yu, C. Bo, Z. Zhang, and L. Li. 2014. Effects of chlorpyrifos on reproductive toxicology of male rats. *Environmental Toxicology* 29(9):1083–1088.

Saillenfait, A.M., J.P. Sabate, F. Denis, G. Antoine, A. Robert, A.C. Roudot, D. Ndiaye, and E. Eljarrat. 2017. Evaluation of the effects of cypermethrin on fetal rat testicular steroidogenesis. *Reproductive Toxicology* 72:106–114.

Saito, K, Y. Tomigahara, N. Ohe, N. Isobe, I. Nakatsuka, and H. Kaneko. 2000. Lack of significant estrogenic or antiestrogenic activity of pyrethroid insecticides in three in vitro assays based on classic estrogen receptor alpha-mediated mechanisms. *Toxicological Sciences* 57(1):54–60.

Salazar-Arredondo, E., M.D. Solis-Heredia, E. Rojas-Garcia, I. Hernandez-Ochoa, and B. Quintanilla-Vega. 2008. Sperm chromatin alteration and DNA damage by methyl-parathion, chlorpyrifos, and diazinon and their oxon metabolites in human spermatozoa. *Reproductive Toxicology* 25(4):455–460.

Sams, C. 2017. Urinary naphthol as a biomarker of exposure: Results from an oral exposure to carbaryl and workers occupationally exposed to naphthalene. *Toxics* 5(3):1–7.

Sánchez-Peña, L.C., B.E. Reyes, L. Lopez-Carrillo, R. Recio, J. Moran-Martinez, M.E. Cebrian, and B. Quintanilla-Vega. 2004. Organophosphorous pesticide exposure alters sperm chromatin structure in Mexican agricultural workers. *Toxicology and Applied Pharmacology* 196:108–113.

Santoni, G., F. Cantalamessa, L. Mazzucca, S. Ramagnoli, and M. Piccoli. 1997. Prenatal exposure to cypermethrin modulates rat NK cell cytotoxic functions. *Toxicology* 120:231–242.

Santoni, G.,F. Cantalamessa, R. Cavagna, S. Romagnoli, E. Spreghini, and M. Piccoli. 1998. Cypermethrin-induced alteration of thymocyte distribution and functions in prenatally-exposed rats. *Toxicology* 125:67–78.

Santoni, G., F. Cantalamessa, E. Spreghini, O. Sagretti, M. Staffolani, and M. Piccoli. 1999. Alterations of T cell distribution and functions in prenatally cypermethrin-exposed rats: Possible involvement of catecholamines. *Toxicology* 138:175–187.

Sarabia, L., I. Maurer, and E. Bustos-Obregón. 2009. Melatonin prevents damage elicited by the organophosphorous pesticide diazinon on mouse sperm DNA. *Ecotoxicology and Environmental Safety* 72(2):663–668.

Savitz, D.A., T. Arbuckle, D. Kaczor, and K.M. Curtis. 1997. Male pesticide exposure and pregnancy outcome. *American Journal of Epidemiology* 146(12):1025–1036.

Schleier, J.J., R.S. Davis, L.M. Barber, P.A. Macedo, and R.K.D. Peterson. 2009. A probabilistic risk assessment for deployed military personnel after the implementation of the "Leishmaniasis Control Program" at Tallil Air Base, Iraq. *Journal of Medical Entomology* 46(3):693–702.

Segal, T., L. Minguez-Alarcon, Y. Chiu, P. Williams, F. Nassan, R. Dadd, M. Ospina, A. Calafat, and R. Hauser. 2017. Urinary concentrations of DEET metabolites and semen parameters among men attending a fertility center. *Fertility and Sterility* 108(3 Suppl 1):e28–e29.

Seiler, P., B. Fischer, A. Lindenau, and H.M. Beier. 1994. Effects of persistent chlorinated hydrocarbons on fertility and embryonic development in the rabbit. *Human Reproduction* 9:1920–1926.

Shafer, T.J., D.A. Meyer, and K.M. Crofton. 2005. Developmental neurotoxicity of pyrethroid insecticides: Critical review and future research needs. *Environmental Health Perspectives* 113(2):123–136.

Sharma, P., I.A. Khan, and R. Singh. 2018. Curcumin and quercetin ameliorated cypermethrin and deltamethrin-induced reproductive system impairment in male Wistar rats by upregulating the activity of pituitary-gonadal hormones and steroidogenic enzymes. *International Journal of Fertility & Sterility* 12(1):72–80.

Shelton, J.F., E.M. Geraghty, D.J. Tancredi, L.D. Delwiche, R.J. Schmidt, B. Ritz, R.L. Hansen, and I. Hertz-Picciotto. 2014. Neurodevelopmental disorders and prenatal residential proximity to agricultural pesticides: The CHARGE study. *Environmental Health Perspectives* 122(10):1103–1109.

Siddiqui, M.K.J., S. Srivastava, S.P. Scrivastava, P.K. Mehrotra, N. Mathur, and I. Tandon. 2003. Persistent chlorinated pesticides and intrauterine foetal growth retardation: A possible solution. *International Archives of Occupational and Environmental Health* 76(1):75–80.

Silva, J.G., A.C. Boareto, A.K. Schreiber, D.D.B. Redivo, E. Gambeta, F. Vergara, H. Morais, J.M. Zanoveli, and P.R. Dalsenter. 2017. Chlorpyrifos induces anxiety-like behavior in offspring rats exposed during pregnancy. *Neuroscience Letters* 641:94–100.

Silver, M.K., J. Shao, B. Zhu, M. Chen, Y. Xia, N. Kaciroti, B. Lozoff, and J. D. Meeker. 2017. Prenatal naled and chlopyrifos exposure is associated with deficits in infant motor function in a cohort of Chinese infants. *Environment International* 106:248–256.

Smalley, H.E., J.M. Curtis, and F.L. Earl. 1968. Teratogenic action of carbaryl in beagle dogs. *Toxicology and Applied Pharmacology* 13(3):392–403.

Smith, A.G. 1991. Chlorinated hydrocarbon insecticides. In: W.J. Hayes, Jr., and E. R. Laws, Jr. (eds). *Handbook of pesticide toxicology, vol. 2*. New York: Academic Press. Pp. 731–915.

Sujatha, R., K.C. Chitra, C. Latchoumycandane, and P.P. Mathur. 2001. Effect of lindane on testicular antioxidant system and steroidogenic enzymes in adult rats. *Asian Journal of Andrology* 3(2):135–138.

Sumida, K., K. Saito, N. Ooe, N. Isobe, H. Kaneko, and I. Nakatsuka. 2001. Evaluation of in vitro methods for detecting the effects of various chemicals on the human progesterone receptor, with a focus on pyrethroid insecticides. *Toxicology Letters* 118(3):147–155.

Suwalsky, M., F. Villena, D. Marcus, and A.M. Ronco. 2000. Plasma absorption and ultrastructural changes of rat testicular cells induced by lindane. *Human and Experimental Toxicology* 19(9):529–533.

Taylor, J.S., B.M. Thomson, C.N. Lang, F.Y. Sin, and E. Podivinsky. 2010. Estrogenic pyrethroid pesticides regulate expression of estrogen receptor transcripts in mouse sertoli cells differently from 17beta-estradiol. *Journal of Toxicology and Environmental Health, Part A* 73(16):1075–1089.

Tomczak, S., K. Baumann, and G. Lehnert. 1981. Occupational exposure to hexachlorocyclohexane. IV. Sex hormone alterations in HCH-exposed workers. *International Archives of Occupational and Environmental Health* 48(3):283–287.

Traina, M.E., M. Rescia, E. Urbani, A. Mantovani, C. Macri, C. Ricciardi, A.V. Stazi, P. Fazzi, E. Cordelli, P. Eleuteri, G. Leter, and M. Spano. 2003. Long-lasting effects of lindane on mouse spermatogenesis induced by in utero exposure. *Reproductive Toxicology* 17(1):25–35.

Trifonova, T.K., I.N. Gladenko, and V.D. Shulyak. 1970. Effect of hexachlorocyclohexane gamma-isomer and Sevin on sexual function. *Veterinariia* (Kiev) 6:91–93 [In Russian]. As cited in: W.J. Hayes, Jr., and E.R. Laws, Jr. (eds.). 1991. *Handbook of pesticide toxicology, vol. 2, Classes of Pesticides*. San Diego: Academic Press, Inc.

Tyagi, V., N. Garg, M.D. Mustafa, B.D. Banerjee, and K.Guleria. 2015. Organochlorine pesticide levels in maternal blood and placental tissue with reference to preterm birth: A recent trend in North Indian population. *Environmental Monitoring and Assessment* 187(7):471.

Umosen, A.J., S.F. Ambali, J.O. Ayo, B. Mohammed, and C. Uchendu. 2012. Alleviating effects of melatonin on oxidative changes in the testes and pituitary glands evoked by subacute chlorpyrifos administration in Wistar rats. *Asian Pacific Journal of Tropical Biomedicine* 2(8):645–650.

Upson, K., A.J. De Roos, M.L. Thompson, S. Sathyanarayana, D. Scholes, D.B. Barr, and V.L. Holt. 2013. Organochlorine pesticides and risk of endometriosis: Findings from a population-based case–control study. *Environmental Health Perspectives* 121:1319–1324.

Uzun, F.G., S. Kalender, D. Durak, F. Demir, and Y. Kalender. 2009. Malathion-induced testicular toxicity in male rats and the protective effect of vitamins C and E. *Food and Chemical Toxicology* 47(8):1903–1908.

VA (Department of Veterans Affairs). 2017. *Pesticides and Gulf War veterans*. https://www.publichealth.va.gov/exposures/gulfwar/sources/pesticides.asp (accessed December 4, 2017).

Venerosi, A., G. Calamandrei, and L. Ricceri. 2006. A social recognition test for female mice reveals behavioral effects of developmental chlorpyrifos exposure. *Neurotoxicology and Teratology* 28:466–471.

Venerosi, A., L. Ricceri, M.L. Scattoni, and G. Calamandrei. 2009. Prenatal chlorpyrifos exposure alters motor behavior and ultrasonic vocalization in CD-1 mouse pups. *Environmental Health* 8:12.

Venerosi, A., L. Ricceri, A. Rungi, V. Sanghez, and G. Calamandrei. 2010. Gestational exposure to the organophosphate chlorpyrifos alters social-emotional behaviour and impairs responsiveness to the serotonin transporter inhibitor fluvoxamine in mice. *Psychopharmacology* (Berl) 208(1):99–107.

Venerosi, A., S. Tait, L. Stecca, F. Chiarotti, A. De Felice, M.F. Cometa, M.T. Volpe, G. Calamandrei, and L. Ricceri. 2015. Effects of maternal chlorpyrifos diet on social investigation and brain neuroendocrine markers in the offspring—A mouse study. *Environmental Health* 14:32.

Viel, J.F., C. Warembourg, G. Le Maner-Idrissi, A. Lacroix, G. Limon, F. Rouget, C. Monfort, G. Durand, S. Cordier, and C. Chevrier. 2015. Pyrethroid insecticide exposure and cognitive developmental disabilities in children: The PELAGIE mother–child cohort. *Environment International* 82:69–75.

Viel, J.F., F. Rouget, C. Warembourg, C. Monfort, G. Limon, S. Cordier, and C. Chevrier. 2017. Behavioural disorders in 6-year-old children and pyrethroid insecticide exposure: The PELAGIE mother–child cohort. *Occupational and Environmental Medicine* 74(4):275–281.

Walker, V.R., A.L. Boyles, K.E. Pelch, S.D. Holmgren, A.J. Shapiro, C.R. Blystone, M.J. Devito, R.R. Newbold, R. Blain, P. Hartman, K.A. Thayer, and A.A. Rooney. 2018. Human and animal evidence of potential transgenerational inheritance of health effects: An evidence map and state-of-the-science evaluation. *Environment International* 115:48–69.

Walsh, L.P., and D. M. Stocco. 2000. Effects of lindane on steroidogenesis and steroidogenic acute regulatory protein expression. *Biology of Reproduction* 63(4):1024–1033.

Wang, P., Y. Tian, X.J. Wang, Y. Gao, R. Shi, G.Q. Wang, G.H. Hu, and X.M. Shen. 2012. Organophosphate pesticide exposure and perinatal outcomes in Shanghai, China. *Environment International* 42:100–104.

Wang, Y., Y. Zhang, L. Ji, Y. Hu, J. Zhang, C. Wang, G. Ding, L. Chen, M. Kamijima, J. Ueyama, Y. Gao, and Y. Tian 2017. Prenatal and postnatal exposure to organophosphate pesticides and childhood neurodevelopment in Shandong, China. *Environment International* 108:119–126.

Ware, G.W. 1989. *The pesticide book, 3rd ed.* Fresno, CA: Thomson Publications.

Watkins, D.J., G.Z. Fortenberry, B.N. Sanchez, D.B. Barr, P. Panuwet, L. Schnaas, E. Osorio-Valencia, M. Solano-Gonzalez, A.S. Ettinger, M. Hernandez-Avila, H. Hu, M.M. Tellez-Rojo, and J.D. Meeker. 2016. Urinary 3-phenoxybenzoic acid (3-PBA) levels among pregnant women in Mexico City: Distribution and relationships with child neurodevelopment. *Environmental Research* 147:307–313.

Wauchope, R.D., T.M. Buttler, A.G. Hornsby, P.W.M. Augustijn-Beckers, and J.P. Burt. 1992. SCS/ARS/CES pesticide properties database for environmental decision making. *Reviews of Environmental Contamination and Toxicology* 123:1–155.

Wessels, D., D.B. Barr, and P. Mendola. 2003. Use of biomarkers to indicate exposure of children to organophosphate pesticides: Implications for a longitudinal study of children's environmental health. *Environmental Health Perspectives* 111(16):1939–1946.

Whorton, M.D., T.H. Milby, H.A. Stubbs, B.H. Avashia, and E.Q. Hull. 1979. Testicular function among carbaryl-exposed employees. *Journal of Toxicology and Environmental Health* 5(5):929–941.

Whyatt, R.M., V. Rauh, D.B. Barr, D.E. Camann, H.F. Andrews, R. Garfinkel, L.A. Hoepner, D. Diaz, J. Dietrich, A. Reyes, D. Tang, P.L. Kinney, and F.P. Perera. 2004. Prenatal insecticide exposures and birth weight and length among an urban minority cohort. *Environmental Health Perspectives* 112(10):1125–1132.

Whyatt, R.M., D. Camann, F.P. Perera, V.A. Rauh, D. Tang, P.L. Kinney, R. Garfinkel, H. Andrews, L. Hoepner, and D.B. Barr. 2005. Biomarkers in assessing residential insecticide exposures during pregnancy and effects on fetal growth. *Toxicology and Applied Pharmacology* 206(2):246–254.

Wickerham, E.L., B. Lozoff, J. Shao, N. Kaciroti, Y. Xia, and J.D. Meeker. 2012. Reduced birth weight in relation to pesticide mixtures detected in cord blood of full-term infants. *Environment International* 47:80–85.

Willis, W.O., A. de Peyster, C.A. Molgaard, C. Walker, and T. MacKendrick. 1993. Pregnancy outcome among women exposed to pesticides through work or residence in an agricultural area. *Journal of Occupational Medicine* 35(9):943–949.

Wylie, B.J., M. Hauptman, A.D. Woolf, and R.H. Goldman. 2016. Insect repellants during pregnancy in the era of the Zika virus. *Obstetrics and Gynecology* 128(5):1111–1115.

Wyrobek, A.J., G. Watchmaker, L. Gordon, K. Wong, D. Moore, II, and D. Whorton. 1981. Sperm shape abnormalities in carbaryl-exposed employees. *Environmental Health Perspectives* 40:255–265.

Xia, Y., S. Cheng, Q. Bian, L. Xu, M.D. Collins, H.C. Chang, L. Song, J. Liu, S. Wang, and X. Wang. 2005. Genotoxic effects on spermatozoa of carbaryl-exposed workers. *Toxicological Sciences* 85(1):615–623.

Xia, Y., Y. Han, B. Wu, S. Wang, A. Gu, N. Lu, J. Bo, L. Song, N. Jin, and X. Wang. 2008. The relation between urinary metabolite of pyrethroid insecticides and semen quality in humans. *Fertility and Sterility* 89(6):1743–1750.

Xue, Z., X. Li, Q. Su, L. Xu, P. Zhang, Z. Kong, J. Xu, and J. Teng. 2013. Effect of synthetic pyrethroid pesticide exposure during pregnancy on the growth and development of infants. *Asia-Pacific Journal of Public Health* 25(4 Suppl):72S–79S.

Yoshinaga, J., K. Imai, H. Shiraishi, S. Nozawa, M. Yoshiike, M.N. Mieno, A.M. Andersson, and T. Iwamoto. 2014. Pyrethroid insecticide exposure and reproductive hormone levels in healthy Japanese male subjects. *Andrology* 2(3):416–420.

Young, H.A., J.D. Meeker, S.E. Martenies, Z.I. Figueroa, D.B. Barr, and M.J. Perry. 2013. Environmental exposure to pyrethroids and sperm sex chromosome disomy: A cross-sectional study. *Environmental Health* 12:111.

Young, J.G., B. Eskenazi, E.A. Gladstone, A. Bradman, L. Pedersen, C. Johnson, D.B. Barr, C.E. Furlong, and N.T. Holland. 2005. Association between in utero organophosphate pesticide exposure and abnormal reflexes in neonates. *NeuroToxicology* 26(2):199–209.

Yu, Y., Y. Yang, X. Zhao, X. Liu, J. Xue, J. Zhang, and A. Yang. 2017. Exposure to the mixture of organophosphorus pesticides is embryotoxic and teratogenic on gestational rats during the sensitive period. *Environmental Toxicology* 32(1):139–146.

Yucra, S., M. Gasco, J. Rubio, and G.F. Gonzales. 2008. Semen quality in Peruvian pesticide applicators: Association between urinary organophosphate metabolites and semen parameters. *Environmental Health* 7:59.

Zhang, S.Y., Y. Ito, O. Yamanoshita, Y. Yanagiba, M. Kobayashi, K. Taya, C. Li, A. Okamura, M. Miyata, J. Ueyama, C.H. Lee, M. Kamijima, and T. Nakajima. 2007. Permethrin may disrupt testosterone biosynthesis via mitochondrial membrane damage of Leydig cells in adult male mouse. *Endocrinology* 148(8):3941–3949.

Zhang, S.Y., J. Ueyama, Y. Ito, Y. Yanagiba, A. Okamura, M. Kamijima, and T. Nakajima. 2008. Permethrin may induce adult male mouse reproductive toxicity due to cis isomer not trans isomer. *Toxicology* 248(2–3):136–141.

Zhang, Y., S. Han, D. Liang, X. Shi, F. Wang, W. Liu, L. Zhang, L. Chen, Y. Gu, and Y. Tian. 2014a. Prenatal exposure to organophosphate pesticides and neurobehavioral development of neonates: A birth cohort study in Shenyang, China. *PLOS ONE* 9(2):e88491.

Zhang, J., J. Yoshinaga, A. Hisada, H. Shiraishi, K. Shimodaira, T. Okai, M. Koyama, N. Watanabe, E. Suzuki, M. Shirakawa, Y. Noda, Y. Komine, N. Ariki, and N. Kato. 2014b. Prenatal pyrethroid insecticide exposure and thyroid hormone levels and birth sizes of neonates. *Science of the Total Environment* 488–489:275–279.

Zidan, N.E.A. 2009. Evaluation of the reproductive toxicity of chlorpyrifos methyl, diazinon, and profenofos pesticides in male rats. *International Journal of Pharmacology* 5(1):51–57.

6

Combustion Products and Fuels

Military personnel in the 1990–1991 Gulf War were exposed to combustion products and fuels from more than 600 burning oil wells in Kuwait, from fueling and exhaust from military vehicles and aircrafts, and from heaters in poorly ventilated tents. Post-9/11 military personnel were potentially also exposed to combustion products from fuels, exhaust, and heaters, but they were also exposed to smoke and emissions from the numerous burn pits used to dispose of waste in Iraq and Afghanistan. Gulf War and Post-9/11 veterans deployed to southwest Asia, including Iraq and Afghanistan, were often exposed to heavily dust-laden environments that contained hazardous airborne particles.

This chapter examines the reproductive, developmental, and generational health effects associated with combustion products—particulate matter (PM), polycyclic aromatic hydrocarbons (PAHs), polychlorinated dibenzo-p-dioxins and dibenzofurans (PCDD/PCDFs), and several studies that looked specifically at exhaust—and fuels. Previous *Gulf War and Health* reports, authoritative reviews, and new literature are summarized below.

COMBUSTION PRODUCTS

Several National Academies of Sciences, Engineering, and Medicine's reports have examined the possible contribution of air pollution to adverse health effects among U.S. military personnel serving in the Middle East. In 2011 a report on the hazards of burn pit emissions identified PM, volatile organic compounds (VOCs, such as benzene and toluene), PAHs, and PCDD/PCDFs as the primary exposures of concerns at Joint Base Balad (JBB) in Iraq (IOM, 2011). The report concluded that

> the greatest pollution concern at JBB may be the mixture of regional background and local sources—other than the burn pit—that contribute to high PM. This PM, which was characterized in a different study and at different locations at JBB, consists of substantial amounts of windblown dust combined with elemental carbon and metals that arise from transportation and industrial activities. On the basis of the

> high concentrations in the previous studies of potentially toxic constituents of ambient PM, the air pollution literature that focused on PM and gaseous pollutant co-exposures was considered relevant to the potential morbidity of military personnel at JBB and at other sites in the Middle East. (IOM, 2011, p. 4)

Based on that report, the Volume 11 committee focused on several specific pollutant categories. The following section explores the literature pertaining to the reproductive, developmental, and transgenerational effects of PM, PAHs, and PCDDs/PCDFs. Given the overlap between VOCs and solvents, relevant VOCs are discussed in the chapter on solvents.

The Volume 3 committee reviewed the literature on combustion products through 2004. It approached its task by identifying the most common components in combustion emissions, including PM, sulfur dioxide (SO_2), ozone (O_3), nitrogen oxide (NO), nitrogen dioxide (NO_2), carbon monoxide (CO), carbon dioxide (CO_2), hydrogen sulfide (H_2S), and VOCs and then assessing the possible health effects associated with each of these agents. The Volume 3 committee considered preterm birth, low birth weight, very low birth weight, intrauterine growth retardation, birth defects, and childhood cancers as relevant outcomes. These outcomes were assessed in epidemiologic studies of ambient air pollution—frequently conducted in or near heavily polluted cities—or in case-control studies based on residence or parental occupation. Generally, these studies were limited by a lack of control for other risk factors, such as smoking, and the use of overly broad exposure classifications. The Volume 3 committee concluded that there was:

- inadequate/insufficient evidence of an association between parental combustion product exposure and any childhood cancers or any birth defects,
- limited/suggestive evidence of an association between combustion product exposure during pregnancy and preterm birth,
- limited/suggestive evidence of an association between combustion product exposure during pregnancy and low birth weight or intrauterine growth retardation, and
- insufficient/inadequate evidence of an association at any specific time during pregnancy (e.g., first trimester) and preterm birth, low birth weight, or intrauterine growth retardation (IOM, 2005).

The 2011 IOM report *Long-Term Health Consequences of Exposure to Burn Pits in Iraq and Afghanistan* examined the epidemiologic literature on firefighters and people living or working near incinerators and health endpoints identified by authoritative reviews (e.g., the Environmental Protection Agency [EPA], the Agency for Toxic Substances and Disease Registry [ATSDR], the National Institute for Occupational Safety and Health, and the Hazardous Substances Database) of the 56 chemicals that were measured above the detection limit in burn pit environmental sampling data. Because data on the health of veterans or active-duty service members who were exposed to burn pits were scant, the committee reviewed studies of firefighters and incinerator workers because of their relatively similar exposure to combustion products. That committee found that there were known reproductive and developmental toxicants among the burn pit chemicals and that they should be further studied. The literature at the time included no "key" studies on reproductive or developmental outcomes, and "supporting" studies presented mixed results or showed no elevated risks. Thus, that committee concluded that there was "inadequate/insufficient evidence to determine whether an association exists between parental exposure to combustion products and adverse effects in their children and other adverse reproductive and perinatal outcomes in veterans, firefighters, or people living/working near incinerators" (IOM, 2011, p. 88).

Particulate Matter

Particulate matter is a general term used to describe a large group of chemically diverse substances that exist as particles in ambient air (Spektor, 1998). The particles are derived from both natural and anthropogenic sources; they may form in the atmosphere from a variety of sources or be emitted to the atmosphere with gaseous emissions. Coarse PM (10 μm or less in diameter; PM_{10}) originates from sources such as mining, construction operations, and the resuspension of soil on roads and streets. Fine PM (less than 2.5 μm; $PM_{2.5}$) and ultrafine PM (less than 0.1 μm) are found in emissions from the combustion of motor-vehicle fuel; smelters and steel mills; the combustion of wood, oil, and coal; and the atmospheric alteration of SO_2, organics, and NO (NRC, 2010). The size of the particles is one of the major determinants of its toxicity. Only inhaled PM_{10} and smaller particles are deposited in the lower respiratory tract (i.e., below the vocal cords). Toxicity concerns are greatest for fine PM and ultrafine PM that may be deposited in smaller airways and alveoli (IOM, 2005). Ultrafine particles may even pass through the alveolar-capillary membrane into the circulatory system.

The daily exposures of service members to windblown dust and frequent dust storms increased their concerns about the possible health effects that might result from these exposures. In response to those concerns, the Department of Defense (DoD) designed and implemented the Enhanced Particulate Matter Surveillance Program to characterize and quantify the PM at 15 sites in the Central Command Area of Operations in the Middle East, beginning in Afghanistan in 2001 and in Iraq in 2003. PM sources in the Middle East included dust storms (which would carry the particles considerable distances), agricultural activities, emissions from vehicles and burn pits, battery-processing facilities, cooking stoves and fires, flaring at natural gas and oil extraction facilities, and fertilizer plants (NRC, 2010). DoD monitoring at JBB in Iraq in 2007 and 2009 found that PM_{10} levels ranged from 2 $\mu g/m^3$ to 9,576 $\mu g/m^3$ (with averages of 126 $\mu g/m^3$ in 2007 and 709 $\mu g/m^3$ in 2009) (IOM, 2011). Another study of three military sites in Kuwait in 2004–2005 found that the average PM_{10} concentrations fluctuated between 66 and 93 $\mu g/m^3$ (Brown et al., 2008). In its review of the DoD Enhanced Particulate Matter Surveillance Program, a National Research Council committee determined that ambient PM_{10} concentrations in most areas of the Middle East exceeded the World Health Organization's annual average air quality guideline of 20 $\mu g/m^3$ (NRC, 2010). As a point of reference, PM exposure in the United States is subject to great variability as well, with some areas such as southern California, southern Arizona, and central New Mexico reporting average annual PM_{10} concentrations >50 $\mu g/m^3$ (EPA, 2009).

In 2009, EPA issued an *Integrated Science Assessment for Particulate Matter* that described the human health effects associated with ambient PM through 2009. EPA concluded that the "epidemiologic and toxicologic evidence is suggestive of a causal relationship between long-term exposures to $PM_{2.5}$ and reproductive and developmental outcomes" (p. 2-13). Epidemiologic data showed effects on birth weight, infant mortality, and fetal growth, with less consistent evidence for preterm birth, growth restriction, birth defects, and decreased sperm quality. The available toxicologic data also supported those associations but added little to the mechanistic understanding. EPA also noted that some PM studies had shown epigenetic effects (i.e., changes in DNA methylation), but their relevance to human health was unclear (EPA, 2009).

Although the data presented in this chapter focus on PM, it is just one of many constituents of air pollution determined by the EPA to cause adverse health effects, a so-called criteria pollutant. Other EPA criteria pollutants include O_3, CO, NO_X, and SO_2 (EPA, 2018). Because air pollution is a mixture whose composition varies depending on the source, with emissions from combustion sources generally regarded as the most toxic, it is difficult to distinguish the contributions of specific pollutants from the effects of the overall mixture. Furthermore, PM concentrations are often correlated with other pollutants emitted during combustion, and so the committee recognizes that PM toxicity does not exclude effects of co-pollutants.

Like the Volume 3 committee, the Volume 11 committee did not examine the chemical and physical composition of particles because of the wide variation in particle components across geographic locations and sources, including differences in the relative amounts of elemental and organic carbon, sulfates, nitrates, pollen, microbial contaminants, and metals. Furthermore, the bioavailability and toxicity of such chemicals is affected by adsorption to the particle so that the toxicity of a chemical alone does not represent its toxicity when adsorbed on the particle (IOM, 2005). Rather, the Volume 11 committee focuses on studies of the toxicity of PM, not studies of the individual chemicals that might be adsorbed onto or incorporated into the PM.

The literature on the reproductive and developmental effects of PM is varied and extensive. The committee's search identified 340 relevant publications of reproductive and developmental effects associated with PM published in 2004 or later (combustion products are reviewed in Volume 3 through 2004). Because EPA conducted an extensive review of the literature on the health effects of PM through 2009, the Volume 11 committee limited its review to studies published in 2009 or later, which totaled about 300 publications. No specific studies were identified on the reproductive or developmental effects of PM exposure in veterans. Given the volume of data, the committee paid special attention to evidence synthesized in systematic reviews and meta-analyses as well as to studies on preconception or first-trimester exposures because they were considered to be most relevant to potential veteran exposures.

Reproductive Effects

Several recent publications have explored possible associations between PM and aspects of reproductive health or fertility in men and women—including endometriosis, fertility and fecundity, offspring sex ratios, and impacts on sperm. With the exception of fertility studies that rely on self-reports of contraception use, most of the studies on reproductive effects in women rely on outcomes documented in birth certificates, hospital discharge records, and registries.

Reproductive Effects in Men

A systematic review by Lafuente et al. (2016) evaluated 17 studies on the impacts of air pollution on sperm quality. Although the studies examined a range of windows of exposure before semen collection, all included the 90 days before sampling. The authors also noted a wide variability in the degree to which confounders such as age, smoking, body mass index (BMI), and socioeconomic status (SES) were controlled for. Thirteen studies measured air pollution exposure, six used biomarkers of air pollution exposure, and two did both. The authors concluded that $PM_{2.5}$ was not associated with sperm DNA fragmentation, decreased sperm count, or alterations in sperm morphology.

Four cross-sectional studies examined the effects of PM exposure within 90 days of semen collection with mixed results, as discussed below (Hansen et al., 2010; Jurewicz et al., 2015; Wu et al., 2017; Zhou et al., 2014). Most of the studies had negative findings.

Significant detrimental effects on sperm count and concentration were reported by Wu et al. (2017) in association with $PM_{2.5}$ exposure 70–90 days before sample collection and with the highest quintile of exposure over the whole exposure period of 0 to 90 days (sperm concentration $\beta = -0.42$, 95% confidence interval [CI] –0.67– –0.16; sperm count $\beta = -0.40$, 95% CI –0.66– –0.14; adjusted p-value for trend=0.018 for both). These data showed that there were no effects on sperm motility. The authors also noted no effect of PM_{10} on sperm centration, count, or morphology. Hansen et al. (2010) found that $PM_{2.5}$

had no effect on sperm morphology, cytoplasmic droplets, DNA fragmentation, or immature sperm in an occupational cohort of 228 fertile men. Zhou et al. (2014) reported a positive association between PM_{10} and sperm concentration (β=0.08, 95% CI 0.02–0.11) and a negative association with sperm morphology (β= –0.21, 95% CI –0.80– –0.003) and some, but not all, measures of motility (motile sperm curve linear velocity β= –0.16, 95% CI –0.80 to 0.68, and motile sperm straight line velocity β= –0.21, 95% CI –0.82– –0.016); PM_{10} was not related to semen volume, progressive motility, total motility, or linearity.

Jurewicz et al. (2015) examined the relationship between PM and the percentage of sperm with chromosome disomy (X, Y, 13, 18, and 21). The authors observed significant relationships between $PM_{2.5}$ and disomy Y (YY18 β=0.68, 95% CI 0.55–0.85), sex chromosome disomy (β=0.78, 95% CI 0.59–0.99), and chromosome 21 disomy (%2121 β=0.78, 95% CI 0.62–0.97), with no relationship to XY18, XX18, %1818, %1313, and total disomy. PM_{10} was also related to chromosome 21 disomy (%2121 β=0.58, 95% CI 0.46–0.72), but not to any of the other chromosome disomies.

Reproductive Effects in Women

One systematic review examined the human and animal literature published through early 2014 on fertility in association with PM (Frutos et al., 2015). Ten studies on live births, miscarriages, pregnancy, implantation, and embryo quality were assessed. The authors identified PM_{10} as having a detrimental effect on live births, implantation rates, and miscarriage, while $PM_{2.5}$ was reported to adversely affect pregnancy rates. The authors also noted that impacts were greatest among sub-fertile women undergoing assisted reproduction.

Three cohort studies examined the association between PM exposure and the ability to conceive. The Nurses' Health Study II, a large prospective cohort study of female nurses, examined associations between fertility (defined as attempted conception for ≥12 months without success) over 10 years and $PM_{2.5}$, $PM_{10-2.5}$, and PM_{10} levels based on residential address. Those investigators reported elevated hazard ratios for all three sizes of PM expressed as 2-year, 4-year, or cumulative averages, but all were nonsignificant after adjustment for confounders (Mahalingaiah et al., 2016). In a study that examined a cohort of 1,916 births in Teplice, Czech Republic, fecundability (the probability of pregnancy among noncontracepting couples each month) was found to be significantly related to local $PM_{2.5}$ levels. Exposure in the previous 30 days was significantly related to decreased fecundability (fecundity ratio=0.86, 95% CI 0.77–0.97 per 10 μg/m^3 increase). Fecundability was slightly reduced with $PM_{2.5}$ exposure in the first month of unprotected intercourse, but not significantly. Both average $PM_{2.5}$ in the previous 30-day period and the 2-month average exposure to $PM_{2.5}$ were significantly related to decreased fecundability (adjusted fecundability ratios per 10 μg/m^3=0.86, [95% CI 0.77–0.97] and 0.78, [95% CI 0.65–0.94], respectively) (Slama et al., 2013). Conversely, Nobles et al. (2018) reported on fecundability, over a year compared to modeled PM 5 days before and 10 days after ovulation in 501 couples living in Michigan and Texas but did not find evidence of adverse effects of $PM_{2.5}$ or PM_{10} on fecundability. Nieuwenhuijsen et al. (2014) compared annual averages of $PM_{2.5}$, $PM_{10-2.5}$, and PM_{10} per interquartile range (IQR) change with birth rates at the census tract level and found a significantly decreased birth rate in association with $PM_{10-2.5}$ that remained after adjustment for multiple covariates (incidence rate ratio [IRR]=0.88, 95% CI 0.83–0.94; $PM_{2.5}$ IRR=0.98, 95% CI 0.95–1.02; PM_{10} IRR=0.99, 95% CI 0.97–1.02).

Endometriosis, which can impair fertility, was investigated in one publication of the Nurses' Health Study II (Mahalingaiah et al., 2014). No associations between $PM_{2.5}$, $PM_{10-2.5}$, or PM_{10} and confirmed cases of endometriosis were reported in this cohort.

Merklinger-Gruchala et al. (2017) reported on associations between pollutants and changes in menstrual cycle length in 133 Polish women as a possible contributing factor to fertility problems. While

PM_{10} was not associated with overall cycle length or follicular phase length, mean PM_{10} was associated with a shortened luteal phase length (β= –0.02 day per 1 μg/m^3, 95% CI –0.04– –0.00).

Sex Ratio

Two studies of sex ratios indicated that increased exposure to PM favors female births. In a Chinese birth cohort study that examined concentrations of PM_{10} in the 13 days before conception versus sex ratios, Lin et al. (2015) found a significantly higher probability of female births with increased PM_{10} exposure 2 days before conception (excess risk = 0.64%, 95% CI 0.35–0.93 for each 10 μg/m^3 increase in PM_{10}), while controlling for confounders such as maternal age, parental education, and weather conditions. One ecologic time-series study found a negative association between the ratio of male to female births and annual average PM_{10} levels at the district level (β= –0.001, p=0.02), although no potential confounders or other pollutants were included as covariates in the analysis (El Khouri Miraglia et al., 2013).

Adverse Pregnancy Outcomes

The relationship between exposure to PM and adverse pregnancy outcomes has been studied by numerous researchers assessing a variety of maternal and fetal outcomes. The Volume 11 committee identified several studies of pregnancy outcomes that affect the health of the mother and child; these include 2 studies of placental problems, 3 studies on gestational diabetes, and 12 studies on preeclampsia[1] and gestational hypertension. Several studies also examined the associations between maternal exposure to PM during pregnancy and effects on the uterus and placenta and also on fetal biomarkers that are thought to represent inflammation at the time of birth.

The Volume 11 committee then focused on the effects of PM on birth outcomes such as preterm birth, low birth weight (less than 2,500 g), and fetal death. In the sections on preterm birth and birth weight, the committee evaluated numerous systematic reviews and meta-analyses. Systematic reviews and meta-analyses were not available for outcomes such as miscarriage, stillbirths (fetal loss after 20 weeks of gestation), and spontaneous abortion (fetal loss before 20 weeks of gestation), and therefore the committee considered individual studies for these events. For the most part, the committee considers studies that include appropriate statistical adjustments for potential confounders and indicates instances when a study may not have accounted for common confounders.

Understanding the effects of prenatal PM on birth outcomes requires an appreciation of several confounding issues, such as SES and maternal health. Erickson et al. (2016) found that 49% of the between-neighborhood differences in birth weight were related to neighborhood SES and the interaction between SES and $PM_{2.5}$. SES modified the effect of $PM_{2.5}$ on birth weight in such a way that the most pronounced effect was in neighborhoods with lower SES. Mendola et al. (2016) reported significantly increased risks of preterm birth among mothers with asthma exposed to PM_{10} in the last 6 weeks of pregnancy but no association between preterm birth and PM_{10} among women without asthma.

Placental Problems Two studies examined placental problems and prenatal PM exposure. In Japan,

[1] *Preeclampsia* is a pregnancy complication related to high blood pressure during pregnancy (gestational hypertension) that can cause damage to organ systems, specifically kidney and liver, and lead to the need for early delivery of the baby and, in extreme cases, seizures (eclampsia) in the mother (Mayo Clinic, 2018d).

Michikawa et al. (2016) found a significantly elevated risk of placenta accreta[2] and placenta previa associated with exposure to suspended PM (equivalent to PM_7) in the first 4 weeks of pregnancy (placenta previa odds ratio [OR]=1.12, 95% CI 1.01–1.23; placenta accreta OR=1.33, 95% CI 1.07–1.66, per 10 $\mu g/m^3$), but no associations were found for exposure during gestation weeks 5–12 or in the second trimester. Ibrahimou et al. (2017) examined placental abruption as recorded on Florida birth certificates (884 placental abruptions among 100,495 births) and found an increased risk was associated with $PM_{2.5}$ exposure throughout pregnancy or during the first trimester. Slightly elevated and significant risks were identified for first-trimester exposure to specific components of $PM_{2.5}$ (aluminum and elemental carbon).

Gestational Diabetes Gestational diabetes was the focus of three U.S. cohort studies. In a large cohort study of 219,952 births, Robledo et al. (2015) found no association between gestational diabetes and $PM_{2.5}$ or PM_{10} in the 3 months before pregnancy or in the first trimester. However, Hu et al. (2015) reported an increased risk of gestational diabetes with $PM_{2.5}$ exposure in the first trimester (OR=1.11, 95% CI 1.06–1.16), but not in the second trimester, after controlling for other pollutants although not for prepregnancy weight, an important risk factor for gestational diabetes. Investigating $PM_{2.5}$ exposure in the second trimester, Fleisch et al. (2014) found a significant increase in impaired glucose tolerance when comparing the highest and lowest quartiles of exposure (OR=2.63, 95% CI 1.15–6.01) but no association with gestational diabetes as a clinical diagnosis.

Preeclampsia and Gestational Hypertension One systematic review and meta-analysis of literature published between 2009 and 2013 examined the association between PM and preeclampsia and gestational hypertension, with seven studies on exposure and five on PM_{10} exposure (Pedersen et al., 2014). Pooled estimates showed significant increases in all hypertensive disorders of pregnancy, combined, with each 5 $\mu g/m^3$ increase of $PM_{2.5}$ (OR=1.57, 95% CI 1.26–1.96) and each 10 $\mu g/m^3$ increase of PM_{10} (OR=1.13, 95% CI 1.02–1.26).

Among the studies discussed below, one found increased risks of preeclampsia with PM_{10} exposure (Lee et al., 2013), while four did not (Dadvand et al., 2013; Mobasher et al., 2013; van den Hooven et al., 2011; Wu et al., 2011). Four studies of $PM_{2.5}$ found positive associations with preeclampsia (Dadvand et al., 2013; Lee et al., 2013; Mobasher et al., 2013; Wu et al., 2011), and two studies did not (Rudra et al., 2011; Savitz et al., 2015). One study of preconception exposure by Rudra et al. (2011) found no relationship between $PM_{2.5}$ and preeclampsia.

Lee et al. (2013) found no significant relationship between preeclampsia and first-trimester PM_{10} or $PM_{2.5}$ exposure. However, among mothers who did not smoke during pregnancy, the risks of gestational hypertension were elevated with PM exposure (PM_{10} OR=1.12, 95% CI 1.01–1.25; $PM_{2.5}$ OR=1.11, 95% CI 0.99–1.24, per IQR change); this elevation was not seen among mothers who smoked during pregnancy.

In a cohort study in Spain of 8,398 pregnancies (including 103 cases of preeclampsia), Dadvand et al. (2013) found no association between first- or second-trimester PM exposures and preeclampsia or between third-trimester PM_{10} exposures and preeclampsia. However, IQR increases of $PM_{2.5}$ in the third trimester (OR=1.51, 95% CI 1.13–2.01) and over the entire pregnancy (OR=1.32, 95% CI 1.02–1.71) were both related to preeclampsia, as were increases among late-onset (OR=1.42, 95% CI 1.01–2.00) but not early-onset cases.

[2] *Placenta accreta* is a serious pregnancy condition that occurs when the placenta grows too deeply into the uterine wall. While the placenta usually detaches from the uterine wall after childbirth, with placenta accreta it remains attached and can cause severe blood loss after delivery. *Placenta previa* is when the placenta partially or totally covers the mother's cervix, requiring a cesarean section to deliver the baby. It can cause severe bleeding during pregnancy and delivery. *Placental abruption* is when the placenta separates from the the uterus before delivery, an action that can decrease the baby's oxygen and nutrient supply and cause heavy bleeding in the mother (Mayo Clinic, 2018a,b,c).

Among 81,186 births in Los Angeles and Orange counties, Wu et al. (2011) found no elevated risks of preeclampsia with $PM_{2.5}$ or PM_{10} exposure throughout the entire pregnancy using regression models and PM measured at air quality monitoring stations. However, when an air dispersion model (CALINE 4 model) was used for $PM_{2.5}$ exposure, significantly elevated risks were found (LA County OR=1.08, 95% CI 1.02–1.15; Orange County OR=1.10, 95% CI 1.04–1.17). Another study in LA County used a case-control design (136 cases, 162 controls) to examine the roles of pollutant exposure and BMI on preeclampsia and found a significant interaction (p=0.02). Results showed an increased risk of preeclampsia with $PM_{2.5}$ exposure in the first trimester among women with BMI <30 (OR=8.63, 95% CI 3.10–24.1) but no significant increase among obese women (BMI >30) or related to PM_{10} exposure (Mobasher et al., 2013). A cohort study of pregnant women in the Netherlands showed no relationship between PM_{10} exposure in any trimester and preeclampsia (van den Hooven et al., 2011).

Rudra et al. (2011) examined $PM_{2.5}$ exposure from prepregnancy through the last month of pregnancy in 3,509 Washington State births and found no association between $PM_{2.5}$ and preeclampsia. Savitz et al. (2015) also examined $PM_{2.5}$ exposure in the first and second trimesters and found no association with gestational hypertension or with mild or severe preeclampsia among 268,601 New York City births.

Several studies discussed below reported a positive association between maternal blood pressure or gestational hypertension and exposure to PM (Lee et al., 2012; van den Hooven et al., 2011; Vinikoor-Imler et al., 2012; Xu et al., 2014); however, one study found no such effects (Hampel et al., 2011).

Xu et al. (2014) reported on the risk of hypertensive disorders of pregnancy (including gestational hypertension, preeclampsia, and eclampsia) among 22,041 pregnancies in Florida. Although there was no association between hypertensive disorders of pregnancy and $PM_{2.5}$ exposure in the first trimester, elevated risks were reported for exposure in the second trimester (OR=1.28, 95% CI 1.13–1.46) and across the entire pregnancy (OR=1.24, 95% CI 1.08–1.43).

In a cohort of 1,684 pregnant women in Pennsylvania, investigators compared blood pressure measurements taken in the first 20 weeks of gestation with those measured late in pregnancy and found increases that were associated with first-trimester $PM_{2.5}$ exposure (systolic β=0.84 mmHg, 95% CI –0.33–2.00, and diastolic β=0.60 mmHg, 95% CI –0.27–1.47, per IQR) and PM_{10} exposure (systolic β=1.88 mmHg, 95% CI 0.84–2.93, and diastolic β=0.63 mmHg, 95% CI –0.50–1.76). No associations were seen with exposures during the second or third trimesters (Lee et al., 2012).

Hampel et al. (2011) measured blood pressure longitudinally in a cohort of 1,500 pregnant French women and assessed associations with PM_{10} exposures in the preceding 7 days. No significant changes for systolic and diastolic pressure changes were associated with exposure on each day in the week before blood pressure was measured. However, a significant decrease in systolic pressure was observed when PM_{10} exposure was averaged across the 7 days before measurement (–0.3 mmHg, 95% CI –0.6–0.0).

Among 7,006 Dutch women, van den Hooven et al. (2011) reported that 10 $\mu g/m^3$ increases in PM_{10} concentrations were associated with a 1.11 mmHg increase in systolic blood pressure in the second trimester (95% CI 0.43–1.79) and a 2.11 mmHg increase in the third trimester (95% CI 1.34–2.89), but there were no associations with first-trimester exposure or diastolic blood pressure. The authors reported a significantly increased risk of pregnancy-related hypertension (OR=1.72, 95% CI 1.12–2.63) for each 10 $\mu g/m^3$ increase in PM_{10}.

Vinikoor-Imler et al. (2012) found increased risks of gestational hypertension with IQR increases in $PM_{2.5}$ and PM_{10} averaged to represent the entire pregnancy in 222,775 North Carolina births ($PM_{2.5}$ RR=1.11, 95% CI 1.08–1.15, and PM_{10} RR=1.07, 95% CI 1.04–1.11). The associations remained significant after adjustments for neighborhood poverty. However, this study did not control for maternal weight gain, prepregnancy weight, or hypertension.

Prenatal exposure to $PM_{2.5}$ has also been associated with an increased systolic blood pressure in the child at birth. Each IQR increase in $PM_{2.5}$ estimated for the 2–90 days before birth was associated with a 1.0 mmHg increase in systolic blood pressure (95% CI 0.1–1.8) (van Rossem et al., 2015).

Most of the studies cited above controlled for prepregnancy weight, BMI, or maternal weight gain, all of which are important risk factors for gestational hypertension and preeclampsia (Dadvand et al., 2013; Hampel et al., 2011; Lee et al., 2012; Mobasher et al., 2013; Rudra et al., 2011; Savitz et al., 2015; van den Hooven et al., 2011). Three studies did not adjust for maternal BMI (Lee et al., 2013; Vinikoor-Imler et al., 2012; Wu et al., 2011), thus limiting their usefulness.

Biomarkers of Oxidative Stress and Inflammation at Birth Thirteen studies identified by the committee investigated various measures and markers of stress and inflammation in the uterus, placenta, and cord blood in relation to prenatal PM exposure. Toxicologic data suggests that adverse health effects in offspring may be mediated by a greater susceptibility of the mother to the oxidative and inflammatory effects of PM during pregnancy; for example, inflammatory or immune response in pregnant mice has been associated with health effects in the offspring (EPA, 2009).

Effects of PM on the uterus and placenta have been studied in four cohorts. In a large cohort of 5,059 mother–child pairs in Boston, increased risks of intrauterine inflammation (intrapartum fever and placental pathology) were reported with the highest quartile of $PM_{2.5}$ exposure compared with the lowest quartile in the 3 months before conception (OR=1.52, 95% CI 1.22–1.89), first trimester (OR=1.93, 95% CI 1.55–2.40), second trimester (OR=1.67, 95% CI 1.35–2.08), and third trimester (OR=1.53, 95% CI 1.24–1.90) (Nachman et al., 2016). Placental 3-nitrotyrosine (3-NTp; a marker of oxidative stress) levels increased with each IQR increase in $PM_{2.5}$ (29%, 95% CI 4.9–58.6) and black carbon (23.6%, 95% CI 4.4–46.4) in the first trimester in a birth cohort in Belgium (N=90) (Saenen et al., 2016). A study of 3,614 Italian women did not find an association between PM_{10} and placental weight (Giovanni et al., 2018).

To investigate whether placental oxidative stress could affect fetal growth and maternal hypertensive complications, van den Hooven et al. (2012b) measured growth factors that are important for placental growth in maternal and cord blood as well as placental vascular resistance and placental weight in 7,801 pregnant women in the Netherlands (known as the Generation R Study). Throughout pregnancy, PM_{10} exposure (10 μg/m^3) was associated with decreased maternal growth factor levels as measured by soluble fms-like tyrosine kinase 1 (sFlt-1= –4.5%, 95% CI –8.4– –0.5) and changes in fetal growth factors (sFlt-1= 35.8%, 95% CI 25.6–45.9; and placental growth factor= –16.3%, 95% CI –21.9– –10.7%). Although PM_{10} was associated with the umbilical artery pulsatility index in the second trimester (difference= –0.10, 95% CI –0.17– –0.03), it was not associated with the uterine artery pulsatility index, uterine artery notching, or placental weight (van den Hooven et al., 2012b). These findings indicate that PM may affect placental and fetal growth.

Several studies documented changes in immune markers in cord blood associated with PM exposure. Ashley-Martin et al. (2016) reported an association between the highest quartile of exposure to $PM_{2.5}$ in the first trimester and immunoglobulin E (IgE) in cord blood among 582 female births (OR=2.37, 95% CI 1.23–4.58) in Canada, although there was no association among 671 male births or with other markers (IL-33 and TSLP). The prevalence ratios of elevated cord serum IgE for each μg/m^3 increase in $PM_{2.5}$ indicated decreased risks in the first month of pregnancy and elevated risks in months 4 through 7 in a study of 459 births in the Czech Republic; the results were modified by maternal IgE levels and cigarette smoke (Herr et al., 2011).

Levels of C-reactive protein, a marker of inflammation, have been studied in association with PM exposure. Lee et al. (2011) found an increased risk of having elevated C-reactive protein (≥8 ng/ml) in maternal blood collected before the 22nd week of gestation and PM in the month before sample collection (PM_{10} 9.2 μg/m^3 increase OR=1.41, 95% CI 0.99–2.00; $PM_{2.5}$ 4.6 μg/m^3 increase OR=1.47, 95% CI

1.05–2.06) in a cohort of nonsmoking pregnant women in Pennsylvania. In the Netherlands, the highest quartile of PM_{10} exposure in the 2 weeks before maternal blood sampling had increased risks of elevated C-reactive protein levels (≥8 ng/ml) among pregnant women (OR=1.32, 95% CI 1.08–1.61), but there was no association at 1 and 4 weeks before sampling. This study also found that high PM_{10} throughout the pregnancy was related to elevated fetal C-reactive protein at delivery (>1 mg/L) (OR=2.18, 95% CI 1.08–4.38) (van den Hooven et al., 2012a).

Changes in newborn cord blood lymphocyte subpopulations associated with PM_{10} exposure before and during pregnancy were reported among 370 women giving birth at a hospital in France (Baiz et al., 2011). Preconception exposure to PM_{10} (per 10 μg/m^3 increase) was associated with increases in CD8+ cells (β=1.52, 95% CI 0.05–2.99) and decreases in CD4+CD25+ cells (β= –0.82, 95% CI –1.45– –0.19). First-trimester exposure was associated with decreases in CD3+ cells (β= –3.10, 95% CI –6.02– –0.18) and increases in natural killer (NK) cells (β=0.22, 95% CI 0.008–0.43), and exposure across all three trimesters was associated with decreases in CD4+CD5+ cells (1st β= –0.71, 95% CI –1.37– –0.05; 2nd β= –0.88, 95% CI –1.30– –0.17; 3rd β= –0.59, 95% CI –1.15– –0.04) (Baiz et al., 2011). Another study of 1,397 births in the Czech Republic also showed changes in lymphocyte subpopulations with PM exposure in early and late pregnancy. First-trimester $PM_{2.5}$ exposure was associated with increases in CD3+ and CD4+ fractions and decreases in CD19+ fraction and NK cells; whereas, third-trimester exposure was associated with decreased CD3+ and CD4+ fractions and increased CD19+ fraction and NK cells (Herr et al., 2010).

In the cord blood of 197 newborns from the Belgian ENVIRONAGE (Environmental influence ON early AGEing) study, Martens et al. (2017a) measured oxylipins as a marker of the oxidation of fatty lipids. The investigators found that oxylipins, representing the lipoxygenase metabolic pathway for inflammation, were significantly associated with $PM_{2.5}$ in the second trimesters for both the 5-LOX and the 12/15-LOX pathways, but only the 5-LOX pathway was significantly associated with $PM_{2.5}$ exposure throughout the pregnancy. Reductions in telomere length, a marker of oxidative stress and inflammation, were studied in 730 newborns from the same cohort study (Martens et al., 2017b). Each 5 μg/m^3 increase in $PM_{2.5}$ in the second trimester was significantly associated with shorter telomere length in cord-blood leukocytes (-9.4%, 95% CI –13.1– –5.6%) and placental tissue (-0.1%, 95% CI –11.6– –2.4%).

Fetal Growth and Preterm Birth There is an extensive literature surrounding birth outcomes (preterm birth, low birth weight, and fetal death) associated with PM, often with conflicting results. The committee's search identified 96 studies on preterm birth and birth weight (70 studies on birth weight, small for gestational age, and intrauterine growth retardation, and 44 studies on preterm birth) published since 2009. To best describe this volume of literature, the committee examined relevant systematic reviews and meta-analyses and selected publications that described special issues of interest such as confounders and preconception exposure. The systematic reviews and meta-analyses reviewed here are summarized in Table 6-1. Fetal death, including stillbirths and miscarriages, associated with PM exposure has been the subject of relatively few extensive reviews and meta-analyses, and those studies are reviewed individually.

Eight systematic reviews and meta-analyses have assessed the consistency of the literature on adverse birth outcomes associated with PM exposure. These assessments cover the literature on preterm birth and birth weight through 2015 and small for gestational age through 2014. All these reviews noted difficulties in assessing the evidence due to the various studies' heterogeneity in study design, exposure assessment methods, windows of exposure assessment (each trimester, only specific trimesters or time periods, or the entire duration of the pregnancy), the ability to adjust for confounders (e.g., SES, smoking, and maternal nutrition), and the level of increase reported in analyses (IQR=1, 10, 50 or 100 μg/m^3; low versus high exposure; distance from an air quality monitoring station, etc.). Furthermore, there are

TABLE 6-1 Meta-Analyses and Systematic Reviews of PM and Preterm Birth, Birth Weight/Low Birth Weight, and Small for Gestational Age

Study	Approach	Exposure/Pooled Result or Positive Studies/Total Studies			Comments
		PTB	Birth Weight	SGA	
Lai et al. (2013)	SR* of Chinese population-based studies, though 2012.	PM_{10}: 1/1			Data on birth outcomes are insufficient for meta-analyses.
Shah et al. (2011)	SR of women exposed to pollutants, through 2009.	$PM_{2.5}$: 1/1 PM_{10}: 1/2	$PM_{2.5}$: 2/4	$PM_{2.5}$: 3/4	Heterogeneity of associations across studies. $PM_{2.5}$ associated with LBW, PTB, and SGA.
Bosetti et al. (2010)	SR of maternal exposure to pollutants, through 2009.	$PM_{2.5}$: 3/4 PM_{10}: 3/9	$PM_{2.5}$: 2/3 PM_{10}: 4/12	$PM_{2.5}$: 3/3 PM_{10}: 1/3	No summary estimates provided due to heterogeneity. Does not provide convincing evidence of association with risk of PTB, LBW, or SGA.
Jacobs et al. (2017)	SR of Chinese studies, through 2015.	PM_{10}: 5/10	PM_{10}: 4/7		Associations between birth weight and PM_{10} are not as consistent as SO_2.
Sun et al. (2015)	MA of prenatal exposure to $PM_{2.5}$, through 2014.	13 studies OR=1.13 (95% CI 1.03–1.24)			Clear association between $PM_{2.5}$ and PTB but with significant heterogeneity. Estimates by trimester were not significant.
Sun et al. (2016)	MA of prenatal exposure to $PM_{2.5}$, through 2015.		32 studies birth weight β= −15.9 (95% CI −26.8– −5.0) LBW OR=1.09 (95% CI 1.03–1.15)		Significant heterogeneity. $PM_{2.5}$ significantly associated with decreased birth weight and risk of LBW with second and third trimesters both significant.

continued

TABLE 6-1 Continued

Study	Approach	Exposure/Pooled Result or Positive Studies/Total Studies			Comments
		PTB	Birth Weight	SGA	
Zhu et al. (2015a)	MA of birth outcomes and $PM_{2.5}$, through 2014.	8 studies OR=1.10 (95% CI 1.03–1.18)	12 studies birth weight β= –14.58 (95% CI –19.31– –9.86) LBW OR=1.05 (95% CI 1.02–1.07)	6 studies OR=1.15 (95% CI 1.10–1.20)	Significant heterogeneity. Effects by trimester not significant for PTB, second and third trimester exposure significant for birth weight, all trimesters significant for SGA.
Sapkota et al. (2012)	MA of birth outcomes and $PM_{2.5}$ or PM_{10}, through 2009.	6 studies on $PM_{2.5}$ and 8 studies on PM_{10}. $PM_{2.5}$: OR=1.15 (95% CI 1.14–1.16) PM_{10}: OR=1.02 (95% CI 0.99–1.04)	4 studies on $PM_{2.5}$ and 11 studies on PM_{10}. $PM_{2.5}$: OR=1.09 (95% CI 0.9–1.32) PM_{10}: OR=1.02 (95% CI 0.99–1.05)		Third trimester exposure significantly related to PTB and LBW. Significant heterogeneity for PM_{10} but not $PM_{2.5}$.
Lamichhane et al. (2015)	MA of birth outcomes and $PM_{2.5}$, or PM_{10}, through 2015.	7 studies on $PM_{2.5}$, 3 studies on PM_{10} $PM_{2.5}$: OR=1.14 (95% CI 1.06–1.22) PM_{10}: OR=1.23 (95% CI 1.04–1.41)	8 studies on $PM_{2.5}$, 16 studies on PM_{10} $PM_{2.5}$: β= –13.88 (95% CI –15.7– –12.06) PM_{10}: β= –6.50 (95% CI –10.94– –2.5)		Analyses stratified by adjustment for smoking. Pooled estimates of studies adjusted for smoking were much higher than those that did not. Pooled trimester estimates not reported.

NOTE: CI=confidence interval; LBW=low birth weight; MA=meta-analysis; OR=odds ratio; PM=particulate matter; PTB=preterm birth; SGA=small for gestational age; SO_2=sulfur dioxide.

* Systematic reviews (SRs) defined as those that reported databases searched, search terms, inclusion and exclusion criteria, and approach for assessing biases. Positive study=any statistically significant results ($p<0.05$) at any level of exposure at any time period during pregnancy (entire pregnancy, first, second or third trimesters).

inconsistencies among trimester-specific results. All the meta-analyses express pooled estimates as ORs per 10 μg/m^3 increases in PM. These inconsistencies make the interpretation of the results challenging and highlight the need for additional work in this area.

Preterm birth associated with $PM_{2.5}$ was the subject of two systematic reviews and four meta-analyses. The two reviews reported significantly elevated risks of preterm birth in association with prenatal $PM_{2.5}$ exposure (Bosetti et al., 2010; Shah et al., 2011). Of the four meta-analyses that reported pooled estimates of preterm birth associated with prenatal exposure to $PM_{2.5}$ throughout the gestational period, all reported slight but significantly elevated ORs (Lamichhane et al., 2015; Sapkota et al., 2012; Sun et al., 2015; Zhu et al., 2015a), which ranged from 1.10 (95% CI 1.03–1.18), based on eight studies (Zhu, et al., 2015a), to 1.15 (95% CI 1.14–1.16), based on six studies (Sapkota et al., 2012). First-, second-, and third-trimester-specific estimates were less consistent. Sapkota et al. (2012) found positive associations in all three trimesters (ORs=1.04, 95% CI 0.73–1.34; 1.07, 95% CI 1.00–1.15; and 1.15, 95% CI 1.15–1.16, respectively), but only the associations for the second and third trimesters were significant. By contrast, Zhu et al. (2015a) found that none of the trimester-specific estimates were elevated (ORs=0.96, 95% CI 0.77–1.21; 0.90, 95% CI 0.79–1.03; and 0.97, 95% CI 0.89–1.05, respectively), and Sun et al. (2015) reported elevated but not statistically significant estimates (ORs=1.08, 95% CI 0.92–1.26; 1.09, 95% CI 0.82–1.44; and 1.08, 95% CI 0.99–1.17, respectively). Lamichhane et al. (2015) did not report trimester-specific estimates for $PM_{2.5}$.

Fewer studies have examined the risk of preterm birth in association with prenatal exposure to PM_{10}. Four systematic reviews reported 1 of 1, 1 of 2, 3 of 9, and 5 of 10 studies that found statistically significant elevated risks (Bosetti et al., 2010; Jacobs et al., 2017; Lai et al., 2013; Shah et al., 2011). Such heterogeneity leaves unanswered questions related to the effects of PM on the risk of preterm birth. Two of the meta-analyses calculated pooled estimates for PM_{10} throughout the gestational period and preterm birth; the first found an OR=1.02 (95% CI 0.99–1.04) based on eight studies (Sapkota et al., 2012), while the second calculated an OR=1.23 (95% CI 1.04–1.41) based on three studies (Lamichhane et al., 2015). Regarding trimester-specific pooled estimates, Sapkota et al. (2012) found significantly increased ORs for the second and third trimesters (OR=1.02, 95% CI 0.97–1.06; OR=1.02 95% CI 1.01–1.03, respectively), whereas Lamichhane et al. (2015) found no significant increase with PM_{10} exposure in the first trimester (OR=0.98, 95% CI 0.94–1.03), a significant decrease in the second trimester (OR=0.97, 95% CI 0.95–0.99), and significant increase in the third trimester (OR=1.03, 95% CI 1.01–1.05).

Two systematic reviews and four meta-analyses assessed decreases in birth weight and low birth weight in association with prenatal exposure to $PM_{2.5}$. The systematic reviews identified two (out of four) and two (out of three) studies that reported effects on birth weight in association with $PM_{2.5}$ (Bosetti et al., 2010; Shah et al., 2011). Three of the meta-analyses calculated pooled estimates of decreases in birth weight associated with 10 μg/m^3 changes in $PM_{2.5}$ exposure throughout gestation with statistically significant results: $\beta = -15.9$ (95% CI –26.8– –5.0), based on 32 studies (Sun et al., 2016); $\beta = -14.58$ (95% CI –19.31– –9.86), based on 12 studies (Zhu et al., 2015a); and $\beta = -13.88$ (95% CI –15.7– –12.06), based on 8 studies (Lamichhane et al., 2015). Of those that reported trimester-specific pooled estimates, Sun et al. (2016) found significant decreases in birth weight for the second and third trimesters (βs= –12.6 and –10.0, respectively) as did Zhu et al. (βs= –8.0 and –14.91, respectively). Pooled estimates of the association between low birth weight and prenatal exposure to $PM_{2.5}$ throughout gestation showed significant increases: OR=1.09 (95% CI 1.03–1.15), based on 19 studies (Sun et al., 2016); OR=1.05 (95% CI 1.02–1.07), based on 6 studies (Zhu et al., 2015a); and OR=1.09 (95% CI 0.9–1.32), based on 4 studies (Sapkota et al., 2012). By trimesters, Sun et al. (2015) reported increased but not statistically significant risks of low birth weight for PM_{10} exposure in all three trimesters (ORs=1.026, 1.035, 1.233, respectively). The Volume 11 committee notes that these findings are mixed and indicate the need for additional work in this area.

Changes in birth weight and low birth weight associated with PM_{10} throughout gestation were examined in two systematic reviews that reported statistically significant effects in 4 out of 12 studies (Bosetti et al., 2010) and four out of seven studies (Jacobs et al., 2017) as well as in two meta-analyses (Lamichhane et al., 2015; Sapkota et al., 2012). Lamichhane et al. (2015) examined changes in birth weight in 16 studies and reported β= –6.50 (95% CI –10.94– –2.5). The authors examined trimester-specific risks stratified by whether the study adjusted for smoking in its analyses and found that among smoking-adjusted studies the risks were significantly elevated for the third trimester (trimester effect sizes –1.43, –6.50, and –5.11), while the opposite was true for smoking-unadjusted studies: the first and second trimesters had significantly elevated risks (trimester effect sizes –3.31, –1.24, 1.36). Residual confounding by smoking was about 6.73%. Sapkota et al. (2012) reported a pooled estimated OR for low birth weight of 1.02 (95% CI 0.99–1.05), based on 11 studies, with trimester-specific estimates close to 1 (ORs=1.0, 1.0, 1.02, respectively).

Small for gestational age was assessed in two systematic reviews, both of which had three studies (out of three and four studies, respectively) finding significant effects associated with $PM_{2.5}$ (Bosetti et al., 2010; Shah et al., 2011); Bosetti et al. (2010) found one (out of three studies) that reported significant effects associated with PM_{10}. The Zhu et al. (2015a) meta-analysis found an association between small for gestational age and $PM_{2.5}$ exposure throughout gestation, with an OR=1.15 (95% CI 1.10–1.20) based on six studies. Trimester-specific estimates were all slightly elevated and statistically significant (ORs 1.07, 1.06, 1.06, respectively). Collectively, the data suggest that PM may have a slight but significant effect on small-for-gestational-age pregnancy outcomes.

One recent publication that reported on 499 participants of the Belgian ENVIRONAGE study found that $PM_{2.5}$ was related to thyroid hormone levels in cord blood, which may mediate effects on birth weight. For an IQR increase in $PM_{2.5}$ (8.2 $\mu g/m^3$) in the third trimester, cord blood levels of thyroid-stimulating hormone (TSH) declined 11.6% (95% CI –21.8––0.1), and the free thyroxin/triiodothyronine ratio (FT_4/FT_3) decreased by 62.7% (95% CI –91.6– –33.8%). Only FT_4 was significantly associated with decreases in birth weight, and the analysis estimated that FT_4 levels explained 21% of the association (-19g, 95% CI –37– –1) between $PM_{2.5}$ and birth weight (Janssen et al., 2017).

Fetal Death, Stillbirth, and Miscarriage Fetal mortality was not adequately captured by the systematic reviews and meta-analyses. Several studies have examined the associations between spontaneous abortion/miscarriage and stillbirth and PM exposure using hospital discharge data or birth records and registries. A number of studies on the relationship between exposure to traffic-related air pollutants (which includes $PM_{2.5}$) and fetal death (spontaneous abortion and stillbirth) have reported significant associations (Arroyo et al., 2016; DeFranco et al., 2015; Enkhmaa et al., 2014; Faiz et al., 2012, 2013; Green et al., 2015; Hwang et al., 2011; Moridi et al., 2014).

Two studies examined the risk of miscarriage/spontaneous abortion with PM exposure. Candela et al. (2015) examined the risk of miscarriage (1,375 miscarriages among 11,875 pregnancies) in association with PM_{10} from local incinerators in Northern Italy. Although ORs reflected an increasing risk of spontaneous abortions with increasing quartiles of PM_{10} exposure (p-value for trend=0.042), none of the estimates were significantly elevated (highest quintile [PM_{10}>1.33 ng/m^3] versus no exposure OR=1.29, 95% CI 0.97–1.72). Although there was no significant interaction (p=0.19), risks of spontaneous abortion with high levels of PM_{10} exposure were observed among women with no history of previous spontaneous abortion (4th quintile OR=1.45, 95% CI 1.08–1.94; 5th quintile OR=1.44, 95% CI 1.06–1.96; p-value for trend=0.009). Enkhmaa et al. (2014) examined the correlations between monthly hospitalizations for spontaneous abortions in 1,219 women and monthly $PM_{2.5}$ and PM_{10} levels in Mongolia and found them to be significantly correlated (R=0.92 and 0.64, respectively, both $p<0.001$).

Stillbirth was reported by five independent studies. Faiz et al. (2013) examined 1,719 stillbirths in New Jersey in a cohort study (n=343,077) using a case-crossover design to investigate the effects of pollutants in the week before delivery; it found no significant associations with $PM_{2.5}$. Green et al. (2015) reported on 13,999 stillbirths in several areas of California (compared with more than 3 million live births) and found no significant association between $PM_{2.5}$ and stillbirths in any trimester. However, stratification by maternal demographic variables revealed significant effects of maternal age (25–34 years OR=1.07, 95% CI 1.0–1.16; ≥35 years OR=1.13, 95% CI 1.03–1.24) and maternal educational level (college or beyond OR=1.32, 95% CI 1.19–1.47). DeFranco et al. (2015) examined Ohio births (349,188 live births, 1,848 still births) within 10 km of an air monitoring station and found that high levels of exposure to $PM_{2.5}$ (≥mean $PM_{2.5}$ + IQR range) were associated with stillbirth in the third trimester (OR=1.42, 95% CI 1.06–1.91), with the association stronger for births within a 5-km radius (OR=1.54, 95% CI 1.08–2.20); however, no significant associations were found for the first or second trimesters or estimates when $PM_{2.5}$ was analyzed as a continuous variable. A case-control study (9,325 cases and 93,250 controls) in Taiwan found that the risk of stillbirth was only associated with first-trimester PM_{10} exposure among preterm births (OR=1.03, 95% CI 1.0–1.07) after controlling for other pollutants (Hwang et al., 2011). Black smoke (PM <4 $\mu g/m^3$) exposure during any trimester of pregnancy, which was studied by Pearce et al. (2010) among 812 stillbirths and 90,537 live births in the United Kingdom, was not associated with stillbirth. One study of cause-specific stillbirths (n=5,377) in California found no association between $PM_{2.5}$ total mass and congenital malformations, fetal disorders, or maternal complications; however, $PM_{2.5}$ was significantly associated with stillbirths caused by fetal growth (OR=1.23, 95% CI 1.06–1.44) and obstetric complications (OR=1.13, 95% CI 1.03–1.24), although not for those caused by maternal complications, congenital malformations, or fetal disorders (Ebisu et al., 2018).

In a study of 385 infant deaths before the age of 1 year among 465,682 births in Massachusetts, no association was found between $PM_{2.5}$ throughout gestation or in each trimester and respiratory death, sudden infant death syndrome, or all causes of death (Son et al., 2017).

Animal Studies

In EPA's review of PM (EPA, 2009), toxicological evidence supported an association between PM and adverse reproductive outcomes. However, there were few data on biological plausibility to explain the link between PM exposure and reproductive outcomes, although systemic inflammation and oxidative stress were implicated. The Volume 11 committee identified several animal studies that examined PM exposure and reproductive effects that have appeared since the 2009 EPA review. These studies provide some additional mechanistic information and are discussed below.

Cao et al. (2015) showed decreased fertility (reduced sperm count, increased rates of sperm abnormalities, and testicular damage by histomorphology) with evidence of oxidative stress mediated by the PI3K/Akt pathway in male rats exposed to $PM_{2.5}$. An additional study by Cao et al. (2017) indicated that $PM_{2.5}$ causes reproductive injury by compromising the blood–testes barrier integrity in such a way that affects mating success, sperm parameters, epididymal morphology, the expression of markers of spermatogenesis, superoxide dismutase levels in testes, and the expression of blood–testes barrier junction proteins. Similarly, Liu et al. (2017a) showed that $PM_{2.5}$, particularly in the winter time, adversely affects sperm motility, sperm malformations, testicular tissue injury, and testicular apoptosis—effects believed to be induced by endoplasmic reticulum stress.

Reduced gestational length and birth weight were reported by Blum et al. (2017) in mice exposed to ambient $PM_{2.5}$ throughout gestation (6h/day on gestational day [GD] 0.5–16.5). This period aligns with milestones in human development.

An in vitro study found that cytotoxicity and genotoxicity differed by the size of the PM (<0.49, 0.49–0.97, 0.97–3 and >3 μm), with the smallest particles having the greatest bioactivity (Velali et al., 2016). Another in vitro study found that the chemical constituents bound to ambient PM, particularly PAHs, affected the cytotoxicity of PM in JEG-3 human placental cells (van Drooge et al., 2017). The PAHs were associated with the burning of biomass in rural areas.

Developmental Effects

The Volume 11 committee considered a wide spectrum of developmental effects that are evident in infants at or after birth and in children as they continue to develop. This section includes any developmental outcomes in infants and children, including birth defects, childhood cancer, autism spectrum disorder (ASD), neurodevelopment and behavioral outcomes, and respiratory effects, in relation to parental preconception or prenatal exposures that were reported in the literature. No studies of outcomes in adult offspring were identified by the committee.

Birth Defects

A number of studies have investigated the associations between in utero exposure to PM and congenital anomalies, with heterogeneous findings (Chen et al., 2014; Vrijheid et al., 2011). Because of the wealth of data on PM exposures and birth defects, the text below summarizes the results of epidemiologic studies; the details about these studies (design, population, and exposures and outcomes) are summarized in Table 6-2.

Among studies that reported on congenital anomalies, two conducted systematic reviews and meta-analyses (Chen et al., 2014; Vrijheid et al., 2011). Vrijheid et al. (2011) conducted a systematic review and meta-analysis of 10 studies of congenital anomalies and air pollution published between 2002 and 2011. The authors reported an elevated summary estimate for atrial septal defects (OR=1.14, 95% CI 1.01–1.28) with continuous exposure to PM_{10}, but the association was not significant in a binary analysis comparing high- to low-exposure groups (OR=1.23, 95% CI 0.91–1.67). Other defects (ventricular septal defects, coarctation of the aorta, and tetralogy of Fallot) were not associated with PM_{10} exposure. A second systematic review and meta-analysis by Chen et al. (2014) of 17 studies published between 2011 and 2014 found no significant association between any congenital anomaly and PM_{10}.

The committee reviewed 25 publications from 22 individual studies that investigated associations between PM exposure and congenital anomalies, particularly congenital heart defects. Most studies examined exposure to PM_{10}, used registries of birth defects, and were large population-based, case-control studies from countries around the world—China (4), Spain, Australia, Israel (2), Italy, Taiwan, and England (4)—as well as from several states in the United States (California [4], Massachusetts, New Jersey, Texas, and North Carolina) and the National Birth Defects Prevention Study (NBDPS) (3). Exposures were modeled on the basis of residential distance to air monitors or roadways, or on land use. Many studies controlled for other risk factors such as SES, maternal smoking, and alcohol use; none of the studies assessed any paternal or occupational exposures. All the studies examined exposure in the first trimester, generally weeks 2 or 3 to week 8 of gestation. Two studies examined preconception exposures (Yao et al., 2016; Zhu et al., 2015b). The results of the studies are briefly summarized below, and the details of the location, study population and size, and other characteristics are presented in Table 6-2.

TABLE 6-2 Characteristics of Studies of Birth Defects

Study	Cohort/ Country	Year	Design	Size	Exposure	Window	Outcomes Examined
Agay-Shay et al. (2013)	Tel-Aviv, Israel	2000–2006	case-control	1,260 cases and 130,402 controls	$PM_{2.5}$ and PM_{10}	1st: weeks 3–8 of pregnancy	Congenital heart defects
Dadvand et al. (2011b)	Northern Congenital Abnormality Survey/England	1985–1996	case-control	2,713 cases and 9,975 controls	Black smoke	1st: weeks 3–8 of pregnancy	Congenital heart defects
Dadvand et al. (2011a)	Northern Congenital Abnormality Survey/England	1993–2003	case-control	2,140 case and 14,256 controls	PM_{10}	1st: weeks 3–8 of pregnancy	Congenital heart defects
Dolk et al. (2010)	Northern Congenital Abnormality Survey/England	1991–1999	ecologic	9,085 cases	PM_{10}—1996 annual mean at census ward level	Not specific	Congenital anomalies
Farhi et al. (2014)	Israel	1997–2004	cohort	216,730 infants	PM_{10}	1st, 2nd, and entire pregnancy	Congenital anomalies
Gianicolo et al. (2014)	Italy	2001–2010	case-control	189 cases and 756 controls	TSP	1st: weeks 3–8 of pregnancy	Congenital anomalies
Girguis et al. (2016)	Massachusetts	2001–2008	case-control	3,461 cases, 7,816 controls	$PM_{2.5}$	1st trimester	Cardiac, neural tube, and orofacial defects
Hansen et al. (2009)	Brisbane, Australia	1998–2004	case-control	150,308 births	PM_{10}	1st: weeks 3–8 of pregnancy	Congenital heart defects and orofacial clefts
Hwang et al. (2015)	Taiwan	2001–2007	case-control	1,087 cases and 10,870 controls	PM_{10}	Entire pregnancy	Cardiac defects
Liang et al. (2014)	Hainan province, China	2009–2011	case-control	509 cases and 63,391 controls	PM_{10}	1st, 2nd, 3rd, and entire pregnancy	Congenital anomalies
Liu et al. (2017b)	Fuzhou, China	2007–2013	case-control	662 cases and 3,972 controls	PM_{10}	1st: days 11–60	Congenital heart defects

continued

TABLE 6-2 Continued

Study	Cohort/ Country	Year	Design	Size	Exposure	Window	Outcomes Examined
Marshall et al. (2010)	New Jersey	1998–2003	case-control	717 cases and 12,925 controls	$PM_{2.5}$ and PM_{10}	1st: weeks 3–8 of pregnancy	Orofacial clefts
Padula et al. (2013a)	San Joaquin Valley, CA	1997–2006	case-control	806 cases and 849 controls	$PM_{2.5}$ and PM_{10}	1st	Neural tube defects, orofacial clefts, gastroschisis
Padula et al. (2013b)	San Joaquin Valley, CA	1997–2006	case-control	822 cases and 849 controls	$PM_{2.5}$ and PM_{10}	1st	Congenital heart defects
Padula et al. (2013c)	San Joaquin Valley, CA	1997–2006	case-control	874 cases and 849 controls	$PM_{2.5}$ and PM_{10}	1st	Congenital anomalies, except congenital heart defects, neural tube defects, orofacial clefts, and gastroschisis
Padula et al. (2015)	San Joaquin Valley, CA	1997–2006	case-control	215 cases and 849 controls	$PM_{2.5}$ and PM_{10}	1st	Neural tube defects
Rankin et al. (2009)	Northern Congenital Abnormality Survey/England	1985–1990	case-control	3,197 cases and 15,000 controls	Black smoke	1st	Congenital anomalies
Schembari et al. (2014)	Barcelona, Spain	1994–2006	case-control	2,247 cases and 2,991 controls	$PM_{2.5}$, PM_{10}, and PMcoarse (10–2.5 μm)	1st: weeks 3–8 of pregnancy	Congenital anomalies
Stingone et al. (2014)	NBDPS	1997–2006	case-control	Not provided	$PM_{2.5}$ and PM_{10}	1st: weeks 2–8 of pregnancy	Congenital heart defects
Vinikoor-Imler et al. (2013)	North Carolina	2003–2005	cohort	322,969 live births	$PM_{2.5}$	1st: weeks 3–8 of pregnancy	Congenital anomalies
Vinikoor-Imler et al. (2015)	Texas	2002–2006	case-control	21,060 cases and 1,401,611 controls	$PM_{2.5}$	1st	Congenital anomalies
Warren et al. (2016)	NBDPS	2001–2006	case-control	1,986 cases and 2,741 controls	$PM_{2.5}$	1st: weeks 2–8 of pregnancy	Congenital heart defects

Study	Cohort/ Country	Year	Design	Size	Exposure	Window	Outcomes Examined
Yao et al. (2016)	Anqing City, China	2010–2012	cohort	16,332	PM_{10}	Preconception, 1st, 2nd, 3rd trimesters, and entire pregnancy	Congenital anomalies
Zhou et al. (2017)	NBDPS	2001–2007	case-control	7,035 cases and 4,697,523 births	$PM_{2.5}$	1st: weeks 5–10 of pregnancy	Orofacial clefts
Zhu et al. (2015b)	Consortium on Safe Labor	2002–2008	retro-spective cohort	188,102 births and fetal deaths	$PM_{2.5}$ and PM_{10}	Preconception and 1st: weeks 3–8 of pregnancy	Orofacial clefts

NOTE: NBDPS=National Birth Defects Prevention Network (Arizona, Florida, New York [excluding New York City], and Texas); PM=particulate matter; TSP=total suspended particulate.

Among studies that examined PM in association with any birth defect, no increase was reported with $PM_{2.5}$, PM_{10}, or black smoke in the first trimester (Liang et al., 2014; Rankin et al., 2009; Schembari et al., 2014). Yao et al. (2016) examined the relationship between 398 children with birth defects among 16,332 births in Anqing City, China, and PM_{10} exposure during preconception and in the first, second, and third trimesters and found no associations. However, Liang et al. (2014) reported that birth defects in Hainan province, China (509 birth defects and 63,391 controls), were associated with PM_{10} exposure in the second and third trimesters (second-trimester OR=1.039, 95% CI 1.016–1.063; third-trimester OR=1.066, 95% CI 1.043–1.090).

Congenital heart defects were the most widely studied group of congenital anomalies, but the results were not consistent across studies. PM_{10} exposure throughout pregnancy was associated with significantly increased risks of all congenital heart defects (OR=1.07, 95% CI 1.0–1.14) (Farhi et al., 2014), ventricular septal defects (OR=1.18, 95% CI 1.01–1.39) (Farhi et al., 2014), and atrial septal defects (OR=2.52, 95% CI 1.44–4.42) (Hwang et al., 2015). Exposure to PM_{10} in the first 3 to 8 weeks of pregnancy was associated with multiple congenital heart defects (OR=1.05, 95% CI 1.01–1.10) (Agay-Shay et al., 2013). Another study that examined 10-day intervals in early pregnancy found significant increased risks of ventricular septal defects, atrial septal defects, and patent ductus arteriosus with the second quartile of PM_{10} exposure, but not the third or fourth quartiles, for days 31–40 and 41–50 (ORs ranging from 1.19 to 2.17) (Liu et al., 2017b), indicating that the response was not monotonic. Other studies reported no significantly increased risk of these outcomes in association with PM_{10} (Agay-Shay et al., 2013; Dadvand et al., 2011a; Gianicolo et al., 2014; Hansen et al., 2009; Hwang et al., 2015; Padula et al., 2013b; Schembari et al., 2014; Stingone et al., 2014; Yao et al., 2016) or a significantly reduced risk of ventricular septal defects with exposure in the first 3 to 8 weeks of pregnancy (OR=0.88, 95% CI 0.81–0.97; Schembari et al., 2014). Thus, the Volume 11 committee found the results to be mixed, and no clear explanation for these increases could be derived from the reports.

For $PM_{2.5}$, seven studies reported no increased risk for any congenital heart defect or for most of the specific heart defects examined (Agay-Shay et al., 2013; Girguis et al., 2016; Padula et al., 2013b; Schembari et al., 2014; Stingone et al., 2014; Vinikoor-Imler et al., 2013, 2015; Warren et al., 2016). However, $PM_{2.5}$ exposure was associated with increased risks of certain specific defects: namely, dextro-transposition of the great arteries with first-trimester exposure (3rd quartile of exposure OR=2.6, 95% CI 1.1–6.5) (Padula et al., 2013b), pulmonary valve stenosis with exposure on day 53 of gestation, and tetralogy of Fallot on days 50–51 of gestation (estimates not reported) (Warren, et al., 2016). $PM_{2.5}$ exposure in the first 3 to 8 weeks of gestation was associated with reduced risks for ventricular septal defects (OR=0.83, 95% CI 0.72–0.97) (Schembari et al., 2014), septal heart defects (OR=0.79, 95% CI 0.76–0.83) (Vinikoor-Imler et al., 2015), obstructive heart defects (OR=0.88, 95% CI 0.79–0.98) (Vinikoor-Imler et al., 2015), and patent ductus arteriosus (OR=0.78, 95% CI 0.68–0.91) (Agay-Shay et al., 2013). Two studies found that exposure to black smoke was not associated with significant risk of congenial heart defects (Dadvand et al., 2011b; Rankin et al., 2009). Together this mixed evidence suggests that additional work on the risk of prenatal exposure PM for heart defects is needed.

Many studies investigated the associations between orofacial clefts and $PM_{2.5}$ or PM_{10}, and most found no significantly elevated risks (Farhi et al., 2014; Girguis et al., 2016; Hansen et al., 2009; Marshall et al., 2010; Padula et al., 2013a; Rankin et al., 2009; Schembari et al., 2014; Vinikoor-Imler et al., 2013, 2015). Two studies noted an association between PM and cleft palate but not cleft lip with or without cleft palate during certain windows of development. Zhou et al. (2017) reported an OR=1.43 (95% CI 1.11–1.86) per 10 $\mu g/m^3$ increase in $PM_{2.5}$ between 5 and 10 weeks of gestation among 2,609 cases and more than 4 million control births in the NBDPS. In a study of 159 cases and 188,102 live birth controls in the Consortium on Safe Labor cohort in the United States, Zhu et al. (2015b) observed an association between cleft palate only and $PM_{2.5}$ exposure in the first 3 to 8 weeks of gestation (OR=1.74, 95% CI 1.15–2.64), but the association did not extend to exposure to $PM_{2.5}$ in the 3 months before conception. Conversely, Hansen et al. (2009) reported a reduced risk of cleft palate with PM_{10} exposure in the first 3 to 8 weeks of gestation (OR=0.69, 95% CI 0.50–0.93) among 145 cases and 150,308 controls in Brisbane, Australia. Yao et al. (2016) found no elevated risk of cleft palate or cleft lip with PM_{10} exposure in the 3 months before pregnancy among 16,332 births in Anqing City, China.

No increased risk of neural tube defects in association with PM has been reported for the U.S. general population. One study in California reported an interaction between PM_{10} and socioeconomic factors for the risk of spina bifida, with the risk elevated among people with low income and low education (Padula et al., 2015). Other studies have reported null findings for PM exposure and neural tube defects (Dolk et al., 2010; Girguis et al., 2016; Padula et al., 2013a; Schembari et al., 2014; Vinikoor-Imler et al., 2013, 2015).

Two studies examined chromosomal defects (specifically, trisomy 21, the cause of Down syndrome) in association with PM_{10}. Farhi et al. (2014) found an increased risk in the first trimester (OR=1.14, 95% CI 1.01–1.28), whereas Dolk et al. (2010) did not. No obvious difference between the two studies has been identified.

Long lists of other congenital anomalies have been studied, with no significant effects reported in more than one study. Increased risks have been reported for abdominal wall defects with both PM_{10} and $PM_{2.5}$ in the first 3 to 8 weeks of gestation ($PM_{2.5}$ OR=1.33, 95% CI 1.0–1.76 and PM_{10} OR=1.36, 95% CI 1.14–1.62) (Schembari et al., 2014); esophageal atresia with quartiles of ambient PM_{10} concentration in the first trimester (2nd quartile OR=4.1, 95% CI 1.2–14.8; 3rd quartile OR=3.9, 95% CI 1.1–14.0; 4th quartile OR=4.9, 95% CI 1.4–17.2) (Padula et al., 2013c); nervous system anomalies with black smoke in the first trimester (OR=1.10, 95% CI 1.03–1.18) (Rankin et al., 2009); and omphalocele (a gastrointestinal defect) with PM_{10} exposure (RR=2.17, 95% CI 1.0–4.71) (Dolk et al., 2010). Padula et al. (2013c) reported decreased risks of hydrocephaly for specific quartiles of both $PM_{2.5}$ and PM_{10} exposure in the first trimester: $PM_{2.5}$ 2nd quartile OR=0.2 (95% CI 0.1–0.7) and PM_{10} 4th quartile OR=0.3 (95% CI 0.1–0.9). Also, a negative association (OR=0.78, 95% CI 0.64–0.96) between craniosynostosis and $PM_{2.5}$ exposure in the first 3 to 8 weeks of gestation was reported by Vinikoor-Imler et al. (2015). Other studies reported no significant associations for these outcomes and others with exposure to PM_{10} (Dolk et al., 2010; Farhi et al., 2014; Padula et al., 2013a,c; Schembari et al., 2014; Yao et al., 2016) and $PM_{2.5}$ (Padula et al., 2013a; Schembari et al., 2014; Vinikoor-Imler et al., 2013, 2015). Yao et al. (2016) investigated a range of birth defects with exposure to PM_{10} in the 3 months before conception and found no significant effects.

Childhood Cancer

Three studies assessed the associations between childhood cancer and prenatal exposures to PM (Badaloni et al., 2013; Heck et al., 2013b; Lavigne et al., 2017). Badaloni et al. (2013) found no association between childhood leukemia and exposure to $PM_{2.5}$ or PM_{10} in an Italian case-control study of 620 cases and 957 controls. Heck et al. (2013b) examined 3,590 cases of childhood cancer from the California Cancer Registry and compared them with 80,224 health children born in California and found no relationship between IQR increases in $PM_{2.5}$ exposure during pregnancy and acute lymphoblastic leukemia (ALL), acute myeloid leukemia (AML), non-Hodgkin lymphoma (NHL), ependymoma, astrocytoma, intracranial and intraspinal embryonal tumors, medulloblastoma, primitive neuroectodermal tumors (PNETs), neuroblastoma, retinoblastoma, Wilms' tumor, or hepatoblastoma in children under 6 years of age.

Another large registry-based study in a population of 2,350,898 children born in Ontario, Canada, also found no significant association between IQR increases in $PM_{2.5}$ during pregnancy and ALL, AML, NHL, ependymoma, astrocytoma, medulloblastoma, PNET, neuroblastoma, retinoblastoma, Wilms' tumor, hepatoblastoma, rhabdomyosarcoma, or germ cell tumor. However, a significant association with astrocytoma was reported for exposure in the first trimester and throughout the entire pregnancy (first-trimester hazard ratio [HR]=1.40, 95% CI 1.0– –1.86; second-trimester HR=1.26, 95% CI 0.95–1.67; third-trimester HR=0.96, 95% CI 0.71–1.28; entire pregnancy HR=1.35, 95% CI 1.0–1.85; first-year HR=1.07, 95% CI 0.79–1.28) (Lavigne et al., 2017).

Neurodevelopmental Outcomes

In recent years, many publications have described studies of neurodevelopmental and behavioral outcomes in children exposed to various air pollutants, many of which have focused on ASDs. Therefore, the committee discussed the literature on ASD together, followed by studies that examined other neurodevelopmental outcomes, such as measures or scores to quantify the effects on intelligence quotient (IQ), cognition, motor skills, attention, memory, and behavior.

Autism Spectrum Disorders Nine studies examined ASDs in association with prenatal PM exposure (Becerra et al., 2013; Gong et al., 2014, 2017; Guxens et al., 2016; Kalkbrenner et al., 2015; Kerin et al., 2018; Raz et al., 2015; Talbott et al., 2015; Volk et al., 2013). Three of these studies considered preconception exposure (Kalkbrenner et al., 2015; Raz et al., 2015; Talbott et al., 2015).

Becerra et al. (2013) conducted a large population-based case-control study in Los Angeles County with 7,603 cases of children with a primary diagnosis of autistic disorder and 76,030 controls. No significant effects were reported in single-pollutant models, but increased risks were found for PM after controlling for NO_2 exposure throughout the entire pregnancy per IQR increases ($PM_{2.5}$ OR=1.07, 95% CI 1.01–1.12; PM_{10} OR=1.08, 95% CI 1.03–1.13). Trimester-specific estimates were inconsistent. Kerin et al. (2018) studied the severity and functioning of 327 children with ASD in California and found that PM_{10} and $PM_{2.5}$ exposure during pregnancy was not associated with greater severity or decreased functioning.

Gong et al. (2017) conducted a large population-based case-control study (5,136 cases and 18,237 controls) in Sweden and found no association between PM_{10} exposure during pregnancy and ASD, either with or without intellectual disabilities. Another study by the same investigators examined ASD and attention deficit–hyperactivity disorder (ADHD) at 9 to 12 years of age among 3,426 Swedish twins and found no associations with PM_{10} exposure during pregnancy, the first year, or the ninth years of life (Gong et al., 2014). Guxens et al. (2016) analyzed four European cohorts totaling 8,079 children and found no association between borderline or clinical ASD and prenatal exposure to $PM_{2.5}$ or PM_{10}.

Kalkbrenner et al. (2015) examined the risk of ASD in 979 cases and 14,666 controls from North Carolina and San Francisco versus PM_{10} exposure starting 80 days before conception through the child's first birthday. The only significantly elevated window of exposure was the third trimester (OR=1.36, 95% CI 1.13–1.63), and this association remained significant after further adjustment for covariates, but only among cases and controls in North Carolina, not San Francisco. No explanation for the site differences was presented. Preconception exposure was not associated with ASD (OR=0.94, 95% CI 0.82–1.08). Raz et al. (2015) conducted a nested case-control study of 245 cases and 1,522 controls using the Nurses' Health Study II cohort to look for associations between ASD and exposures to $PM_{2.5}$ and $PM_{10–2.5}$. No significant association with $PM_{10–2.5}$ exposure was found, but ASD was found to be related to IQR changes in $PM_{2.5}$ exposure in all three trimesters (first-trimester OR=1.23, 95% CI 1.01–1.49; second-trimester OR=1.27, 95% CI 1.05–1.54; third-trimester OR=1.49, 95% CI 1.20–1.85). When comparing exposures during the 9 months before pregnancy, during pregnancy, and after pregnancy, the authors found that exposures to $PM_{2.5}$ during the preconception period or during the postnatal period were not related to ASD.

Talbott et al. (2015) reported a case-control study of 217 cases and 226 controls in Pennsylvania that assessed $PM_{2.5}$ exposure from preconception through the second year of life. They found elevated, but not significant, risks for ASD per IQR changes for windows of exposure that reflected preconception through the first year of life (ORs ranged from 1.07 to 1.37), but only exposures in the second year of life were significantly associated with ASD (OR=1.45, 95% CI 1.01–2.08).

All of the studies described above measured exposure based on maternal residence at birth, except Volk et al. (2013), who collected data on the place of residence beginning 3 months before pregnancy until the time of assessment in order to account for residential mobility and better examine risk by trimester. In the study of 279 cases with full syndrome autism in California compared to 245 children with typical development, increased risks of autism were associated with elevated PM throughout pregnancy and the first year of life ($PM_{2.5}$ per 8.7 μg/m^3 increase: first-trimester OR=1.22. 95% CI 0.96–1.53; second-trimester OR=1.48, 95% CI 1.40–1.57; third-trimester OR=1.40, 95% CI 1.11–1.77; first-year OR=2.12, 95% CI 1.45–3.10; and PM_{10} per 14.6 μg/m^3 increase: first-trimester OR=1.44, 95% CI 1.07–1.96; second-trimester OR=1.83, 95% CI 1.35–2.47; third-trimester OR=1.61, 95% CI 1.20–2.14; first-year OR=2.14, 95% CI 1.46–3.12). Volk et al. (2013) used two approaches to assigning exposure—regional air quality monitoring data and dispersion modeling—and found elevated risks with both approaches.

Of the three studies that considered preconception exposure, none reported an increased risk of ASD in association with $PM_{2.5}$ or PM_{10} (Kalkbrenner et al., 2015; Raz et al., 2015; Talbott et al., 2015).

A meta-analysis of the studies summarized above reported a high degree of heterogeneity among the studies (Flores-Pajot et al., 2016). Still, the authors concluded that $PM_{2.5}$ in the first trimester and in the postnatal period was significantly associated with ASD, although prenatal PM_{10} exposure was not. Pooled estimates for $PM_{2.5}$ and PM_{10} for each window of exposure are reported in Table 6-3, derived from Flores-Pajot et al. (2016). A systematic review by Suades-Gonzalez et al. (2015) found an association between prenatal and postnatal $PM_{2.5}$ exposure and ASD based on several high-quality studies. The significant impact of postnatal exposure on later ASD development is an important consideration when weighing the evidence on prenatal exposures.

TABLE 6-3 Pooled Estimates (95% CI) for Risk of Autism per 10 μg/m^3 Increases in $PM_{2.5}$ or PM_{10} Exposure

Window of Exposure	OR $PM_{2.5}$ (95% CI)	P-Value for Heterogeneity	OR PM_{10} (95% CI)	P-Value for Heterogeneity
Entire pregnancy	1.34 (0.83–2.17)*	0.000	1.03 (0.77–1.37)*	0.003
1st trimester	1.10 (1.02–1.19)	0.717	1.01 (0.86–1.20)*	0.008
2nd trimester	1.21 (0.88–1.66)*	0.000	1.12 (0.90–1.40)*	0.001
3rd trimester	1.33 (0.99–1.77)*	0.022	1.23 (0.97–1.55)*	0.000
Postnatal (1–4 yrs)	2.43 (1.61–3.68)	0.723	1.33 (0.86–2.05)*	0.002

NOTE: A significant p value for heterogeneity (*$p<0.05$) indicates the presence of heterogeneity among the studies in the meta-analysis.
SOURCE: Flores-Pajot et al., 2016.

Other Neurodevelopmental Outcomes The committee identified nine studies that reported on associations between exposure to PM and a variety of neurodevelopmental and behavioral outcomes (Chiu et al., 2016; Eenhuizen et al., 2013; Guxens et al., 2014; Harris et al., 2016; Kim et al., 2014; Lertxundi et al., 2015; Lin et al., 2014; Stingone et al., 2016; Yorifuji et al., 2016). This section focuses on all neurodevelopmental and behavioral outcomes other than ASD. A systematic review by Suades-Gonzalez et al. (2015) evaluated 16 studies on PM and neuropsychological development and concluded that there was insufficient evidence of associations with cognitive and psychomotor development.

Lertxundi et al. (2015) studied cognitive and psychomotor development in 438 15-month-old Spanish children and found that reductions in motor scale scores were significantly associated with 1 $\mu g/m^3$ increases in $PM_{2.5}$ throughout pregnancy (β= –1.15, 95% CI –1.76– –0.54), but there was no association with mental-scale scores after adjustment for confounders and NO_2 exposure. No adjustments were made for postnatal exposures, but results stratified by residential distance to metal processing plants showed significant relationships. Guxens et al. (2014) examined cognitive and psychomotor development among 1- to 6-year-olds in six European birth cohorts (n=9,482) and found no relationship between prenatal $PM_{2.5}$, PM_{10}, or $PM_{10-2.5}$ exposure and either cognitive or psychomotor development.

Kim et al. (2014) conducted a cohort study (n=520) of cognitive and psychomotor development in South Korea. Using a general linear model, they found that a 10 $\mu g/m^3$ increase in PM_{10} was significantly associated with decreased cognitive scores (β= –4.60, 95% CI –6.71– –2.49) and psychomotor scores (β= –7.24, 95% CI –9.79– –4.69) at 6 months, but not at 12 or 24 months. General estimating equations showed significant associations for both measures across 6 to 24 months of age (cognitive β= –2.83, 95% CI –4.71– –0.94; psychomotor β= –3.00, 95% CI –4.86– –1.14). Lin et al. (2014) conducted a cohort study of 533 Taiwanese children exposed to PM_{10} throughout pregnancy and up to 18 months of age and found that prenatal PM_{10} exposure was not associated with gross motor, fine motor, language, or social-personal scores at 6 and 18 months of age.

Yorifuji et al. (2016) examined motor and verbal developmental milestones in 2.5-year-olds and behavioral milestones in 5.5-year-olds in Japan in association with PM (<7 μm) exposure estimated for the entire pregnancy (n=46,039). Parents responded to questions about their children's attention, self-regulation, and socially appropriate behavior as part of the national Longitudinal Survey of Babies in the 21st Century. Exposure in the 9 months before conception was adjusted for using regression models, but no adjustments were made for any exposures after birth. While no significant associations were found for milestones at age 2.5, there were several significant associations with 5.5-year milestones per IQR increases in prenatal PM (inability to listen without fidgeting OR=1.10, 95% CI 1.04–1.17; inability to focus on one task OR=1.06, 95% CI 1.00–1.13; inability to express emotions OR=1.10, 95% CI 1.05–1.16; and inability to keep promises OR=1.08, 95% CI 1.02–1.14).

Chiu et al. (2016) reported on IQ, attention, and memory in a cohort of 267 children (average age 6.5 yrs) in Boston and found differences between specific prenatal windows of exposure by sex. Children were administered the Wechsler Intelligence Scale for Children (WISC)-IV, the Conners' Continuous Performance Test-II, and the Wide Range Assessment of Memory and Learning, 2nd Edition. While $PM_{2.5}$ was not associated with these outcomes overall, among the boys significant associations were found between $PM_{2.5}$ and lower IQ scores at 31–38 weeks of age, errors of omission at 20–26 weeks, slower reaction time at 32–36 weeks, and variability in response time at 22–40 weeks. Significant associations with $PM_{2.5}$ among girls included decreased visual memory index at 18–26 weeks, decreased attention/concentration index at 8–18 weeks, and decreased general memory index scores at 12–20 weeks.

Harris et al. (2016) conducted a cohort study (Project Viva in Massachusetts) and reported on executive functioning and behavioral problems in 1,212 children around 8 years old in relation to $PM_{2.5}$ and black carbon exposures estimated for the third trimester, first 3 years, and first 6 years of life. Although some problems were associated with mid-childhood exposure, no executive functioning or behavioral problems were associated with prenatal exposure.

Immune Outcomes

The association between exposure to PM and eczema in children was studied by Jedrychowski et al. (2011a,b) and Lu et al. (2017), while Orione et al. (2014) examined juvenile dermatomyositis, an autoimmune disease.

Jedrychowski et al. (2011a,b) used personal monitors to measure $PM_{2.5}$ for 2 days in the second trimester of pregnancy. The risk of infantile eczema in a cohort of 469 Polish children was associated with a variety of risk factors (Jedrychowski et al., 2011a). While prenatal $PM_{2.5}$ exposure alone was not significantly associated with eczema, elevated risks were reported among children exposed to high levels of $PM_{2.5}$ and environmental tobacco smoke. In a follow-up study of 322 children through age 5, prenatal $PM_{2.5}$ exposure alone was not associated with eczema, but when combined with maternal acetaminophen use during pregnancy, the risk of eczema symptoms doubled (HR=2.7, 95% CI 1.01–4.34) (Jedrychowski et al., 2011b).

Lu et al. (2017) reported on eczema in a cohort of 2,598 Chinese children ages 3 to 6 years and found no association with PM_{10} exposure in the 6 months before pregnancy or at any time in the prenatal period. Exposure measures for both mother and father in the 6 months before pregnancy were calculated based on air pollution monitoring results for the time period of interest, but they were not related to parental reports of eczema on their children.

Orione et al. (2014) conducted a small case-control study of 20 cases of juvenile dermatomyositis and 56 controls in Brazil to identify environmental risk factors, including those experienced during the prenatal period. There was no association between prenatal PM_{10} exposure and a diagnosis of juvenile dermatomyositis.

Asthma and Other Respiratory Outcomes

The Volume 11 committee considered 16 studies of PM and respiratory outcomes in children, most of which predominantly focused on asthma, but there were also explorations of wheeze, allergy, and lung function. Asthma was assessed in five cohort studies (Clark et al., 2010; Deng et al., 2015, 2016; Hsu et al., 2015; Tetreault et al., 2016; Yang et al., 2016) and one cross-sectional study (Liu et al., 2016b). Positive associations between prenatal exposure to $PM_{2.5}$ and asthma were reported in three of the cohort studies (Clark et al., 2010; Hsu et al., 2015; Tetreault et al., 2016), and one of those reported an association with PM_{10} (Clark et al., 2010), although two did not observe an association between PM_{10} and asthma (Deng et al., 2015, 2016; Liu et al., 2016b). One meta-analysis examined prenatal exposure to pollutants and asthma or wheezing in children up to 14 years old and found no association between prenatal $PM_{2.5}$ exposures and either outcome. However, the pooled estimate for PM_{10} was significant for childhood asthma (OR=1.08, 95% CI 1.05–1.12) (Hehua et al., 2017).

Hsu et al. (2015) studied a cohort of 736 children in Boston and found that prenatal $PM_{2.5}$ exposure between 16 and 25 weeks of gestation was associated with a diagnosis of asthma in boys up to age 6, but not in girls. There was a significant difference between the sexes and a significant interaction between prenatal $PM_{2.5}$ exposure and sex (p=0.01; ORs not reported). The sex differences were not explained.

Tetreault et al. (2016) reported a significant association between time-varying prenatal $PM_{2.5}$ exposure and diagnosed asthma in children up to 12 years of age (per IQR increase HR=1.33, 95% CI

1.31–1.34). This large cohort of more than 1 million children in Quebec included 162,752 cases of diagnosed asthma. A subgroup analysis indirectly adjusted for secondhand smoke and found a much smaller effect of $PM_{2.5}$ (per IQR, HR=1.04, 95% CI 1.02–1.06).

Clark et al. (2010) examined the incidence of asthma in 37,401 children ages 3–4 years in British Columbia in association with $PM_{2.5}$, PM_{10}, and black carbon. Two methods were used to estimate prenatal exposures. Regulatory air monitoring data and land use regression models for temporal variability were used to estimate individual exposures. $PM_{2.5}$ was significantly associated with asthma incidence (per 1 $\mu g/m^3$ increase, OR=1.02, 95% CI 1.0–1.03), as was black carbon (per 10^{-5}/m increase in filter absorbance, OR=1.08, 95% CI 1.02–1.15); PM_{10} was not analyzed. Exposure, as determined by the inverse distance-weight summation of emissions from point sources, showed no association between $PM_{2.5}$ and asthma incidence (per 1 $\mu g/m^3$ increase, OR=0.95, 95% CI 0.91–1.0), but there was a significant association with PM_{10} (per 1 $\mu g/m^3$ increase, OR=1.09, 95% CI 1.05–1.13); black smoke was not analyzed using this model.

Yang et al. (2016) studied 3,701 Dutch children through age 14. Those investigators found that exposure to $PM_{2.5}$ estimated at the time of birth using a land use regression model was not associated with asthma or asthma symptoms in childhood.

In China, Deng et al. (2015, 2016) reported no association between prenatal PM_{10} exposure and asthma among 2,490 children ages 3 to 6 years. A separate Chinese cross-sectional study by Liu et al. (2016b) also found no association between asthma in 4- to 8-year-old children and prenatal PM_{10} exposure (n=3,358).

Yang et al. (2016), Liu et al. (2016b), and Deng et al. (2015, 2016) also assessed respiratory allergy. Yang et al. did not find any relationship between $PM_{2.5}$ concentrations at a child's birth address and hay fever, rhinitis, or allergic sensitization in a cohort of Dutch children up to 14 years old. Liu et al. (2016b) found no association between allergic rhinitis and prenatal PM_{10} exposure in Chinese children who were around 5 years old. Deng et al. (2015) reported no association between prenatal PM_{10} and allergic rhinitis or eczema throughout pregnancy or in any specific trimester among Chinese children ages 3–6 years old (Deng et al., 2016).

Chiu et al. (2014) reported significant associations between repeated wheezing among 708 Boston children up to 2 years of age and high prenatal exposure to $PM_{2.5}$ and black carbon versus low exposure to these two pollutants ($PM_{2.5}$ OR=2.02, 95% CI 1.20–3.40; black carbon OR=1.84, 95% CI 1.08–3.12). These investigators also reported that psychosocial stressors such as community violence were important contributors to the occurrence of wheezing. Jedrychowski et al. (2010b) found a significant effect of prenatal $PM_{2.5}$ exposure on wheezing at 2 years of age (high versus low IRR=1.377, 95% CI 1.252–1.514) but not at 4 years of age (high versus low IRR=1.063, 95% CI 0.923–1.223) among a cohort of 339 Polish children. Exposures were determined by mothers using personal monitors for 2 days in the second trimester. Rosa et al. (2017a) studied wheezing in 552 children in Mexico City in association with prenatal $PM_{2.5}$ exposure and maternal stress and found a significant interaction. $PM_{2.5}$ exposure in the first trimester was associated with the risk of current wheezing in children in the presence of high maternal stress (per IQR increase RR=1.35, 95% CI 1.00–1.83), but not in the case of low maternal stress. No associations were noted for other trimesters.

Respiratory system infections were examined in four studies. Liu et al. (2016b) found no association between pneumonia in 4- to 8-year-old Chinese children and prenatal PM_{10} exposure. MacIntyre et al. (2014) conducted a meta-analysis of 16,059 children from 10 European cohorts (ESCAPE project) and found significant associations between pneumonia in the first 2 years of life and PM_{10} (per 10 $\mu g/m^3$ increases, OR=1.76, 95% CI 1.00–3.09) and $PM_{2.5-10}$ (OR=1.24, 95% CI 1.03–1.5), but not for $PM_{2.5}$. No associations between PM and croup or otitis media were found. In a study of 1,617 children ages 3–4 years in Changsha, China, prenatal PM_{10} exposure was found to have no association with otitis media (Deng et al., 2017). Recurrent broncho-pulmonary infections (≥5 episodes) in 214 children through age 7 were associated with prenatal $PM_{2.5}$ exposure (OR=2.08, 95% CI 1.08–4.06) (Jedrychowski et al., 2013). Exposures were determined by mothers using personal monitors for 2 days in the second trimester.

Lung function was reported on by six studies. Liu et al. (2016b) found no association between prenatal PM_{10} exposure and lung function in 4- to 8-year-old Chinese children (n=3,358). Gehring et al. (2013) analyzed the lung function of children age 6 or 8 years from five European cohorts and found no association with $PM_{2.5}$, PM_{10}, or $PM_{10-2.5}$ at the birth address (n=5,921).

Among healthy 5-week-old newborns in Switzerland (n=265), Latzin et al. (2009) found that maternal exposure to PM_{10} during pregnancy had affected tidal breathing (minute ventilation β=24.9, 95% CI 9.3–0.5), but not multiple breath washout or inflammatory markers; no effect was found for postnatal exposure. Jedyrchowski et al. (2010a) reported decrements in lung function in a cohort of 176 Polish children with maternal personal monitoring conducted in the second trimester. Lung function was significantly reduced at 5 years of age among children exposed prenatally to the highest quartile (>52.6 $\mu g/m^3$) compared to the lowest quartile of $PM_{2.5}$ (FVC β= –91.92, 95% CI –159.60– –24.24; and FEV_1 β= –87.71, 95% CI –151.85– –23.57). Although there was a step-wise trend across the quartiles, the lung function of children in the second- and third-exposure quartiles were not significantly lower than in the first quartile.

Prenatal exposure to PM_{10} reduced respiratory function in 232 children with asthma ages 6–11 years in the San Joaquin Valley. Notably, the subgroups most affected by prenatal exposure to pollutants were children who were African American, diagnosed before age 2, and exposed to maternal smoking during pregnancy (Mortimer et al., 2008).

Other Outcomes Studied in Children

Single studies have reported on vitamin D levels, metabolic function, body weight, and pubertal development in children with prenatal exposure to PM.

In a French birth cohort of 370 pregnant women (EDEN study), Baiz et al. (2012) found that decreased vitamin D levels in cord blood were associated with maternal exposure to PM_{10} in the first trimester (10 $\mu g/m^3$ PM_{10}; β= –0.35, 95% CI –0.78– –0.03) and in the third trimester (β= –0.43, 95% CI –0.72– –0.14). In a Canadian cohort (MIREC) study of 1,257 mother–child pairs, researchers examined the correlation of maternal $PM_{2.5}$ exposure with the levels of leptin and adiponectic—two measures of metabolic function—in cord blood (Lavigne et al., 2016). IQR increases of 3.2 $\mu g/m^3$ in $PM_{2.5}$ exposure throughout pregnancy were associated with increased adiponectin levels (β=11%, 95% CI 4–17%) and leptin levels (β=11%, 95% CI 1–21%); however, when birth weight was included in the adjustments, the increases in leptin levels ceased to be significant, although the increases in apiponectin levels retained significance.

Kim et al. (2016) studied changes in body weight measured from birth to age 5 in relation to prenatal PM_{10} exposure in 1,129 South Korean children. They did not find a relationship between prenatal PM_{10} exposure and changes in weight-for-age. However, a significant association was found in Bangladeshi children under 5 years old between the second, third, and fourth quartiles of mean $PM_{2.5}$ exposure throughout pregnancy and stunting, wasting, and underweight (RRs ranged from 1.109 to 1.272). Exposures after birth were not significantly related to the outcomes studied (Goyal and Canning, 2017).

A few studies have reported increases in markers of obesity with PM exposure. A study of 239 children about 4 years old in the Boston area reported increased anthropometric measures associated with prenatal $PM_{2.5}$ exposure estimated weekly. In boys, increased $PM_{2.5}$ during gestational weeks 8–17 was significantly associated with increased BMI z-scores, and $PM_{2.5}$ in weeks 15–22 was significantly associated with fat mass. In girls, increased waist-to-hip ratio was significantly associated with increased $PM_{2.5}$ in gestational weeks 10–29 (relative risks not reported) (Chiu et al., 2017). Mao et al. (2017) reported increased risks of childhood overweight or obesity among 1,446 children ages 2–9 years in the Boston area as a function of $PM_{2.5}$ in each trimester (per IQR increases RR=1.1, 95% CI 1.0–1.2 for each trimester). Significant associations were also reported for exposure in the prenatal period (per IQR increase RR=1.1, 95% CI 1.0–1.2) and the first 2 years of life (per IQR increase RR=1.1, 95% CI 1.0–1.2).

Thiering et al. (2013) examined the relationship between estimated PM_{10} and $PM_{2.5}$ concentrations at the mother's residential address and insulin resistance in children at age 10 in two German birth cohorts (n=397). A two-standard-deviation increase in PM_{10} was associated with a 17.5% increase in insulin resistance (95% CI 1.9–35.6).

In a study of 4,074 children about 11 years old in Hong Kong, China, prenatal PM_{10} exposure was significantly related to later pubertal development in girls (Tanner stage [a measure of puberty] mean difference= –0.05, 95% CI –0.08– –0.02), but no differences were noted in boys (Huang et al., 2017).

Animal Studies

In EPA's 2009 review of PM, toxicological evidence was found to support an association between PM and adverse developmental outcomes. However, there were few data on biological plausibility to explain the link between PM exposure and developmental outcomes, although developmental windows of susceptibility and systemic inflammation and oxidative stress were implicated. The Volume 11 committee identified a few animal studies published since that 2009 review that examined PM exposure and developmental or generational effects.

Tang et al. (2017) found decreased lung volume parameters, compliance, and airflow on expiration and also lung damage related to oxidative stress in rat pups on postnatal day 28 after in utero exposure to $PM_{2.5}$ (0.1, 0.5, 2.5, or 7.5 mg/kg once every 3 days from GD 0–18).

In rats exposed in utero to $PM_{2.5}$ (0.375, 1.5, or 6.0 mg/kg on GD 10, 12, 14, and 16) researchers found various signs of cardiotoxicity, including a disordered arrangement of myocardial fibers, irregular-shaped cardiomyocytes, increased apoptotic rates in myocardium, and altered expression of mitochondrial fusion/fissure genes (Wang et al., 2017b). The exposure of pregnant rats to $PM_{2.5}$ at levels corresponding to ambient levels in an urban Chinese environment for 24 hours per day throughout gestation and lactation resulted in changes related to cardiac development in the offspring. $PM_{2.5}$ was associated with reduced levels of messenger ribonucleic acid (mRNA) and the proteins associated with cardiac precursor cells and cardiac development (GATA4 and Nkx2-5) and increased levels of TNF-α and IL-1β (inflammatory cytokines) in plasma, and it exacerbated the negative effects of homocysteine on cardiac development (myocardial apoptosis and structural abnormalities) (Chen et al., 2017a). Cardiac dysfunction was observed in adult rats after in utero exposure to $PM_{2.5}$ (average 73.61 $\mu g/m^3$ for 6 h/day throughout pregnancy), including an acute inflammatory response, chronic matrix remodeling, and an altered expression of Ca^{2+} handling proteins (Tanwar et al., 2017a). In mice, exposure to $PM_{2.5}$ throughout gestation (average 91.78 $\mu g/m^3$ for 6h/day, 5 days/week) resulted in adverse functional cardiac changes in early adolescence, including fractional shortening, impaired cardiomyocyte functioning, and reduced calcium transport amplitude and fluorescence decay rate. The authors stated that gestational exposure to $PM_{2.5}$ alters calcium-handling proteins, which is responsible for the cardiac dysfunction observed in neonatal nice (Tanwar et al., 2017b).

An in vitro study found that cytotoxicity and genotoxicity differed by the size of PM (<0.49, 0.49–0.97, 0.97–3 and >3 μm), with the smallest particles having the greatest bioactivity (Velali et al.,

2016). Another in vitro study emphasized the important role of chemical constituents on the cytotoxicity of PM in placental cells (van Drooge et al., 2017).

Epigenetic and Other Effects on DNA

Studies that focused on the genetic and epigenetic effects of prenatal PM exposure are summarized in Table 6-4. The section below provides an overview of the studies, and Table 6-4 provides additional study details, such as the tissue and cell type examined.

The epigenetic literature on PM has relied on relatively large sets of samples and studies, including ENVIRONAGE (Grevendonk et al., 2016; Janssen et al., 2012, 2013, 2015; Saenen et al., 2015, 2017; Wincklemans et al., 2017), the Children's Health Study (Breton et al., 2016; Salam et al., 2012), PROGRESS (Programming Research in Obesity, Growth, Environment and Social Stressors) (Rosa et al., 2017b), and various consortiums and group studies (Pedersen et al., 2015; Silva da Silva et al., 2015). Three tissue types—cord blood, placenta, and peripheral blood lymphocytes—have generally been evaluated. These tissues represent a collection of different cell types, each with very different epigenomes, including different DNA methylation profiles. These studies of PM epigenetic effects have not accounted for the variability associated with heterogeneous cell types in samples. Differences in cell composition across different samples may result in what appear to be methylation differences but which actually are reflections of differences in cell purity or differences induced by immune responses (Houseman et al., 2012, 2015). Such complexities were interpreted by the Volume 11 committee to result in equivocal results.

Another challenge in interpreting results from these observational studies is that estimates of exposure are often confounded with other potential modifiers of the epigenome, as PM is frequently estimated longitudinally through source-distance models. Potential confounders, such as smoking or other environmental exposures that have been reported to be associated with altered DNA methylation (Jenkins et al., 2017; Knopik et al., 2012), are often not accounted for in these analyses, illustrating the complexity of the problem. Furthermore, the mutagenic activity of organic extracts from $PM_{2.5}$ has been associated with increases in genomic DNA fragmentation (Silva da Silva et al., 2015) and higher DNA adduct levels as $PM_{2.5}$ exposure increases (Pedersen et al., 2015).

Effects that change with the developmental timing of the exposure have also been reported, as different tissues are susceptible in different developmental periods. For example, during the last month of pregnancy a 16.1% decrease in the placental DNA content of cord blood (95% CI –25.2– –6.0%, p=0.003) has been reported, but no such decrease in the mitochondrial DNA content (Janssen et al., 2012). In that particular study, $PM_{2.5}$ exposure over the entire pregnancy was positively associated with mitochondrial DNA methylation (MT-RNR1: +0.91%, p=0.01 and D-loop: +0.21%, p=0.05), but the exposure was inversely associated with the mitochondrial DNA content (relative change of –15.60%, p=0.001) in placental tissue (Janssen et al., 2015). Others have measured levels of oxidative stress induced by PM_{10} and $PM_{2.5}$, as measured by 8-hydroxy2′-deoxyguanosine (8-OHdG) in mitochondria. Maternal PM_{10} and $PM_{2.5}$ exposures are both associated with increased 8-OHdG through the entire pregnancy (18.3%, 95% CI 5.6–33.4%, p=0.004; and 13.9%, 95% CI 0.4–29.4%, p=0.04, respectively), which is heightened in the third trimester (28.1%, 95% CI 8.6–51.2%, p=0.004; and 28.1%, 95% CI 3.6–58.4%, p=0.004, respectively) (Grevendonk et al., 2016). An association between 8-OHdG in cord blood and PM_{10} was observed only in the first and second trimesters (23.0%, 95% CI 5.9–42.8%, p=0.007; and 16.6%, 95% CI 1.8–33.5%, p=0.03, respectively). The Volume 11 committee notes that those statistically significant results do not account for the presence of multiple comparisons, nor were any sensitivity analyses performed.

TABLE 6-4 Summary of Genetic and Epigenetic Effects of Particulate Matter

Study	Design/Population	Exposure	Results
Janssen et al. (2012)	Cohort—ENVIRONAGE 178 newborns born at a Belgium hospital 2010–2011.	Modeled PM_{10} based on mother's residence.	mtDNA content in placenta and cord blood. No association between PM_{10} and mtDNA in cord blood. PM_{10} (10 μg/m³ increments) associated with decreased mtDNA in third trimester (–17.4%, 95% CI –31.8– –0.1%), last month of pregnancy (–16.1%, 95% CI –25.2– –6.0%), and last week of pregnancy (–10.1%, 95% CI –17.6– –1.9%).
Janssen et al. (2013)	Cohort—ENVIRONAGE 240 newborns born at a Belgium hospital.	Modeled $PM_{2.5}$ based on mother's residence. Exposure estimates accounted for mother's change of address during pregnancy.	Global DNA methylation in placenta. Reduced global methylation per 5 μg/m³ increase in $PM_{2.5}$ in first trimester (–2.13%, 95% CI –3.71– –0.54%) and through entire pregnancy (–2.19, 95% CI –3.65– –0.73%) associated with DNA global methylation. Indicates that fertilization through implantation is a susceptible window.
Janssen et al. (2015)	Cohort—ENVIRONAGE 381 newborns born at a Belgium hospital.	Modeled $PM_{2.5}$ based on mother's residence.	mtDNA methylation in placenta. IQR increases in $PM_{2.5}$ associated with increased methylation at MT-RNR1 (0.91%, p=0.01) and D-loop (0.21%, p=0.05), and decreased mtDNA content (–15.6%, p=0.001).
Winckelmans et al. (2017)	Cohort—ENVIRONAGE 142 newborns born at a Belgium hospital.	Modeled $PM_{2.5}$ based on mother's residence. Short-term exposure = exposure in the last month of pregnancy; long-term exposure = annual average before delivery.	Whole-genome gene expression (RNA) in cord blood. Differences in gene expression differed by duration of exposure (short- versus long-term) and infant sex.
Grevendonk et al. (2016)	Cohort—ENVIRONAGE 224 mothers and 293 newborns born at a Belgium hospital.	Modeled $PM_{2.5}$ and PM_{10} based on mother's residence.	Mitochondrial 8-OHdG and mtDNA content in maternal and cord blood. Maternal mitochondrial 8-OHdG associated with third trimester PM_{10} (28.1% change/IQR, 95% CI 8.6–51.2%) and $PM_{2.5}$ (28.1% change/IQR, 95% CI 3.6–58.4%); first and second trimesters not significant. Cord blood mitochondrial 8-OHdG associated with first and second trimester PM_{10} (23.0% change/IQR, 95% CI 5.9–42.8%; and 16.6% change/IQR, 95% CI 1.8–33.5, respectively); third trimester PM_{10} and $PM_{2.5}$ not significant. Levels of 8-OHdG positively correlated with mtDNA content in maternal blood (β=0.38, 95% CI 0.28–0.49) and cord blood (β=0.52, 95% CI 0.43–0.61).

Study	Design/Population	Exposure	Results
Saenen et al. (2015)	Cohort—ENVIRONAGE 90 mother–newborn pairs at a hospital in Belgium 2010–2012.	Modeled $PM_{2.5}$ based on mother's residence. Estimated exposure for pre-implantation period (5 days).	Fetal brain development measured by placental expression of *BDNF*, and associated pathways (% change per 5 µg/m^3 $PM_{2.5}$). In first trimester of pregnancy, –25.9% change *BNDF* (–28.7– –0.2%), specifically in the first month and around the time of implantation. Not significant for second and third trimesters. *SOS2* and *SYN1* also significant decreased expression in early pregnancy (data not reported). *SOS* and *PLCG* signaling cascades reduced in first month. *SOS* β= –0.1, 95% CI –0.2– –0.07; *PLCG* β= –0.08, 95% CI –0.1– –0.03.
Saenen et al. (2017)	Cohort—ENVIRONAGE 361 mother–newborn pairs at a hospital in Belgium 2010–2013.	Modeled $PM_{2.5}$ based on mother's residence, accounting for residential mobility during pregnancy.	*LEP* methylation status in the placenta was negatively associated with $PM_{2.5}$ exposure during the second trimester. An interquartile range increase (7.5 µg/m^3) in second-trimester $PM_{2.5}$ exposure was associated with 1.4% (95% CI –2.7– –0.19%) decrease in *LEP* methylation.
Breton et al. (2016)	Cohort—Children's Health Study 392 children ages 11–12 years with newborn blood spot tests.	Prenatal PM exposure estimated from community monitors based on address at birth.	Newborn *LINE1* and Alu methylation, and blood pressure and carotid intima-media thickness in childhood. $PM_{2.5}$ and PM_{10} had no association with blood pressure or intima-media thickness, *LINE1* Alu methylation. PM_{10} associated with *LINE1* methylation in first trimester only (β= –0.66, 95% CI –1.22– –0.09).
Rosa et al. (2017b)	Cross-sectional—PROGRESS 456 pregnant women in Mexico City 2007–2011.	$PM_{2.5}$ modeled based on maternal home address at birth.	mtDNA in cord blood leukocytes. Significant reduction in mtDNA content per 10 µg/m^3 increase in $PM_{2.5}$ in weeks 35–40 only. No data reported.
Cai et al. (2017)	Case-control 80 newborns with grown restriction and 101 healthy newborns in China 2011–2013.	PM_{10} averages based on nearby air monitoring station during pregnancy.	Placental DNA methylation of *LINE1*, *HSD11B2*, and *NR3C1* In cases, *LINE1* methylation decreased with first trimester PM_{10} (10 µg/m^3) (β= –1.78%, 95% CI –3.35– –0.22%); *HSD11B2* methylation increased with first and second trimester PM_{10} exposure (β=1.03%, 95% CI 0.07–1.98%; β=2.23%, 95% CI 0.69–3.76%); No associations in health controls and *NR3C1* methylation not associated with PM_{10} in cases or controls.

continued

TABLE 6-4 Continued

Study	Design/Population	Exposure	Results
Pedersen et al. (2015)	Cross-sectional—NewGeneris 511 pregnant women from 5 European countries 2006–2010.	Modeled $PM_{2.5}$ based on maternal home address.	Bulky DNA adducts in cord blood. Mean ratio of bulky DNA adduct levels per 5 μg/m^3 increment of $PM_{2.5}$=1.14 (95% CI 0.99–1.32; p=0.07).

NOTE: 8-OHdG=8-hydroxy-2′-deoxyguanosine; CI=confidence interval; DNA=deoxyribonucleic acid; ENVIRONAGE=Environmental Influence ON Early AGEing; HSD11B2=11β-hydroxysteroid dehydrogenase type 2; IQR=interquartile range; LEP=leptin; mtDNA=mitochondrial DNA; PM=particulate matter; PROGRESS=Programming Research in Obesity, Growth, Environment and Social Stressors; RNA=ribonucleic acid.

In principle, DNA methylation can also vary depending on temporal and spatial measurements. For example, global changes in genome methylation in placental tissue and $PM_{2.5}$ exposure during pregnancy are correlated, particularly with first-trimester exposure. A multi-lag model found significant associations between lower levels of global DNA methylation and $PM_{2.5}$ exposure in the first trimester (–2.13% per 5 μg/m^3 increase, 95% CI –3.71– –0.54%, p=0.009), and exposure during implantation (6–21d) showed an even stronger association (–1.08% per 5 μg/m^3 increase, 95% CI –1.80– –0.36%, p=0.004); both of them led to an increased hypomethylated state (Janssen et al., 2013). During the first trimester of pregnancy, each 5 μg/m^3 increase in $PM_{2.5}$ was associated with a 15.9% decrease (95% CI –28.7– –3.2%, p=0.015) in the expression of placental *brain-derived neurotrophic factor* (*BDNF*) at birth and a 24.3% decrease (95% CI –42.8 – –5.8%, p=0.011) in *synapsin-1* (Saenen et al., 2015), two genes involved in neurodevelopment. Using newborn blood spots, Breton et al. (2016) found that $PM_{2.5}$ exposure during the first trimester was associated with a reduction in repetitive element methylation (i.e., *LINE1*, *AluYb8*). The degree of methylation was found to be genotype-dependent when 11 SNPs for DNA methyltransferase 1(*DNMT1*), DNA methyltransferase 3 Beta (*DNMT3B*), Tet methylcytosine dioxygenase 2 (*TET2*), and thymine DNA glycosylase (*TDG*) genes were assayed (Breton et al., 2016). Furthermore, differences in response have been reported with differences in the duration of exposure and infant sex. Wincklemans et al. (2017) reported differential gene expression to be associated with $PM_{2.5}$ exposure—in particular, whether the exposure was short or long term (a month or a year before birth)—and also sex. For example, RNA expression reflecting DNA damage was altered in infants of both sexes with both short- and long-term exposure, whereas expression of RhoA pathways was affected in boys with short-term exposure, and defensin expression was altered in girls with long-term exposure.

The impacts of in utero PM exposure on gene expression in placenta have been studied in several populations (ENVIRONAGE, Rhode Island, and China) focusing on different genes. $PM_{2.5}$ has been reported to affect the expression of *LEP* (leptin, an energy-regulating hormone) (Saenen et al., 2017), insulin-like growth factor-2 *(IGF2)*, *MEG3*, *MEST*, and *PLAG1* (all associated with infant birth weight); PM_{10} decreased the placental methylation of *LINE1* (to represent global methylation) and increased the methylation of *HSD11B2* (which encodes for 11β-hydroxysteroid dehydrogenase type 2, involved in glucocorticoid metabolism) (Cai et al., 2017).

These reports of changes in the methylation status of both the nuclear and the mitochondrial genomes, globally as well as at specific sites, in response to PM stress during pregnancy are intriguing and provide possible basis for the impact of PM on early development (Soto-Martinez and Sly, 2010; Teng et al., 2016). However, this body of evidence has several limitations, including small sample sizes and the heterogeneity of cell types, which affect both the reliability and the interpretation of the data. Biochemical mechanisms for how these exposures result in methylation changes have not been fully described, nor have these findings been confirmed in animals.

Although some research has shown that PM has epigenetic effects, including DNA methylation and mitochondrial DNA methylation, the impacts of those changes on the health of children are not clear, and the understanding of the mechanisms is incomplete. Research in animals has emphasized the role of gene–environment interactions, the modulation of effect as a function of development (Soto-Martinez and Sly, 2010), and exposure to multiple mixtures (Silva da Silva et al., 2015). In utero PM exposure has been reported to play a role in early cardio, orofacial, and other defects (Teng et al., 2016); the transgenerational inheritance of ovarian disease (Nilsson et al., 2012); cardiovascular disease in adulthood (Tanwar et al., 2017a); brain defects (Chao et al., 2017); and many pathways, including antioxidant response, xenobiotic metabolism, inflammatory signaling, and endothelial dysfunction (Thomson et al., 2013). While using animal models makes it possible to control exposures and permits the study of defined compositions of multiple elements and tissues from multiple organ sources, it lacks the temporal resolution and cumulative exposures that are observed in humans and their individualized responses.

Synthesis and Conclusions

This literature for PM includes data on populations from around the world, often with relatively high exposures as a result of traffic or industrial pollution. Most studies examined environmental exposures, with only a few of them assessing occupational exposures.

The relevance of any of these studies to the exposures likely experienced by veterans is unclear. Exposures described in this literature are primarily continuous environmental exposures, whereas some veterans' exposures ceased upon their return from deployment, such as exposure to burn pits, while others may have continued, such as exposure to diesel exhaust and PM. Thus, the studies reviewed here do not necessarily address the long-term effects of concern to veterans. There is also a lack of data on the reproductive or developmental outcomes that may be expected following male or female exposures to combustion products prior to conception or, in the case of female service members, exposures in early pregnancy before they would have left the war zone. Because there are so few data on preconception and first-trimester exposures, particularly in humans, the committee's conclusions are based on prenatal exposures in general and not specifically on preconception or first-trimester exposures.

Several methodological issues make interpretation of the studies difficult: the heterogeneity of study designs and exposure assessment methods, the complexity of pollutant mixtures, and a limited mechanistic understanding. Exposure is frequently estimated rather than measured, using methods such as the distance between maternal residences at birth and an air monitoring station or modeling based on satellite data and land use regression at varying units of area, such as zip code or census tract. The potential for exposure misclassification using such approaches is of concern, particularly as compared with studies that conduct air monitoring for each individual in a prospective manner. Studies that adjust for changes in a subject's residence or the sources of pollution over time (such as increased traffic or the discontinuation of industrial sources) are more helpful than those that do not. Studies that measure outcomes in children, sometimes many years after exposure was estimated in pregnancy, often do not account for the expected changes in exposures that occur after birth.

Reproductive Effects

Reproductive Effects in Men and Women Adverse effects on female fertility were noted for both $PM_{2.5}$ and PM_{10} (Frutos et al., 2015; Nieuwenhuijsen et al., 2014; Slama et al., 2013). However, no effects on fertility and endometriosis were found in the Nurses' Health Study (Mahalingaiah et al., 2014, 2016). The effects of both $PM_{2.5}$ and PM_{10} on sperm count, concentration, motility, and morphology have been inconsistently reported (Hansen et al., 2010; Jurewicz et al., 2015; Lafuente et al., 2016; Wu et al., 2017; Zhou et al., 2014).

The Volume 11 committee concludes that there is inadequate/insufficient evidence to determine whether an association exists between PM exposure and reproductive effects in men or women.

Adverse Pregnancy Outcomes The Volume 3 committee concluded that there was "limited/suggestive evidence of an association" between prenatal exposure to combustion products and low birth weight and preterm birth. However, they also found that the evidence was insufficient/inadequate to determine whether any association existed between reproductive outcomes and exposure during specific time periods (e.g., trimesters).

EPA (2009) concluded that the evidence was "suggestive of a causal relationship between long-term exposures to $PM_{2.5}$ and reproductive . . . outcomes" but that the evidence was inadequate for $PM_{10-2.5}$.

EPA justified its conclusion based on reports that $PM_{2.5}$ had a greater impact on birth weight than did PM_{10} and on the consistent findings in epidemiologic studies of significant associations between $PM_{2.5}$ and preterm birth and growth restriction. Animal studies also reported these effects but provided little information on the mechanisms or biologic plausibility.

Since 2009 the epidemiologic literature has grown, and it now supports associations between maternal exposure to PM during pregnancy and adverse pregnancy outcomes, including low birth weight, preterm birth, and small for gestational age (Shah et al., 2011; Zhu et al., 2015a). In this literature, the relationship between exposure to air pollution, especially $PM_{2.5}$, and low birth weight is the most robust (Shah et al., 2011; Sun et al., 2016; Zhu et al., 2015a). Associations between exposure to $PM_{2.5}$ and preterm birth and small for gestational age have been reported in systematic reviews and meta-analyses (Shah et al., 2011; Sun et al., 2015; Zhu et al., 2015a). Preterm birth, low birth weight, and small for gestational age are known to increase a child's risk for subsequent health problems later in the life-course (Hack et al., 1995; Saigal and Doyle, 2008). Data on trimester-specific risks are inconsistent, but increased risks of preterm birth and decreases in birth weight associated with PM exposure in the third trimester are consistently reported. Exposure to PM during pregnancy has been associated with changes in biomarkers that are indicative of oxidative stress and inflammation processes, both of which may contribute to preterm birth and low birth weight.

Exposure to PM was also associated with miscarriage in two studies (Candela et al., 2015; Enkhmaa et al., 2014). The association between PM and stillbirth is inconsistent, with one study reporting increased risks with high levels of $PM_{2.5}$ exposure in the third trimester (DeFranco et al., 2015) and another reporting increased risks with PM_{10} exposure in the first trimester (Hwang et al., 2011). Three other studies considered by the committee showed no such effect of $PM_{2.5}$ (Faiz et al., 2012, 2013; Green et al., 2015; Pearce et al., 2010).

The risk of gestational diabetes and PM exposure was studied in three cohorts, but the results were mixed (Fleisch et al., 2014; Hu et al., 2015; Robledo et al., 2015). Preeclampsia and gestational hypertension were more extensively studied. Although PM_{10} was generally not associated with preeclampsia (Dadvand et al., 2013; Mobasher et al., 2013; van den Hooven et al., 2011; Wu et al., 2011), one study found increased risks of preeclampsia associated with PM_{10} exposure in mothers who did not smoke (Lee et al., 2013). Four studies of $PM_{2.5}$ found some positive association with preeclampsia (Dadvand et al., 2013; Lee et al., 2013; Mobasher et al., 2013; Wu et al., 2011), but the timing of exposure was variable, and two studies did not find any association (Rudra et al., 2011; Savitz et al., 2015). Preconception exposure was considered by Rudra et al. (2011), who found no relationship between preconception exposure to $PM_{2.5}$ and preeclampsia. Additionally, four studies reported increased blood pressure or gestational hypertension (a characteristic of preeclampsia) with PM exposure (Lee et al., 2012; van den Hooven et al., 2011; Vinikoor-Imler et al., 2012; Xu et al., 2014), and one study found no such effects (Hampel et al., 2011).

The Volume 11 committee concludes that there is sufficient evidence of an association between prenatal exposure to PM and adverse pregnancy outcomes—low birth weight and preterm birth.

The Volume 11 committee also concludes that there is limited/suggestive evidence of an association between exposure to PM during pregnancy and pregnancy-induced hypertensive disorders.

Developmental Effects

The committee found the literature on respiratory outcomes and neurodevelopmental effects to be relatively robust and convincing of associations with prenatal exposure to PM. The literature on other outcomes in children did not show any clear or consistent associations with PM exposure.

Respiratory Outcomes The Volume 3 committee concluded that there was "inadequate/insufficient evidence to determine whether an association exists" between combustion products or fuels and developmental effects in children (IOM, 2005). EPA concluded that the evidence was "suggestive of a causal relationship between long-term exposures to $PM_{2.5}$ and . . . developmental outcomes" based on associations between PM exposure and infant mortality. This conclusion was based on studies of respiratory conditions in children with supporting studies on lung development (EPA, 2009).

Sixteen recent studies examined the relationship between prenatal PM exposure and asthma and respiratory outcomes in childhood. There is a robust epidemiologic literature, including several large cohort studies from various locations, that supports an association between prenatal exposure to traffic-related air pollutants (including $PM_{2.5}$) and an increased risk of childhood asthma (Clark et al., 2010; Hsu et al., 2015; Tetreault et al., 2016; Voynow and Auten, 2015). Associations with other allergic diseases (atopic dermatitis and allergic rhinitis) (Deng et al., 2016; Huang et al., 2015; Liu et al., 2016b; Lu et al., 2017) and lung function growth (Eenhuizen et al., 2013; Jedrychowski et al., 2010a; Latzin et al., 2009; Morales et al., 2015; Mortimer et al., 2008) have also been reported. Interactive effects with combined prenatal exposure to community violence (Chiu et al., 2014) and traffic-related air pollution have been reported.

EPA (2009) found associations between $PM_{2.5}$ and increased infant mortality (<1 year) especially due to respiratory diseases that occur during the neonatal period. EPA emphasized that the susceptibility of the developing lung from embryogenesis into adult life allows for a long period of vulnerability to stressors, including exposures to air pollutants such as PM. Because biological detoxification systems are not fully developed until after birth, the disruption of cell signaling during development can have long-term effects on lung growth.

The Volume 11 committee concludes that there is limited/suggestive evidence of an association between prenatal exposure to PM and respiratory effects in children.

Neurodevelopmental Outcomes A variety of neurodevelopmental, cognitive, and behavioral deficits and ASD up to age 12 have been associated with prenatal PM exposure. Few of these studies, however, controlled for postnatal exposures that contribute to neurobehavioral changes.

Eight studies of ASD and PM were reviewed. Several studies found that ASD was associated with prenatal $PM_{2.5}$ (Becerra et al., 2013; Raz et al., 2015; Volk et al., 2013) and prenatal PM_{10} exposure (Kalkbrenner et al., 2015), although trimester-specific estimates of risk were inconsistent, and several studies showed no such effects (Gong et al., 2014, 2017; Guxens et al., 2016). A meta-analysis reported increased risks of ASD with $PM_{2.5}$ exposure in the first trimester and the postnatal period. None of the studies that examined preconception exposure found any association between $PM_{2.5}$ or PM_{10} and ASD (Kalkbrenner et al., 2015; Raz et al., 2015; Talbott et al., 2015).

While two studies reported significant associations between prenatal PM exposure and cognitive or psychomotor development in children up to 2 years old (Kim et al., 2014; Lertxundi et al., 2015), these results were not corroborated in other populations of children (Guxens et al., 2014; Lin et al., 2014). In children ages 5 to 6 years, attention, IQ, and memory problems were associated with prenatal exposure to PM, but there were clear gender differences (Chiu et al., 2016; Yorifuji et al., 2016). One study found that problems with executive functioning and behavior were associated with childhood PM exposure but not prenatal exposure (Harris et al., 2016).

Based on the positive results from several large studies and some well-conducted studies of ASD (Becerra et al., 2013; Raz et al., 2015; Volk et al., 2013) on consistent decrements in measures of neurodevelopment (although measures differed between studies), and on support from animal studies and mechanistic data that identify in utero exposure as a particularly susceptible window of development for neurodevelopmental effects associated with air pollutants and PM (Allen et al., 2017; Block et al., 2012; EPA, 2009), the committee had concerns about possible neurodevelopmental effects. The committee identified neurobehavioral effects in children of veterans as a priority area for future research, as discussed in later chapters.

The Volume 11 committee concludes that there is limited/suggestive evidence of an association between prenatal exposure to PM and neurodevelopmental effects.

Other Developmental Effects Twenty-one studies have examined the association of birth defects with PM exposure. Most are population-based case-control studies using registries to assess a list of congenital defects and modeling exposures based on maternal residence at time of birth to represent prenatal exposure. The majority of the studies reported equivocal results, although differences between the studies (i.e., in the specificity of outcomes examined and the time frame of the exposures) makes this hard to interpret. Two meta-analyses that examined PM_{10} exposure and congenital anomalies did not find increased risk. Although the majority of studies that assessed the risks of congenital heart defects did not find any associations with prenatal $PM_{2.5}$ or PM_{10}, a few studies did. For PM_{10}, associations were found for ventricular septal defects and atrial septal defects (Farhi et al., 2014) as well as multiple congenital heart defects and exposure in the first 3–8 weeks of pregnancy (Agay-Shay et al., 2013). For $PM_{2.5}$, there were associations with dextro-transposition of the great arteries (Padula et al., 2013b), pulmonary valve stenosis, and tetralogy of Fallot (Warren et al., 2016). Two studies found an increased risk of cleft palate associated with $PM_{2.5}$ exposure (Zhou et al., 2017; Zhu et al., 2015b), whereas 10 studies did not find increased risk of orofacial clefts with PM exposure. No increased risk of neural tube defects was reported in 7 studies. There were significantly increased risks of chromosomal defects (Farhi et al., 2014), abdominal wall defects (Schembari et al., 2014), omphalocele (Dolk et al., 2010), esophageal atresia (Padula et al., 2013c), and nervous system anomalies (Rankin et al., 2009) found in single studies.

Two studies reported analyses that included preconception exposures to explain the risk of orofacial clefts. Zhu et al. (2015b) observed a significantly increased risk of cleft palate with increased PM_{10} exposure through the 3 months before conception. Yao et al. (2016) found no association between $PM_{2.5}$ exposure in the 3 months before conception and cleft palate or cleft lip.

Childhood cancers were not associated with PM in two studies (Badaloni et al., 2013; Heck et al., 2013b), but a third study found a significantly elevated risk of astrocytoma, although no other cancer, in children in Ontario (Lavigne et al., 2017).

Several other outcomes were reported in the literature, but none of them had enough data on which to base any conclusions.

A few studies examined immune effects in children following prenatal PM exposure, but no associations with childhood eczema or dermatomyositis were found (Jedrychowski et al., 2011a,b; Lu et al., 2017; Orione et al., 2014). Associations between prenatal exposure to air pollution and abnormal immunological parameters in neonates have been reported (Ashley-Martin et al., 2016; Baiz et al., 2011; Herr et al., 2010, 2011); however, the long-term significance of these effects is not known. One study found that higher exposures to NO_2 and PM_{10} during pregnancy were both associated with increased maternal and fetal cord blood levels of C-reactive protein, which is indicative of inflammation, but the significance of this association is unclear (van den Hooven et al., 2012a).

There is some evidence of an association between prenatal exposure to air pollution and cardiovascular and metabolic dysfunction later in childhood (Breton et al., 2016; Poursafa et al., 2016; Thiering et al., 2013; van Rossem et al., 2015).

Although some animal studies support the associations observed in epidemiologic studies, a lack of mechanistic understanding remains. The induction of oxidative stress, of DNA damage, and of the alteration of molecular signaling or epigenetic events have all been proposed as possible mechanisms (Saenen et al., 2015, 2016; Teng et al., 2016). Several studies support an effect of exposure to air pollutants (e.g., NO_2 or PM_{10}) and damage to fetal mitochondrial DNA from oxidative stress (Clemente et al., 2016; Grevendonk et al., 2016; Janssen et al., 2012). In a Boston birth cohort, exposure to relatively low levels of $PM_{2.5}$ was associated with intrauterine inflammation (Nachman et al., 2016). Preexisting asthma and gestational diabetes in mothers may be effect modifiers of the association between air pollution and adverse birth outcomes (Erickson et al., 2016; Mendola et al., 2016).

Although some evidence has associated epigenetic changes with PM exposure, the impact of those changes on the health of children or the potential for such changes to be inherited by subsequent generations to cause generational health effects has not been demonstrated in either human or animal studies.

The Volume 11 committee concludes that there is inadequate/insufficient evidence to determine whether an association exists between prenatal exposure to PM and other developmental effects.

Polycyclic Aromatic Hydrocarbons

PAHs are chemicals formed as a result of the incomplete burning of organic substances (such as coal, oil, gasoline, diesel and jet fuel, wood, garbage, and tobacco). There are more than 100 different PAHs, and they generally are found as components of complex mixtures of chemicals. Some PAHs are used in medicines and to make dyes, plastics, and pesticides; others are in asphalt, and they are present in such substances as crude oil, coal, coal tar pitch, creosote, and roofing tar (ATSDR, 1995). Certain PAHs are carcinogenic and can cause other health effects (IOM, 2011). Benzo[a]pyrene (BaP) has been well studied in both epidemiologic studies and in the laboratory. It has been characterized as both a female reproductive toxicant and a developmental toxicant by EPA and the European Chemicals Agency in recent reviews (ECHA, 2017; EPA, 2017). BaP has been used as a sentinel of PAH exposure in some epidemiology studies (Guo et al., 2012; Herbstman et al., 2012; Perera et al., 2005a,b, 2007, 2012, 2014, 2015; Tang et al., 2006, 2012; Wu et al., 2010; Yin et al., 2017).

Gulf War personnel were exposed to PAHs as a result of the burning of over 600 oil wells in Kuwait. However, it was determined at that time that, based on the available air monitoring data, PAH exposure in soldiers deployed to Kuwait was relatively low to moderate when compared to the U.S. reference population. In addition, data from 61 soldiers indicated that the soldiers actually had lower concentrations of PAH-DNA adducts measured while in Kuwait than they had post-deployment, after spending a month at their base in Germany (Poirier et al., 1998). Post-9/11 personnel may have been exposed to PAHs as a result of burn pit use. PAH levels on military bases have been monitored as part of efforts to investigate the health hazards of burn pits (IOM, 2011). At JBB, a U.S. airbase in Iraq with a large burn pit, air sampling showed that vehicle and aircraft emissions were the primary sources of PAHs (Masiol et al., 2016a,b). In 2007, the average total PAH concentration across JBB was 379 ng/m^3, with the average concentration of BaP being 1.4 ng/m^3 (average total BaP-toxic equivalent=2.9 ng/m^3) (Masiol et al., 2016a). For comparison, total PAH and BaP concentrations from four of the cohorts discussed below are shown in Table 6-5.

Because PAHs were not specifically examined in any of the prior *Gulf War and Health* or other IOM volumes, the Volume 11 committee used the 1995 ATSDR toxicological profile on PAHs as the starting point for the literature to be considered in this report—that is, literature published after 1994. The committee identified more than 140 papers that report on reproductive, developmental, or generational effects in association with exposure to PAHs. Most studies investigated environmental exposures to PAHs. There were multiple publications for many cohorts—for example, there were 12 publications from the Columbia Center for Childrens' Health (CCCEH) study in New York City (Bocskay et al., 2005; Choi et al., 2008; Herbstman et al., 2012; Perera et al., 2009a,b, 2012, 2014; Peterson et al., 2015; Rundle et al., 2012; Tang et al., 2012; Vishnevetsky et al., 2015). The committee reviewed three publications on occupational exposure to PAHs among Taiwanese coke oven workers (Hsu et al., 2006; Jeng et al., 2013a,b). Recent epidemiologic studies describing the reproductive and developmental effects of PAHs reviewed by the committee are summarized in Table 6-6 at the end of this section.

None of the studies reported on preconception exposures except for analyses of the National Birth Defects Prevention Study. Some studies used personal air monitoring during pregnancy (such as the CCCEH-run studies in New York and Poland). Many more estimated ambient PAH levels by modeling residential proximity to specific PAH sources (e.g., the World Trade Center disaster) or to ambient air monitoring stations. Others measured PAHs, PAH metabolites, or PAH-DNA adducts in blood, serum, urine, or placental tissue. For most studies of the effects seen in children after birth, the exposures were determined for the prenatal period and assumed to be consistent or representative of exposures through childhood. A few studies conducted follow-ups of exposure during childhood (Jedrychowski et al., 2014, 2015a,b,c; Perera et al., 2014). The only studies of ambient exposure to consider parental occupation were reported from the National Birth Defects Prevention Study (Langlois et al., 2012, 2013; Lupo et al., 2012a,b; O'Brien et al., 2016).

TABLE 6-5 Examples of PAH and BaP Exposure Levels (ng/m^3) in Ambient Air in Cohort Studies

Cohort	Mean Level (SD)	Range	Study
California Cancer Registry	PAH=1.48 (1.13) BaP=0.21 (0.23)	0.16–12.89 0.02–2.45	Heck et al. (2013a)
Columbia Center for Children's Environmental Health Study (New York)	PAH=2.39 (2.12)	0.27–36.47	Rundle et al. (2012)
	PAH=3.212 (3.40) BaP=0.368 (0.46)	0.27–36.47 0.02–6.20	Choi et al. (2008)
Krakow, Poland	PAH=20.2 (95% CI 17.6–23.1)		Jedrychowski et al. (2015b)
Tongliang, China	BaP in 2002=13.14 BaP in 2005=9.14		Tang et al. (2014)

Reproductive Effects

Reproductive Effects in Men

Several studies assessed the effects of PAHs on male reproduction. Many of these studies were conducted in China and Taiwan, with a handful conducted in populations in Europe and the United States. Many of the studies presented below measured the presence of urinary metabolites of PAHs, particularly 1-hydroxypyrene (1-OHP), a metabolite of pyrene. 1-OHP has been consistently detected in urine and has been used as a biological marker for assessing an internal dose of activated PAHs (Jeng et al., 2013a). Other urinary metabolites of PAHs include 1-hydroxynaphthalene (1-OHNa), 2-hydroxynaphthalene (2-OHNa), 2-hydroxyfluorene (2-OHF) (Xia et al., 2009), 9-hydroxyphenanthrene (9-OHPh), 4-hydroxyphenanthrene (4-OHPh), and 9-hydroxyfluorene (9-OHFlu) (Yang et al., 2017b).

The three publications on exposure to PAHs for a cohort of 65 coke oven workers in Taiwan (Hsu et al., 2006; Jeng et al., 2013a,b) measured effects on sperm quality. Workers wore personal monitors to assess PAH exposure; 1-OHP was measured in urine after shifts (Jeng et al., 2013a). Men who smoked and had jobs that involved working close to the coke ovens, which are sources of PAH exposure, had reduced sperm quality and DNA damage (Hsu et al., 2006; Jeng et al., 2013a), but PAHs and 1-OHP did not affect sperm concentration or count or DNA fragmentation. The three papers reported conflicting results regarding the associations between ambient PAHs and sperm normal morphology, motility, and vitality and between 1-OHP and sperm motility. 1-OHP was negatively associated with normal morphology in all three publications. 1-OHP and some PAH species were significantly correlated with DNA adducts (Jeng et al., 2013b), and 1-OHP was significantly associated with measures of chromatin structure and mitochondrial membrane potential, although PAHs were not (Hsu et al., 2006).

Of the studies that examined semen parameters and sperm DNA integrity, most measured exposure based on urinary PAH metabolites (Gu et al., 2010; Han et al., 2011; Jurewicz et al., 2013b; Radwan et al., 2016; Xia et al., 2009; Yang et al., 2017b). Jurewicz et al. (2013b) and Xia et al. (2009) investigated the relationship between urinary PAH metabolites and sperm quality. Jurewicz et al. (2013b) reported that sperm neck abnormalities, volume, motility, and movement were significantly associated with increased urinary 1-OHP in 277 Polish men attending an infertility clinic; no associations were observed between 1-OHP and the DNA fragmentation index (DFI), sperm head or tail morphological abnormalities, semen concentration, the percent of atypical sperm, or measures of motility. Xia et al. (2009) compared levels of urinary PAH metabolites among 222 infertile men with abnormal semen quality, 291 infertile men with normal semen quality, and 273 fertile men in Nanjing, China, in a case-control study. Men in the highest tertile of exposure were more likely to have abnormal sperm than those in the lowest tertile (1-OHP OR=1.49, 95% CI 1.03–2.15; 2-OHF OR=1.52, 95% CI 1.06–2.17; and all metabolites OR=1.53, 95% CI 1.06–2.20). In 405 men in Wuhan, China, Yang et al. (2017b) reported no associations between urinary PAH metabolites and tail % or tail distributed moment, and only 9-OHFlu was associated with increased tail length and comet length (mean differences first versus third tertiles: 8.65%, 95% CI 2.53–15.03%, and 7.14%, 95% CI 2.33–12.19%, respectively). A significant association was observed between 9-OHPh and decreased Annexin V–/PI– spermatozoa (mean difference first versus third tertiles –5.38%, 95% CI –8.92– –1.86), but there were no other associations between metabolites and sperm apoptosis parameters. These data indicate that exposure to PAH may result in decreased sperm function.

Han et al. (2011), Gu et al. (2010), and Radwan et al. (2016) examined the association between effects on sperm DNA and urinary PAH metabolites. Han et al. (2011) noted increased DNA damage in sperm, but no effect on semen parameters in a cross-sectional study of 232 men in Chongqing, China. Total PAH metabolites were associated with the tail % (β=15.96, 95% CI 8.86–23.07), but not with the tail length or tail distributed movement. Significant associations were also reported between 2-OHNa and tail %, tail length, and tail distributed moment (ORs=13.26, 12.25, 7.55, all $p<0.05$). Gu et al. (2010) reported the joint effects of PAH exposure and specific polymorphisms on sperm DNA integrity among 620 infertile couples in Nanjing, China, in a nested case-control study; they found that men with high levels of 1-OHP and certain DNA nucleotide excision repair genotypes (*XPA* and *XPD*) were at higher risk of sperm DNA damage. In a Polish cross-sectional study of 181 men with normal semen attending an infertility clinic, urinary 1-OHP levels were associated with sperm aneuploidy, specifically increased risks of total sex-chromosome disomy (β=1.46, 95% CI 1.05–2.03) and disomy 18 (β=1.22, 95% CI 1.02–1.63), but not other kinds of disomy for sex chromosomes or chromosomes 13 and 18 (Radwan et al., 2016).

Five additional studies reported on semen quality (Conti et al., 2017; Gaspari et al., 2003; Rubes et al., 2005; Song et al., 2013; Yang et al., 2017a). In a group of 182 Italian men, PAH adducts in sperm were found to be correlated with physiologic forms (r= –0.18, p=0.016; terminology undefined), abnormal head morphology (r=0.30, p=0.0001), and abnormal neck morphology (r= –0.21, p=0.009), but not with sperm count or tail morphology. PAH adduct levels were higher among those with any abnormality (p=0.04) (but not among men with asthenospermia, oligospermia, or teratospermia) and among infertile men than among fertile men (with fertility based on the pregnancy status of partners) at a 1-year follow-up (p=0.04), suggesting that PAH adducts might be a marker of infertility (Gaspari et al., 2003). Another study of 86 Italian men compared BaP–DNA adducts in sperm cells to semen parameters and found that BaP–DNA adducts were inversely associated with sperm motility (Conti et al., 2017). Among 53 men attending a fertility clinic in Guangzhou, China, Song et al. (2013) found that total PAHs in blood correlated with semen volume, concentration, progressive motility, and nonlinear motility (r= –0.07, 0.10, 0.07, –0.10, all $p<0.05$) but were not associated with motility. In the only study that reported ambient air PAHs, a study that took place in the Czech Republic, exposure in the 90 days before sample collection was not associated with sperm count or concentration, volume, motility, morphology, velocity, linearity, or aneuploidy; only sperm chromatin abnormalities (%DFI) were related to PAH exposure (β=0.19, 95% CI 0.02–0.36) among 36 men who were followed over 2 years (Rubes et al., 2005). A group of 933 men visiting an infertility clinic in Wuhan, China, showed significant inverse associations between urinary PAH metabolites and sperm parameters (Yang et al., 2017a). Among the 10 metabolites analyzed, significant decreases in sperm concentration (–22.66%, 95% CI –34.49– –8.70%), sperm count (–19.99, 95% CI –33.83– –3.34%), and percentage of sperm with normal morphology (–2.35, 95% CI –4.24– –0.46%) were found between the first and the fourth quartiles of exposure to 1-OHNa. Adverse associations were also seen for semen volume and exposure to 4-OHPh (–0.31 mL, 95% CI –0.61– –0.01) and 9-OHPh (–0.43 mL, 95% CI –0.74– –0.12). Decreased motility was associated with 9-OHPh exposure (straight-line velocity –1.34 μm/sec, 95% CI –2.37– –0.31; curvilinear velocity –2.30 μm/sec, 95% CI –4.06– –0.54). No associations were noted between individual metabolites and sperm motility.

Han et al. (2010) examined the effect of PAH exposure on reproductive hormones in 562 men being evaluated for unexplained male factor infertility in Nanjing, China. An analysis by tertiles of metabolites and trisections of hormones showed both increased risks of higher hormone levels and significant trends between the following hormone–metabolite pairs: luteinizing hormone (LH) and both 1-naphthol (1-N) and 2-OHF (p-trend=0.025 and 0.019); follicle-stimulating hormone (FSH) and 2-OHF (p-trend=0.027); and estradiol and both 2-OHF and 1-OHP (p-trend=0.047 and 0.025). An analysis conducted using continuous variables showed only one significant relationship—between LH and 1-OHP (p=0.01).

Reproductive Effects in Women

Three studies examined the reproductive effects of PAHs in women. Slama et al. (2013) found that PAH exposure in the 2 months prior to the start of unprotected intercourse did not affect fecundability in a cohort of 1,916 Czech births between 1994 and 1999. In a prospective cohort study of 51 fertile women in California, Luderer et al. (2017a) found that higher PAH levels, as assessed by urinary concentrations of nine different PAHs, were associated with changes in follicular phase length, follicular phase LH, estrone 3-glucuronide (E13G) levels, pre-ovulatory LH surge concentrations, and peri-ovulatory E13G slope and concentration. In a separate case-control study conducted in China among 80 women (50 with polycystic ovary syndrome [PCOS] and 30 without this condition), individuals with PCOS had higher concentrations of serum PAHs and their metabolites. Total serum PAHs were associated with a significant risk of PCOS with PAH exposure (aOR=4.04, 95% CI 1.16–14.0). Higher levels of certain metabolites, hydroxyl-phenanthrenes (aOR=2.34, 95% CI 0.73–7.49) and hydroxyl-biphenyls (aOR=2.01, 95% CI 0.64–6.35), were associated with a twofold increased risk of PCOS; however, these findings did not reach statistical significance. This study was limited due to its sample size and power limitations (Yang et al., 2015).

Adverse Pregnancy Outcomes

Although many studies have examined the effects of air pollution and air quality on birth outcomes, such as preterm birth and birth weight, few have specifically assessed PAHs. The committee's literature search identified eight publications on birth size, two studies on preterm birth, one study of missed abortion (embryo died but miscarriage has not occurred in early pregnancy), and one study of reproductive hormones in umbilical cord serum.

Perera et al. (2005b) did not find any association between BaP adducts in maternal or cord blood—a proxy for prenatal PAH exposure—and birth weight, length, or head circumference among 186 women living near the World Trade Center in New York City at the time of the 9/11 disaster and delivering within 41 weeks of September 11, 2001. However, there was a significant interaction between cord blood adduct levels and environmental tobacco smoke exposure, with significantly lower birth weight and head circumference. Conversely, in the CCCEH cohort of pregnant women in New York City, total PAHs measured by personal monitor in the third trimester were significantly associated with increased risks of small for gestational age (OR=2.43, 95% CI 1.05–5.62, per 1 ln PAH unit increase), preterm births (OR=4.68, 95% CI 1.84–11.89), and reduced fetal growth ratio (<85%; OR=1.93, 95% CI 1.04–3.56) among African American mothers (n=224) but not for Dominican mothers (n=392) (Choi et al., 2008).

In a Chinese cohort of 183 births, Guo et al. (2012) did not observe any adverse effects of prenatal PAH exposure on birth height, weight, gestational age, Apgar score, or BMI, although some specific PAHs were significantly and negatively associated with height. A study of another Chinese cohort, this one consisting of 106 pregnant women in Wuhan, China, found that certain urinary metabolites measured in the third trimester were associated with decreased birth length, but none of the metabolites measured were associated with birth weight or gestational age. In a comparison of the first and third tertiles of exposure, 2-OHNa was found to be associated with a 0.80% reduction (95% CI –1.39– –0.20%) in mean birth length; neither Alu nor LINE-1 methylation (used as markers of global methylation) correlated with this association (Yang et al., 2018). Associations between higher PAH levels in the first gestational month and small for gestational age were seen in a Czech Republic study of 3,378 birth, suggesting that early exposure to PAH conferred a modest 20% increase in the odds of intrauterine growth restriction (aOR=1.22, 95% CI 1.07–1.39, per 10 ng increase in ambient PAH exposure) (Dejmek et al., 2000).

In a cohort of 344 pregnant Polish women, PAHs assessed by personal monitors in each trimester of pregnancy were associated with markers of growth restriction in the first trimester (fetal growth ratio= –3%, 95% CI –5%–0%, per 1 ln change in PAH exposure) (Choi et al., 2012) and with reduced birth weight and height for first and third trimesters (Wang and Choi, 2014). In a different cohort of 449

Polish women, urinary 1-OHP—used to represent PAH exposure—measured at 20–24 weeks of gestation was not related to birth weight, cephalization index (head circumference to body weight ratio), chest circumference, length, head circumference, or ponderal index (fetal weight to height). Only a reduction in chest circumference associated with 1-HP remained significant in the fully adjusted model, which accounted for salivary cotinine levels (Polanska et al., 2010, 2014). The authors reported a modest association between the interaction of hydroxyphenanthrene and cotinine levels on the cephalization index (p=0.04) (Polanska et al., 2014). Some studies have reported a significant interaction effect of PAH exposure and environmental tobacco smoke (Perera et al., 2005b; Polanska et al., 2014). In the same Polish birth cohort (n=455), personal monitoring for PAHs and PM was conducted in the second trimester to examine the impact of $PM_{2.5}$ and PAHs together. Although $PM_{2.5}$ alone was significantly associated with birth weight, birth length, and head circumferences, it was not significantly associated with these outcomes with co-pollutant models with PAH exposure. PAH exposure was strongly associated with all three measures on its own, but in the co-pollutant model PAH exposure was significantly associated only with birth weight (β= –0.20, p=0.004) and birth length (β= –0.17, p=0.025), not with head circumference (β= –0.13, p=0.086). The authors interpreted the results to indicate that PAH exposure is more biologically relevant for fetal development than PM exposure (Jedyrchowski et al., 2017). The Volume 11 committee notes that metabolic interactions between PM and PAHs were not considered in this study, but it is possible that they play some role in the observed health effects.

A Japanese study of 149 mother–child pairs found 1-OHP to be related to reductions in birth weight (β= –0.15, p=0.053), birth length (β= –0.18, p=0.022), and head circumference (β= –0.17, p=0.052), but the findings were not significant after smokers had been excluded (Suzuki et al., 2010). A cross-sectional study of 1,578 Saudi births found associations between PAH concentrations in cord blood and birth outcomes. BaP was associated with placental thickness (β= –0.071, p=0.017) and cord length (β= –0.075, p=0.012), and a summary measure of 4 PAHs was associated with decreased cord length (β= –0.077, p=0.003). Short cord length has been used as an indicator of fetal movement and developmental abnormalities. However, neither BaP nor the sum of 4 PAHs nor 1-OHP was associated with numerous other anthropometric birth outcome measures (Al-Saleh et al., 2013). This study also found an association between 1-OHP in cord blood and a marker of oxidative stress, 8-OHdG levels (β=0.303, p<0.001), which suggests that oxidative stress is a potential mechanism by which PAHs may produce adverse pregnancy outcomes. In the Generation R study, a population-based prospective cohort study of 4,680 births in the Netherlands between 2002 and 2006, investigators found inverse associations between maternal occupational exposure to PAH and fetal growth measures, with significantly lower associations between prenatal PAH exposure and relative change in fetal weight across pregnancy (β= –0.0166, SE=0.0080, p<0.05) (Snijder et al., 2012).

Langlois et al. (2014) reported on small for gestational age among births selected as controls from a series of case-control studies using the National Birth Defect Prevention Study (2,803 births). Parental occupational PAH exposure, as determined by an industrial hygienist, from the month before pregnancy through the first trimester had a significant effect on small for gestational age, although the result was based on only 17 small-for-gestational-age births with PAH exposure (OR=2.2, 95% CI 1.3–3.8).

In addition to fetal growth measures, researchers have assessed the effects of PAH exposure on preterm births. A study conducted in California of 42,904 mother–child pairs living within range of an EPA air monitoring site in Fresno, California, between 2001 and 2006, evaluated preterm births (Padula et al., 2014). This study used geocoding and modeling techniques to estimate the exposure to individual PAHs and the sum of PAHs. The model explained 81% of the between-residence variability and 18% of the within-residence variability, with the main sources of these PAHs in this area being roadways, agriculture, and residential fireplaces, stoves, and heating. In this study, PAH exposures during the last 6 weeks of pregnancy were found to be associated with a nearly threefold increase in early preterm birth (i.e., delivery at 20–27 weeks gestation) (OR=2.74, 95% CI 2.24–3.34) when comparing the highest quartile to the lower three quartiles. Quartiles of PAH exposure were also significantly related to preterm births, with a dose–response pattern (compared to lowest exposure: 2nd quartile OR=1.49, 95% CI 1.08–2.06; 3rd quartile OR=2.63, 95% CI 1.93–3.59; 4th quartile OR=3.94, 95% CI 3.03–5.12). The associations were similar across gradations of SES, but the associations were affected by the season of conception, with the strongest associations seen for pregnancies conceived during the summer (June–August) and inverse associations observed for pregnancies conceived in March–May (Padula et al., 2014). The authors were unable to determine the cause of these inconsistencies.

A case-control study of 29 preterm births and 31 full-term births conducted in India between 2005 and 2006 found that placental PAH levels were significantly higher in samples taken from women who had experienced preterm births than from those with full-term births, with significantly higher concentrations of fluoranthene and benzo(b)fluroanthene (both $p<0.05$). When considering the distribution of the PAHs in the placental tissue, the three-ringed PAHs made up more of the mixture in the preterm birth group (41%) than in the control group (31%) (Singh et al., 2008). Although this was a small study of only 60 women with limited power, it provides some suggestive evidence that PAHs may affect gestation length.

Missed abortion was studied by Wu et al. (2010) in a study of 81 cases and 81 controls in China; the researchers found no association between missed abortion and BaP–DNA adducts in fetal tissue. However, higher levels of BaP–DNA adducts in maternal blood (per 10^8 nucleotides) increased the risk of missed abortion (OR=1.35, 95% CI 1.11–1.64). Although adduct levels in maternal blood and fetal tissue were not correlated, maternal-blood BaP–DNA adduct levels did correlate with a survey on PAH exposure from common sources; 26% of the variance in missed abortion was explained by maternal blood BaP–DNA adduct levels. Also associated with missed abortion were other self-reported proxies for PAH exposure: residence near traffic congestion (OR=3.07, 95% CI 1.31–7.16), commute by walking (OR=3.52, 95% CI 1.44–8.57), and routinely cooking during pregnancy (OR=3.78, 95% CI 1.11–12.87).

Another study conducted in the Shendsi Islands of China cross-sectionally evaluated the association between umbilical-cord-blood PAH levels and umbilical-cord-blood hormone levels in mothers among 109 births. An inverse association was found between PAH levels and estradiol and anti-Müllerian hormone (AMH), and a positive association was found between PAH levels and FSH in women at the time of delivery (Yin et al., 2017). No significant associations were reported between testosterone, luteotropic hormone (prolactin), or estradiol and any specific PAH species or between acenaphthylene, benzo(*b*)fluoranthene (BbF), benzo(*k*)fluoranthene (BkF), or BaP and any hormone. Several significant positive associations were reported between FSH and fluorine, phenanthrene, anthracene, fluoranthene, benz(a)anthracene, and chrysene (β=0.47, 0.44, 0.51, 0.38, 0.42, 0.35, all $p<0.05$), and significant negative associations were reported between AMH and naphthalene, acenaphthene, fluorine, and fluoranthene (β= –0.33, –0.33, –0.44, –0.35, all $p<0.05$) after adjusting for confounders. Because a number of childhood and later life conditions in offspring are theorized to be associated with hormonal changes in pregnancy, this finding may provide a pathway by which higher concentrations of PAH could operate through a hormonally mediated mechanisms to affect pregnancy loss as well as pregnancy complications and fetal outcomes (Yin et al., 2017).

Developmental Effects

Developmental outcomes assessed after birth—including childhood cancers, neurobehavioral outcomes, growth, and respiratory outcomes—are discussed here. Few studies assessed the same outcome or measure in different populations, making it difficult to assess consistency across studies. None of these studies specifically assessed preconception exposures, and many of these studies assessed outcomes in children without consideration for the continuous nature of exposures throughout childhood—for example, investigating prenatal PAH exposure with an outcome at 9 years of age without factoring in PAH exposures between birth and age 9.

Birth Defects

As with pregnancy complications, birth defects may be the downstream effects of exposures to PAHs in utero. Several epidemiologic studies have evaluated the associations between PAHs and birth defects. These studies are mostly case-control study designs using data from national or regional registries. Most studies were conducted in China or the United States. The U.S. studies were primarily analyses based on the NBDPS, a large population-based case-control study that assessed about 30 different birth defects in 10 states over 14 years (CDC, 2017). Data on birth defects and live births were collected as part of state surveillance systems in Arkansas, California, Georgia, Iowa, Massachusetts, New Jersey, New York, and Texas, with data including live births. Controls came from the same areas as the cases and were randomly selected by birth certificate or hospital birth records. Various birth defects were considered, such as neural tube defects, cleft palate, gastroschisis, craniosyntosis, and congenital heart defects. All the U.S. studies based their exposure information on maternal occupational exposures, with most of them evaluating exposure to PAHs on the basis of retrospective data collected on direct or indirect exposures as well as on the duration and intensity of exposures for each job. Preconception exposure was not distinguished from prenatal exposure. Only inhalation was considered, and skin and ingestion exposure routes were not accounted for in these studies. On the other hand, the Chinese studies mainly looked at the relationship between PAHs—examined in a variety of tissues, including maternal blood, cord blood, and placenta—and neural tube defects.

Analyses of the NBDPS have all used a case-control design with nearly 3,000 healthy controls. Significantly elevated risks were reported for cleft lip, with or without cleft palate (n=805; OR=1.47, 95% CI 1.02–2.12), but not cleft palate alone (n=439; OR=1.24, 95% CI 0.76–2.13) (Langlois et al., 2013). The risk of gastroschisis was also elevated (n=299; OR=1.75, 95% CI 1.05–2.92), specifically among mothers 20 years of age and older (OR=2.53, 95% CI 1.27–5.04) (Lupo et al., 2012a). No significant associations with congenital heart defects were observed (n=1,907), including for conotruncal defects, left ventricular outflow tract defects, right ventricular outflow tract defects, or septal defects (Lupo et al., 2012b). However, the risk of craniosynostosis was significantly elevated (OR=1.75, 95% CI 1.01–3.05), although only 16 of the 3,016 cases had reported PAH exposure (O'Brien et al., 2016). No significant risks of neural tube defects were observed (n=520) (Langlois et al., 2012).

Two separate case-control studies in Shanxi Province, China, reported on the relationship between neural tube defects and PAH exposure (Yi et al., 2015; Yuan et al., 2013). Among 80 cases and 50 controls born in 2005–2007, investigators found a significant inverse relationship between PAH adducts in placental tissue and neural tube defects, with the controls having significantly higher concentrations of PAHs than the cases. No significant differences were found for spina bifida or anencephaly subtypes. When stratified by PAHs and PAH–DNA adducts, significantly elevated risks remained only among those with high PAH exposure and low PAH adducts (OR=8.2, 95% CI 2.1–32.7) (Yuan et al., 2013). Among 60 cases and 60 controls born in 2010–2012, Yi et al. (2015) reported a significant dose–response relationship for neural tube defects, spina bifida, and anencephaly with tertiles of PAH–DNA adducts in umbilical cord tissue and blood (p-trend <0.05 for all). Risks at the highest tertiles of exposure were significantly increased for neural tube defects (OR=2.96, 95% 1.16–7.58), spina bifida (OR=2.97, 95% CI 1.18–7.49), and anencephaly (OR=3.12, 95% CI 1.14–8.55).

Childhood Cancer

Several case-control studies (Heck et al., 2013a, 2014; Shrestha et al., 2014; von Ehrenstein et al., 2016) have used the California Cancer Registry to examine the risks of cancer among children younger than 6 years of age; data from birth certificates were used to identify population-based controls to match with the cases of children with cancer. Heck et al. (2013a) estimated exposure to PAHs for each trimester of pregnancy at the mother's residence using data collected from nearby community-based air pollution monitors. There was no significant association of PAH levels with an increased risk of neuroblastoma for children within 5 km of a monitor (75 cases and 14,602 controls); however, those living within 2.5 km showed an increased risk of neuroblastoma associated with total PAHs (OR=1.39, 95% CI 1.01–1.91). Among children of mothers living within 5 miles of a monitor, there was no increase in the risk of primary neuroectodermal tumors (43 cases) or astrocytoma (106 cases), but the risk of medulloblastoma (in 34 cases versus 30,569 controls) was correlated with total PAH exposure (OR=1.44, 95% CI 1.15–1.80), particularly for benzo(k)fluoranthene, benzo(a)pyrene, benzo(b)fluoranthene, indeno(1,2,3-cd)pyrene, dibenzo(a,h)anthracene, and benzo(g,h,i)perylene (von Ehrenstein et al., 2016). Risk of Wilms' tumor, a type of kidney cancer of embryonic origin, among 337 cases and 96,514 controls living within 15 miles of a monitor was associated with PAH exposures throughout pregnancy (OR=1.15, 95% CI 1.02–1.31), but the estimates were not significant for individual trimesters (Shrestha et al., 2014). For children living within 6 km of an air monitor, there was an increased, but not significant, risk of ALL (69 cases and 2,994 controls) and AML (46 cases and 19,209 controls) with exposure to PAHs throughout pregnancy. Third-trimester exposure to PAHs was associated with a modest increase in ALL (OR=1.16, 95% CI 1.04–1.29), including significantly increased associations with individual PAH species in the third trimester, with ORs ranging from 1.06 to 1.27. Several other exposures, including arsenic, 1,3-butadiene, and lead, also showed significant associations (Heck et al., 2014).

Using data from children diagnosed with retinoblastoma from a private medical practice in Philadelphia or at a U.S. or Canadian institution of the Children's Oncology Group (more than 200 medical centers) between June 2006 and 2012, investigators examined 187 unilateral and 95 bilateral cases of retinoblastoma (Omidakhsh et al., 2018). Controls (n=155) were identified through cases by identifying friends or a relative of the case child who was less than 15 years of age. Exposure data were assessed on the basis of paternal occupational exposure to PAHs in the 10 years before conception. Maternal occupational exposures were assessed 1 month before as well as during pregnancy. Increased, but not significant, associations were noted for unilateral (OR=1.34, 95% CI 0.48–3.72) and bilateral (OR=1.51, 95% CI 0.36–6.38) neuroblastoma, but the analyses were limited by the relatively few PAH-exposed cases (n=22) and controls (n=18). (Omidakhsh et al., 2018).

In a subset of 60 infants born to African American and Dominican women participating in the CCCEH cohort study, investigators measured chromosomal aberration frequencies in cord blood as markers of cancer risk. Prenatal exposures to PAHs measured in air were positively associated with stable chromosomal aberrations ($r=0.35$, $p<0.01$, and $\beta=0.14$, $p=0.006$), but not with PAH–DNA adducts. This finding suggests that PAHs have the potential to cause cytogenic damage related to an increased risk of cancer (Bocskay et al., 2005).

Neurobehavioral Outcomes

The associations between prenatal exposures to PAHs and childhood neurological conditions have been the subject of multiple investigations. Most studies come from two countries—the United States and Poland. A total of 11 epidemiological studies have been conducted, with 4 of the studies from Poland and 7 from the United States. Most of the U.S. studies are of the CCCEH cohort conducted in the northern Manhattan section of New York City among Dominican and African American mother–child pairs. A range of neurological outcomes were assessed, including IQ and cognitive dysfunction as assessed by the WISC, behavioral development evaluated by a 118-item Child Behavior Checklist for children ages 6–9 years, and cognitive and psychomotor development evaluated by Bayley-II Scales of Infant Development (BSID-II). Other neurological conditions were assessed, including ADHD, as well as white matter function, cognition, and behavior in later childhood.

Three reviews sought to summarize the literature base regarding the impacts of exposure to environmental toxicants, including PAHs, on children's neurodevelopment and behavior. Polanska et al. (2012) studied risk factors for ADHD in the literature published between 2000 and 2012 and cited one study on the risk of ADHD with PAH. Polanska et al. (2012) concluded that the ADHD risk associated with tobacco smoke, a source of PAH exposure, was consistent but that the evidence regarding environmental exposures, including PAHs, was insufficient to reach any conclusions about ADHD and environmental exposures, specifically PAHs. Regarding cognitive development and behavioral problems, Jurewicz et al. (2013a) cited eight studies and noted the possible adverse impact of PAHs on children's neurodevelopment. Suades-Gonzalez et al. (2015) summarized the literature on air pollutants and neuropsychological development and found seven publications that reported on prenatal PAH exposure. The authors concluded that there was sufficient evidence to show an association between pre- or postnatal PAH exposure and decreased global IQ scores, but that there was inadequate evidence to support associations with academic skills or ADHD.

Neurobehavioral outcomes in children have been well studied in the CCCEH cohort study. This study measured environmental PAH exposure in mothers who wore personal monitors in the third trimester; determined PAH–DNA adducts in maternal and cord blood and in children's urine at ages 3 and 5 years; and assessed neurodevelopmental indicators at age 7 (brain development, behavior, and IQ) (Perera et al., 2009b, 2012, 2014, 2015; Peterson et al., 2015; Vishnevetsky et al., 2015).

Two publications based on the CCCEH cohort examined measures of brain physiology and development. Brain development, as assessed by brain-derived neurotrophic factor in cord blood and the BSID-II Mental Development Index (MDI) scores at age 2 years, was negatively correlated with PAH–DNA adducts in cord blood ($\beta = -0.11$, $p=0.02$) and with MDI scores ($\beta = -2.07$, $p=0.04$). These associations were not observed in a model that included all three variables, at age 3, or when using BaP–DNA adducts to represent exposure (n=505; Perera et al., 2015). Prenatal PAH exposure was inversely correlated with white matter surface measures, especially in the left hemisphere, in 40 children assessed between ages 7 to 9, and high exposure was associated with reduced processing speed during intelligence testing (mediated by white matter disturbances). Such an effect could help explain the reductions in verbal IQ and information processing and the increases in attention and behavioral problems reported in other studies (Peterson et al., 2015).

Publications from the CCCEH study also reported differences in behavior. In children 6 or 7 years of age, ambient prenatal PAH exposures were associated with anxiety and depression scores (continuous exposure OR=1.2, 95% CI 1.06–1.37), attention problems (high/low OR=3.79, 95% CI 1.14–12.66), anxiety disorder (high/low OR=4.59, 95% CI 1.46–14.27), and ADHD (high/low OR=2.3, 95% CI 0.79–6.7), but none of the behaviors were significantly associated with maternal or cord blood PAH–DNA adduct measurements taken at the time of delivery (n=253) (Perera et al., 2012). DNA adducts in maternal blood were correlated with ADHD at age 9 in 250 children, after adjusting for prior childhood exposure (using urinary PAH metabolites at ages 3 and 5), with significantly increased risk for the DSM-IV inattentive subtype (OR=5.06, 95% CI 1.43–17.93). Adducts in cord blood were not related to ADHD (Perera et al., 2014).

Multiple publications from the CCCEH study reported on the relationship between PAH exposure and IQ measures performed using the Wechsler Preschool and Primary Scale of Intelligence-Revised.

Perera et al. (2009b) studied a group of 249 children and reported that high levels of prenatal PAHs were significantly associated at age 5 with IQ decrements on verbal performance (β= –3.53 points, p=0.002) and full-scale IQ scores (β= –3.0 points, p=0.009). Children exposed to high PAHs had IQ scores about 4 points lower than children with lower exposure (above versus below the median). Vishnevetsky et al. (2015) measured IQ at age 7 using the WISC and noted a significant interaction between material hardship (unmet basic needs in the areas of food, housing, and clothing) and PAH–DNA adducts on working memory (β= –8.07 points, 95% CI –14.48– –1.66), such that children with high prenatal hardship and high levels of PAH-DNA adducts had lower working memory scores (β= –6.67 points, 95% CI –11.38– –1.95). Children who experienced high prenatal hardship and had high PAH-DNA adducts also had significant decrements in full-scale and perceptual reasoning scores (β= –5.81 points, 95% CI –10.35– –1.26 and β= –5.44 points, 95% CI –10.27– –0.61, respectively), but there was no significant effect of the interaction term on full-scale IQ, verbal comprehension, processing speed, and perceptual reasoning scores in 276 children with low prenatal material hardship. In another analysis, PAH–DNA adducts measured in cord blood were found to be associated with depressed verbal IQ scores among 170 children at 7 years of age (RR=3.00, 95% CI 1.32–6.79) but not with other IQ scores. However, breastfeeding exclusively for at least 6 months had a protective effect on verbal IQ scores attributed to PAH exposure (RR=0.31, 95% CI 0.11–0.89) (Jedyrchowski et al., 2015a).

IQ and neurodevelopment were also studied in cohorts of children in New York, China, and Poland. Edwards et al. (2010) observed a cohort of 214 Polish children whose mothers were monitored for PAH exposure. Decrements in neurodevelopment at age 5 were associated with second-trimester exposure when comparing high to low exposure (above or below the median of 17.96 ng/m^3) (β= –1.36 points, 95% CI –2.48– –0.23, p=0.02) and continuous exposure (β= –0.56 points, 95% CI –1.00– –0.11, p=0.02). Perera et al. (2007) assessed a cohort of 98 children born in New York City to mothers who resided within 1 kilometer of the World Trade Center and had exposure to PAHs during pregnancy as a result of the towers burning. In a multivariate analysis, BaP–DNA adducts in cord blood at the time of delivery were not associated with the BSID psychomotor development index or MDI scores at age 3 years (Perera et al., 2007).

Other studies of neurobehavioral development include those of cohorts of children from China and of two Polish cohorts. In a study of Chinese children, Tang et al. (2014a) found a significantly increased percentage of children who had developmental delays among 2-year-old children with higher PAH exposure (n=150; expressed as plasma BDNF=1,266.56 pg/mL) when compared with those with lower PAH exposure (n=158; expressed as plasma BDNF=752.87 pg/mL), such that a unit increase in cord blood PAH–DNA adducts was negatively associated with average (β=212.11, p=0.01), motor (β=210.70, p=0.05), and adaptive (β=216.47, p=0.02) Gesell Developmental Schedule developmental quotient scores. No differences in language delays were noted. In another study of 604 Polish children 1 or 2 years of age, Polanska et al. (2013) found that prenatal PAH exposure, determined by urinary 1-OHP collected between 20 and 24 weeks of pregnancy, was not associated with cognitive, language, or motor development, although exposure to environmental tobacco smoke had a significant effect on cognitive and motor development. In a 2015 study evaluating behavioral development in 151 children ages 6–9 years old who were born to mothers living in Krakow, Poland, data on PAH exposure were collected from personal air monitors worn for 48-hours during the second trimester of pregnancy. Associations varied based on the micronutrients (retinol, alpha (α)-tocopherol, gamma (γ)-tocopherol, and a composite variable for carotenoids) in maternal and cord blood. Higher PAH concentrations were associated with higher scores in anxious/depressed domains as well as with being withdrawn/depressed and having social problems, attention problems, and aggressive behaviors on the basis of scores from the Child Behavior Checklist. The strongest associations were seen for low retinol intake and higher PAH levels with withdrawn/depressed behavior, with a 0.41 increase in this score for every unit increase in PAH levels (p=0.0008) (Genkinger et al., 2015).

Neurodevelopmental effects were significantly affected by factors such as breast-feeding (Jedyrchowski et al., 2015a), maternal hardship (Vishnevetsky et al., 2015), nutrition/antioxidant levels (Grenkinger et al., 2015), and environmental tobacco smoke (Polanska et al., 2013).

Growth

Given that a number of studies have suggested that prenatal PAH exposure relative to growth restriction and other measures of newborn and early infancy growth measures, it is plausible that prenatal exposure could affect later childhood measures of growth. The impacts of prenatal PAH exposure on growth in childhood were reported in three studies. A cohort of 150 children born in 2002 and a second cohort of 158 unexposed children born in 2005, both living near a power plant that ceased operation in 2004 in China, were studied for effects on growth at birth, 18, 24, and 30 months (Tang et al., 2006, 2014b). Exposure was estimated based on environmental sampling and PAH–DNA adducts in maternal and cord blood. Growth rates did not differ between the two cohorts, although the 2005 cohort had significantly lower BaP exposure (according to both environmental sampling and measures of DNA adducts, p<0.001). In the 2002 cohort, PAH–DNA adducts were significantly related to a smaller head circumference at birth and lower weight at 18, 24, and 30 months (Tang et al., 2014b).

Jedrychowski et al. (2015b) assessed the height through age 9 of 379 Polish children and compared that with prenatal PAH exposures (measured by personal monitors in the second trimester) and indoor and outdoor PAH exposure measured at age 3. Researchers found that a higher prenatal exposure to PAHs measured in the second trimester was associated with modest but significantly lower height gain between the ages of 3 and 9 years than in children who were not exposed ($\beta = -1.07$ cm, 95% CI –2.01––0.05); however, the decrements in height gain were mediated by shorter birth lengths that were also associated with prenatal PAH exposure.

Among the children of women residing in New York City who were assessed for PAH exposure during their third trimesters by personal ambient air monitors over a 48-hour period, prenatal PAH exposure was found to be associated with BMI at both 5 years (n=453) and 7 years (n=371) of age. At both ages, children in the second and third tertiles of exposure had increased risks of obesity compared with children in the first tertile of exposure (at age 5, PAH 2nd tertile [1.73-3.07 ng/m^3] RR= 1.79, 95% CI 1.08–2.98 and PAH 3rd tertile [≥3.08 ng/m^3] RR=1.79, 95% CI 1.09–2.96; at age 7, PAH 2nd tertile RR=2.25, 95% CI 1.27–4.01 and PAH 3rd tertile RR= 2.26, 95% CI 1.28–4.00). Furthermore, higher ambient prenatal PAH exposure was associated with higher fat mass (Rundle et al., 2012).

Respiratory Outcomes

A series of publications on a cohort of Polish mothers and children examined the respiratory effects of prenatal PAH exposure measured by personal monitor in the second trimester. In the two studies that distinguished between prenatal and postnatal exposure, significant effects of postnatal exposure were reported (Jedrychowski et al., 2014, 2015c).

Prenatal PAH exposure was significantly associated with the number of respiratory symptom episodes in the first year of life, including ear infection (RR=1.82, 95% CI 1.03–3.23), cough (RR=1.27, 95% CI 1.07–1.52), cough without cold (RR=1.72, 95% CI 1.02–2.92), barking cough (RR=4.80, 95% CI 2.73–8.44), wheezing without cold (RR=3.83, 95% CI 1.18–12.43), and sore throat (RR=1.96, 95% CI 1.38–2.78). The durations of respiratory episodes were similar to the number of occurrences. In addition, a significant interaction between prenatal PAH exposure and postnatal environmental tobacco smoke exposure smoking was observed for these associations (n=333) (Jedyrchowski et al., 2005). At age 4, the severity of wheezing was associated with prenatal PAH exposure (IRR=1.12, 95% CI 1.07–1.18) and also with PAH exposure measured at age 3 (IRR=1.08, 95% CI 1.02–1.14). Recurrent wheezing was associated with postnatal PAH exposure (OR=1.61, 95% CI 1.16–2.24) but not with prenatal exposure (OR=1.40, 95% CI 0.97–2.03) (n=257) (Jedyrchowski et al., 2014). Lung function (FEV_{05}, FEV_1, $FEF_{25–75}$) measured between the ages of 5 and 9 years was significantly reduced among children who had been in the highest tertiles of prenatal PAH exposure. Postnatal indoor and outdoor PAH exposure measured at age 3 was also related to decreased lung function between the ages of 5 and 9 (n=195) (Jedrychowski, et al., 2015c). Based on PAH–DNA adducts measured in cord blood in this cohort, prenatal PAH exposure was significantly related to fractional exhaled nitric oxide (FeNO) (β=0.32, p=0.006) at 7 years old in a subset of 82 children. Atopy and maternal allergy were also significantly related to FeNO, but PAH exposure explained 11% of the variance in FeNO levels (all three variables together explained 21% of the variance). FeNO was used as an indicator of airway inflammation (Jedrychowski et al., 2012). One meta-analysis of six studies reporting on childhood wheezing and prenatal PAH exposure reported a nonsignificant increased association (OR=1.04, 95% CI 0.94–1.15) (Hehua et al., 2017).

One exploratory study evaluated the mechanisms involved in prenatal PAH exposure and the DNA methylation of the acyl-CoA synthetase long-chain family member (*ACSL3*) as it related to parental report of asthma symptoms. The *ACSL3* gene is associated with fatty acid metabolism and is expressed in the lung (Perera et al., 2009a). As such, this exploratory study may provide an epigenetic mechanism by which PAH exposure could affect lung function.

Animal Studies

There is a large literature that specifically examines BaP with rodent and in vitro studies. EPA's 2017 *Toxicologic Review of BaP* stated: "Animal studies demonstrate that exposure to benzo[a]pyrene is associated with developmental (including developmental neurotoxicity), reproductive, and immunological effects" (EPA, 2017).

The EPA review found that animal models indicated that BaP exposure prior to mating and during pregnancy can decrease the ability of females to maintain pregnancy (including embryo/fetal resorptions, decreased litter size, and decreases in ovulation rate); one study found decreased litter size after a single exposure prior to mating (Mattison et al., 1980). Multigenerational studies of BaP exposure have shown effects on fertility and the development of reproductive organs (decreased ovary and testes weight, decreased sperm quality, the destruction of primordial follicles, decreased corpora lutea, the stimulation of oocyte apoptosis, decreased sensitivity to FSH-stimulated follicle growth) in offspring exposed in utero.

The Volume 11 committee identified several animal studies on BaP exposure that were not cited in EPA's review. These studies are briefly summarized below.

In one study, alterations in male reproductive parameters were evaluated after repeated exposure to BaP (Jeng et al., 2015). Young, adult male Hsd: ICR (CD1) mice (n=8) were administered BaP by oral gavage at doses of 0, 1, 10, 50 or 100 mg/kg/day for 30 or 60 days. Body weight was not affected by the treatment. In mice treated for 60 days with 100 mg/kg/day, the weights of the testes, seminal vesicle, and epididymis were significantly less (p<0.05) than those of the controls. With 60 days of treatment, sperm motility and vitality were significantly decreased at 100 mg/kg/day, while sperm morphology was significantly altered at both 50 and 100 mg/kg/day. DNA strand breaks in spermatozoa were significantly increased at doses of ≥50 mg/kg/day for 30 days and ≥10 mg/kg/day for 60 days. Microscopic lesions of the testes and a loss of integrity of the seminiferous tubule and epithelium were observed at ≥50 mg/kg/

day. Another study of the effects of BaP exposure (25, 50, 100 mg/kg/day orally for 28 days) on male germ cells 42 days after the end of exposure found that there were twice as many mutations in dividing spermatagonia at the 50 and 100 mg/kg doses than in control mice (Rowan-Carrol et al., 2017).

Other PAHs have also been known to affect male reproductive function. For example, in mice exposed in utero, low-dose exposure to BbF was associated with altered sperm function, with more apoptotic cell death at higher concentrations (Kim et al., 2011). Other studies have shown associations between certain PAHs and effects on sperm parameters, including decreased motility, abnormal head morphology, vitality, and concentration of mature spermatozoa as well as alterations in DNA repair genes in animal models (Jeng et al., 2015).

Li et al. (2017) reported that BaP impaired endometrial decidualization and decidual angiogenesis (which is related to embryo implantation and maintenance of pregnancy) in pregnant mice. BaP (0, 0.2, 2, and 20 mg/kg/day by gavage on GD 1–8) was associated with several adverse reproductive effects, including smaller and more irregular uterine implantation sites; impaired response to artificial decidualization stimulus; decreased estradiol and progesterone steroid levels in serum and a reduced expression of estradiol and progesterone hormone receptors in the uteri; reduced levels of key molecules related to decidualization; and the disruption of progesterone and vascular endothelial growth factor signaling mechanisms.

One in vitro study found that BaP (50, 100 or 250 μM) was associated with meiotic failure and the impaired fertilization of oocytes from pigs by increasing reactive oxygen species and apoptosis (Miao et al., 2018).

A study of the ovarian effects of prenatal exposure to BaP (2 mg/kg/day orally on GD 6.5–15.5) on female offspring found that exposed female F1 mice reached puberty earlier than controls (5 days) and showed a depletion of ovarian follicles. Maternal glutamase cysteine ligase modifier subunit (*Glcm*) deficiency did not modify the ovarian effects of prenatal BaP exposure. Neither BaP exposure nor *Glcm* genotype were related to *Kras* mutations in F1 mice (Luderer et al., 2017b).

Increased mutation rates and mosaicism in the brain, bone marrow, liver, and sperm of mice exposed to BaP in utero (10, 20, or 40 mg/kg/day by gavage on GD 7–16) were reported by Meier et al. (2017). F1 mice also showed decreased sperm count and motility compared to controls.

Learning deficits following in utero exposure to BaP were assessed by McCallister et al. (2016). Pregnant Long Evans Hooded rats were administered 0, 150, 300, 600, or 1200 μg/kg/day on GD 14–17. Metabolites were measured in blood and cortex samples from pups on PNDs 0–15. Beginning on PND 40, selected offspring were tested in a spatial discrimination and reversal task using operant chambers. Treatment with BaP had no effect on maternal and offspring body weight or on reproductive parameters, and no clinical signs of toxicity were observed. Total metabolites showed a dose-dependent increase and a time-dependent decrease in offspring blood and brain tissue during lactation; the most common metabolites were -diol and -epoxide derivatives. Offspring from treated and control dams showed no differences in the total number of correct or incorrect lever presses or omissions throughout behavioral testing, exhibiting a similar ability to acquire original discrimination and reach criterion. However, on the first day of reversal, a dose-related decrease in correct responses and increase in incorrect responses was observed in offspring exposed to 600 and 1200 μg/kg/day. Response acquisition for the second reversal was not affected by treatment and was similar to the original discrimination for the treated groups.

In vitro studies have demonstrated the mechanistic plausibility of early embryo loss due to BaP. The migration and invasion of HTR-8/SVneo trophoblast cells were inhibited at BaP concentrations ≥1 μM (Liu et al., 2016a), suggesting an adverse effect on implantation. BaP caused cell cycle arrest in the JEG-3 human trophoblast cancer cell line but not in ex vivo human trophoblasts from term placentas (Wakx et al., 2016). An increase in reactive oxygen species and in the percentage of apoptotic cells was observed in mouse preimplantation embryos exposed to ≥5 nM BaP (Zhan et al., 2015). Another in vitro study showed that benzo[a]pyrene-7,8-diol-9,10-epoxide, a metabolite of BaP, can adversely affect embryo implantation by the induction of apoptosis of trophoblast cells, which create the outer layer of the embryo and develop into part of the placenta in human cell lines (Wang et al., 2017d, 2018).

In an in vitro study using rat cells, researchers showed the importance of the timing of exposure on the sensitivity of neurodifferentiation, presumably resulting in neurodevelopmental effects and behavioral effects. The differentiation of neurotypic PC12 cells (already set to become neural cells) was more sensitive to BaP, but embryonic stem cells (not yet determined to become neural cells) were more sensitive to the PAH mixture (Slotkin et al., 2017).

Although the routes of exposure studied in animal studies are not always identical to the major routes of exposure relevant to human populations, it is important to note that these findings align with the findings from epidemiological studies.

Epigenetic Effects

Three CCCEH studies assessed the epigenetic effects of PAHs by measuring DNA methylation in cord blood (Herbstman et al., 2012; Perera et al., 2009a; Tang et al., 2012). Herbstman et al. (2012) analyzed umbilical cord white blood cells from 164 newborns and reported that decreased global methylation was associated with prenatal PAH exposure ($\beta = -0.11$, 95% CI –0.21–0.0), there were no associations between methylation and urinary metabolites, and increased global methylation was associated with BaP adducts in cord blood (OR=2.35, 95% CI 1.35–4.09). In an in vitro study, Tang et al. (2012) found that prenatal PAH exposure was associated with an increased methylation of the interferon gamma (*IFNγ*) promoter region in umbilical cord blood white blood cells from 53 CCCEH participants (low PAH 88.7% methylation versus high PAH 97.1% methylation, $p<0.01$). There was no association with *IL4* promoter methylation. The *IFNγ* gene is related to asthma risk. An analysis by Perera et al. (2009a) examined the methylation of *ACSL3* 5′CGI because hypermethylation at this location and the degree of gene expression were strongly correlated with PAH exposure. Among 56 children in the CCCEH cohort, prenatal PAH exposure (above or below 2.41ng/m^3) was associated with the methylation of *ACSL3* 5′CGI (OR=13.8, 95% CI 3.8–50.2) and methylation was associated with asthma diagnosed before the age of 5 years (OR=3.9, 95% CI 1.1–14.3).

In a cohort of 106 pregnant Chinese women, urinary PAH metabolites were found to be significantly associated with birth outcomes, although global methylation (as represented by LINE-1 and Alu repetitive elements) in cord DNA was not found to mediate the association between urinary PAHs and birth outcomes. Specifically, two PAH metabolites (2-OHNa and 1-OHPh) out of the 10 that were measured were associated with lower Alu methylation, with no significant relationships between PAH metabolites and LINE-1 methylation (Yang et al., 2018).

In a small case control study of 20 children with neural tube defects and 20 controls, PAH content in fetal neural tissue and maternal serum was positively correlated with methylation at two CpG sites (*CTNNA1* and *MYH2*), with the correlation confirmed in a mouse model using in utero exposure to BaP. The results led researchers to conclude that the hypermethylation of those two genes is associated with an increased risk of neural tube defects (Wang et al., 2017c).

Godschalk et al. (2015) investigated BaP mutations in the germ lines of male mice that were deficient for nucleotide excision repair gene *Xpc* ($Xpc^{-/-}$) as well as in the germ lines of their wild-type littermates. Males were bred 6 weeks after exposure ceased (13 mg/kg BaP, 3 days/week for 6 weeks by gavage). Although DNA adducts in the testes of F0 mice were unaffected, the litters fathered by treated $Xpc^{-/-}$ males were significantly smaller ($p=0.014$) than the controls, but the litter size of exposed wild-type males was only slightly smaller than that of controls, and the difference was not significant. Significant testicular

DNA hypomethylation was found in the wild-type treated males but not in the *Xpc*$^{-/-}$ treated males, compared with their respective controls. The global methylation of retrotransposons in liver samples of offspring was not affected by paternal treatment. The mutation rates of paternal origin were increased only in offspring from repair-deficient sires treated with BaP (0.056±0.020 versus 0.017±0.013 for controls; p=0.034), and there was no effect of exposure on mutation rates in wild-type males.

An animal study found changes in adult weight gain and increased adult adipocyte size in males and females in the F1 and F2 generations as well as increased expression of peroxisome proliferator-activated receptor γ, Cox2, and C/EPBα in white and brown adipose tissue. Sex and tissue differences were also present for certain adipogenic genes (i.e., Adipoq and Fas expression) (Yan et al., 2014).

Taken together, the human and animal studies suggest that prenatal PAH exposure can elicit changes in the methylation status of coding and noncoding segments of genes and the repetitive elements associated with prenatal PAH exposure.

Synthesis and Conclusions

Reproductive Effects

Reproductive Effects in Men and Women In general, higher PAH levels, assessed using a number of different markers, were found to be associated with significantly higher sperm DNA damage and genetic alterations (Gaspari et al., 2003; Gu et al., 2010; Han et al., 2010; Hsu et al., 2006; Jeng et al., 2013a,b; Jurewicz et al., 2013b; Radwan et al., 2016; Rubes et al., 2005; Song et al., 2013; Xia et al., 2009), including polymorphisms in the xeroderma pigmentosum group A gene, which have been shown to have deleterious effects on spermatogenesis in mice (Gu et al., 2010). Higher concentrations of PAH biomarkers were associated with polymorphisms in the nucleotide excision repair pathway linked to sperm DNA damage, which could provide critical information about the mechanisms involved (Gu et al., 2010).

Other associations with PAH exposure include altered hormone levels, including abnormal and "super" normal LH levels and abnormal levels of FSH and estradiol (Han et al., 2010). Other studies show associations between urinary 1-OHP concentrations and sperm neck abnormalities and decreased semen volume and sperm motility (Jeng et al., 2013a, 2015; Jurewicz et al., 2013b). Associations were stronger in smokers and had some seasonal variation. In addition, associations were seen for total sex chromosome disomy and sperm aneuploidy (Radwan et al., 2016). Occupational studies also show associations between higher PAH levels and male reproductive outcomes, including sperm dysfunction (Hsu et al., 2006; Jeng et al., 2013b, 2015).

The committee noted that research based in several populations shows sperm dysfunction and effects on DNA integrity in epidemiologic studies from a variety of populations and that these effects are supported by results from animal studies. However, because most of the studies on sperm effects assessed exposure using PAH metabolites sampled at the same time as sperm was collected, and PAHs are quickly metabolized, it is unclear if these results reflect long-term effects.

The known effects of PAH exposure on female reproduction are few, with only one study each having been done on fecundability, hormone changes, and PCOS (Luderer et al., 2017a; Slama et al., 2013; Yang et al., 2015). While the evidence of female preconception reproductive outcomes is based on a small number of limited-power epidemiological studies, toxicology and animal-based studies have found mechanistic associations between PAHs and decreased fertility, ovarian effects, decreased estradiol levels, and uterine inflammation (EPA, 2017).

The Volume 11 committee concludes that there is limited/suggestive evidence of an association between exposure to PAHs and reproductive effects in men.

The Volume 11 committee also concludes that there is inadequate/insufficient evidence to determine whether an association exists between exposure to PAHs and reproductive effects in women.

Adverse Pregnancy Outcomes Birth weight and prenatal PAH exposure were assessed in five cohorts, with significant associations reported in two (Choi et al., 2008, 2012; Guo et al., 2012; Langlois et al., 2014; Perera et al., 2005b; Polanska et al., 2010, 2014; Wang and Choi, 2014). Two studies found associations between prenatal PAH exposure and preterm birth (Padula et al., 2014a; Singh et al., 2008). Some measures of BaP and PAH exposure were associated with missed abortion (Wu et al., 2010), and one study reported the effects of certain species of PAHs on the levels of FSH and AMH in umbilical cord serum (Yin et al., 2017). Additionally, the ability of BaP to cause reproductive and developmental effects, including reduced birth weight, had been previously described by EPA (2009). Animal models also suggest that BaP exposure in the second trimester has a dose-dependent effect on fetal survival in pregnant rats and mice. Furthermore, animal studies have reported accumulations of PAHs in the placenta, umbilical cord, and endothelium as well as in neonatal white blood cells (Bocskay et al., 2005).

Together, these epidemiologic and animal studies provide limited/suggestive evidence that PAHs may have an association with adverse birth outcomes.

The Volume 11 committee concludes that there is limited/suggestive evidence of an association between prenatal PAH exposure and adverse birth outcomes—specifically, low birth weight and preterm birth.

Developmental Effects

Associations between prenatal PAH exposure and birth defects were investigated in the NBDPS in the United States and in birth cohorts in China. In the United States, increased risks were found for cleft lip, gastroschisis, and craniosynostosis but not for congenital heart defects or neural tube defects (Langlois et al., 2012, 2013; Lupo et al., 2012a,b; O'Brien et al., 2016). These analyses relied on an industrial hygienist's assessment of the maternal self-reported exposures, including occupational exposures, with no assessment of paternal exposures. No associations were seen between maternal occupations that have higher levels of PAH exposure and congenital heart defects (Lupo et al., 2012b). Studies conducted in one region of China at different times showed an inverse association between PAH exposure in 2005–2007 and neural tube defects, and by 2010–2012 there was a significant dose–response relationship between risk of neural tube defects and PAH–DNA adducts (Yi et al., 2015; Yuan et al., 2013). However, the Chinese studies failed to control for confounding factors, including cigarette smoking. The associations with neural tube defects were relatively consistent across study populations and exposure assessment methods.

Prenatal PAH exposure was associated with some childhood cancers, including ALL, neuroblastoma, medulloblastoma, and Wilms' tumor. However, studies used various distances to air monitoring stations (ranging from 2.5 km to 15 miles) to represent PAH exposure, which may have introduced exposure misclassification, and the associations with trimesters of exposure and specific species of PAHs were inconsistent.

Given that some PAHs are known carcinogens, and considering the recent data showing that prenatal exposure to PAHs is associated with an increased risk of certain tumors, the evidence suggests that these chemicals could affect cancer risk in offspring.

A variety of neurodevelopmental, cognitive, and behavioral deficits have been associated with prenatal PAH exposure up to age 9 years. Few of these studies, however, controlled for postnatal exposures that might contribute to neurobehavioral changes.

Studies of neurobehavioral effects and PAH exposure have used several proxies for exposure, including DNA adducts in cord blood, maternal urinary metabolites, personal sampling, and residential location in polluted areas. Systematic reviews have indicated that prenatal PAH exposure have an impact on neurodevelopment and IQ scores but have also noted the difficulties involved in distinguishing the effects of PAHs from other pollutants (Perera et al., 2011; Polanska et al., 2012; Suades-Gonzalez et al., 2015). The studies reviewed by the committee reported decrements for many different outcomes and measures in association with prenatal PAH exposure, including brain development (BDNF, white matter surface disturbances), MDI scores, mental health scores, and IQ scores; delays in developing motor skills and adaptive and social capabilities (Edwards et al., 2010; Perera et al., 2009b, 2014, 2015; Peterson et al., 2015; Tang et al., 2014b; Vishnevetsky et al., 2015) were also reported in assocation with prenatal PAH exposure. Two studies found no effects on psychomotor or mental development (Perera et al., 2007; Polanska et al., 2013). However, those studies of neurodevelopment were limited to maternal exposures assessed during second and third trimesters of pregnancy, and no studies examined the effects of preconception or first-trimester exposure, or paternal exposure. Neurodevelopmental effects were significantly influenced by factors such as breast-feeding (Jedrychowski et al., 2015a), maternal hardship (Vishnevetsky et al., 2015), nutrition/antioxidant levels (Genkinger et al., 2015), and environmental tobacco smoke (Polanska et al., 2013). None of these studies adjusted for the effects of PAH exposure between birth and the time of the assessment. EPA's review of BaP did describe supporting evidence for the neurodevelopmental toxicity that has been observed in animal studies (EPA, 2017).

Respiratory effects associated with prenatal PAH exposure were studied in one cohort that assessed prenatal PAH exposure with personal monitors in the second trimester as well as by measuring adducts in maternal and cord blood and maternal urinary metabolites. Significant associations were found between those measures and respiratory symptoms in the first year of life (Jedrychowski et al., 2005). Both prenatal exposure and exposure at 3 years were associated with lung function between the ages of 5 and 9 (Jedrychowski et al., 2015c). In analyses that considered postnatal exposure (measured at age 3), PAH exposure in childhood was found to have a significant effect on respiratory conditions (Jedrychowski et al., 2014). Exposure to cigarette smoking and maternal atopy were significant factors associated with respiratory symptoms (Jedyrchowski et al., 2005, 2012). Additionally, some evidence suggests that respiratory symptoms caused by maternal exposure are mediated by epigenetic changes (Perera et al., 2009a).

The Volume 11 committee concludes that there is limited/suggestive evidence of an association between prenatal exposure to PAHs and developmental effects—specifically, birth defects, childhood cancer, neurodevelopmental effects, and respiratory outcomes—in childhood.

Some studies examined the effect of prenatal PAH exposure on child growth. The growth outcomes associated with that exposure include decreased head circumference, decreased rate of growth (height), and obesity (Jedrychowski et al., 2015b; Rundle et al., 2012; Tang et al., 2006, 2014b). The evidence from this limited number of studies suggests that PAHs could affect growth and metabolic health, but the possibility that the observed associations are related to unknown confounders limits interpretation.

The Volume 11 committee concludes that there is inadequate/insufficient evidence to determine whether an association exists between prenatal PAH exposure and other developmental effects.

TABLE 6-6 Summary of Reproductive and Developmental Effects of Polycyclic Aromatic Hydrocarbons

Study	Design/Population	Exposure	Results
Reproductive Effects			
Reproductive Effects in Men			
Gaspari et al. (2003)	Cross-sectional 182 men recruited from an infertility clinic (75 followed up for fertility status 1 year later) in Milan, Italy. 2001	PAH adducts measured in semen, self-reported occupational and lifestyle exposures.	Sperm abnormalities and fertility. PAH adducts correlated with physiologic forms (r= –0.18, p=0.016), abnormal head morphology (r=0.30, p=0.0001), and abnormal neck morphology (r= –0.21, p=0.009), but not sperm count or tail morphology. PAH adducts greater among those with any abnormality (p=0.04) but not among those with asthenospermia, oligospermia, or teratospermia. PAH adducts were greater in infertile men compared with fertile men (based on pregnancy status) after 1 year of follow-up (p=0.04). Associations were observed between alcohol and PAH adducts but not smoking and PAH adducts.
Gu et al. (2010)	Nested case control 620 infertile men and 273 fertile controls seeking care at a fertility clinic in Nanjing, China. 2005–2009	Urinary 1-OHP and four functional genotypes.	Sperm DNA integrity. No significant associations between 1-OHP and genotypes for *ERCC1* 8092C/A or *XPF* Ser835Ser. Significant associations between *XPA-4* G/A genotypes and *XPD* Lys751Gln genotypes and DNA damage among men with high 1-OHP (p<0.05) but not low 1-OHP. Interaction effects: 1-OHP × *XPA-4* G/A, p=0.02; 1-OHP × *XPD* Lys751Gln, p=0.08. Shows joint effects of PAH exposure and DNA repair gene polymorphisms on male reproductive capacity.
Han et al. (2010)	Cohort 562 men with unexplained male factor infertility, in Nanjing, China. 2004–2007	Urinary PAH metabolites 1-N, 2-N, 2-OHF, and 1-OHP.	Reproductive hormone levels in blood (FSH, LH, E2, T, PRL). Analysis as continuous variables: significant negative correlation between 1-OHP and LH (p=0.01), no other associations found. Analysis by tertiles of metabolites and trisections of hormones: Increased ORs and significant trends between LH and 1-N (p-trend=0.025); LH and 2-OF (p-trend = 0.019); FSH and 2-OF (p-trend=0.027); E2 and 2-OF (p-trend=0.047); E2 and 1-OP (p-trend= 0.025).

Study	Design/Population	Exposure	Results
Han et al. (2011)	Cross-sectional 232 men ages 20–40 years residing in Chongqing, China. 2007	Urinary hydroxylated PAH metabolites (2-OHNa, 9-OHPh, 2-OHF, 1-OHP).	Sperm DNA damage. No association between metabolites and semen parameters. Total PAH metabolites associated with PI+ cells (β=12.59, 95% CI 4.15–21.02) and Annexin V-/PI- (β= –13.02, 95% CI –21.55– –4.5), but not Annexin V+/PI- (β=0.03, 95% CI –0.11–0.17). Significant associations between 2-OHNa and Tail%, tail length, and TDM (ORs=13.26, 12.25, 7.55, all $p<0.05$). Total PAH metabolites associated with Tail% (β=15.96, 95% CI 8.86–23.07); but not tail length (β=16.56, 95% CI –0.39–33.52) or TDM (β=6.29, 95% CI –2.36–14.95). Adjusted for age, abstinence, smoking status.
Hsu et al. (2006)	Cross-sectional 48 coke oven workers in Taiwan. 2003	PAHs in personal breathing zone on first and third days after 2 days off; and urinary 1-OHP in urine collected post-shift on days when air monitoring was conducted.	Semen quality and DNA damage. Among smokers, topside-oven workers had significantly more individuals with oligospermia and asthenospermia, a greater percent of abnormal morphology, and less motility ($p<0.05$). No significant differences between nonsmoking side-oven and topside-oven workers. No association between air PAH and sperm quality. Significantly greater DNA denaturation (COMP αT, αT) among smoking topside-oven workers than nonsmoking and smoking side-oven workers ($p<0.05$). Urinary 1-OHP significantly related to abnormal morphology (β=0.107, p=0.012), chromatin structure integrity (COMP αT and αT, β=0.235 and 0.078, both $p<0.01$).
Jeng et al. (2013b)	Cross-sectional 36 coke oven workers and 15 administrative and security staff as controls, in Taiwan, ages 25–50.	PAHs in personal breathing zone air sampling on first and sixth days after a 2-day break; and urinary 1-OHP in urine collected before and after shifts on the first and sixth workdays and at the time of semen collection.	Semen quality and DNA integrity. No differences between exposed workers and controls for semen concentration, oligospermia, volume, pH, motility (progressive, nonlinear, non-progressive), morphology (total head defects, total coiled tail), vitality, and DNA fragmentation. Significant increases in immotile sperm, asthenospermia, and decreases in normal morphology, and bulky DNA adducts among exposed workers, especially those highly exposed.

continued

TABLE 6-6 Continued

Study	Design/Population	Exposure	Results
Jeng et al. (2013a)	Cohort 65 coke oven workers ages 25–60, in Taiwan.	Occupational exposure measured as urinary 1-OHP levels (pyrene metabolite); and personal breathing zone sampling for 16 PAHs.	Semen quality and DNA integrity. 1-OHP level not correlated with semen concentration, motility, vitality or DNA fragmentation; significantly correlated with morphology ($\beta = -0.28$, $p<0.05$), 8-oxodGuo ($\beta=0.37$, $p<0.05$), and bulky DNA adducts ($\beta=0.45$, $p<0.05$). Some PAH species were significantly correlated with sperm morphology (14 of 16), motility (4 of 16), 8-oxodGuo (2 of 16), and bulky DNA adducts (2 of 16).
Jurewicz et al. (2013b)	Cross-sectional 277 men attending an infertility clinic with normal semen concentration or slight oligozoospermia (15–300 mLn/mL), in Poland.	Urinary 1-OHP, collected at the same time as sperm and questionnaire.	Semen quality parameters: Sperm neck abnormalities (%) $\beta=2.12$, $p=0.001$; Volume (ml) $\beta= -0.06$, $p=0.014$; Motility (%) $\beta= -8.33$, $p=0.0001$; Static (%) $\beta= 0.16$, $p=0.018$. No significant association between 1-OHP and DFI, sperm head or tail abnormalities, semen concentration, atypical %, or measures of motility. Adjusted for age, smoking, past diseases, season, sexual abstinence.
Radwan et al. (2016)	Cross-sectional 181 men attending an infertility clinic with normal semen concentration or slight oligozoospermia (20–300mLn/mL), in Poland. 2008–2011	Urinary 1-OHP, collected at the same time as sperm and questionnaire.	Sperm aneuploidy. Total sex-chromosome disomy: $\beta=1.46$, 95% CI 1.05–2.03; Disomy 18: $\beta=1.22$, 95% CI 1.02–1.63. Nonsignificant results for other kinds of disomy (X-Y-18, X-X-18, Y-Y-18, 13-13, 18-18, 21-21, or total chromosome disomy). Adjusted for abstinence, age, smoking, season of year, past diseases.
Rubes et al. 2005	Cohort 36 men born 1974–1976, sampled 7 times between 1995–1997, in the Czech Republic.	Average ambient PAHs in the 90 days before sample collection based on a monitoring site.	Sperm DNA damage. No association between PAH/air pollution and sperm count or concentration, volume, motility, morphology, velocity, linearity, or aneuploidy. Only sperm chromatin abnormalities (%DFI) were related to PAHs/air pollution ($\beta=0.19$, 95% CI 0.02–0.36, adjusted for smoking and briefs).
Song et al. (2013)	Cross-sectional 53 men attending a fertility clinic, in Guangzhou, China. 2010–2011	PAHs in blood.	Semen quality. Total PAHs correlated with semen volume, concentration, progressive motility, and nonlinear motility ($r= -0.07$, 0.10, 0.07, -0.10, all $p<0.05$). Total PAHs not associated with motility ($\exp\beta=0.96$, 95% CI 0.85–1.81). Adjusted for age and BMI.

Study	Design/Population	Exposure	Results
Xia et al. (2009)	Case-control 513 infertile men (291 with normal semen quality, 222 with abnormal semen quality) and 273 fertile men, in Nanjing, China. 2004–2007	Urinary PAH metabolites (1-N, 2-N, 1-OHP, 2-OHF, sum PAHs).	Idiopathic infertility defined by semen quality. Mean PAH metabolite levels were lowest in controls and highest in cases with abnormal sperm (except for 1-N). Dose–response relationship by tertile of metabolites present for all 5 measures of PAHs, significant for 1-OHP, 2-OHF, and sum PAHs (p-value for trend=0.034, 0.022, and 0.022). Sum PAHs 2nd tertile OR=1.2, 95% CI 0.84–1.71; 3rd tertile OR=1.53, 95% CI 1.06–2.20; compared to 1st tertile, adjusted for age and abstinence time.
Yang et al. (2017b)	Cross-sectional 405 men visiting an infertility clinic in Wuhan, China. 2013 (See Yang et al., 2017a)	PAH metabolites in urine.	Sperm DNA damage. 9-OHF, highest versus lowest tertile, was associated with increased tail length and comet length (mean increases of 8.65%, 95% CI 2.53%–15.03%, p-value for trend=0.05; and 7.14%, 95% CI 2.33%–12.19%, p-value for trend=0.01, respectively). 9-OHPh, highest versus lowest tertile, was associated with decreased percentage of Annexin V–/PI–spermatozoa (mean decrease 5.38%, 95% CI –8.92– –1.86, p-value for trend=0.04). No significant associations for other metabolites or measures of DNA damage.
Yang et al. (2017a)	Cross-sectional 933 men visiting an infertility clinic in Wuhan, China. 2013 (See Yang et al., 2017b)	PAH metabolites in urine.	Semen quality. 1-OHNa, highest versus lowest quartiles, associated with decreased sperm count (–19.99%, 95% CI –33.83%– –3.34%), sperm concentration (–22.66% (95% CI –34.49%– –8.70%), and percentage of normal morphology (–2.35%, 95% CI –4.24%– –0.46%) (all p-value for trends <0.05). 9-OHPh associated with decreased semen volume (0.43 mL, 95% CI –0.74– –0.12) and sperm straight-line velocity (–1.34 μm/sec, 95% CI –2.37– –0.31) (both p for trends <0.05). 4-OHPh associated with decreased semen volume (0.31 mL, 95% CI –0.61– –0.01). No associations between the urinary PAH metabolites and the total sperm motility to progressive sperm motility. Suggests that naphthalene and phenanthrene are related to decreased semen quality.

continued

TABLE 6-6 Continued

Study	Design/Population	Exposure	Results
Conti et al. (2017)	Cross-sectional 86 men in Italy.	BaP adducts in sperm DNA, and BaP–metabolite adducts [anti--BPDE hydrolyzed DNA adducts or Tetrol I-1 (r-7,c-10t-8,t-9-tetrahydroxy-7,8,9, 10-tetrahydrobenzo(a)pyrene) and syn-BPDE hydrolyzed DNA adducts or Tetrol II-2 (8r-7,t-9,t--10,t-8-tetrahydroxy-7,8,9,10-tetrahydrobenzo(a)pyrene)]	Semen quality. Tetrol I-1 and Tetrol II-2 adducts were associated with decreased progressive motility (r= –0.26, p=0.014; r= –0.22, p=0.040), but not sperm concentration, normal forms, or count.
Reproductive Effects in Women			
Luderer et al. (2017a)	Cohort—California, Orange County, National Children's Study. 51 fertile women not intending to become pregnant/not using hormonal contraception, ages 18–44. Convenience sample. 2010–2012	Urinary hydroxylated PAH metabolites collected on the 10th day after menses onset for two or three cycles.	Endocrine endpoints: cycle length, follicular phase length, ovulatory status, LH, and estrone 3-glucuronide levels. Positive associations of fluorene metabolites and negative associations of naphthalene metabolites with two measures of LH surge amplitude. Positive associations of 2-OHNa and 1-OHP and negative association of phenanthrene metabolites with average follicular LH. Follicular phase length was positively associated with 3-OHF and 11-OHP.
Slama et al. (2013)	Cohort 1,916 births in the Czech Republic. 1994–1999	Average monthly concentrations of total carcinogenic PAHs at an air-monitoring site.	Self-reported time to pregnancy. Probability of pregnancy during first month of unprotected intercourse not related to average total PAH concentration in fully adjusted model. Excluded unplanned pregnancies, 12 months of infertility, and fertility treatments.
Yang et al. (2015)	Case-control 50 cases of PCOS and 30 controls recruited from a hospital in Northern China. 2012	EDCs in blood (PCBs, organochlorine pesticides, and PAHs).	Polycystic ovary syndrome. dl-PCBs OR=5.52, 95% CI 1.51–20.2 and all PCBs OR=3.34, 95% CI 0.9–11.6. Organochlorine pesticides OR=14.8, 95% CI 3.2–68.8; PAHs OR=4.04, 95% CI 1.16–14.0; hydroxyl-PAHs OR=1.12, 95% CI 0.37–3.41. Octylphenol, nonylphenol, and BPA all nonsignificant. Adjusted for triglycerides, cholesterol, age, education, occupation.

Study	Design/Population	Exposure	Results
Adverse Pregnancy Outcomes			
Choi et al. (2008)	Prospective cohort—CCCEH. 616 children of African American and Dominican women living in Washington Heights, Harlem, or South Bronx, NY, recruited 1998–2005.	Personal monitoring in third trimester for PAHs. Total PAHs expressed as ln.	Gestational age: African American mothers $\beta = -0.35$, 95% CI –0.71–0.006 Dominican mothers $\beta = -0.006$, 95% CI –0.19–0.18 Preterm delivery: African American mothers OR=4.68, 95% CI 1.84–11.89 Dominican mothers OR=0.52, 95% CI 0.18–1.50 Adjusted for BMI, sex, parity, delivery season, ETS exposure. SGA: African American mothers OR=2.43, 95% CI 1.05–5.62 Dominican mothers OR=0.87, 95% CI 0.51–1.47 Adjusted for BMI, ETS exposure, parity, winter delivery. Fetal growth ratio <85%: African American mothers OR=1.93, 95% CI 1.04–3.56 Dominican mothers OR=0.82, 95% CI 0.51–1.33 Adjusted for BMI, gestational weight gain, ETS exposure, parity.
Choi et al. (2012)	Prospective cohort 344 pregnant women in Krakow, Poland, recruited 2000–2003. (See Wang and Choi, 2014)	Personal monitoring of PAHs for 48 hours in each trimester.	Birth size. PAH exposure in the first trimester is associated with a reduction of markers for growth restriction.
Guo et al. (2012)	Cohort: 183 pregnant women from Guiya, where there was open combustion of e-waste, and 80 pregnant women from Chaonan, China. 2008–2009	PAH concentrations in cord blood.	Adverse birth outcomes. Total PAHs not related to birth height, weight, gestational age, APGAR score, or BMI. Height negatively associated with BaA ($\beta = -0.23$, $p=0.006$); gestational age negatively associated with chrysene ($\beta = -0.20$, $p=0.013$) and BaP ($\beta = -0.17$, $p=0.042$).

continued

TABLE 6-6 Continued

Study	Design/Population	Exposure	Results
Langlois et al. (2014)	Cross-sectional—NBDPS. 2803 births without birth defects (221 were SGA).	Any self-reported maternal occupational PAH exposure in the month before conception through third month of pregnancy, assigned by an industrial hygienist.	SGA. OR=2.2 (95% CI 1.3–3.8) (adjusted for maternal age). 17 SGA births had PAH exposure.
Padula et al. (2014)	Cohort—SAGE study, Fresno, CA. 42,904 births to women living within 20 km of a monitoring site. 2001–2006	Prenatal exposure is the modeled sum of semi-volatile PAHs based on maternal residence on birth certificate.	PTB on birth certificates. No association between gestational ages 34–36 weeks, 32–33 weeks, 28–31 weeks and PAHs in any trimester. PTB 20–27 weeks gestation associated with PAHs in the 6 weeks before birth OR=2.74 (95% CI 2.24–3.34). Dose response for quartiles of exposure, compared to lowest exposure: 2nd quartile OR=1.49 (95% CI 1.08–2.06); 3rd quartile OR=2.63 (95% CI 1.93–3.59); 4th quartile OR=3.94 (95% CI 3.03–5.12). Stratification by month conceived: greatest association between PTBs and PAHs in the last 6 weeks of pregnancy for births conceived in June–August (20–27 weeks gestation OR=10.2, 95% CI 7.8–13.4). All adjusted for maternal age, education, race/ethnicity, first trimester prenatal care, payment of birth expenses.
Perera et al. (2005b)	Cohort—WTC. 186 women pregnant as of 9/11/01 who delivered at hospitals near the WTC, NY in December 2001–June 2002.	BaP–DNA adducts in maternal and/or cord blood samples at delivery; residential and work addresses in relationship to WTC.	Birth outcomes in medical records. No significant relationship between BaP adducts and birth weight, length, or head circumference. Significant effect of BaP adduct x ETS interaction on head circumference.

Study	Design/Population	Exposure	Results
Polanska et al. (2010)	Prospective cohort—REPRO_PR. 449 mother–child pairs recruited at 8–12 weeks of pregnancy, in Poland.	PAH exposure determined by urinary 1-OHP collected at 20–24 weeks pregnancy.	Size at birth as reported by gynecologist or neonatologist. Birthweight (g) $\beta = -105.40$, $p=0.10$; Length (cm) $\beta = -0.40$, $p=0.30$; Head circumference (cm) $\beta = -0.30$, $p=0.20$; Chest circumference (cm) $\beta = -0.40$, $p=0.07$; Ponderal index (g/cm^3) $\beta = -0.003$, $p=0.40$; and Cephalization index (cm/g) $\beta=3.0$, $p=0.09$. Adjusted for gestational age, gender, marital status, education level, season of last menstruation period, prepregnancy BMI, weight gain in pregnancy, saliva cotinine level.
Polanska et al. (2014)	Prospective cohort—REPRO_PR. 210 mother–child pairs recruited at 8–12 weeks of pregnancy, in Poland.	PAH exposure determined by urinary metabolites collected at 20–24 weeks pregnancy.	Size at birth as reported by gynecologist/neonatologist. None of the metabolites were significantly associated with birth weight, cephalization index, chest circumference, length, head circumference, or ponderal index, adjusted for gestational age and gender. Interaction of OH-PHE and environmental tobacco smoke associated with cephalization index ($p=0.04$).
Singh et al. (2008)	Case-control 29 preterm deliveries versus 31 full-term deliveries, in India. 2005–2006	Prenatal exposure; placental concentration of 10 PAHs.	PTBs. Concentrations for almost all PAHs higher among PTBs; fluoranthene (mean: 208.6 versus 325.91) and benzo(b) fluoranthrene (mean: 23.84 versus 61.91) were significantly higher ($p<0.05$).
Wang and Choi (2014)	Prospective cohort 344 nonasthmatic children of pregnant women in Krakow, Poland, recruited 2000–2003. (See Choi et al., 2012)	Personal monitoring of PAHs for 48 hours in the second trimester.	Birth weight, height, and head circumference. Reduced head circumference associated with PAHs across the pregnancy but not significant. Reduced birth weight and height associated with PAHs, but only significant in the first and third trimesters. Adjusted for season of birth, gestational age at birth, gender, parity, c-section, prepregnancy weight, and maternal height.

continued

TABLE 6-6 Continued

Study	Design/Population	Exposure	Results
Yang et al. (2018)	Cohort 106 pregnant women in China. 2011–2012	PAH metabolites in urine of pregnant women during late pregnancy.	Birth outcomes and DNA methylation of *LINE1* and Alu repetitive elements to represent global DNA methylation in cord blood. Decreased birth length associated with 2-OHNa and ΣOH-PAHs, first versus third tertiles (-0.80%, 95% CI –1.39%– –0.20%; and –0.70%, 95% CI –1.39%– –0.10%). No associations between PAH metabolites and birth weight or gestational age. Decreased Alu methylation associated with 1-OHPh and 2-OHNa (2.57%, 95% CI –4.30%– –0.80%; and 1.88%, 95% CI –3.73%– –0.10%). No significant associations between *LINE-1* methylation and PAH metabolites. Alu and *LINE-1* methylation were not mediators of the associations between PAH metabolites and birth outcomes.
Dejmek et al. (2000)	Cohort 4854 births (446 IUGR births) in Teplice and Prachatice, Czech Republic. 1994–1998	Modeled PAHs based on air monitors.	IUGR; birthweight <10th percentile. For births in Teplice, levels of PAH exposure in the first gestation month was associated with IUGR: medium levels OR=1.60 (95% CI 1.06–2.15) and high levels OR=2.15 (95% CI 1.27–3.63), per 10 ng increase of PAH, OR=1.22 (95% CI 1.07–1.39). Adjusted for parity, maternal age and height, prepregnancy weight, education, marital status, month-specific maternal smoking, season, rhythm, and year of the study. Similar results for births from Prachatice. No clear associations for exposure during other months of gestation.
Jedrychowski et al. (2017)	Cohort 455 infants in Krakow, Poland. 2002–2004	PAHs measured by personal monitor for 48 hours in the second trimester.	Birth outcomes (weight, length, and head circumference). Analyses also considered PM exposure; PAH exposure was more strongly related to birth outcomes than PM. Birth weight: $\beta= -0.20$, $p=0.004$ Birth length: $\beta= -0.17$, $p=0.025$ Head circumference: $\beta= -0.13$, $p=0.086$ Adjusted for maternal education (years), child sex, parity, maternal prepregnancy weight (kg), weight gain in pregnancy (kg), gestational age (weeks), exposure to environmental tobacco smoke (yes versus no), and birth season.

Study	Design/Population	Exposure	Results
Suzuki. et al (2010)	Cohort 149 pregnant women in Tokyo, Japan. 2005–2008	Metabolite of pyrene (1-OHP) in urine collected between gestational weeks 9 and 40.	Birth outcomes (weight, height, head circumference, gestational age). Statistically significant negative associations were observed between 1-OHP and birth weight ($\beta = -0.15$, $p=0.05$), birth length ($\beta = -0.18$, $p=0.02$) and head circumstances ($\beta = -0.17$, $p=0.05$). Analyses of nonsmokers only found no associations.
Al-Saleh et al. (2013)	Cross-sectional 1578 births in Saudi Arabia. 2005–2006	PAHs in placenta, maternal blood, and cord blood (BaP, and sum of benzo(a)anthracene, chrysene, benzo(b)fluoranthene, dibenzo(a,h)anthracene; and 1-OHP in maternal urine.	Birth outcomes (birth size, APGAR scores, placental weight and thickness, ponderal index, cephalization index) and markers of oxidative stress (malondialdehyde in cord and maternal serum and 8-hydroxy-2-deoxyquanosine in maternal urine). None of the tested PAHs was found in maternal or cord blood. All five PAH compounds were detected in placentas. Placental BaP associated with placental thickness ($\beta = -0.071$ cm, $p=0.018$) and cord length ($\beta = -0.074$ cm, $p=0.013$); sum of other placental PAHs associated with cord length ($\beta = -0.074$ cm, $p=0.013$); and urinary 1-OHP was not associated with any birth outcomes.
Snijder et al. (2012)	Cohort—Generation R Study. 4,680 births in the Netherlands.	Maternal occupational PAH exposure assessed by questionnaire and industrial hygiene assessment.	Fetal growth and birth outcomes. Placental weight: $\beta = -7.64$, 95% CI –52.03–36.76; Fetal weight: $\beta = -0.017$, SE=0.0080, $p<0.05$; Head circumference: $\beta = -0.011$, SE=0.011, $p>0.05$; Fetal length: $\beta = -0.0031$, SE=0.010, $p>0.05$.
Wu et al. (2010)	Case-control 81 cases of missed abortion and 81 controls (elective abortions) matched on hospital, maternal age, gravidity, gestational age, in Tianjin, China. 2007	BaP adducts in fetal tissue and maternal blood. Proxy measures of PAH exposure based on self-report.	Missed abortion (embryo has died but miscarriage has not occurred, in early pregnancy). No association between BaP adducts in fetal tissue and missed abortion. BaP adducts in maternal blood (per 10^8 nucleotides) increased risk of missed abortion—OR=1.35, 95% CI 1.11–1.64. Also associated with residence near traffic congestion (OR=3.07, 95% CI 1.31–7.16), commute by walking (OR=3.52, 95% CI 1.44–8.57), and routinely cooking during preganancy (OR=3.78, 95% CI 1.11–12.87). Adjusted for maternal education and household income.

continued

TABLE 6-6 Continued

Study	Design/Population	Exposure	Results
Yin et al. (2017)	109 pregnant women, in the Shendsi Islands, China. 2011–2012	16 PAHs in umbilical cord serum.	Reproductive hormones in umbilical cord serum. No significant associations between testosterone, luteotropic hormone, or estradiol and any PAHs; or between acenaphthylene, benzo(b)fluoranthene, benzo(k)fluoranthene, or BaP and any hormone. Significant positive associations between FSH and fluorine, phenanthrene, anthracene, fluoranthene, BaA, chrysene (β=0.47, 0.44, 0.51, 0.38, 0.42, 0.35, all $p<0.05$). Significant negative associations between anti-Müllerian hormones and naphthalene, acenaphthene, fluorine, and fluoranthene (β= –0.33, –0.33, –0.44, –0.35, all $p<0.05$). Adjusted for neonate gender, maternal age, prepregnancy BMI, gestational age, parity, number of abortions, education, pregnancy weight gain.
Developmental Effects			
Birth Defects			
Yi et al. (2015)	Case-control 60 cases of NTD and 60 controls matched on birth hospital, sex, mother's county of residence, mother's date of last menstrual period; born in northern Shanxi province, China. 2010–2012.	PAH adducts in umbilical cord tissue and blood.	Significant dose response for NTD, spina bifida, and anencephaly with tertiles of PAH adducts in cord tissue (p-value for trend<0.05 for each). NTDs at highest tertile of PAH adducts in tissue OR=2.96, 95% 1.16–7.58; Spina bifida at highest tertile OR=2.97, 95% CI 1.18–7.49; Anencephaly OR=3.12, 95% CI 1.14–8.55. Adjusted for maternal age, education, occupation, parity, hyperthermia during pregnancy, obesity, periconceptional folate supplement.

Study	Design/Population	Exposure	Results
Yuan et al. (2013)	Case-control 80 NTD-affected pregnancies and 50 uncomplicated pregnancies in Shanxi Province, China, 2005–2007.	PAHs and PAH adducts in placental tissue.	Controls had greater median concentration of PAH adducts than cases (9.92 versus 8.12 adducts/10^8 nucleotides, $p<0.05$). Dose response by PAH adduct tertiles showed inverse relationship: 1st tertile OR=1.48, 95% CI 0.59–3.75 and 2nd tertile OR=2.67, 95% CI 1.07–6.64, compared to the 3rd (highest) tertile (p trend=0.029). Trend also noted for spina bifida and anencephaly subtypes (p trend=0.054 and 0.081). Stratified by PAH and PAH adducts, only significantly elevated risks remained among those with high PAH exposure and low PAH adducts (OR=8.2, 95% CI 2.1–32.7). Adjusted for maternal age and hyperthermia.
Langlois et al. (2012)	Case-control—NBDPS 520 cases of NTD versus 2,989 controls. 1997–2002	Any self-reported maternal occupational PAH exposure in the month before conception through third month of pregnancy, assigned by an industrial hygienist.	NTDs. OR=1.01 (95% CI 0.61–1.66) (adjusted for BMI, second-hand smoke, study center). All adjusted ORs for subanalyses were close to 1.0 and not significant.
Langlois et al. (2013)	Case-control—NBDPS 805 cases of cleft lip with or without cleft palate, 439 cases of cleft palate versus 2,989 controls. 1997–2002	Any self-reported maternal occupational PAH exposure in the month before conception through third month of pregnancy, assigned by an industrial hygienist.	Cleft lip, with or without cleft palate. OR=1.47 (95% CI 1.02–2.12) (adjusted for maternal education). Cleft palate. OR=1.24 (95% CI 0.76–2.03) (adjusted for maternal secondhand smoke exposure).
Lupo et al. (2012a)	Case-control—NBDPS 299 cases of gastroschisis versus 2,993 controls. 1997–2002	Any self-reported maternal occupational PAH exposure in the month before conception through third month of pregnancy, assigned by an industrial hygienist.	Gastroschisis. OR=1.75, (95% CI 1.05–2.92) (adjusted for maternal age, BMI, education, gestational diabetes, maternal smoking, study center). Mothers <20 years old: OR=1.14 (95% CI 0.55–2.33); Mothers ≥20 years old: OR=2.53 (95% CI 1.27–5.04).
Lupo et al. (2012b)	Case-control—NBDPS 1,907 cases of congenital heart defects versus 2,853 controls. 1997–2002	Any self-reported maternal occupational PAH exposure in the month before conception through third month of pregnancy, assigned by an industrial hygienist.	Congenital heart defects. Conotruncal defects: OR=0.98 (95% CI 0.58–1.67); Left ventricular outflow tract defects: OR=1.31 (95% CI 0.74–2.30); Right ventricular outflow tract defects: OR=0.54 (95% CI 0.23–1.24); and Septal defects: OR=1.28 (95% CI 0.86–1.90). All adjusted for maternal age, race or ethnicity, education, smoking, folic acid supplement, study center.

continued

TABLE 6-6 Continued

Study	Design/Population	Exposure	Results
O'Brien et al. (2016)	Case-control—NBDPS 316 cases of craniosynstosis versus 2,993 controls. 1997–2002	Any self-reported maternal occupational PAH exposure in the month before conception through third month of pregnancy, assigned by an industrial hygienist.	Craniosynostosis. 16 cases exposed. OR=1.75 (95% CI 1.01–3.05) (adjusted for maternal age and education).
Childhood Cancer			
Bocskay et al. (2005)	Nested cohort—CCCEH 60 newborns of African American and Dominican women living in Washington Heights, Harlem, or South Bronx, NY, recruited, randomly selected.	Personal monitoring in third trimester for PAHs; PAH adducts in cord blood.	Chromosomal aberrations as markers of cancer risk. No associations between PAH air exposure or adducts and unstable aberrations. Stable aberrations associated with PAH air exposure, $r=0.35$, $p<0.0$, and $\beta=0.14$, $p=0.006$.
Heck et al. (2013a)	Case-control—California Cancer Registry, APCC 75 cases of childhood neuroblastoma younger than 6 years old versus 14,602 matched, randomly selected controls, within 5 km of an air monitor. 1990–2007	Modeled PAH exposure based on home address listed on birth certificate for each trimester of pregnancy.	Neuroblastoma. All nonsignificant at 5 km. At 2.5 km: Total PAHs OR=1.39 (95% CI 1.01–1.91); Benzo(k)fluoranthene OR=1.18 (95% CI 0.91–1.51); Benzo(a)pyrene OR=1.15 (95% CI0.91–1.46); Benzo(b)fluoranthene OR=1.19 (95% CI 0.91–1.58); Indeno(1,2,3-cd)pyrene OR=1.39 (95% CI 1.05–1.84); Dibenzo(a,h)anthracene OR=1.11 (95% CI 1.03–1.20); and Benzo(g,h,i)perylene OR=1.62 (95% CI 0.84–3.13). Adjusted for birth year, mother's age, mother's race/ethnicity, method of payment for prenatal care.
Omidakhsh et al. (2018)	Case-control 282 cases of retinoblastoma and 155 friend-controls recruited from multiple medical centers. 2006–2012	Paternal occupational PAH exposure in 10 years before conception, and maternal occupational PAH exposure in the month before conception ascertained by questionnaire.	Retinoblastoma in children up to 15 years old. Paternal PAH exposure 10 years before conception, unilateral retinoblastoma OR=1.34, 95% CI 0.48–3.72; bilateral retinoblastoma OR=1.51, 95% CI 0.36–6.38. Analyses of paternal PAH exposure 6 months before conception showed no association. Associations were stronger among fathers >30 years of age, fathers who had exposure to any hazardous agent, and a higher income bracket.

Study	Design/Population	Exposure	Results
Heck et al. (2014)	Case-control—California Cancer Registry, APCC Cases of childhood cancer younger than 6 years old matched with randomly selected controls based on data from birth certificates. 69 cases ALL versus 2,994 controls, within 2 km of an air monitor; 46 cases of AML versus 19,209 controls, within 6 km of an air monitor. 1990–2007	Modeled PAH exposure based on home address listed on birth certificate for each trimester of pregnancy.	ALL: Total PAHs through entire pregnancy OR=1.17 (95% CI 0.94–1.45); Total PAHs in 1st trimester OR=0.95 (95% CI 0.82–1.11); Total PAHs in 2nd trimester OR=1.04 (95% CI 0.94–1.14); and Total PAHs in 3rd trimester OR=1.16 (95% CI 1.04–1.29). Exposure to each individual PAH in 3rd trimester statistically significant, ORs range 1.06–1.27. AML: Total PAHs through entire pregnancy OR=1.07 (95% CI 0.69–1.65); Total PAHs in 1st trimester OR=0.88 (95% CI 0.63–1.21); Total PAHs in 2nd trimester OR=0.96 (95% CI 0.74–1.24); and Total PAHs in 3rd trimester OR=1.13 (95% CI 0.93–1.36). Adjusted for maternal race/ethnicity, birth year, parity, maternal birth place, neighborhood SES estimated by census block.
Shrestha et al. (2014)	Case-control—California Cancer Registry, APCC 337 cases of childhood Wilms' tumor younger than 6 years old versus 96,514 matched, randomly selected controls based on data from birth certificates, within 15 mi of an air monitor. 1990–2007	Modeled PAH exposure based on home address listed on birth certificate for each trimester of pregnancy.	Wilms' tumor. Total PAHs 1st trimester OR=0.99 (95% CI 0.88–1.12) 2nd trimester OR=1.06 (95% CI 0.98–1.15) 3rd trimester OR=1.10 (95% CI 0.99–1.22) Entire pregnancy OR=1.15 (95% CI 1.02–1.31) Adjusted for birth year, mother's age, mother's race/ethnicity, parity, SES estimated by census block.

continued

TABLE 6-6 Continued

Study	Design/Population	Exposure	Results
von Ehrenstein et al. (2016)	Case-control—California Cancer Registry, APCC Cases of childhood cancer younger than 6 years old matched, randomly selected controls. 43 cases of PNET, 34 cases of medulloblastoma, 106 cases of astrocytoma versus 30,569 controls, within 5 mi of an air monitor. 1990–2007	Modeled PAH exposure based on home address listed on birth certificate for each trimester of pregnancy.	PNET: Total PAHs OR=1.06 (95% CI 0.73–1.55); and All individual PAHs nonsignificant, ORs range 0.81–1.58. Medulloblastoma: Total PAHs OR=1.44 (95% CI 1.15–1.80); Benzo(k)fluoranthene OR=1.44 (95% CI 1.07–1.52); Benzo(a)pyrene OR=1.25 (95% CI 1.06–1.46); Benzo(b)fluoranthene OR=1.33 (95% CI 1.10–1.61); Indeno(1,2,3-cd)pyrene OR=1.38 (95% CI 1.13–1.69); Dibenzo(a,h)anthracene OR=1.07 (95% CI 1.01–1.14); and Benzo(g,h,i)perylene OR=1.94 (95% CI 1.20–3.14). Astrocytoma: Total PAHs OR=1.06 (95% CI 0.85–1.33). All individual PAHs nonsignificant, ORs range 0.96–1.09. Adjusted for maternal race/ethnicity, age, education, birth place, and birth year.
Neurobehavioral Outcomes			
Edwards et al. (2010)	Prospective cohort 214 children of pregnant women in Krakow, Poland. 2000–2006	Personal monitoring of PAHs for 48 hours in the second or third trimester.	Neurodevelopment (Raven Coloured Progressive Matrices score) at age 5. PAHs associated with significantly reduced neurodevelopmental scores. PAH (high versus low) $\beta = -1.36$, p=0.02 ln(PAH) $\beta = -0.56$, p=0.02 Both models adjusted for environmental tobacco smoke, sex of child, maternal education.

Study	Design/Population	Exposure	Results
Jedrychowski et al. (2015a)	Prospective cohort 170 children of pregnant women in Krakow, Poland, recruited 2000–2003.	PAH adducts in cord blood at birth; and household air monitoring for 48 hours at age 3.	IQ at age 7. 17 children had a depressed verbal IQ score. No significant IQ or covariate differences between detectable and non-detectable levels of PAH–DNA adducts in cord blood. To predict depressed verbal IQ scores ≥22 points below: Cord blood adducts RR=3.0 (95% CI 1.32–6.79); Postnatal PAH RR=1.63 (95% CI 1.03–2.53). Exclusive breast feeding (6+ months) RR=0.31 (95% CI 0.11–089). Adjusted for birth season, birth season × PAH–DNA adducts interaction, maternal education, gender, parity.
Perera et al. (2007)	Prospective cohort 98 children of women pregnant as of 9/11/01 who delivered at hospitals near the WTC, NY in December 2001–June 2002.	BaP–DNA adducts in maternal and/or cord blood samples at delivery; residential and work addresses in relationship to WTC.	Development at age 3 documented in medical records. No significant effect of BaP adducts on psychomotor development index or MDI. Significant interaction of BaP adducts × ETS on mental development index (β= −12.25, p=0.02).
Perera et al. (2009b)	Prospective cohort—CCCEH 249 children of African American and Dominican women living in Washington Heights, Harlem, or South Bronx, NY, recruited 1998–2003.	Personal monitoring in third trimester for PAHs. Does not distinguish between prenatal and postnatal exposures.	IQ (Wechsler Preschool and Primary Scale of Intelligence-Revised) at age 5. IQ versus high or low PAH exposure (< or >2.26ng/m^3): Full-scale IQ β= −4.31, p=0.007; Verbal IQ β= −4.67, p=0.003; Performance IQ β= −2.37, p=0.17. Adjusted for ETS exposure, gender, maternal education, ethnicity, HOME score, Test of Maternal Nonverbal Intelligence, Third Edition score. IQ versus ln(PAH): Full-scale IQ β= −3.0, p=0.009; Verbal IQ β= −3.53, p=0.002; and Performance IQ β= −1.47, p=0.24.

continued

TABLE 6-6 Continued

Study	Design/Population	Exposure	Results
Perera et al. (2012)	Prospective cohort—CCCEH 253 children of African American and Dominican women living in Washington Heights, Harlem, or South Bronx, NY, recruited 1998–2003.	Personal monitoring in third trimester for PAHs; BaP adducts in maternal and cord blood at delivery. BaP used as proxy for PAHs. Does not distinguish between prenatal and postnatal exposures.	Behavior at ages 6–7 (CBCL). Anxious/Depressed Scale: Environmental PAH (high/low) OR=8.89, 95% CI 1.7–46.51 and PAH (continuous) OR=1.2, 95% CI 1.06–1.37); Maternal and cord adducts ORs=1.42 and 2.56, both non-significant. Attention problems scale: Environmental PAH (high/low) OR=3.79, 95% CI 1.14–12.66; Maternal and cord adducts ORs=2.24 and 4.06, both non-significant. Anxiety disorder DSM-IV: Environmental PAH (high/low) OR=4.59, 95% CI 1.46–14.27 and PAH (continuous) OR=2.03, 95% CI 0.97–4.26; Maternal and cord adducts ORs=2.19 and 2.53, both non-significant. ADHD DSM-IV: Environmental PAH (high/low) OR=2.3, 95% CI 0.79–6.7 and PAH (continuous) OR=1.54, 95% CI 0.7–3.4; Maternal and cord adducts, ORs=1.84 and 2.64, both non-significant. Adjusted for prenatal ETS, sex of child, gestational age, maternal IQ, HOME inventory, maternal education, ethnicity, prenatal demoralization, age at assessment, season.

Study	Design/Population	Exposure	Results
Perera et al. (2014)	Prospective cohort—CCCEH 250 children of African American and Dominican women living in Washington Heights, Harlem, or South Bronx, NY, recruited 1998–2006.	BaP adducts in maternal and cord blood at delivery; urinary PAH metabolites at ages 3 or 5 years.	ADHD and behavior at age 9 (CBCL and CPRS). Cord blood adducts not related to any ADHA outcome. CBCL ADHD not related to PAH exposure. Maternal BaP adducts related to CPRS scales: ADHD index β=0.14, 95% CI 0.03–0.25, OR=1.83, 95% CI 0.61–5.54; DSM-IV hyperactive-impulsive β=0.16, 95% CI 0.03–0.29, OR=1.58, 95% CI 0.55–4.52; DSM-IV inattentive β=0.17, 95% CI 0.04–0.31, OR=5.06, 95% CI 1.43–17.93. Adjusted for postnatal PAH exposure by urinary metabolites at age 3 or 5, prenatal ETS, child sex, maternal education, ethnicity, gestational age, maternal demoralization, season, HOME caretaking environment, maternal intelligence, age at assessment, maternal ADHD, child anxiety/depression at age 9.
Perera et al. (2015)	Prospective cohort—CCCEH 505 children of African American and Dominican women living in Washington Heights, Harlem, or South Bronx, NY, recruited 1998–2006.	^{32}P post-labeling assay for PAH adducts in cord blood and BaP adducts in maternal and cord blood at delivery. Does not distinguish between prenatal and postnatal exposures.	BNDF in cord blood; MDI (using the Bayley Scales of Infant Development-Revised) at age 2. BaP-adducts not related to BNDF or MDI. Effect of ^{32}P adducts on MDI: β= –2.07, p=0.04; Effect of ^{32}P adducts on BDNF: β= –0.11, p=0.02; Effect of BNDF on MDI: β=2.69, p=0.003; Effect of ^{32}P adducts (and BNDF) on MDI: β= –1.92, p=0.07. Conclusion: PAHs affect development by reducing BNDF; BNDF plays a role in early brain development.
Peterson et al. (2015)	Prospective cohort—CCCEH 40 children of African American and Dominican women living in Washington Heights, Harlem, or South Bronx, NY, recruited 1998–2006.	Personal monitoring in third trimester for PAHs.	Brain white matter, cognition, and behavior (WISC-IV) at 7–9 years old. Prenatal PAH inversely correlated with white matter surface measures, especially the left hemisphere. Reduced white matter associated with externalizing problems and externalizing symptoms. High prenatal PAH associated with reduced processing speed during intelligence testing (mediated by white matter disturbances). Prenatal PAH not correlated with PAHs at age 5.

continued

TABLE 6-6 Continued

Study	Design/Population	Exposure	Results
Tang et al. (2014a)	Prospective cohort 150 newborns born March–June 2002 and 158 newborns born March–May 2005, residing within 2.5 km of operational Tongliang power plant in China (power plant shut down in 2004). (see Tang et al., 2014b)	Environmental air sampling at 3 sites in 2002–2003 and 2005–2006; BaP–DNA adducts (as proxy for PAH–DNA adducts) in maternal and cord blood at birth.	Development at age 2 (Gesell Developmental Schedule) and BDNF, a protein involved in neuronal growth, in umbilical cord blood. Lower mean levels of PAH–DNA adducts (0.204 versus 0.324 adducts/10^8 nucleotides), higher concentrations of BDNF (1266.57 versus 752.87 μg/dL) and higher DQ scores (100.3 versus 99.42) were in the 2005 cohort enrolled after closure of the power plant (all $p<0.05$). Among both groups combined, PAH–DNA adducts were correlated with BDNF ($r= -0.23$, $p<0.01$) as well as the change in motor scores ($\beta= -10.70$, $p = 0.05$), adaptive scores ($\beta= -16.48$, $p=0.022$), and average score ($\beta= -12.11$, $p=0.014$), after adjusting for cord blood lead, cord mercury, ETS, mother's education, mother's age, gestational age, and gender. BDNF levels (log BNDF) were associated with changes in motor ($\beta=2.12$, $p=0.018$), social ($\beta=3.22$, $p=0.001$), and average score ($\beta=2.50$, $p=0.017$), adjusted for cord PAH–DNA adducts, prenatal ETS, cord lead, cord mercury, gender, gestational age, mother's education, mother's age, and income.
Polanska et al. (2013)	Prospective cohort—REPRO_PR. 411 mother–child pairs examined at 1 year of age in Poland, 198 mother–child pairs examined at 2 years of age, recruited at 0–12 weeks of pregnancy in 2007.	PAH exposure determined by urinary 1-OHP collected at 20–24 weeks pregnancy.	Neurodevelopment at 1 or 2 years. 1-OHP levels not associated with psychomotor scores at 1 or 2 years.

Study	Design/Population	Exposure	Results
Vishnevetsky et al. (2015)	Prospective cohort—CCCEH 276 children of African American and Dominican women living in Washington Heights, Harlem, or South Bronx, NY, recruited 1998–2006.	PAH adducts in maternal and cord blood at delivery, PAH metabolites in urine at age 5.	IQ at age 7 using the WISC-IV. Effect of prenatal material hardship × adducts interaction on working memory $\beta = -8.07$, 95% CI –14.48– –1.66. Non-significant for full scale, verbal comprehension, processing speed, and perceptual reasoning. No associations between IQ components and PAH-adducts among low prenatal material hardship subjects. Among high prenatal material hardship subjects, PAH adducts associated with the full scale $\beta = -5.81$, 95% CI –10.35– –1.26; verbal comprehension $\beta = -3.36$, 95% CI –7.61–0.90; processing speed $\beta = -4.17$, 95% CI –9.75–1.41; perceptual reasoning $\beta = -5.44$, 95% CI –10.27– –0.61; and working memory $\beta = -6.67$, 95% CI –11.38– –1.95. Adjusted for ETS, sex, maternal education and intelligence, ethnicity, HOME caretaking.
Genkinger et al. (2015)	Cohort—CCCEH 151 children of African American and Dominican women living in Washington Heights, Harlem, or South Bronx, NY, recruited 1998–2006.	PAH exposure measured by personal air monitoring for 48 hours in the third trimester.	Behavior between 6 and 9 years of age modified by micronutrients measured in cord blood. Interactions were observed between the effects of prenatal micronutrients and PAH exposure on childhood behavior/symptoms. α-tocopheroland PAH: withdrawn/depressed $\beta=0.25$, $p=0.02$; aggressive behavior $\beta=0.15$, $p=0.02$; internalizing problems $\beta=0.11$, $p=0.03$; externalizing problems $\beta=0.11$, $p=0.04$. γ-tocopheroland PAH: internalizing problems $\beta=0.14$, $p=0.007$. Carotenoids and PAH: somatic complaints $\beta = -0.23$, $p=0.05$; aggressive behavior $\beta=0.14$, $p=0.02$; externalizing problems $\beta=0.12$, $p=0.02$. Retinol and PAH: no significant interaction effects. Adjusted for sex of the newborn, maternal gestational age, maternal years of education, maternal psychological distress, the age of the child at the time of the CBCL assessment, heating season, lead exposure, prenatal and postnatal environmental tobacco smoke, and dietary PAH.

continued

TABLE 6-6 Continued

Study	Design/Population	Exposure	Results
Growth			
Rundle et al. (2012)	Prospective cohort—CCCEH 702 children of African American and Dominican women living in Washington Heights, Harlem, or South Bronx, NY, in 1998–2006 (453 at age 5; 371 at age 7).	Personal monitoring in third trimester for PAHs. Does not distinguish between prenatal and postnatal exposures.	Obesity at ages 5 and 7. At age 5, compared to lowest tertile of PAH exposure (>1.73ng/m^3): PAH 2nd tertile (1.73–3.07 ng/m^3) RR= 1.79, 95% CI 1.08–2.98. PAH 3rd tertile (≥3.08 ng/m^3) RR=1.79, 95% CI 1.09–2.96. At age 7: PAH 2nd tertile RR=2.25, 95% CI 1.27–4.01. PAH 3rd tertile RR=2.26, 95% CI 1.28–4.00. Adjusted for birth weight, ethnicity, child's sex, maternal prepregnancy obesity, child age at measurement.
Tang et al. (2006)	Prospective cohort 150 newborns born March–June 2002 residing within 2.5 km of Tongliang power plant in China.	Environmental exposure estimated from number of months of gestation during power plant operation; PAH adducts in maternal and cord blood at birth.	Growth at birth, 18, 24, and 30 months. Maternal adducts not related to growth. High cord blood adducts (0.36 adducts/10^{-8} nucleotides) significantly associated with lower weight (p=0.023), smaller head circumference (p=0.056), but not height. Duration of exposure associated with height (p<0.001) but not weight or head circumference. Adjusted for ETS, sex, maternal height and weight.
Tang et al. (2014b)	Prospective cohort 150 newborns born March–June 2002 and 158 newborns born March–May 2005, residing within 2.5 km of operational Tongliang power plant in China (power plant shut down in 2004).	Environmental air sampling at 3 sites in 2002–2003 and 2005–2006; BaP adducts in maternal and cord blood at birth.	Growth at birth, 18, 24, and 30 months and IQ (Gesnel Developmental Scale) at age 2. The 2005 cohort had significantly lower environmental BaP and lower BaP adducts (p<0.001). Growth rates in the 2005 cohort were not greater than the 2002 cohort. Cord adducts significantly negatively associated with motor developmental quotient in the 2002 cohort, β= −16.01, p=0.043 (but not for adaptive, language, or social measures or any measures in the 2005 cohort).

Study	Design/Population	Exposure	Results
Jedrychowski et al. (2015b)	Prospective cohort 379 children of pregnant women in Krakow, Poland, recruited 2000–2004.	Personal monitoring of PAHs for 48 hours in the second trimester; and household air monitoring for 48 hours at age 3 years.	Height gain at age 9. Prenatal PAH exposure correlated with birth length ($r = -0.092$, $p<0.05$), but not height at older ages. Postnatal household PAHs not related to height. Height decreased 1cm for children exposed to PAHs >34.7 ng/m^3 ($p=0.04$), adjusted for cord blood Hg, cord blood Pb, prepregnancy maternal weight, maternal height, maternal weight gain in pregnancy, maternal education, sex of child, age of child, parity. Birth length and maternal height were the strongest predictors of child's height.
Respiratory Outcomes			
Jedrychowski et al. (2005)	Prospective cohort 333 pregnant women in Krakow, Poland, recruited 2000–2002.	Personal monitoring of PAHs for 48 hours in the second or third trimesters. Does not distinguish effects of prenatal from postnatal exposure.	Respiratory symptoms in first year of life—runny or stuffy nose, ear infection, cough, cough without cold, barking cough, difficult breathing, wheezing, wheezing without cold, sore throat. Statistically significant positive associations between either number of episodes and/or the duration for all the symptoms. Highest OR=4.8 (95% CI 2.73–8.44) for number of episodes of barking cough. Adjusted for child gender, birth weight, season of birth, postnatal ETS, mother's allergy, mother's education, and molds at home.
Jedrychowski et al. (2012)	Prospective cohort 82 nonasthmatic children of pregnant women in Krakow, Poland, recruited 2000–2002.	PAH adducts in cord blood at birth. Does not distinguish effects of prenatal from postnatal exposure.	Fractional exhaled nitric oxide at age 7. Regression model predicting fractional exhaled nitric oxide: Prenatal PAH exposure $\beta=0.32$, $p=0.006$; maternal atopy $\beta=0.25$, $p=0.03$; atopy $\beta=0.23$, $p=0.4$.
Jedrychowski et al. (2014)	Prospective cohort 257 children to pregnant women in Krakow, Poland, recruited 2000–2002.	Personal monitoring of PAHs for 48 hours in the second trimester; and survey of home and outdoor air pollution at age 3 years.	Wheezing (20 or more days in the follow-up period) up to age 4. Prenatal PAH OR=1.40 (95% CI 0.97–2.03); Postnatal PAH OR=1.61 (95% CI 1.16–2.24). Prenatal exposure modifies effect of postnatal exposure on wheezing. Adjusted for asthma and number of older siblings.

continued

TABLE 6-6 Continued

Study	Design/Population	Exposure	Results
Jedrychowski et al. (2015c)	Prospective cohort 195 nonasthmatic children of pregnant women in Krakow, Poland.	Personal monitoring of PAHs for 48 hours in the second trimester; and household air monitoring for 48 hours at age 3 years.	Lung function at ages 5–9; and atopy (skin prick) at ages 5–8. Highest tertiles of exposure for prenatal PAHs, indoor PAHs at age 3, and outdoor PAHs at age 3 significantly related to reduced FEV_{05}, FEV_1, FEF_{25-75} (only outdoor PAHs at age 3 related to reduced FVC). Adjusted for gestational age, gender, height, parity, atopic status, ETS, and season of residential air pollution survey.
Perera et al. (2009a)	Sub-cohort—CCCEH Children of African American and Dominican women living in Washington Heights, Harlem, or South Bronx, New York, recruited 1998–2006. 20 children sampled for DNAm and PAH analyses; 56 children sampled for analyses of DNAm and asthma.	Personal air monitoring for 48 hours in the third trimester.	Asthma and DNAm in cord blood and placental tissue. More than 30 DNA sequences were identified whose methylation status was associated with maternal PAH exposure; 6 sequences were related to genes with ≥1 5'CpG islands; and acyl-CoA synthetase long-chain family member 3 (*ACSL3*) had the highest concordance between methylation of 5'-CpG islands in umbilical cord white blood cells and the level of gene expression in matched fetal placental tissue in the initial 20 cohort children (tau= –0.45, 95% CI –0.76– –0.15). *ACSL3* is related to asthma and was then investigated in the sample of 56 children. *ACSL3* 59-CpG island methylation was significantly associated with high maternal airborne PAH exposure (>0.41 ng/m^3; OR=13.8; $p<0.001$; sensitivity=75%; specificity=82%) and with a parental report of asthma symptoms in children prior to age 5 (OR=3.9, 95% CI 1.1–14.3, $p<0.05$).

NOTE: ADHD=attention deficit–hyperactivity disorder; ALL=acute lymphoblastic leukemia; AML=acute myeloid leukemia; APCC=Air Pollution and Childhood Cancer Study; APGAR=Appearance, Pulse, Grimace, Activity, and Respiration; BaA=benzo[a]anthracene; BaP=benzo[a]pyrene; BMI=body mass index; BNDF= brain-derived neurotrophic factor; BPA=bisphenol; BPDE=benzo[a]pyrene diol-epoxide-DNA adducts; BSID=Bayley Scales of Infant Development II; CBCL=Child Behavioral Checklist; CCCEH=Columbia Center for Children's Environmental Health study; CI=confidence interval; COMP αT=cells falling outside of the main population; CTRS=Conner's parent rating scale-revised; DFI=DNA fragmentation index; DNA=deoxyribonucleic acid; DNAm=DNA methylation; DQ=development quotient; DSM-IV=*Diagnostic and Statistical Manual of Mental Disorders, Fourth Edition*; E2=estradiol; EDC=endocrine disrupting chemical; ETS=environmental tobacco smoke; FEF_{25-75}=forced expiratory flow 25–75%; $FEV_{0.5}$=forced expiratory volume in 0.5 s; FEV_1=forced expiratory volume in 1 s; FSH=follicle-stimulating hormone; FVC=forced volume capacity; HOME=Home Observation for Measurement of the Environment; IQ=intelligence quotient; IUGR=intrauterine growth restriction; LH=luteinizing hormone; MDI=mental development index; 1-N=1-naphthol; 2-N=2-naphthol; NBDPS=National Birth Defects Prevention Study; NTD=neural tube defect; 2-OF=2-hydroxyfluorene; OHNa=hydroxynaphtha¬lene; 1-OHP=1 hydroxypyrene; OHPh=hydroxyphenanthrene; OR=odds ratio; PAH=polycyclic aromatic hydrocarbon; PCB=polycyclic biphenyl; PCOS=polycystic ovary syndrome; PM=particulate matter; PNET=primitive neuroectodermal tumors; PRL=prolactin; PTB=preterm birth; RR=relative risk; SE=standard error; SES=socioeconomic status; SGA=small for gestational age; T=testosterone; TDM=tail distributed moment; WISC-IV=Wechsler Intelligence Scale for Children-IV; WTC=World Trade Center.

Polychlorinated Dibenzodioxins and Polychlorinated Dibenzofurans

PCDD/PCDFs are products of combustion that have been measured in the emissions from burn pits on military bases (IOM, 2011; Masiol et al., 2016a,b). Air monitoring at JBB in 2007 and 2009 showed that at some sampling locations PCDD/PCDFs concentrations were relatively high compared to urban and industrial areas, such as Beijing, with average concentrations reaching 1,309 fg I-TEQ/m^3 (IOM, 2011).[3] A pilot study showed that 400 Post-9/11 military personnel who had been deployed to bases operating burn pits or other regions had higher serum concentrations of PCDD/PCDFs congeners than the general U.S. population. For example, 2,3,7,8-tetrachlorodibenzo-*p*-dioxin (TCDD) was detected in 8 out of 800 serum samples, with a mean of 0.2 pg/mL (200 ppt[4]), compared to a geometric mean of <0.0038 pg/mL (3.8 ppt) in the general population, as reported in the 2003–2004 National Health and Nutrition Examination Survey. Pre- versus post-deployment samples indicated that exposures during deployment did not lead to increases in congener levels (Xia et al., 2016). Estimates of Vietnam veterans' exposures to PCDD/PCDFs as a result of the TCDD contamination of Agent Orange are also problematic because of the lack of data on individual behaviors and locations, of an understanding of the chemicals' behavior in the environment, and of contemporaneous chemical measurements. However, TCDD exposure estimates based on serum samples indicate that Vietnam veterans who sprayed Agent Orange (Ranch Hands, the most highly exposed group of veterans) were exposed to levels in the ppt range (about 10–20 ppt), which although higher than for ground troops, were an order of magnitude lower than exposure levels for occupational cohorts (20–300 ppt) and three orders of magnitude lower than exposure levels associated with the Seveso, Italy, industrial explosion (4,540–16,600 ppt) (NASEM, 2016; Pirkle et al., 1995).

Like PAHs, PCDD/PCDFs exist as part of a variable mixture of many species, the toxicity of which is usually presented based on the levels of the most toxic species (TCDD). Even though there are many species of PCDD/PCDFs, TCDD has been the most extensively studied species because of its high toxicity and its common occurrence in herbicides, including Agent Orange, during the Vietnam War. TCDD is a persistent compound with a biological half-life that in human studies has ranged from 3 months to more than 10 years depending on BMI, age, sex, and TCDD concentration (NASEM, 2016).

There is extensive information available about the health effects of TCDD from authoritative bodies such as EPA, ATSDR, and the National Academies, all of which have described studies on the health of children born to exposed parents. Specifically, in 2012 EPA released an assessment of TCDD and ATSDR released an assessment of the larger class of chemicals—chlorinated dibenzodioxins—both of which included literature published through 2011 (ATSDR, 2012; EPA, 2012). The most recent review, conducted by the National Academies in 2016, is the 10th update in the *Veterans and Agent Orange* (VAO) series on the health effects of Agent Orange in Vietnam veterans (NASEM, 2016). The Gulf War and Health Volume 11 committee relied on the 2016 VAO report and any new data published since that review's cutoff in 2014.

The 10th VAO report reviewed the literature on TCDD and other chemical constituents present in the herbicide mixtures used in Vietnam, through 2014, and found that

---

[3] *TEQs* are a weighted quantity measure based on the toxicity of each member of the dioxin and dioxin-like compounds category relative to the most toxic members of the category. TEQs are used to account for how dioxin and dioxin-like compounds vary in toxicity and to better understand the cumulative toxicity of mixtures of dioxin and dioxin-like compounds (EPA, 2016).

[4] 1 pg/mL=1,000 ppt; 1 ppt=0.001 pg/mL.

- The studies linking dioxin exposure with endometriosis are few and inconsistent. Although animal studies support the biologic plausibility of an association, contemporary human exposures may be too low to show an association consistently.
- Regarding fertility, although there was relative consistency in reports of reduced testosterone with the highest exposure and increased gonadotropins, levels were still within the normal ranges and clinical consequences were not expected. Only one study examined, and observed, the relationship between dioxin exposure in women and time to pregnancy and infertility, and no data were available regarding effects on menstrual cycle function in humans, thus data were insufficient.
- A single study concerning dioxin and spontaneous abortion, stillbirth, neonatal death, or infant death has been published since the previous volume, but it did not provide supporting evidence of an association between dioxin and these outcomes, nor do toxicologic studies provide clear evidence for the biologic plausibility of an association (p. 741).
- Although the animal literature does support an effect of TCDD exposure at high doses on birth weight, the epidemiologic literature is insufficiently robust to allow a final determination (p. 735).

Based on these findings, the VAO committee concluded that

> there is limited or suggestive evidence that paternal exposure to TCDD is *not* associated with risk of spontaneous abortion and that insufficient information is available to determine whether there is an association between maternal exposure to TCDD or either maternal or paternal exposure to 2,4-D, 2,4,5-T, picloram, or cacodylic acid and the risk of spontaneous abortion. The committee concludes that there is inadequate or insufficient evidence to determine whether there is an association between exposure to the COIs [chemicals of interest] and stillbirth, neonatal death, or infant death.

That same committee also gave special consideration to the possibility of adverse health outcomes at any time during the lives of all progeny of Vietnam veterans. Regarding the potential health effects in the children of Vietnam veterans, that committee found that

- It is clear that the fetal rodent is more sensitive to the adverse effects of TCDD than the adult rodent. Human data are generally lacking, however, and the sensitivity to developmental disruption in humans is less apparent, in part because contemporary studies of environmental dioxin exposure and birth defects have involved extremely low exposures. Human population-based studies have provided mixed results in attempts to link TCDD exposures to birth defects.
- No associations were observed in the two case-control studies that considered childhood ALL [acute lymphoblastic leukemia] and exposure to phenoxy herbicides and to 2,4-D in particular. Furthermore, evidence is sparse that exposure to dioxin increases the risk for childhood cancers.
- The animal literature contains evidence that environmental agents mediated by maternal exposure affect later generations through fetal and germ line modifications, but in the case of adult male exposures before conception of the next generation, there is insufficient evidence of transgenerational effects. Although it may be physiologically possible for paternal exposure to cause changes in offspring that are manifested later in life, none of the published epidemiologic studies assessed such potential. Thus, the observation of any changes reported in studies should be applicable only to children born to female Vietnam veterans during or after their deployment in Vietnam. Thus, no transgenerational studies have been reported to date.

The committee concluded that no adverse outcomes in future generations had sufficient evidence of an association with dioxin and that there was inadequate or insufficient evidence to determine whether there is an association between parental exposure to the chemicals of interest and birth defects, childhood cancers, or disease in the children of Vietnam veterans as they mature or in later generations (NASEM, 2016).

An 11th update in the *VAO* series is scheduled to be released in fall 2018. Like the previous volumes, it reviews any reproductive and developmental outcomes in Vietnam veterans and their descendants.

Because of the extensive volume of research conducted on dioxins, the Volume 11 committee limited its review to studies on reproductive, developmental, and generational effects published since the most recent NASEM review (see Table 6-7). The results include 26 human studies and 21 animal studies published since 2014.

Reproductive Effects

Reproductive Effects in Men and Women

In a case-control study in Belgium, subfertility was found to be not related to PCDD/PCDF exposure (OR=1.59, 95% CI 0.96–2.65) among 40 infertile men and 80 controls (Den Hond et al., 2015). A Russian study, however, identified levels of PCDD/PCDFs in the semen of 105 infertile men (both with and without abnormal sperm) that were more than twice as high as those in fertile men (n=63), but the results were not adjusted for any potential confounders (Galimova et al., 2015). Among 251 men living near a municipal waste facility in France, semen parameters were largely unaffected by PCDD/PCDF exposure except for a reduced multiple anomalies index (β= –0.013, 95% CI –0.023– –0.004) and fewer abnormal mid-pieces (β= –0.010, 95% CI –0.018– –0.002) by year as emissions decreased (Faure et al., 2014).

In a small case-control study of 30 women with deep infiltrating endometriosis and 30 controls, adipose samples from the cases contained higher median TEQs for 3 out of the 17 PCDD/PCDFs that were quantified. However, any differences disappeared after the results were adjusted for BMI, age, and smoking (Martinez-Zamora et al., 2015).

In an in vitro study, estradiol-17β production was decreased in human luteinizing granulosa cells that had been cultured in the presence of TCDD (Baldridge et al., 2015), but clear effects on ovulation and fertility have not been seen in humans (NASEM, 2016).

Adverse Pregnancy Outcomes

The sex ratios of children born to workers at a New Zealand herbicide production plant were compared with back-calculated TCDD serum concentrations at the time of birth. Although there was no relationship between the sex ratios and TCDD levels among exposed mothers, the probability of having a male child was significantly reduced for fathers with serum levels ≥20 pg TCDD/g lipid (sex ratio=0.47, OR=0.49, 95% CI 0.30–0.79) (Mannetje et al., 2016).

A systematic review and meta-analysis that included 15 studies on dioxin exposure and birth outcomes found associations between dioxins in food and LBW and between maternal exposure to dioxin in solid contaminants (residing near hazardous waste sites or a solid waste incinerator) and birth defects, but dioxin exposure was not associated with other outcomes, including spontaneous abortion, SGA, and stillbirth (Pan et al., 2015). Researchers have examined birth outcomes from 1996 through 2009 among women exposed to TCDD as a result of the 1976 chemical explosion in Seveso, Italy. In that study, no associations were found between exposure and spontaneous abortion, fetal growth, gestational length, or birth weight (Wesselink et al., 2014). However, specific genotypes can also affect the impact of PCDD/

PCDF exposure on birth outcomes. For example, a strong association between PCDD/PCDF exposure and reduced birth weight was reported for women with glutathione S-transferase mu 1(*GSTM1*) null genotype (β= –345, 95% CI –584– –105), but not women with aromatic hydrocarbon receptor (*AHR*), cytochrome P450 1A1 (*CYP1A1*), or *GSTM1* non-null genotypes (Kobayashi et al., 2017).

An ecological study in Guam of infant deaths in 1970–1989 due to congenital anomalies found that deaths were more likely among mothers who lived in areas that had been sprayed with Agent Orange (β=2.02, 95% CI 0.08–3.96) (Noel et al., 2015).

Developmental Effects

In the latest VAO review (NASEM, 2016), there was no available epidemiologic evidence that convincingly demonstrated a relationship between paternal exposure to dioxins before conception and outcomes in offspring. The committee found that although some evidence showed effects in offspring related to maternal exposure, there was no evidence to support the transmission of effects from father to offspring.

Most new epidemiologic studies published since 2014 of children exposed to PCDD/PCDFs prenatally or perinatally, as represented by concentrations in breast milk, have assessed growth and neurocognitive development. The environmental exposures that have been studied represent continuous exposures, which may have limited applicability to veteran exposures. One study examined the children of Vietnam veterans (Grufferman et al., 2014), and several studies examined Vietnamese children born after the war. One study relied on dioxin in maternal serum measured soon after a chemical plant explosion in Seveso, Italy, to study atopy and asthma (Ye et al., 2018).

A case-control study of rhabdomyosarcoma in children of Vietnam veterans (295 cases of rhabdomyosarcoma diagnosed between 1982 and 1988, and 295 controls) found that although increased risks were observed with maternal military service (OR=2.75, 95% CI 0.71–10.62) and paternal exposure to Agent Orange (OR=1.72, 95% CI 0.55–5.41), paternal military service was not associated with an increased risk (OR=0.85, 95% CI 0.58–1.25); none of the associations were statistically significant (Grufferman et al., 2014).

A pooled analysis of three European cohorts (n=367) found that prenatal/perinatal exposure to dioxins as measured in maternal cord blood and breast milk was related to the growth of the children. Changes in z-scores for weight-for-age measurements in children 0–24 months of age were non-significantly associated with dioxin exposure (β=0.07, 95% CI –0.01– 0.14) with no sex differences. Among children assessed for BMI at age 7 years, dioxin exposure was significantly associated with increased BMI among girls (β=0.49, 95% CI 0.07–0.91), but not among boys (β= –0.03, 95% CI –0.55–0.49). The interaction between dioxin exposure and sex was significant (p=0.044). No associations between growth and dioxin exposure were found in any single cohort, and all three cohorts differed substantially (p<0.05) (Iszatt et al., 2016).

Immune function as represented by allergies and infections at ages 3.5 and 7 years was investigated among the children of 514 Japanese women. Prenatal/perinatal exposure to dioxin-like chemicals (DLCs) was measured in maternal blood and compared to IgE in cord blood as well as to reports of food allergies, eczema, wheezing, otitis media, and respiratory infections in the children. Maternal DLC concentration was related to decreased cord blood IgE in boys (β= –0.87, 95% CI –1.68– –0.06) but not in girls (β=0.27, 95% CI –0.38–0.91). Cord blood IgE levels were not associated with an increased risk of allergies or infections at either age. At 3.5 years, girls had a nonsignificantly increased risk of wheezing with DLC exposure (OR=2.52, 95% CI 0.10–60.34), but not boys (OR=0.03, 95% CI 0.00–0.94). At 7 years, wheezing was significantly increased among all DLC-exposed children (OR=7.81, 95% CI 1.42–42.94), but not for boys alone (OR=12.05, 95% CI 0.99–146.37) or girls alone (OR=4.49, 95% CI

0.33–60.44). No patterns were noted for allergy, food allergy, eczema, or infections (Miyashita et al., 2018). These findings are further supported by the lack of positive associations found between maternal dioxin exposure from the Seveso, Italy, chemical plant explosion in 1976 and asthma, hay fever, or eczema in 676 children born since 1976 and assessed in 2014 (Ye et al., 2018).

Among a cohort of 161 11-year-old children born in Hong Kong, researchers found no associations between dioxins in breast milk (representing prenatal dioxin exposure) and measures of neurocognitive and intellectual function (IQ, fine motor coordination, verbal and nonverbal reasoning, learning, and attention) (Hui et al., 2016).

Some deficits in attention in German children ages 7–11 years were associated with prenatal PCDD/PCDF exposure as measured in maternal blood and breast milk (n=117). Distractibility (measured by reaction time) was significantly associated with the levels of PCDD/PCDFs in breast milk (geometric mean ratio=1.05, 95% CI 1.0–1.11), and divided attention (measured by number of omissions) was significantly associated with the levels of PCDD/PCDFs in maternal blood (geometric mean ratio=1.47, 95% CI 1.08–2.0). Other measures of distractability and divided attention were not significantly associated with PCDD/PCDF exposure, nor were measures of performance speed or performance quality. ADHD scores were negatively associated with PCDD/PCDFs in blood, although not significantly (Neugebauer et al., 2015).

In the same German birth cohort (n=136), maternal blood levels of PCDD/PCDFs assessed during pregnancy were found to be inversely associated with sex-typical behaviors at age 9, significantly among girls (social responsiveness scale $\beta = -10.98$, 95% CI –19.43– –2.53), but not among boys. Measures of empathy or systemizing were also inversely associated with PCDD/PCDF levels. The results indicated a significant interaction effect of sex and exposure for all three measures of behavior. Maternal blood levels of PCDD/PCDFs were not above background levels (Nowack et al., 2015).

A series of publications have examined the growth and development of 241 Vietnamese children living in a high TCDD/PCDD/PCDF exposure area near Da Nang Air Base[5] (Boda et al., 2018; Nishijo et al., 2014, 2015; Pham et al., 2015; Tai et al., 2016; Tran et al., 2016; Van Tung et al., 2016). Exposure was measured in cord blood at birth and in breast milk collected 28–33 days after birth. Assessments on the children were conducted at 1 month, 4 months, 1 year, and 3 years of age. Using cord blood samples available for 162 infants, investigators found decreases in estradiol and testosterone that varied by sex. Among female infants, dioxin levels in breast milk were inversely associated with testosterone levels in cord blood for certain measures (1,2,3,6,7,8-HxCDD $\beta = -0.32$, 95% CI –0.54– –0.10; TEQ-PCDD $\beta = -0.23$, 95% CI –0.45– –0.01), although this was not seen with male infants. No associations with estradiol were found (Boda et al., 2018). At 1 year of age, TCDD and total PCDD/PCDF exposure were not associated with cognitive, language, or motor function, but social-emotional scores were significantly reduced among those with high PCDD/PCDF and TCDD exposure (Pham et al., 2015). Growth and development through 3 years of age was associated with TCDD and PCDD/PCDFs in a sex-specific manner. Among boys, high PCDD/PCDF exposure was significantly associated with decreased expressive communication scores, and neither TCDD nor PCDD/PCDF exposure was associated with reduced body size. No association between PCDD/PCDFs and neurodevelopment was observed for girls, but girls with high exposure had greater head and abdominal circumferences (Tai et al., 2016).

---

[5] Dioxin concentrations in the environment and in humans living there remained elevated in areas sprayed with herbicides, including Agent Orange, during the Vietnam War (1961–1971). Several decades after the Vietnam war, total PCDD/PCDF TEQ remained high around Da Nang Airbase, with measurements up to 365,000 pg/g. A survey of 520 nursing mothers in 2008–2009 showed that primiparae women living in hot spots (14.10 pg/g lipid) and sprayed areas (10.89 pg/g lipid) had higher total TEQ of 2,3,7,8-subsitituted dioxin concentrations in breast milk than women residing in unsprayed areas (4.09 pg/g lipid) (Tai et al., 2011).

In this Vietnamese cohort, greater rates of autistic traits were associated with high TCDD exposure in both boys and girls, but not with total PCDD/PCDFs. High exposure to total PCDD/PCDFs, but not to TCDD, was associated with significantly lower neurodevelopmental scores in boys, but not in girls (Nishijo et al., 2014). A nested case-control study within this cohort investigated changes in urinary amino acid profiles to identify alterations in amino acids that function as neurotransmitters in the developing brain. The authors noted that urinary levels of the amino acids histidine and tryptophan were significantly lower among children highly exposed to total PCDD/PCDFs, and the histidine-to-glycine ratio was significantly lower among children with high exposure to both total PCDD/PCDFs and TCDD. Histidine and the histidine-to-glycine ratio were also correlated with neurodevelopmental scores for language and fine motor skills (Nishijo et al., 2015). A follow-up assessment at 5 years of age showed decrements in movement and neurodevelopment among boys but not girls. Compared with boys with lower mean PCDD/PCDF exposure, boys with higher exposure had lower mean scores for total movement (7.7 versus 9.7, $p<0.01$), balance (7.3 versus 9.3, $p<0.01$), nonverbal index (78.9 versus 90.1, $p=0.01$), and pattern reasoning (5.3 versus 7.1, $p=0.041$) (Tran et al., 2016). The investigators suggested that TCDD acts differently than other PCDD/PCDFs and that there are sex differences in responses that last into childhood.

Nearly 45 years after the Vietnam War, Van Tung et al. (2016) assessed the birth weight of 58 babies born to mothers living in another Agent Orange–contaminated area of Vietnam compared with 62 control babies born in another community that was not sprayed with herbicides during the war. The PCDD/PCDF levels in breast milk were three to four times higher in exposed children (means 12.31 versus 3.51 pg/g lipid total TEQ PCDD/PCDFs). Two congeners were significantly correlated with birth weight (2,3,7,8-TeCDD $r=-0.18$; 2,3,4,7,8-PeCDF $r=-0.21$, both $p<0.05$), but no congeners were correlated with infant size at 8–9 or 12–14 weeks of age. Maternal salivary cortisol levels collected at the same time as breast milk, as a marker of an adverse intrauterine environment, were not related to PCDD/PCDF exposure.

Animal Studies

The Volume 11 committee identified more than 20 animal studies published since 2014 on the reproductive, developmental, and generational effects of PCDD/PCDFs, all of which reported on TCDD specifically.

Two studies provided additional support for the adverse effects of TCDD on male reproduction. Rats treated with TCDD (100 ng/kg bw/day) for 15 days had reduced testicular steroidogenesis and increased oxidative stress (Dhanabalan et al., 2015). A day after exposure to TCDD (4 μg/kg bw), significant changes in gene expression and in the levels of nine genes related to AhR expression in testicular or epididymal tissue (caput, corpus, and cauda) were reported. AhR expression was greater in the epididymis than in the testes, and AhR protein levels were affected in epididymal epithelial cells but not Sertoli or Leydig cells. The authors interpreted these results as showing that TCDD can cause male infertility by affecting AhR expression and proper sperm development (Wajda et al., 2017).

Effects of prenatal exposure to TCDD were assessed in 15 studies. Wu et al. (2014) found that an oral dose of TCDD (1.6 or 8.0 μg/kg bw) on GD 15 was associated with suppressed placental vascular remodeling at GD 20. Although there was no relationship with fetal capillary density, changes in the expression of angiogenic growth factors were also observed. An in vitro study showed that TCDD decreased the viability of human umbilical cord vein and artery cells (Li et al., 2015).

Although in utero TCDD is widely used to induce cleft palate in animal models in order to study mechanisms, humans are much less sensitive to this endpoint than rodents and other species (Abbott et al., 1999; EPA, 2012; NASEM, 2016). Therefore, although there continues to be work done with this model endpoint, this committee did not delve further into the data on TCDD-induced cleft palate in animal models. One study showed a possible role of TCDD in the development of other congenital defects. Sholts et al. (2015) reported that rats exposed to TCDD at 1,000 ng/kg on GD 11 had reduced cranium size and fluctuating asymmetry at 1 year of age.

Immune effects were observed by Ahrenhoerster et al. (2014) in an in vitro study, which showed that relatively low levels of TCDD (3 μg/kg) on GDs 0.5 and 7.5 inhibited lymphocyte differentiation by altering hematopoietic stem and progenitor cell homeostasis in such a way that B- and T-lymphocyte differentiation decreased 2.5-fold at GD 14.5. Van Esterik et al. (2015) reported that prenatal exposure to TCDD (10–10,000 pg/kg) was associated with altered immune homeostasis in mouse offspring; dams were exposed via their feed for up to 10 weeks prior to mating and through PND 14. At 1 year of age decreased fat pad and spleen weights and an increase in IL-4 production by splenic immune cells were observed in the male offspring, while increased fat pad weights and production of IFNγ were seen in the female offspring. Laiosa et al. (2016) showed that TCDD's effects on the developing hematopoietic system are mediated through fetal activation of the AhR.

A variety of endocrine effects have been studied in association with prenatal TCDD exposure. Takeda et al. (2014b) examined the impact of prenatal TCDD exposure on hormones and sexual maturity. TCDD (0.2–20 μg/kg) administered on GD 12 reduced the pituitary expression of mRNAs for LH, FSH, and glycoprotein hormone α-subunit (αGSU) and of growth hormone measured on GD 18, PND 2, and PND 4 in mice. TCDD also reduced the gonadal expression of steroidogenic proteins and had adverse effects on litter size and pup body weight. Mouse strains that express high or low AhR affinity for dioxins respond to TCDD exposure differently, which emphasizes the role of AhR activation in causing these effects (Takeda et al., 2014b). In another study by Takeda et al. (2014a), 1 μg TCDD/kg on GD 15 affected the levels of hypothalamic gonadotropin-releasing hormone (GnRH) and sexual behaviors in rats. Deficits in GnRH levels and sexual behaviors were remedied by equine chorionic gonadotropin at GD 15, and an intracerebroventricular infusion of GnRH after sexual maturity restored sexual behaviors (Takeda et al., 2014a). The effect of the TCDD was subsequently shown to be due, in part, to an altered energy status (decreased ATP) in the fetal whole brain and hypothalamus (Takeda et al., 2017).

Schneider et al. (2014) studied the effect of prenatal TCDD (5 μg/kg, po, on embryonic day 15.5) on mouse prostate development and found that ventral prostatic budding in the embryonic urogenital sinus had been prevented as a result of β-catenin signaling at embryonic day 16.5.

Sugai et al. (2014) studied the effects of prenatal TCDD exposure in mice (3 μg/kg on GD 12.5) and then assigned the offspring to either regular or high-calorie diets. Unexposed mice eating high-calorie diets were obese and showed signs of lipid dysregulation at 26 weeks, whereas TCDD-exposed mice eating the same high-calorie diet did not, suggesting that TCDD attenuated the effects of a high-calorie diet on obesity and related adult diseases.

Brain development was the subject of three recent studies. Kobayashi et al. (2015) showed that an oral dose of TCDD (20–5,000 ng/kg) at 8.5 days post coitus had significant impacts on brain development at embryonic day 18.5. Mice exposed to the highest dose showed reduced glial fibrillary acidic protein (GFAP) immunoreactivity in the dentate gyrus and hippocampal fimbria and reduced immunoreactive fimbria; all doses were associated with decreased proliferating cell nuclear antigen-positive cells. Rats administered TCDD and TBDD (2,3,7,8-tetrabromodibenzo-*p*-dioxin) at 0, 200, or 800 ng/kg on GD 15 exhibited impaired paired-associated learning in adulthood for both compounds at 200 ng/kg, but not at 800 ng/kg. Similarly, rats exposed to 200 ng/kg of TCDD or TBDD showed greater anxiety-like behaviors than controls or highly exposed animals (Kakeyama et al., 2014). Safe and Luebke (2016) considered auditory neuropathy among three strains of mice exposed prenatally to TCDD (500 ng/kg) on embryonic day 12 by oral gavage. At 1.5 months of age, the cochlear threshold sensitivity was significantly elevated in mice with certain AhR alleles. The authors concluded that prenatal TCDD exposure may be a risk factor for auditory neuropathy.

Muenyi et al. (2014) found that prenatal TCDD (10 μg/kg on GD 12) accelerated the development of abnormal epidermal permeability barrier with acanthosis and hyperkeratosis and also epidermal tight junction function as measured through PND 1 in mice. Such changes have been linked to atopic diseases.

Adult mice (up to 4 months old) exposed to a single dose of TCDD in utero (13 μg/kg on day 13 post-coitus) and slow release implants of testosterone and 17 β-estradiol at 8 weeks old had increased bladder, kidney, prostate, and seminal vesicle weights. They also had more hydronephrosis, prostate epithelial cell proliferation, thickened prostate periductal smooth muscle, and altered collagen fiber distribution in their prostate and bladder tissue. Mice exposed to in utero TCDD but not exogenous hormones had few changes from controls. The authors interpreted these data as showing that early life exposure to TCDD alters susceptibility to adult urinary tract dysfunction (Ricke et al., 2016).

Studies have also reported effects in subsequent generations. ATSDR (2012) reported examples of intergenerational effects in hamsters and mice in which reproductive effects were observed in F2 or F3 offspring after the gestational exposure of the F0 female, and transgenerational effects have been the subject of a recent systematic review. That review of the evidence of inherited transgenerational effects found that although there is no human evidence concerning the transgenerational effects of dioxin, there have been eight studies in animals, from five groups of investigators, that examined the transgenerational effects of gestational dioxin exposure on offspring, including its effects on growth and development, its reproductive effects in offspring, and its hepatic, immune, and renal effects (Walker et al., 2018). Four studies reported transgenerational effects on male reproductive endpoints (Bruner-Tran et al., 2014; Manikkam et al., 2012a,b; Sanabria et al., 2016). Although dioxin exposure had no reported effects on the traditional measures of male reproductive endpoints (sperm concentration and motility, apoptosis of testes germ cells, prostate or testes disease, LH concentration, reproductive organ weights, or puberty), one study found an increase in abnormal sperm morphology (Bruner-Tran et al., 2014), and two studies from the same researchers found age-dependent changes in testosterone concentrations (decreased at 3–4 months of age and increased at 12 months of age) (Manikkam et al., 2012a,b). Five studies reported on female reproductive outcomes (Bruner-Tran and Osteen, 2011; Bruner-Tran et al., 2016; Manikkam et al., 2012a,b; Nilsson et al., 2012). One group of researchers reported decreased primordial follicles and increased ovarian cysts (Manikkam et al., 2012a,b; Nilsson et al., 2012) and early onset of puberty (Manikkam et al., 2012a,b) associated with dioxin exposure. One study investigated adenomyosis (similar to endometriosis) and found increased uterine microvessel density in the offspring of exposed rats (Bruner-Tran et al., 2016). Other endpoints that have been studied but were not affected by exposure include fertility, sex ratio, tumor development, and reproductive organ weight. Two studies reported growth and developmental outcomes (Manikkam et al., 2012a,b) and found that dioxin was associated with an increased body weight among males at weaning and at 12 months of age, but no effect was observed in females (Manikkam et al., 2012a,b). Additionally, kidney disease (Manikkam et al., 2012b), effects on liver function (Ma et al., 2015), and increased immune response (Bruner-Tran et al., 2014) were all observed in males. Inconsistencies across studies (heterogeneity in endpoints selected and in the measurement of endpoints), a lack of information about the age of animals when observations were made, and a lack of analysis using the litter as the unit of analysis limit confidence in these findings.

Since 2014, three groups of researchers have reported on transgenerational effects observed in rodents, all of them cited in the systematic review described above (Bruner-Tran et al., 2014, 2016; Ma et al., 2015; Sanabria et al., 2016; Walker et al., 2018).

Epigenetic Effects

Ma et al. (2015) studied TCDD's epigenetic effect on the *IGF2* gene in rats through three generations. Only the F0 dams were treated, and the F2 generation was used for production of the F3 but was not further evaluated. Prenatal exposure (200 or 800 ng/kg TCDD on GD 2-14) was associated with increased *IGF2* expression, hypermethylation of the *IGF2* imprinted control region, hypomethylation of the differentially methylated region 2, and altered expression of DNA methyltransferases in F1 and F3 mice compared with control mice.

In studies on mice, Bruner-Tran and colleagues (2017) observed an endometriosis-like phenotype and other reproductive effects in the female offspring (F1–F4) after in utero exposure to TCDD, and they reported reduced endometrial progesterone receptor (PR) protein expression in uterine tissue in F1–F3 mice. They also reported partial methylation of the PR in 60% of tissues from F1 females and 40% of tissues of F3 females, leading them to conclude that there was transgenerational inheritance of epigenetic silencing of the PR.

In reporting results from a mouse model of TCDD-induced palatogenesis, researchers suggested that TCDD caused the upregulation of DNA methyltransferase 3a in fetal palate tissue and increased global DNA methylation and caused palate malformation. However, the association was only observed in fetal mice at GD 13.5, but not GD 14.5 or 15.5 (Wang et al., 2017a).

Synthesis and Conclusions

The effects of PCDD/PCDFs have been studied extensively, with much attention given to the effects of exposures in Vietnam veterans. Although some studies have shown reproductive or developmental effects at very high doses, such as those experienced in the Seveso, Italy, accident, those associations have not been shown—or, in some cases, even studied—in other populations. Therefore, associations at lower levels of exposure cannot be assessed. For example, studies in Seveso found associations between women with TCDD levels >100 ppt and time to pregnancy (Eskenazi et al., 2010), but other studies of similar endpoints have not been conducted, so it is not possible to assess the consistency of this association (NASEM, 2016). Similarly, the developmental effects of early life exposure in the Seveso cohort included reduced semen quality among adult men who had been breast-fed by exposed mothers, but because of questions about the reliability of the data and covariates, these results require further validation or support (IOM, 2014; Mocarelli et al., 2011).

Since the last VAO review of the literature on the health effects of dioxins (NASEM, 2016), numerous studies have reported on dioxin's effects on male fertility (Den Hond et al., 2015; Galimova et al., 2015), endometriosis (Martinez-Zamora et al., 2015), estradiol production (Baldridge et al., 2015), the sex ratios of children (Mannetje et al., 2016), adverse birth and pregnancy outcomes (Pan et al., 2015; Wesselink et al., 2014), and birth defects (Noel et al., 2015), but the Volume 11 committee found no consistent patterns for reproductive outcomes when considering the entirety of the evidence base, including reviews by the National Academies (2016), EPA (2012), and ATSDR (2012).

Studies of adverse pregnancy outcomes show some evidence of effects of prenatal exposure, but there is much variability among the studies. Kobayashi et al. (2017) provides a mechanistic rationale for differences among exposed individuals with certain genotypes.

Developmental outcomes that have been studied include rhabdomyosarcoma in the children of Vietnam veterans (Grufferman et al., 2014), infant and child growth (Iszatt et al., 2016; Tai et al., 2016; Van Tung et al., 2016), allergies and infections in childhood (Miyashita et al., 2018), language development (Caspersen et al., 2016), neurocognitive development and intellectual function (Hui et al.,

2016), attention measures (Neugebauer et al., 2015), sex-typical behaviors (Nowack et al., 2015), and neurodevelopment (Nishijo et al., 2014, 2015; Pham et al., 2015; Tran et al., 2016). Some studies support associations between dioxin exposure and effects that are mediated by genotype (Kobayashi et al., 2017) and sex (Miyashita et al., 2018; Nishijo et al., 2014, 2015; Nowack et al., 2015; Tai et al., 2016; Tran et al., 2016). The results of these studies are inconsistent, and few outcomes were studied in more than one population.

The Volume 11 committee identified more than 20 animal studies on the reproductive and developmental effects of prenatal TCDD exposure. The studies generally support the conclusions reached in recent reviews by EPA (2012), ATSDR (2012), and the National Academies (2016) that TCDD may result in adverse male reproductive effects and a variety of developmental effects, including endocrine, immune, and neurodevelopmental changes. Animal models point to oxidative stress and AhR-activation as the mechanisms by which TCDD causes these effects (Dhanabalan et al., 2015; Laiosa et al., 2016). However, the doses used in the animal studies are much higher than expected human exposures. Additionally, there is great variability in species sensitivity to PCDD/PCDFs, depending on AhR binding ability, and humans are much less sensitive than laboratory rodents (ATSDR, 2012; EPA, 2012; NASEM, 2016). Thus, the relevance to human health outcomes of the large evidence base derived from animal studies is unclear.

Although there is some evidence from animal studies that maternal exposure to dioxins may result in epigenetic effects and transgenerational health effects (ATSDR, 2012; Bruner-Tran et al., 2014, 2016; NASEM, 2016; Walker et al., 2018), there is no evidence of such effects in humans.

There is a large evidence base describing human health effects in populations exposed occupationally, environmentally, and as a result of the Vietnam war and a similarly robust evidence base in animal models (many thousands of publications have been reviewed by the VAO series), but there are few consistencies across cohorts, and the ability to use animal studies to support associations noted in humans studies is limited by the ability to extrapolate outcomes in animals to humans.

The Volume 11 committee discussed the association between dioxins and reproductive effects at length. The committee was challenged by the large volume of literature describing a wide range of effects in particular populations with very high levels of exposure (e.g., Seveso). The studies included a number of effects, but few of them examined the same effects or found the same results. The committee's discussion differed in focus from those of other committees, such as VAO and prior Gulf War and Health committees. Those committees focused on diagnosed clinical outcomes such as fertility and endometriosis. Although those committees considered effects such as abnormal semen parameters, these effects alone did not justify a conclusion of adverse clinical outcomes. By contrast, the Volume 11 committee, given its task of assessing generation effects in veterans and their descendants and also assessing animal models, considered the broader range of biological effects, such as changes in semen parameters, to be indicative of potential adverse reproductive outcomes regardless of the level of exposure. The committee finds that, taken as a whole, the literature it reviewed above for both humans and animals demonstrates that biological effects on the reproductive system may be possible at high levels of exposure and represents a residual level of concern. Therefore, the committee identified reproductive effects of dioxins as a major priority for future monitoring and research as discussed in the following chapters.

The Volume 11 committee concludes that there is inadequate/insufficient evidence to determine whether an association exists between exposure to PCDDs/PCDFs and reproductive or developmental effects.

TABLE 6-7 Summary of Reproductive and Developmental Effects of Polychlorinated Dibenzodioxins

Study	Design/Population	Exposure	Results
Reproductive Effects			
Den Hond et al. (2015)	Case-control 40 cases of male infertility and 80 controls, recruited from fertility clinics in Belgium.	PCDD/PCDFs measured in serum.	Semen parameters and sex hormones in serum. No association between PCDD/PCDFs and subfertility (OR=1.59, 95% CI 0.96–2.65) or hormone levels.
Faure et al. (2014)	Ecological 251 men living near a municipal waste incinerator in France where exhaust controls were implemented in 1998, semen samples collected in 2001–2007.	Modeled exposure to PCDD/PCDFs from incinerator emissions by year as surrogate for exposure.	Semen parameters by year. Abnormal mid-piece: β= –0.010, 95% CI –0.018– –0.002; multiple anomalies index: Symbol = –0.013, 95% CI –0.023– –0.004. Other parameters not significant.
Galimova et al. (2015)	Case-control 105 men with pathospermia and 63 men with normal sperm seen at a fertility clinic, and 49 fertile controls, living near a chemical plant in Russia.	PCDD/PCDFs in semen.	Semen parameters. Higher PCDD/PCDF content TEQ among infertile normospermia and pathospermia men than fertile men (total TEQ pg/g lipids: 466.6, 482.1, 212.5, respectively). No statistical testing conducted.
Martinez-Zamora et al. (2015)	Case-control 30 cases of deep infiltrating endometriosis and 30 controls, in Catalonia, Spain.	17 PCDD/PCDFs measured in adipose tissue.	Significantly higher median TEQ among endometriosis cases than controls for TCDD: OR=1.41, 95% CI 1.12–2.10; 1,2,3,7,8-PeCDD: OR=1.82, 95% CI 1.36–7.14; 2,3,4,7,8-PeCDF: OR=2.13, 95% CI 1.97–6.42. Also, 4 PCB congeners were significantly associated with endometriosis. All other congeners not significant.
Adverse Pregnancy Outcomes			
Mannetje et al. (2016)	Cohort 355 children born to parents (127 fathers and 21 mothers) employed at a chemical plant in New Zealand.	TCDD in parental serum back-calculated to estimate exposure at the time of birth.	Sex ratio. Overall ratio=0.55. Any maternal exposure not significant. Paternal exposure ≤4pg/g: SR=0.60 (ref); 4–20 pg/g SR=0.62, OR=1.0, 95% CI 0.50–2.02; 20–100 pg/g SR=0.47, OR=0.52, 95% CI 0.29–0.92; ≥100 pg/g SR=0.46, OR=0.45, 95% CI 0.23–0.89; p trend=0.007.

continued

TABLE 6-7 Continued

Study	Design/Population	Exposure	Results
Wesselink et al. (2014)	Cohort 1,211 pregnancies between 1976 (chemical plant explosion) and 2009, in Seveso, Italy.	TCDD in serum collected in 1976 or 1996.	Adverse birth outcomes. TCDD measured in 1976 or estimated at birth was not related to spontaneous abortion, fetal growth, gestational length, or birth weight.
Kobayashi et al. (2017)	Cohort—Hokkaido Study 421 pregnant women in Japan. 2002–2005	17 PCDD/PCDFs measured in maternal blood in third trimester or within a week of birth; *AHR*, *CYP1A1*, and *GSTM1* genotypes.	Birth size. No association between *AHR* and *CYP1A1*, and *GSTM1* non-null genotypes and PCDD/Fs on birth weight, height, or head circumference. Among women with the GSTM1 null genotype, PCDD/Fs associated with reduced birth weight (β= –345, 95% CI –584– –105).
Noel et al. (2015)	Ecological All live births in Guam 1970–1989 (N=49,841); 121 infant deaths due to congenital anomalies.	Maternal residence in areas sprayed with Agent Orange (high risk) versus areas not sprayed (low risk).	Infant mortality due to congenital anomalies. Deaths associated with maternal residence in a high-risk area: β=2.02, 95% CI 0.08–3.96.
Developmental Effects			
Gufferman et al. (2014)	Case-control 295 cases of rhabdomyosarcoma and 295 matched random controls, from U.S. births 1982–1988.	Parental military service and reported Agent Orange exposure.	Rhabdomyosarcoma. Maternal military service: OR=2.75, 95% CI 0.71–10.62. Paternal military service: OR=0.85, 95% CI 0.58–1.25. Paternal Agent Orange exposure: OR=1.72, 95% CI 0.55–5.41. Not significant for paternal deployment periods, exposure to radiation, radar or microwaves, and nuclear, chemical, or biological weapons. Adjustment for drug use, but no assessment for alcohol or smoking.
Iszatt et al. (2016)	3 Cohorts 96 Belgian children, 207 Slovak children, and 64 Norwegian children. 2002–2009	PCDD/PCDFs in cord blood and breast milk.	Infant growth 0–24 months and BMI at 7 years. Change in infant weight-for-age z-scores β=0.07, 95% CI –0.01– 0.2. BMI at 7 years old for girls β=0.49, 95% CI 0.07–0.91; not significant for boys. Significant interaction dioxin × sex (p=0.044). Significant differences between cohorts for most demographic and outcome measures.

Study	Design/Population	Exposure	Results
Miyashita et al. (2018)	Cohort-Hokkaido Study 514 pregnant women at a hospital in Japan. 2002–2005	Dioxin-like compounds in maternal blood and in cord blood	Cord blood IgE and allergies at ages 3.5 and 7 years. Maternal dioxin-like compounds associated with decreased cord blood IgE in boys (β= –0.87, 95% CI –1.68– –0.06); not significant for girls. At 3.5 years, reduced risk of wheezing associated with dioxin-like compounds exposure among boys (OR=0.03, 95% CI 0.0–0.94); not significant for girls. At 7 years, risk of wheezing increased for all children (OR=7.81, 95% CI 1.42–42.94); not significant for boys and girls individually. No association btw cord blood IgE and allergies at 3.5 or 7 years of age. No associations with food allergy, eczema, or infections.
Ye et al. (2018)	Cohort-Seveso Women's Health Study 677 children born to TCCD exposed mothers 1976–2016.	TCDD in maternal serum measured following the explosion of a chemical plant in 1976.	Atopic conditions (eczema, hay fever, asthma) in children ascertained by mothers' self-report. Eczema: RR=0.63, 95% CI 0.40–0.99; Hay fever: RR=0.99, 95% CI 0.76–1.27; and Asthma: RR=0.93, 95% CI 0.61–1.40. Adjustments for maternal age at explosion, atopic history, age at pregnancy, BMI closest to birth year, smoking during pregnancy, birth order, child sex, child age, and primary wage earner education.
Hui et al. (2016)	Cohort 161 mother–child pairs in Hong Kong. 2002	Dioxins in breast milk measured 2–6 weeks post-partum.	Neurocognitive development at 11 years old. No associations found with full-scale IQ, verbal comprehension, perceptual reasoning, processing speed, working memory, learning, intrusion error, preservation error scores, or tests of attention. No sex × breast-feeding interactions note.

continued

TABLE 6-7 Continued

Study	Design/Population	Exposure	Results
Neugebauer et al. (2015)	Cohort-Duisburg Birth Cohort 117 mother–child pairs in Germany. 2000–2011	PCDD/PCDFs in maternal blood at 32nd week of pregnancy and breast milk collected within 2 weeks of birth.	Attention performance (using KITAP, a computerized test battery for attentional performance for children) and attention behavior (FBB-ADHD, a parent rating scale for ADHD) in school-age children. Distractability: slower reaction time associated with total PCDD/PCDFs TEQ in breast milk (geometric mean ratio=1.05, 95% CI 1.0–1.11), but not omissions or false alarm rates. Divided attention: increased number of omissions associated with PCDD/PCDFs TEQ in maternal blood (geometric mean ratio=1.47, 95% CI 1.08–2.0), but not false alarm rates or reaction time. Negative but not significant associations between maternal blood or breast milk PCDD/PCDFs with performance speed or quality or ADHD.
Nowack et al. (2015)	Cohort-Duisburg Birth Cohort 136 mother–child pairs in Germany. 2000–2011	PCDD/PCDFs in maternal serum during pregnancy.	Empathizing, systemizing, and autistic traits at 9–10 years. Empathizing and systemizing quotients not related to PCDD/PCDF exposure in boys or girls. Social responsiveness scale for autistic traits associated with PCDD/F exposure among girls (β= –10.98, 95% CI –19.43– –2.53) but not boys (β= –2.37, 95% CI –9.18–4.45).
Van Tung et al. (2016)	Case-control 58 mother–infant pairs from an Agent Orange contaminated region in Vietnam and 62 pairs from a region with no contamination. 2007	PCDD/PCDFs and TCDD in breast milk and maternal cortisol levels. Infants were 7–16 weeks old at time of sampling.	Birth weight. Average PCDD/PCDFs higher in breast milk of exposed mothers than controls (12.3 versus 3.5 pg/g lipid, $p<0.001$). Two congeners correlated with birth weight (TCDD r= –0.18; 2,3,4,7,8-PeCDF r= –0.21; both $p<0.05$). Mean cortisol was higher in mothers of low birth weight babies than normal weight (6.52 versus 3.2, $p<0.05$), not related to total PCDD/PCDFs or specific congeners. No difference in body size at 8–9 weeks or 12–14 weeks of age.

Study	Design/Population	Exposure	Results
Boda et al. (2018)	Cohort 162 mother–infant pairs in Da Nang, Vietnam. 2012 (See Pham et al., 2015)	PCDD/PCDFs in breast milk collected 1 month after birth.	Estradiol and testosterone in cord blood. No association between estradiol and PCDD/PCDFs in breast milk. Decreased testosterone associated with PCDD/PCDFs in breast milk among girls (1,2,3,6,7,8-HxCDD β= –0.32, 95% CI –0.54– –0.10; and TEQ-PCDD β= –0.23, 95% CI –0.45– –0.01, other congeners not significant). No dose–response relationship found. No association among boys.
Pham et al. (2015)	Cohort 214 mother–infant pairs in Da Nang, Vietnam. 2008–2009	PCDD/PCDFs in breast milk collected 28–33 days after birth (low: ≤7.4 pg/g lipid TEQ; mild: 7.4–11.5; moderate: 11.5–17.6; high: ≥17.6). Daily dioxin intake (low: ≤49.8 pg TEQ/kg/day; mild: 49.8–77.8; moderate: 77.8–118.2; high: ≥118.2). TCDD (low: ≤ 0.9 pg/g lipid; mild: 0.9–1.8; moderate: 1.8–3.5; high: ≥3.5).	Neurodevelopment at 1 year (Bayley-III scores). Mean cognitive, language, and motor scores not related to PCDD/PCDFs or TCDD exposure. Cognitive scores were significantly lower in the low daily dioxin intake exposure group than mild, moderate, or high groups (mean scores 97.4 versus 102.8, 102.1, and 102.4, $p<0.042$ for all three). Social emotional scores significantly lower among those with high PCDD/PCDFs exposure (89.9 versus 93.4, $p=0.049$) and high TCDD exposure (88.4 versus 90.8, $p=0.019$) than low exposure. No association for adaptive behavior scores.
Tai et al. (2016)	Cohort 217 mother–infant pairs in Da Nang, Vietnam. (See Pham et al., 2015)	PCDD/PCDFs in breast milk collected 28–33 days after birth.	Neurodevelopment at 3 years (Bayley-III scores and growth expressed by z-scores to show marginal means). Boys with high PCDD/PCDF exposure had low mean expressive communication scores (8.4 versus 9.0, $p=0.03$); boys with high TCDD exposure had low mean composite motor scores (94.9 versus 100.5, $p=0.049$) and gross motor scores (9.1 versus 10.4, $p=0.036$). Boys with high PCDD/PCDF exposure had reduced mean weight growth (–0.38 versus –0.08, $p=0.01$) and BMI (–0.43 versus –0.14, $p=0.02$). No neurodevelopmental differences among girls. Girls with high TCDD exposure had greater mean head circumference growth (0.18 versus –0.28, $p=0.00$), and high PCDD/PCDFs exposures had greater chest circumference growth (0.17 versus –0.12, $p=0.02$).

continued

TABLE 6-7 Continued

Study	Design/Population	Exposure	Results
Nishijo et al. (2014)	Cohort 153 mother–infant pairs in Da Nang, Vietnam. (See Pham et al., 2015)	PCDD/PCDFs in breast milk collected 28–33 days after birth (high versus low exposure: ≥ or <3.5 pg/g fat). TCDD exposure (high versus low: ≥ or <17.9 pg/g fat).	Autistic traits using the Autism Spectrum Rating Scale and neurodevelopment (Bailey-III scales) at 3 years. Children with high TCDD exposure had higher mean autism score than low exposure (boys: 61.5 versus 55.0, p=0.042; girls: 58.2 versus 54.3, p=0.012) but no difference in neurocognitive scores. Children with high PCDD/PCDF exposure had similar autism scores as low exposure children, but highly exposed boys had lower cognitive scores (93.0 versus 96.8, p=0.023).
Nishijo et al. (2015)	Nested case-control 26 children in Da Nang, Vietnam. (See Pham et al., 2015)	PCDD/PCDFs in breast milk collected 28–33 days after birth in 4 groups: (1) low PCDD/PCDFs and well-developed controls; (2) low PCDD/PCDFs and poorly developed controls (3) high PCDD/PCDFs and low TCDD; and (4) high PCDD/PCDFs and high TCDD.	Urinary amino acids in children with neurodevelopmental deficits at 3 years. Mean histidine levels of group 4 significantly lower than group 1 (18.58 versus 187.93, p=0.004) and tryptophan (0.69 versus 2.99, p=0.007). Ratio of histidine/glysine significantly lower in groups 4, 3, and 2, than 1 (1.37, 2.73, 1.70 versus 7.5; p<0.006 for all). Histidine levels associated with neurodevelopmental scores (cognitive β=11.8; receptive communication β=2.7; expressive communication β=1.5; language β=18.7; fine motor β=2.1; motor β=13.4; all p<0.05) same pattern shown by histidine/glysine ratio.
Tran et al. (2016)	Cohort 176 mother–infant pairs in Da Nang, Vietnam. (See Pham et al., 2015)	PCDD/PCDFs in breast milk collected 28–33 days after birth.	Cognitive development (using the Kaufman Assessment Battery for Children, 2nd ed.) and motor coordination (using the Movement Assessment Battery for Children, 2nd ed.) at 5 years. Boys with high exposure had lower mean scores than low exposure groups for total movement (7.7 versus 9.7, p<0.01) and balance scores (7.3 versus 9.3, p<0.01); nonverbal index scores (78.9 versus 90.1, p=0.01); and pattern reasoning scores (5.3 versus 7.1, p=0.041). No associations between exposure and motor coordination or cognitive development in girls.

NOTE: ADHD=attention deficit–hyperactivity disorder; AhR=aryl hydrocarbon receptor; Bayley-III=Bayley Scales of Infant and Toddler Development, Third Edition; BMI=body mass index; CI=confidence interval; CYP1A1=cytochrome P450 1A1; GSTM1=glutathione S-transferase mu 1; IgE=immunoglobulin E; IQ=intelligence quotient; OR=odds ratio; PCB=polychlorinated biphenyl; PCDD=polychlorinated dibenzo-p-dioxin; PCDF=polychlorinated dibenzofuran; RR=relative risk; SR=sex ratio; TCDD=2,3,7,8-tetrachlorodibenzo-*p*-dioxin; TEQ=toxic equivalent.

Exhaust

The Volume 11 committee identified a few studies pertaining specifically to combustion engine exhaust that have been published since the last review by the Volume 3 committee in 2004 (see Table 6-8). Exhaust is a mixture that includes PM, PAHs, PCDD/PCDFs, and VOCs in addition to numerous other compounds that may result from the combustion of fuels such as gasoline, diesel, or jet fuel. No studies were conducted in veteran populations, and there were no studies that investigated possible generational effects.

Reproductive Effects

Reproductive Effects in Men and Women

In an epidemiologic study, Guven et al. (2008) provided a cross-sectional look at the semen quality of 38 toll collectors and 35 office workers at the same company. Toll collectors had lower sperm density ($p=0.002$) and motility ($p=0.003$) and higher percentages of abnormal sperm morphology (head abnormalities $p=0.01$, mixed abnormalities $p=0.04$) than the office workers. No data relating these sperm effects to fecundity were reported.

In an animal study, gasoline exhaust was shown to have reproductive effects in male mice, including significant dose-dependent increases ($p<0.05$) in malondialdehyde and carbonyl protein in testes and DNA damage as measured by comet assay. Significant dose-dependent decreases ($p<0.05$) in superoxide dismutase and glutathione peroxidase in testicles were also reported (Che et al., 2009). Biodiesel fuel exhaust particles caused adverse effects on male reproductive function in mice, including having significant impacts ($p<0.05$) on sperm integrity, testosterone levels in testes, LH in serum, sperm DNA fragmentation, inflammatory cytokines in serum and testes, interstitial edema, degenerating spermatocytes, and dystrophic seminiferous tubules with arrested spermatogenesis (Kisin et al., 2015).

Adverse Pregnancy Outcomes

No new epidemiologic studies that specifically examined exposure to exhaust reported on preterm birth, birth weight, or other birth outcomes. Weldy et al. (2014) reported that diesel exhaust air pollution promotes significant placental injury ($p<0.05$), as manifested by hemorrhage, vascular compromise, focal necrosis, embryo resorption, inflammation, and oxidative stress in mice exposed in utero.

Developmental Effects

A prospective cohort study in eastern Massachusetts examined the effect of living near gasoline filling stations on growth and weight from birth through early childhood (Fleisch et al., 2015, 2017). The study (Project Viva) recruited more than 2,000 pregnant women from a medical practice and estimated third-trimester exposure based on modeled $PM_{2.5}$, carbon black, traffic density, and residence distance to roadway. The highest levels of third-trimester carbon black and neighborhood traffic density were associated with lower mean fetal growth (–0.13 units, 95% CI –0.25– –0.01) and rapid mean weight gain to 6 months of age (0.25 units, 95% CI 0.01–0.49) (Fleisch et al., 2015). Living within 50 m (compared with greater than 200 m) of a major roadway at birth was significantly associated with greater BMI 0.3 kg/m^2 (95% CI 0.0–0.7), 1.7 cm larger waist circumference (95% CI 0.6–2.8), 1.9 mm larger sum of skinfold thickness (95% CI 0.6–3.2), and 40.7% higher leptin concentration (95% CI 5.2–88.1) in early childhood (mean age 3.3 years), but other indicators of exposure were not related to growth (Fleisch et al., 2017). This study did account for changes in address during the follow-up period, but it did not differentiate between prenatal or postnatal exposure.

Mice exposed prenatally to exhaust have demonstrated a variety of effects. Exposure to diesel exhaust $PM_{2.5}$ particles can affect mothering by dams, resulting in altered energy metabolism in offspring. Prenatal mothering by exposed dams increased the mass of epididymal adipose tissue through hyperplasia, and postnatal mothering by diesel exhaust particle–exposed dams increased the mass of all tested fat pads through hypertrophy (Chen et al., 2017b). Reduced primordial and primary follicles in the offspring of diesel-exhaust-exposed mice were reported by Ogliari et al. (2013). Thirtamara Rajamani et al. (2013) reported that mice demonstrated increased locomotor activity, rearing behaviors, and repetitive self-grooming but no changes in social interaction or anxiety-like behaviors. Weldy et al. (2014) reported increased body weight, altered blood pressure, and increased susceptibility to pressure-overload-induced heart failure among adult mice with prenatal exposure to diesel exhaust.

One review inventoried the developmental effects of prenatal diesel exhaust, diesel exhaust particles, and carbon black that had been reported in 39 toxicologic studies (Ema et al., 2013). Male reproductive system effects included changes in the weight of the testes and accessory reproductive organs, in serum hormone levels, in spermatogenesis, in the histopathology of the testes, and in gene expression for male gonadal development. Female offspring had reproductive effects, including changes in postnatal behavior, in the histopathology of the cerebral cortex and hippocampus, in the development of the central dopaminergic system, in monoaminergic neurochemistry in the brain, and in the expression of steroid hormone–related and thyroid hormone–related genes in the brain. The reported changes in immune response in offspring were sometimes contradictory with regard to prenatal sensitization, but the effects included decreased thymus and spleen weight, an accelerated production of IgE against pollen, modified expression of immune-related genes, increased allergic susceptibility, altered inflammatory indices in the lung, and increased airway hyper reactivity. The authors noted that the data on genotoxicity were inconsistent (Ema et al., 2013).

Synthesis and Conclusions

Several studies have examined the reproductive or developmental effects of exposure to exhaust. The effects on sperm have been reported in a cross-sectional study of toll collectors, which showed adverse effects on sperm, and in studies of the effects of biodiesel and diesel exhaust in mice and rats (Che et al., 2009; Guven et al., 2008; Kisin et al., 2015). Prenatal exposure to high levels of exhaust from traffic has been associated with decreased growth at 6 months of age and a high BMI in childhood, although the analyses did not adjust for postnatal exposures (Fleisch et al., 2015, 2017). Studies in mice have found associations between prenatal exposures and adverse pregnancy outcomes as well as obesity, behavior changes, and reduced primordial germ cells and primary follicles in offspring (Chen et al., 2017b; Ogliari et al., 2013; Thirtamara Rajamani et al., 2013; Weldy et al., 2013). These studies demonstrate in utero susceptibility to exhaust. No studies examined effects following parental preconception exposure to exhaust. These studies on exhaust are limited by the lack of adjustment for PM, a major component of exhaust, in most studies.

The Volume 11 committee concludes that there is inadequate/insufficient evidence to determine whether an association exists between exposure to exhaust and reproductive or developmental effects.

TABLE 6-8 Summary of Reproductive and Developmental Effects of Exhaust

Study	Design/Population	Exposure	Results
Guven et al. (2008)	Cross-sectional 38 healthy toll collectors and 35 healthy controls working as office personnel at the same company.	Exposure categorized by job title.	Semen quality. Toll collectors had lower sperm density ($p=0.002$) and motility ($p=0.003$) and higher percents of abnormal morphology (head abnormalities $p=0.01$, mixed abnormalities $p=0.04$).
Fleisch et al. (2015)	Prospective cohort (Project Viva) 2,115 pregnant women from a medical practice in Boston.	Estimated third-trimester exposure based on modeled $PM_{2.5}$, carbon black, traffic density, and residence distance to roadway. Exposure estimates accounted for changes in address.	Fetal growth and infant growth at 6 months Black carbon and $PM_{2.5}$ not related to outcome measures. Lower fetal growth and rapid weight gain to 6 months of age associated with the highest quartiles of exposure for third trimester carbon black (OR=2.0, 95% CI 0.82–4.84) and traffic density (OR=3.01, 95% CI 1.08–8.44). Adjustments for household income, paternal BMI, maternal education, race/ethnicity, prepregnancy BMI, gestational weight gain, gestational diabetes, smoking, gestational age. Did not adjust for any postnatal factors.
Fleisch et al. (2017)	Prospective cohort (Project Viva) 1,418 pregnant women from a medical practice in Boston.	Estimated prenatal through mid-childhood exposure based on modeled $PM_{2.5}$, carbon black, traffic density, and residence distance to roadway. Exposure estimates accounted for changes in address after birth.	Early and mid-childhood BMI and metabolic measures (median ages 3.3 and 7.7). Prenatal exposures to carbon black, $PM_{2.5}$, or high traffic density not associated with increased BMI or cardiometabolic measures in early or mid-childhood. Living within 50 m of a major roadway at birth was significantly associated with increased BMI, waist circumference, skinfold thickness, and leptin change in childhood.

NOTE: BMI=body mass index; CI=confidence interval; OR=odds ratio; PM=particulate matter.

FUELS

Several petroleum-based fuels were used by the U.S. military in the Persian Gulf region during Operation Desert Shield and Operation Desert Storm, including gasoline, kerosene, diesel, and the jet-propulsion fuels JP-4, JP-5, and JP-8. Those fuels powered aircraft, ground vehicles, tent heaters, and cooking stoves. They were also used for less conventional purposes, such as suppressing sand, cleaning equipment, and burning trash. Military personnel serving in the Gulf War theater of operations could have been exposed to uncombusted fuels, the combustion products from burning those fuels, or a combination of uncombusted and combusted materials (IOM, 2005).

The Volume 3 committee found several studies of parental exposure to fuel that examined adverse reproductive outcomes which may result from genetic alterations in either sperm or egg, including infertility, spontaneous abortion, childhood leukemia, neuroblastoma, and Prader-Willi syndrome. The committee found that it was difficult to come to conclusions about the health outcomes because of the small number of studies that were available for each health outcome, the possibility of recall bias, and the lack of specificity of exposure to the agents of concern in this report. Thus, the Volume 3 committee concluded that there was inadequate/insufficient evidence to determine whether an association exists between exposure to fuels and adverse reproductive or developmental outcomes, including infertility, spontaneous abortion, childhood leukemia, central nervous system tumors, neuroblastoma, and Prader-Willi syndrome (IOM, 2005).

The Volume 11 committee's assessment of the reproductive and developmental effects of fuels was augmented by a 2017 ATSDR profile that described the extensive literature on jet fuels. The committee identified only one additional study on jet fuels not assessed by ATSDR (Tracey et al., 2013). Because the ATSDR profile is recent and broad, the committee did not re-review those materials and instead cites the profile to describe the reproductive and developmental effects of jet fuels.

The remainder of the literature in this section pertains to exposure to automotive gasoline and additives (see Table 6-9). No new studies describing the effects of diesel or kerosene exposure on reproductive or developmental effects were identified. A handful of studies on diesel exhaust are discussed in the previous section on exposure to exhaust. Other than the ATSDR profile on jet fuels, no systematic reviews or meta-analyses of fuels were identified.

Reproductive Effects

ATSDR's review of jet fuels reported a lack of data showing clear reproductive effects in humans. It included one study of military and civilian personnel working at a U.S. Air Force base with occupational exposure to fuels in which the exposed women were found to be not at increased risk for menstrual disorders but did have decreased LH levels before ovulation. However, the authors noted that the effects could have been related to jet fuel, other fuels, or products of complete or incomplete combustion (ATSDR, 2017; Reutman et al., 2002; U.S. Army, 2001).

Animal studies on mice, rats, and dogs have examined the reproductive effects of jet fuels using inhalation, dermal, or oral exposures that ranged from 14 days to 103 weeks. No gross, microscopic, or histological changes in reproductive organs or effects on sperm parameters were reported. One study of preconception exposure for 90 days before mating and throughout gestation, with doses of up to 1,500 mg/kg/day JP-8 by gavage to female rats, did not find any significant effect on pregnancy rate, gestation length, or litter size (ATSDR, 2017; Mattie et al., 2000).

Exposure to jet fuels has not been associated with changes in pregnancy rate, gestation length, or litter size in animal models (ATSDR, 2017).

Reproductive Effects in Men and Women

One epidemiologic study compared the levels of reproductive hormones in filling station workers with office workers, matched by age and by glutathione S-transferase T1 and glutathione S-transferase M1 genotypes (*GSTT1* and *GSTM1*; genes that code for enzymes that detoxify some of the toxic chemical compounds found in petrochemicals) in order to investigate potential genetic sensitivity (Saadat and Monzavi, 2008; Saadat et al., 2013). The first analysis found lower testosterone and higher LH levels in the filling station workers. The authors reported a significant statistical interaction between the *GSTT1* genotype and occupation for LH levels, but not for testosterone or FSH levels (Saadat and Monzavi, 2008). In the second analysis, lower testosterone levels were reported for filling station workers with the *GSTM1* genotype, regardless of *GSTT1* genotype, but no other significant differences were seen (Saadat et al., 2013). Both analyses compared mean hormone levels and did not report any ORs.

One ecological study of birth weight among live births in Montreal found no impact of living near gasoline filling stations based on maternal residence at birth (Huppe et al., 2013).

Animal Studies

In a study of male rats exposed to gasoline fumes for 0, 1, 3, 5, or 9 hours per day for 12 weeks, investigators observed significant dose-dependent effects on serum reproductive hormones, oxidative parameters in testicular tissue, sperm parameters (including motility, count, and morphology), and testicular histopathological changes. The authors attributed these changes to oxidative stress (Owagboriaye et al., 2017).

Leachates from gasoline-, diesel-, and kerosene-dispensing sites (0.5 mL of 0%, 1%, 5%, 10%, 25%, or 50% leachate by intraperitoneal injection) were found to adversely affect sperm parameters (morphology and count) 30 days after exposure in mice. Significant effects were noted at 5% for gasoline and 10% for diesel and kerosene. However, the leachate contained high concentrations of heavy metals, PAHs, and benzene, which may be responsible for the observed effects (Alabi et al., 2017).

In recent animal studies, exposure to gasoline during pregnancy did not affect maternal weight gain or food consumption, litter size, pup weight, or pup loss (Bushnell et al., 2015), except at the highest doses (Roberts et al., 2014a,b).

Developmental Effects

ATSDR did not report on any studies of developmental effects in humans, and it concluded that JP-8 was not embryotoxic or teratogenic according to standard developmental endpoints in animal models. However, several studies in animals have shown other developmental effects of jet fuels after in utero exposure, including decreased fetal weight and average litter size, suppressed immune function, decreased thymus and spleen weight, and transient motor delay (ATSDR, 2017).

Two case-control studies examined the relationship between parental vehicle refueling and childhood cancer (Bailey et al., 2011; Greenop et al., 2015). Vehicle refueling from a year before pregnancy up to the time of the child's cancer diagnosis was assessed. No association was reported between refueling and childhood ALL (Bailey et al., 2011). Childhood brain cancers were related to paternal refueling (≥4 times/month OR=1.59, 95% CI 1.11–2.29), but not to maternal exposure (Greenop et al., 2015). Neither study differentiated among preconception, prenatal, and postnatal exposures.

Animal Studies

Adult rats exposed to gasoline in utero through GD 20 were tested for a variety of outcomes, including being given a series of cognitive and neuropsychological tests, tests of immune function, and physiologic assessments; they showed no effect for any of the outcomes (Bushnell et al., 2015; Herr et al., 2016; Oshiro et al., 2015). Even at very high exposure levels (20,000 mg/m^3) adverse maternal and developmental effects were not observed in mice and rats (Roberts et al., 2014a,b).

A two-generation rat study of gasoline evaluated neuropathology and regional brain glial fibrillary acidic protein content. Parental males and females were exposed, as were F1 animals through lactation, to high doses of gasoline (up to 20,000 mg/m^3). No adverse reproductive or developmental effects were noted in any of the three generations (Gray et al., 2014).

An in vitro study of mouse embryonic stem cells (ES-D3) exposed to petroleum substances (containing varying concentrations of PAHs) showed an inhibition of cell differentiation into cardiomyocytes that was dose-dependent and related to PAH concentration. By contrast, gas-to-liquid products (without PAHs) had no effect on viability or cell differentiation. Because the results correlated with those of in vivo studies, the authors concluded that the prenatal developmental toxicity of petroleum substances is due to their PAH components (Kamelia et al., 2017).

A systematic review of the evidence for inherited transgenerational effects found that although there is no human evidence concerning the transgenerational effects of JP-8, there are four studies in rats, all from the same group of investigators, that examined the transgenerational effects of a gestational exposure to JP-8. The effects the studies examined included growth and development, reproductive effects in offspring, and renal effects in offspring (Walker et al., 2018). The observed effects on body weight were inconsistent with one study that had reported an increase (Tracey et al., 2013) and another that reported no change (Manikkam et al., 2012c). Results suggest that the effects of JP-8 exposure are related to increased apoptosis of germ cells in male offspring, but not to reproductive organ weight, prostate disease, or puberty (Manikkam et al., 2012c; Tracey et al., 2013). In female offspring, JP-8 exposure was associated with decreased follicle number and increased ovarian cysts in female offspring, but its effects on puberty were inconsistent, and no effects on fertility or reproductive organ weight were observed (Manikkam et al., 2012c; Nilsson et al., 2012; Tracey et al., 2013). Transgenerational effects on kidney disease were not observed with JP-8 exposure, even though such effects were observed in earlier generations (Tracey et al., 2013). Inconsistencies across studies (heterogeneity of endpoints, differences in measurement of endpoints, and age at observation), a lack of studies from other researchers, and a lack of analysis using the litter as the unit of analysis limit the confidence in these findings.

Epigenetic Effects

Epigenetic effects were associated with exposure to JP-8 in rats (Tracey et al., 2013). No new studies were found that reported epigenetic or transgenerational effects of gasoline, diesel, or kerosene. Rodent and cell-line models suggest that alterations in genome methylation during critical developmental windows, in part through repetitive regions, have profound effects on both the offspring and the subsequent generations at least to the F3. These effects include immediate F1 toxicity which is later followed by an increase in disease frequency. Of note, F3 females exposed to plastics, dioxin, or jet fuel exhibit an increased rate of polycystic ovary syndrome, with 100% affected with exposure to jet fuel. The rate of F3 male obesity increased 10–15% following exposure to jet fuel (Tracey et al., 2013). However, these outcomes were not correlated with genome methylation.

Synthesis and Conclusions

Since the Volume 3 review in 2004 and the ATSDR review in 2017, little new information has been published regarding the reproductive, developmental, and generational effects of fuels. There are no new high-quality epidemiologic studies that provide evidence of additional effects. The Volume 3 committee concluded that there was "inadequate/insufficient evidence" to permit a conclusion regarding an association between exposure to "fuels and reproductive or developmental effects (including infertility, spontaneous abortion, childhood leukemia, CNS [central nervous system] tumors, neuroblastoma, and Prader-Willi syndrome)" (IOM, 2005). ATSDR's review similarly notes a dearth of data pertaining to the reproductive and developmental effects of jet fuel in humans. Although a few animal studies have shown a variety of developmental effects associated with prenatal JP-8 exposure (decreased fetal and pup weight, suppressed immune function, delayed motor coordination), this fuel is not embryotoxic or teratogenic by standard endpoints, and there are no data on the developmental effects of JP-5 (ATSDR, 2017). Animal studies have shown that epigenetic and transgenerational effects are possible (Walker et al., 2018).

Between the three case-control studies (Bailey et al., 2011; Greenop et al., 2015; Saadat and Monzavi, 2008; Sadaat et al., 2013) and one ecological study (Huppe et al., 2013) that studied reproductive hormone levels, PTB, childhood ALL, and brain tumors, few associations have been reported. Animal studies have shown a few effects, mostly at very high doses, that are of questionable relevance to humans.

The Volume 11 committee concludes that there is inadequate/insufficient evidence to determine whether an association exists between exposure to fuels and reproductive or developmental effects.

TABLE 6-9 Summary of Reproductive and Developmental Effects of Fuels

Study	Design/Population	Exposure	Outcome/Result
Reproductive Effects			
Saadat and Monzavi (2008)	Case-control 114 filling station workers and 112 office workers as age-matched controls in Iran, 2006.	Exposure categorized by job title; *GSTT1* genotype.	Testosterone, LH, and FSH in serum by job and *GSTT1* genotype. Testosterone: levels lower in filling station workers than for office workers for *GSTT1*-present (mean=4.23 versus 4.67, p=0.54) and *GSTT1*-null genotypes (mean=4.26 versus 5.48, p=0.001); no interaction. LH: levels higher in filling station workers than for office workers for *GSTT1*-present (mean=2.82 versus 1.17, p=0.50) and the *GSTT1*-null genotype (mean=3.52 versus 1.07, p=0.025); significant interaction between *GSTT1* genotype and exposure (p=0.003). FSH: no differences between exposure groups or genotypes; no interaction. No ORs reported.
Saadat et al. (2013)	Case-control 114 filling station workers and 100 office workers as age- and sex-matched controls in Iran, 2006.	Exposure categorized by job title; *GSTM1* and *GSTT1* genotype.	Testosterone, LH, and FSH in serum by job and *GSTM1* and *GSTT1* genotypes. Among workers with the null *GSTM1* genotypes, levels of testosterone were higher in unexposed workers than filling station works (p<0.001), regardless of *GSTT1* genotype. No other differences noted among exposure, genotypes, or hormones. No ORs reported.
Adverse Pregnancy Outcomes			
Huppe et al. (2013)	Ecological 267,478 live births on the Island of Montreal, 1994–2006.	Distance from gasoline filling stations based on residential zip code at birth.	PTB (<37weeks gestation) determined from administrative live birth file. No association between residential distance to gasoline filling stations and PTB (adjusted for maternal education, country of birth, marital status, age, parity, infant sex, unemployment rate, renters' proportion paying 30% or more of income on rent, and mean street-block income). Adjusted for SES as estimated by census tract and postal code.

Study	Design/Population	Exposure	Outcome/Result
Developmental Effects			
Bailey et al. (2011)	Case-control 389 cases of ALL and 876 controls matched by age, sex, and state of residence, <15 years old. 2003–2007 in Australia	Self-reported exposures by questionnaire and computer-assisted telephone interview about vehicle refueling in the year before and during pregnancy. Does not distinguish among preconception, prenatal, or postnatal exposure.	Childhood ALL. No association between childhood ALL and parental vehicle refueling in the year before or during pregnancy.
Greenop et al. (2015)	Case-control 306 cases of cases of childhood brain cancer and 950 controls matched by age, sex, and state of residence, <15 years old. 2005–2010 in Australia. Same controls as Bailey et al. (2011).	Self-reported exposures by questionnaire and computer-assisted telephone interview about vehicle refueling in the year before, during pregnancy, and to the time of diagnosis. Does not distinguish among preconception, prenatal, or postnatal exposure.	Childhood brain tumors. No association between maternal refueling before or during pregnancy and brain tumors. Paternal refueling ≥4 times/month OR=1.59, 95% CI 1.11–2.29; adjusted for matching variables, father's age, education, occupational exposure to solvents and diesel exhaust.

NOTE: ALL=acute lymphoblastic leukemia; CI=confidence interval; FSH=follicle-stimulating hormone; GSTM1=glutathione S-transferase mu 1; GSTT1=glutathione S-transferase theta 1; LH=luteinizing hormone; OR=odds ratio; PTB=preterm birth; SES=socioeconomic status.

REFERENCES

Abbott, B.D., G.A. Held, C.R. Wood, A.R. Buckalew, J.G. Brown, and J. Schmid. 1999. AhR, ARNT, and CYP1A1 mRNA quantitation in cultured human embryonic palates exposed to TCDD and comparison with mouse palate in vivo and in culture. *Toxicological Sciences* 47:62–75.

Agay-Shay, K., M. Friger, S. Linn, A. Peled, Y. Amitai, and C. Peretz. 2013. Air pollution and congenital heart defects. *Environmental Research* 124:28–34.

Ahrenhoerster, L.S., E.R. Tate, P.A. Lakatos, X. Wang, and M.D. Laiosa. 2014. Developmental exposure to 2,3,7,8 tetrachlorodibenzo-*p*-dioxin attenuates capacity of hematopoietic stem cells to undergo lymphocyte differentiation. *Toxicology and Applied Pharmacology* 277(2):172–182.

Alabi, O.A., B.E. Esan, and A.A. Sorungbe. 2017. Genetic, reproductive and hematological toxicity induced in mice exposed to leachates from petrol, diesel and kerosene dispensing sites. *Journal of Health and Pollution* 7(16):58–70.

Allen, J.L., G. Oberdorster, K. Morris-Schafer, C. Wong, C. Klocke, M. Sobolewski, K. Conrad, M. Mayer-Proschel, D.A. Cory-Slechta. 2017. Developmental neurotoxicity of inhaled ambient ultrafine particle air pollution: Parallels with neuropathological and behavioral features of autism and other neurodevelopmental disorders. *Neurotoxicology* 59:140–154.

Al-Saleh, I., A. Alsabbahen, N. Shinwari, G. Billedo, A. Mashhour, Y. Al-Sarraj, D. Mohamed Gel, and A. Rabbah. 2013. Polycyclic aromatic hydrocarbons (PAHs) as determinants of various anthropometric measures of birth outcome. *Science of the Total Environment* 444:565–578.

Arroyo, V., J. Diaz, R. Carmona, C. Ortiz, and C. Linares. 2016. Impact of air pollution and temperature on adverse birth outcomes: Madrid, 2001–2009. *Environmental Pollution* 218:1154–1161.

Ashley-Martin, J., E. Lavigne, T.E. Arbuckle, M. Johnson, P. Hystad, D.L. Crouse, J.S. Marshall, and L. Dodds. 2016. Air pollution during pregnancy and cord blood immune system biomarkers. *Journal of Occupational and Environmental Medicine* 58(10):979–986.

ATSDR (Agency for Toxic Substances and Disease Registry). 1995. *Toxicological profile for polycyclic aromatic hydrocarbons*. Atlanta, Georgia: U.S. Department of Health and Human Services.

ATSDR. 2012. Addendum to the toxicological profile for chlorinated dibenzo-*p*-dioxins (CDDs). Atlanta, Georgia: U.S. Department of Health and Human Services.

ATSDR. 2017. *Toxicological profile for JP-5, JP-8, and jet A fuels*. Atlanta, GA: U.S. Department of Health and Human Services.

Badaloni, C., A. Ranucci, G. Cesaroni, G. Zanini, D. Vienneau, F. Al-Aidrous, K. De Hoogh, C. Magnani, F. Forastiere, and SETIL Study Group. 2013. Air pollution and childhood leukaemia: A nationwide case-control study in Italy. *Occupational and Environmental Medicine* 70(12):876–883.

Bailey, H.D., N.H. de Klerk, L. Fritschi, J. Attia, J.D. Daubenton, B.K. Armstrong, E. Milne, and Australia ALL Consortium. 2011. Refuelling of vehicles, the use of wood burners and the risk of acute lymphoblastic leukaemia in childhood. *Paediatric and Perinatal Epidemiology* 25(6):528–539.

Baiz, N., R. Slama, M.C. Bene, M.A. Charles, M.N. Kolopp-Sarda, A. Magnan, O. Thiebaugeorges, G. Faure, and I. Annesi-Maesano. 2011. Maternal exposure to air pollution before and during pregnancy related to changes in newborn's cord blood lymphocyte subpopulations. The EDEN study cohort. *BMC Pregnancy and Childbirth* 11:87.

Baiz, N., P. Dargent-Molina, J.D. Wark, J.C. Souberbielle, R. Slama, and I. Annesi-Maesano. 2012. Gestational exposure to urban air pollution related to a decrease in cord blood vitamin D levels. *Journal of Clinical Endocrinology and Metabolism* 97(11):4087–4095.

Baldridge, M.G., G.T. Marks, R.G. Rawlins, and R.J. Hutz. 2015. Very low-dose (femtomolar) 2,3,7,8-tetrachlorodibenzo-*p*-dioxin (TCDD) disrupts steroidogenic enzyme mRNAs and steroid secretion by human luteinizing granulosa cells. *Reproductive Toxicology* 52:57–61.

Becerra, T.A., M. Wilhelm, J. Olsen, M. Cockburn, and B. Ritz. 2013. Ambient air pollution and autism in Los Angeles County, California. *Environmental Health Perspectives* 121(3):380–386.

Block, M.L., A. Elder, R.L. Auten, S.D. Bilbo, H. Chen, J.C. Chen, D. Cory-Slechta, D. Costa, D. Diaz-Sanchez, D.C. Dorman, D. Gold, K. Gray, H.A. Jeng, J.D. Kaufman, M.T. Kleinman, A. Kirshner, C. Lawler, D.S. Miller, S. Nadadur, B. Ritz, E.O. Semmens, L.H. Tonelli, B. Veronesi, R.O. Wright, and R. Wright. 2012. The Outdoor Air Pollution and Brain Health Workshop. *Neurotoxicology* 33(5):972–984.

Blum, J.L., L.C. Chen, and J.T. Zelikoff. 2017. Exposure to ambient particulate matter during specific gestational periods produces adverse obstetric consequences in mice. *Environmental Health Perspectives* 125(7):077020-1–077020-13.

Bocskay, K.A., D. Tang, M.A. Orjuela, X. Liu, D.P. Warburton, and F.P. Perera. 2005. Chromosomal aberrations in cord blood are associated with prenatal exposure to carcinogenic polycyclic aromatic hydrocarbons. *Cancer Epidemiology Biomarkers & Prevention* 14(2):506–511.

Boda, H., T.N. Nghi, M. Nishijo, P.N. Thao, P.T. Tai, H. Van Luong, T.H. Anh, Y. Morikawa, Y. Nishino, and H. Nishijo. 2018. Prenatal dioxin exposure estimated from dioxins in breast milk and sex hormone levels in umbilical cord blood in Vietnamese newborn infants. *Science of the Total Environment* 615:1312–1318.

Bosetti, C., M.J. Nieuwenhuijsen, S. Gallus, S. Cipriani, C. La Vecchia, and F. Parazzini. 2010. Ambient particulate matter and preterm birth or birth weight: A review of the literature. *Archives of Toxicology* 84(6):447–460.

Breton, C.V., J. Yao, J. Millstein, L. Gao, K.D. Siegmund, W. Mack, L. Whitfield-Maxwell, F. Lurmann, H. Hodis, E. Avol, and F.D. Gilliland. 2016. Prenatal air pollution exposures, DNA methyl transferase genotypes, and associations with newborn LINE1 and Alu methylation and childhood blood pressure and carotid intima-media thickness in the Children's Health Study. *Environmental Health Perspectives* 124(12):1905–1912.

Brown, K.W., W. Bouhamra, D.P. Lamoureux, J.S. Evans, and P. Koutrakis. 2008. Characterization of particulate matter for three sites in Kuwait. *Journal of the Air & Waste Management Association* 58(8):994–1003.

Bruner-Tran, K.L., and K.G. Osteen, 2011. Developmental exposure to TCDD reduces fertility and negatively affects pregnancy outcomes across multiple generations. *Reproductive Toxicology* 31:344–350.

Bruner-Tran, K.L., T. Ding, K.B. Yeoman, A. Archibong, J.A. Arosh, and K.G. Osteen. 2014. Developmental exposure of mice to dioxin promotes transgenerational testicular inflammation and an increased risk of preterm birth in unexposed mating partners. *PLOS ONE* 9(8):e105084.

Bruner-Tran, K.L., A.J. Duleba, H.S. Taylor, and K.G. Osteen. 2016. Developmental toxicant exposure is associated with transgenerational adenomyosis in a murine model. *Biology of Reproduction* 95(4):73.

Bruner-Tran, K.L., J. Gnecco, T.B. Ding, D.R. Glore, V. Pensabene, and K.G. Osteen. 2017. Exposure to the environmental endocrine disruptor TCDD and human reproductive dysfunction: Translating lessons from murine models. *Reproductive Toxicology* 68:59–71.

Bushnell, P.J., T.E. Beasley, P.A. Evansky, S.A. Martin, K.L. McDaniel, V.C. Moser, R.W. Luebke, J. Norwood, Jr., C.B. Copeland, T.E. Kleindienst, W.A. Lonneman, and J.M. Rogers. 2015. Toxicological assessments of rats exposed prenatally to inhaled vapors of gasoline and gasoline-ethanol blends. *Neurotoxicology and Teratology* 49:19–30.

Cai, J., Y. Zhao, P. Liu, B. Xia, Q. Zhu, X. Wang, Q. Song, H. Kan, and Y. Zhang. 2017. Exposure to particulate air pollution during early pregnancy is associated with placental DNA methylation. *Science of the Total Environment* 607–608:1103–1108.

Candela, S., L. Bonvicini, A. Ranzi, F. Baldacchini, S. Broccoli, M. Cordioli, E. Carretta, F. Luberto, P. Angelini, A. Evangelista, P. Marzaroli, P. Giorgi Rossi, and F. Forastiere. 2015. Exposure to emissions from municipal solid waste incinerators and miscarriages: A multisite study of the MONITER Project. *Environment International* 78:51–60.

Cao, X.N., C. Yan, D.Y. Liu, J.P. Peng, J.J. Chen, Y. Zhou, C.L. Long, D.W. He, T. Lin, L.J. Shen, and G.H. Wei. 2015. Fine particulate matter leads to reproductive impairment in male rats by overexpressing phosphatidylinositol 3-kinase (PI3K)/protein kinase B (Akt) signaling pathway. *Toxicology Letters* 237(3):181–190.

Cao, X.N., L.J. Shen, S.D. Wu, C. Yan, Y. Zhou, G. Xiong, Y.C. Wang, Y. Liu, B. Liu, X.L. Tang, M. Guo, D.Y. Liu, C.L. Long, M. Sun, D.W. He, T. Lin, and G.H. Wei. 2017. Urban fine particulate matter exposure causes male reproductive injury through destroying blood–testis barrier (BTB) integrity. *Toxicology Letters* 266:1–12.

Caspersen, I.H., M. Haugen, S. Schjolberg, K. Vejrup, H.K. Knutsen, A.L. Brantsaeter, H.M. Meltzer, J. Alexander, P. Magnus, and H.E. Kvalem. 2016. Maternal dietary exposure to dioxins and polychlorinated biphenyls (PCBs) is associated with language delay in 3-year-old Norwegian children. *Environment International* 91:180–187.

CDC (Centers for Disease Control and Prevention). 2017. *National Birth Defects Prevention Study (NBDPS)*. https://www.cdc.gov/ncbddd/birthdefects/nbdps.html (accessed July 11, 2018).

Chao, M.W., C.H. Yang, P.T. Lin, Y.H. Yang, Y.C. Chuang, M.C. Chung, and C.Y. Tseng. 2017. Exposure to $PM_{2.5}$ causes genetic changes in fetal rat cerebral cortex and hippocampus. *Environmental Toxicology* 32(4):1412–1425.

Che, W., H. Qiu, G. Liu, Y. Ran, H. Zhang, L. Zhang, and W. Wen. 2009. Oxidative damage of the extracts of condensate, particulate and semivolatile organic compounds from gasoline engine exhausts on testicles of rats. *Bulletin of Environmental Contamination and Toxicology* 83(1):42–47.

Chen, E.K.C., D. Zmirou-Navier, C. Padilla, and S. Deguen. 2014. Effects of air pollution on the risk of congenital anomalies: A systematic review and meta-analysis. *International Journal of Environmental Research and Public Health* 11(8):7642–7668.

Chen, M.-J., S. Liang, H. Zhou, Y. Xu, X. Qin, Z. Hu, X. Wang, L. Qiu, W. Wang, Y. Zhang, and Z. Ying. 2017a. Prenatal and postnatal mothering by diesel exhaust $PM_{2.5}$-exposed dams differentially program mouse energy metabolism. *Particle and Fibre Toxicology* 14(1):3.

Chen, H., X. Chen, X. Hong, C. Liu, H. Huang, Q. Wang, S. Chen, H. Chen, K. Yang, and Q. Sun. 2017b. Maternal exposure to ambient $PM_{2.5}$ exaggerates fetal cardiovascular maldevelopment induced by homocysteine in rats. *Environmental Toxicology* 32(3):877–889.

Chiu, Y.H.M., B.A. Coull, M.J. Sternthal, I. Kloog, J. Schwartz, S. Cohen, and R.J. Wright. 2014. Effects of prenatal community violence and ambient air pollution on childhood wheeze in an urban population. *Journal of Allergy and Clinical Immunology* 133(3):713–722.

Chiu, Y.H.M., H.H.L. Hsu, B.A. Coull, D.C. Bellinger, I. Kloog, J. Schwartz, R.O. Wright, and R.J. Wright. 2016. Prenatal particulate air pollution and neurodevelopment in urban children: Examining sensitive windows and sex-specific associations. *Environment International* 87:56–65.

Chiu, Y.H., H.H. Hsu, A. Wilson, B.A. Coull, M.P. Pendo, A. Baccarelli, I. Kloog, J. Schwartz, R.O. Wright, E.M. Taveras, and R.J. Wright. 2017. Prenatal particulate air pollution exposure and body composition in urban preschool children: Examining sensitive windows and sex-specific associations. *Environmental Research* 158:798–805.

Choi, H., V. Rauh, R. Garfinkel, Y. Tu, and F.P. Perera. 2008. Prenatal exposure to airborne polycyclic aromatic hydrocarbons and risk of intrauterine growth restriction. *Environmental Health Perspectives* 116(5):658–665.

Choi, H., L. Wang, X. Lin, J.D. Spengler, and F.P. Perera. 2012. Fetal window of vulnerability to airborne polycyclic aromatic hydrocarbons on proportional intrauterine growth restriction. *PLOS ONE* 7(4):e35464.

Clark, N.A., P.A. Demers, C.J. Karr, M. Koehoorn, C. Lencar, L. Tamburic, and M. Brauer. 2010. Effect of early life exposure to air pollution on development of childhood asthma. *Environmental Health Perspectives* 118(2):284–290.

Clemente, D.B.P., M. Casas, N. Vilahur, H. Begiristain, M. Bustamante, A. Carsin, M.F. Fernandez, F. Fierens, W. Gyselaers, C. Iniguez, B.G. Janssen, W. Lefebvre, S. Llop, N. Olea, M. Pedersen, N. Pieters, L.S. Marina, A. Souto, A. Tardon, C. Vanpoucke, M. Vrijheid, J. Sunyer, and T.S. Nawrot. 2016. Prenatal ambient air pollution, placental mitochondrial DNA content, and birth weight in the INMA (Spain) and ENVIRONAGE (Belgium) birth cohorts. *Environmental Health Perspectives* 124(5):659–665.

Conti, C.O., A.E. Calogero, F. Giacone, M. Fiore, M. Barchitta, A. Agodi, and M. Ferrante. 2017. B(a)P adduct levels and fertility: A cross-sectional study in a Sicilian population. *Molecular Medicine Reports* 15(5):3398–3404.

Dadvand, P., J. Rankin, S. Rushton, and T. Pless-Mulloli. 2011a. Ambient air pollution and congenital heart disease: A register-based study. *Environmental Research* 111(3):435–441.

Dadvand, P., J. Rankin, S. Rushton, and T. Pless-Mulloli. 2011b. Association between maternal exposure to ambient air pollution and congenital heart disease: A register-based spatiotemporal analysis. *American Journal of Epidemiology* 173(2):171–182.

Dadvand, P., F. Figueras, X. Basagana, R. Beelen, D. Martinez, M. Cirach, A. Schembari, G. Hoek, B. Brunekreef, and M.J. Nieuwenhuijsen. 2013. Ambient air pollution and preeclampsia: A spatiotemporal analysis. *Environmental Health Perspectives* 121(11–12):1365–1371.

DeFranco, E., E. Hall, M. Hossain, A. Chen, E.N. Haynes, D. Jones, S. Ren, L. Lu, and L. Muglia. 2015. Air pollution and stillbirth risk: Exposure to airborne particulate matter during pregnancy is associated with fetal death. *PLOS ONE* 10(3):e0120594.

Dejmek J., I. Solanský, I. Benes, J. Lenícek, and R.J. Srám. 2000. The impact of polycyclic aromatic hydrocarbons and fine particles on pregnancy outcome. *Environmental Health Perspectives* 108(12):1159–1164.

Den Hond, E., H. Tournaye, P. De Sutter, W. Ombelet, W. Baeyens, A. Covaci, B. Cox, T.S. Nawrot, N. Van Larebeke, and T. D'Hooghe. 2015. Human exposure to endocrine disrupting chemicals and fertility: A case-control study in male subfertility patients. *Environment International* 84:154–160.

Deng, Q., C. Lu, D. Norback, C.G. Bornehag, Y. Zhang, W. Liu, H. Yuan, and J. Sundell. 2015. Early life exposure to ambient air pollution and childhood asthma in China. *Environmental Research* 143(Pt A):83–92.

Deng, Q., C. Lu, Y. Li, J. Sundell, and N. Dan. 2016. Exposure to outdoor air pollution during trimesters of pregnancy and childhood asthma, allergic rhinitis, and eczema. *Environmental Research* 150:119–127.

Deng, Q., C. Lu, Y. Li, L. Chen, Y. He, J. Sundell, and D. Norback. 2017. Association between prenatal exposure to industrial air pollution and onset of early childhood ear infection in China. *Atmospheric Environment* 157:18–26.

Dhanabalan, S., P.P. Mathur, and P. Latha. 2015. TCDD and corticosterone on testicular steroidogenesis and antioxidant system of epididymal sperm in rats. *Toxicology and Industrial Health* 31(9):811–822.

Dolk, H., B. Armstrong, K. Lachowycz, M. Vrijheid, J. Rankin, L. Abramsky, P.A. Boyd, and D. Wellesley. 2010. Ambient air pollution and risk of congenital anomalies in England, 1991–1999. *Occupational and Environmental Medicine* 67(4):223–227.

Ebisu, K., B. Malig, S. Hasheminassab, C. Sioutas, and R. Basu. 2018. Cause-specific stillbirth and exposure to chemical constituents and sources of fine particulate matter. *Environmental Research* 160:358–364.

ECHA (European Chemicals Agency). 2017. *Substance information: Benzo[def]chrysene*. European Union. https://echa.europa.eu/substance-information/-/substanceinfo/100.000.026 (accessed January 30, 2018).

Edwards, S.C., W. Jedrychowski, M. Butscher, D. Camann, A. Kieltyka, E. Mroz, E. Flak, Z. Li, S. Wang, V. Rauh, and F. Perera. 2010. Prenatal exposure to airborne polycyclic aromatic hydrocarbons and children's intelligence at 5 years of age in a prospective cohort study in Poland. *Environmental Health Perspectives* 118(9):1326–1331.

Eenhuizen, E., U. Gehring, A.H. Wijga, H.A. Smit, P.H. Fischer, M. Brauer, G.H. Koppelman, M. Kerkhof, J.C. de Jongste, B. Brunekreef, and G. Hoek. 2013. Traffic-related air pollution is related to interrupter resistance in 4-year-old children. *European Respiratory Journal* 41(6):1257–1263.

El Khouri Miraglia, S.G., M.M. Veras, L.F. Amato-Lourenco, F. Rodrigues-Silva, and P.H.N. Saldiva. 2013. Follow-up of the air pollution and the human male-to-female ratio analysis in Sao Paulo, Brazil: A times series study. *British Medical Journal Open* 3(7):e002552.

Ema, M., M. Naya, M. Horimoto, and H. Kato. 2013. Developmental toxicity of diesel exhaust: A review of studies in experimental animals. *Reproductive Toxicology* 42:1–17.

Enkhmaa, D., N. Warburton, B. Javzandulam, J. Uyanga, Y. Khishigsuren, S. Lodoysamba, S. Enkhtur, and D. Warburton. 2014. Seasonal ambient air pollution correlates strongly with spontaneous abortion in Mongolia. *BMC Pregnancy Childbirth* 14:146.

EPA (U.S. Environmental Protection Agency). 2009. *Integrated science assessment (ISA) for particulate matter (Final report).* EPA/600/R-08/139F. Washington, DC: U.S. Environmental Protection Agency.

EPA. 2012. *EPA's reanalysis of key issues related to dioxin toxicity and response to NAS comments, Volume 1.* (CAS No. 1746-01-6) In support of the summary information on the Integrated Risk Information System (IRIS). EPA/600/R-10/038F. Washington, DC: U.S. Environmental Protection Agency.

EPA. 2016. Dioxin and dioxin-like compounds toxic equivalency information. https://www.epa.gov/toxics-release-inventory-tri-program/dioxin-and-dioxin-compounds-toxic-equivalency-information (accessed April 19, 2018).

EPA. 2017. *Toxicological review of benzo[a]pyrene [CASRN 50-32-8].* EPA/635/R-17/003Fa. Washington, DC: Integrated Risk Information System, National Center for Environmental Assessment, Office of Research and Development, U.S. Environmental Protection Agency.

EPA. 2018. *Regulatory information by topic: Air.* https://www.epa.gov/regulatory-information-topic/regulatory-information-topic-air (accessed July 21, 2018).

Erickson, A.C., A. Ostry, L.H. Chan, and L. Arbour. 2016. The reduction of birth weight by fine particulate matter and its modification by maternal and neighbourhood-level factors: A multilevel analysis in British Columbia, Canada. *Environmental Health* 15:51.

Eskenazi, B., K. Huen, A. Marks, K.G. Harley, A. Bradman, D.B. Barr, and N. Holland. 2010. PON1 and neurodevelopment in children from the CHAMACOS study exposed to organophosphate pesticides in utero. *Environmental Health Perspectives* 118(12):1775–1781.

Faiz, A.S., G.G. Rhoads, K. Demissie, L. Kruse, Y. Lin, and D.Q. Rich. 2012. Ambient air pollution and the risk of stillbirth. *American Journal of Epidemiology* 176(4):308–316.

Faiz, A.S., G.G. Rhoads, K. Demissie, Y. Lin, L. Kruse, and D.Q. Rich. 2013. Does ambient air pollution trigger stillbirth? *Epidemiology* 24(4):538–544.

Farhi, A., V. Boyko, J. Almagor, I. Benenson, E. Segre, Y. Rudich, E. Stern, and L. Lerner-Geva. 2014. The possible association between exposure to air pollution and the risk for congenital malformations. *Environmental Research* 135:173–180.

Faure, A.C., J.F. Viel, A. Bailly, O. Blagosklonov, C. Amiot, and C. Roux. 2014. Evolution of sperm quality in men living in the vicinity of a municipal solid waste incinerator possibly correlated with decreasing dioxins emission levels. *Andrologia* 46(7):744–752.

Fleisch, A.F., D.R. Gold, S.L. Rifas-Shiman, P. Koutrakis, J.D. Schwartz, I. Kloog, S. Melly, B.A. Coull, A. Zanobetti, M.W. Gillman, and E. Oken. 2014. Air pollution exposure and abnormal glucose tolerance during pregnancy: The Project Viva cohort. *Environmental Health Perspectives* 122(4):378–383.

Fleisch, A.F., S.L. Rifas-Shiman, P. Koutrakis, J.D. Schwartz, I. Kloog, S. Melly, B.A. Coull, A. Zanobetti, M.W. Gillman, D.R. Gold, and E. Oken. 2015. Prenatal exposure to traffic pollution: Associations with reduced fetal growth and rapid infant weight gain. *Epidemiology* 26(1):43–50.

Fleisch, A.F., H. Luttmann-Gibson, W. Perng, S.L. Rifas-Shiman, B.A. Coull, I. Kloog, P. Koutrakis, J.D. Schwartz, A. Zanobetti, C.S. Mantzoros, M.W. Gillman, D.R. Gold, and E. Oken. 2017. Prenatal and early life exposure to traffic pollution and cardiometabolic health in childhood. *Pediatric Obesity* 12(1):48–57.

Flores-Pajot, M.C., M. Ofner, M.T. Do, E. Lavigne, and P.J. Villeneuve. 2016. Childhood autism spectrum disorders and exposure to nitrogen dioxide, and particulate matter air pollution: A review and meta-analysis. *Environmental Research* 151:763–776.

Frutos, V., M. Gonzalez-Comadran, I. Sola, B. Jacquemin, R. Carreras, and M.A. Checa Vizcaino. 2015. Impact of air pollution on fertility: A systematic review. *Gynecological Endocrinology* 31(1):7–13.

Galimova, E.F., Z.K. Amirova, and Sh. N. Galimov. 2015. Dioxins in the semen of men with infertility. *Environmental Science and Pollution Research* 22(19):14566–14569.

Gaspari, L., S.S. Chang, R.M. Santella, S. Garte, P. Pedotti, and E. Taioli. 2003. Polycyclic aromatic hydrocarbon-DNA adducts in human sperm as a marker of DNA damage and infertility. *Mutation Research—Genetic Toxicology and Environmental Mutagenesis* 535(2):155–160.

Gehring, U., O. Gruzieva, R.M. Agius, R. Beelen, A. Custovic, J. Cyrys, M. Eeftens, C. Flexeder, E. Fuertes, J. Heinrich, B. Hoffmann, J.C. de Jongste, M. Kerkhof, C. Klumper, M. Korek, A. Molter, E.S. Schultz, A. Simpson, D. Sugiri, M. Svartengren, A. von Berg, A.H. Wijga, G. Pershagen, and B. Brunekreef. 2013. Air pollution exposure and lung function in children: The ESCAPE project. *Environmental Health Perspectives* 121(11–12):1357–1364.

Genkinger, J.M., L. Stigler, W. Jedrychowski, T. Huang, S. Wang, E. Roen, R. Majewska, A. Kieltyka, E. Mroz, and F. Perera. 2015. Prenatal polycyclic aromatic hydrocarbon (PAH) exposure, antioxidant levels and behavioral development of children ages 6–9. *Environmental Research* 140:136–144.

Gianicolo, E.A., C. Mangia, M. Cervino, A. Bruni, M.G. Andreassi, and G. Latini. 2014. Congenital anomalies among live births in a high environmental risk area—A case-control study in Brindisi (southern Italy). *Environmental Research* 128:9–14.

Giovannini, N., L. Schwartz, S. Cipriani, F. Parazzini, I. Baini, V. Signorelli, and I. Cetin. 2018. Particulate matter (PM_{10}) exposure, birth and fetal–placental weight and umbilical arterial pH: Results from a prospective study. *Journal of Maternal–Fetal and Neonatal Medicine* 31(5):651–655.

Girguis, M.S., M.J. Strickland, X. Hu, Y. Liu, S.M. Bartell, and V.M. Vieira. 2016. Maternal exposure to traffic-related air pollution and birth defects in Massachusetts. *Environmental Research* 146:1–9.

Godschalk, R.W.L., N. Verhofstad, M. Verheijen, C.L. Yauk, J.O. Linschooten, H. van Steeg, C.T. van Oostrom, J. van Benthem, and F.J. van Schooten. 2015. Effects of benzo[a]pyrene on mouse germ cells: Heritable DNA mutation, testicular cell hypomethylation and their interaction with nucleotide excision repair. *Toxicology Research* 4(3):718–724.

Gong, T., C. Almqvist, S. Bolte, P. Lichtenstein, H. Anckarsater, T. Lind, C. Lundholm, and G. Pershagen. 2014. Exposure to air pollution from traffic and neurodevelopmental disorders in Swedish twins. *Twin Research and Human Genetics* 17(6):553–562.

Gong, T., C. Dalman, S. Wicks, H. Dal, C. Magnusson, C. Lundholm, C. Almqvist, and G. Pershagen. 2017. Perinatal exposure to traffic-related air pollution and autism spectrum disorders. *Environmental Health Perspectives* 125(1):119–126.

Goyal, N., and D. Canning. 2017. Exposure to ambient fine particulate air pollution in utero as a risk factor for child stunting in Bangladesh. *International Journal of Environmental Research and Public Health* 15(1):23.

Gray, T.M., D. Steup, L.G. Roberts, J.P. O'Callaghan, G. Hoffman, C.A. Schreiner, and C.R. Clark. 2014. Health assessment of gasoline and fuel oxygenate vapors: Reproductive toxicity assessment. *Regulatory Toxicology and Pharmacology* 70(2 Suppl):S48–S57.

Green, R., V. Sarovar, B. Malig, and R. Basu. 2015. Association of stillbirth with ambient air pollution in a California cohort study. *American Journal of Epidemiology* 181(11):874–882.

Greenop, K.R., A.L. Hinwood, L. Fritschi, R.J. Scott, J. Attia, L.J. Ashton, J.A. Heath, B.K. Armstrong, and E. Milne. 2015. Vehicle refuelling, use of domestic wood heaters and the risk of childhood brain tumours: Results from an Australian case-control study. *Pediatric Blood and Cancer* 62(2):229–234.

Grevendonk, L., B.G. Janssen, C. Vanpoucke, W. Lefebvre, M. Hoxha, V. Bollati, and T.S. Nawrot. 2016. Mitochondrial oxidative DNA damage and exposure to particulate air pollution in mother–newborn pairs. *Environmental Health* 15:10.

Grufferman, S., P.J. Lupo, R.I. Vogel, H.E. Danysh, E.B. Erhardt, and S. Ognjanovic. 2014. Parental military service, Agent Orange exposure, and the risk of rhabdomyosarcoma in offspring. *Journal of Pediatrics* 165(6):1216–1221.

Gu, A., G. Ji, P. Zhu, Y. Zhou, G. Fu, Y. Xia, L. Song, S. Wang, and X. Wang. 2010. Nucleotide excision repair polymorphisms, polycyclic aromatic hydrocarbon exposure, and their effects on sperm deoxyribonucleic acid damage and male factor infertility. *Fertility and Sterility* 94(7):2620–2625.

Guo, Y., X. Huo, K. Wu, J. Liu, Y. Zhang, and X. Xu. 2012. Carcinogenic polycyclic aromatic hydrocarbons in umbilical cord blood of human neonates from Guiyu, China. *Science of the Total Environment* 427–428:35–40.

Guven, A., A. Kayikci, K. Cam, P. Arbak, O. Balbay, and M. Cam. 2008. Alterations in semen parameters of toll collectors working at motorways: Does diesel exposure induce detrimental effects on semen? *Andrologia* 40(6):346–351.

Guxens, M., R. Garcia-Esteban, L. Giorgis-Allemand, J. Forns, C. Badaloni, F. Ballester, R. Beelen, G. Cesaroni, L. Chatzi, M. De Agostini, A. De Nazelle, M. Eeftens, M.F. Fernandez, A. Fernandez-Somoano, F. Forastiere, U. Gehring, A. Ghassabian, B. Heude, V.W.V. Jaddoe, C. Klumper, M. Kogevinas, U. Kramer, B. Larroque, A. Lertxundi, N. Lertxuni, M. Murcia, V. Navel, M. Nieuwenhuijsen, D. Porta, R. Ramos, T. Roumeliotaki, R. Slama, M. Sorensen, E.G. Stephanou, D. Sugiri, A. Tardon, H. Tiemeier, C.M.T. Tiesler, F.C. Verhulst, T. Vrijkotte, M. Wilhelm, B. Brunekreef, G. Pershagen, and J. Sunyer. 2014. Air pollution during pregnancy and childhood cognitive and psychomotor development: Six European birth cohorts. *Epidemiology* 25(5):636–647.

Guxens, M., A. Ghassabian, T. Gong, R. Garcia-Esteban, D. Porta, L. Giorgis-Allemand, C. Almqvist, A. Aranbarri, R. Beelen, C. Badaloni, G. Cesaroni, A. de Nazelle, M. Estarlich, F. Forastiere, J. Forns, U. Gehring, J. Ibarluzea, V.W. Jaddoe, M. Korek, P. Lichtenstein, M.J. Nieuwenhuijsen, M. Rebagliato, R. Slama, H. Tiemeier, F.C. Verhulst, H.E. Volk, G. Pershagen, B. Brunekreef, and J. Sunyer. 2016. Air pollution exposure during pregnancy and childhood autistic traits in four European population-based cohort studies: The ESCAPE project. *Environmental Health Perspectives* 124(1):133–140.

Hack, M., N.K. Klein, and H.G. Taylor. 1995. Long-term developmental outcomes of low birth weight infants. *The Future of Children* 5(1):176–196.

Hampel, R., J. Lepeule, A. Schneider, S. Bottagisi, M.A. Charles, P. Ducimetiere, A. Peters, and R. Slama. 2011. Short-term impact of ambient air pollution and air temperature on blood pressure among pregnant women. *Epidemiology* 22(5):671–679.

Han, X., N. Zhou, Z. Cui, M. Ma, L. Li, M. Cai, H. Lin, Y. Li, L. Ao, J. Liu, and J. Cao. 2011. Association between urinary polycyclic aromatic hydrocarbon metabolites and sperm DNA damage: A population study in Chongqing, China. *Environmental Health Perspectives* 119(5):652–657.

Han, Y., Y. Xia, P. Zhu, S. Qiao, R. Zhao, N. Jin, S. Wang, L. Song, G. Fu, and X. Wang. 2010. Reproductive hormones in relation to polycyclic aromatic hydrocarbon (PAH) metabolites among non-occupational exposure of males. *Science of the Total Environment* 408(4):768–773.

Hansen, C.A., A.G. Barnett, B.B. Jalaludin, and G.G. Morgan. 2009. Ambient air pollution and birth defects in Brisbane, Australia. *PLOS ONE* 4(4):e5408.

Hansen, C., T.J. Luben, J.D. Sacks, A. Olshan, S. Jeffay, L. Strader, and S.D. Perreault. 2010. The effect of ambient air pollution on sperm quality. *Environmental Health Perspectives* 118(2):203–209.

Harris, M.H., D.R. Gold, S.L. Rifas-Shiman, S.J. Melly, A. Zanobetti, B.A. Coull, J.D. Schwartz, A. Gryparis, I. Kloog, P. Koutrakis, D.C. Bellinger, M.B. Belfort, T.F. Webster, R.F. White, S.K. Sagiv, and E. Oken. 2016. Prenatal and childhood traffic-related air pollution exposure and childhood executive function and behavior. *Neurotoxicology and Teratology* 57:60–70.

Heck, J.E., A.S. Park, J. Qiu, M. Cockburn, and B. Ritz. 2013a. An exploratory study of ambient air toxics exposure in pregnancy and the risk of neuroblastoma in offspring. *Environmental Research* 127:1–6.

Heck, J.E., J. Wu, C. Lombardi, J. Qiu, T.J. Meyers, M. Wilhelm, M. Cockburn, and B. Ritz. 2013b. Childhood cancer and traffic-related air pollution exposure in pregnancy and early life. *Environmental Health Perspectives* 121(11–12):1385–1391.

Heck, J.E., A.S. Park, J. Qiu, M. Cockburn, and B. Ritz. 2014. Risk of leukemia in relation to exposure to ambient air toxics in pregnancy and early childhood. *International Journal of Hygiene and Environmental Health* 217(6):662–668.

Hehua, Z., C. Qing, G. Shanyan, W. Qijun, and Z. Yuhong. 2017. The impact of prenatal exposure to air pollution on childhood wheezing and asthma: A systematic review. *Environmental Research* 159:519–530.

Herbstman, J.B., D. Tang, D. Zhu, L. Qu, A. Sjodin, Z. Li, D. Camann, and F.P. Perera. 2012. Prenatal exposure to polycyclic aromatic hydrocarbons, benzo[a]pyrene-DNA adducts, and genomic DNA methylation in cord blood. *Environmental Health Perspectives* 120(5):733–738.

Herr, C.E.W., M. Dostal, R. Ghosh, P. Ashwood, M. Lipsett, K.E. Pinkerton, R. Sram, and I. Hertz-Picciotto. 2010. Air pollution exposure during critical time periods in gestation and alterations in cord blood lymphocyte distribution: A cohort of livebirths. *Environmental Health* 9(1):46.

Herr, C.E.W., R. Ghosh, M. Dostal, V. Skokanova, P. Ashwood, M. Lipsett, J.P. Joad, K.E. Pinkerton, P.S. Yap, J.D. Frost, R. Sram, and I. Hertz-Picciotto. 2011. Exposure to air pollution in critical prenatal time windows and IgE levels in newborns. *Pediatric Allergy and Immunology* 22(1 PART 1):75–84.

Herr, D.W., D.L. Freeborn, L. Degn, S.A. Martin, J. Ortenzio, L. Pantlin, C.W. Hamm, and W.K. Boyes. 2016. Neurophysiological assessment of auditory, peripheral nerve, somatosensory, and visual system function after developmental exposure to gasoline, E15, and E85 vapors. *Neurotoxicology and Teratology* 54:78–88.

Houseman, E.A., W.P. Accomando, D.C. Koestler, B.C. Christensen, C.J. Marsit, H.H. Nelson, J.K. Wiencke, and K.T. Kelsey. 2012. DNA methylation arrays as surrogate measures of cell mixture distribution. *BMC Bioinformatics* 13:86.

Houseman, E.A., S. Kim, K.T. Kelsey, and J.K. Wiencke. 2015. DNA methylation in whole blood: Uses and challenges. *Current Environmental Health Reports* 2(2):145–154.

Hsu, H.H., Y.H. Chiu, B.A. Coull, I. Kloog, J. Schwartz, A. Lee, R.O. Wright, and R.J. Wright. 2015. Prenatal particulate air pollution and asthma onset in urban children: Identifying sensitive windows and sex differences. *American Journal of Respiratory and Critical Care Medicine* 192(9):1052–1059.

Hsu, P.C., I.Y. Chen, C.H. Pan, K.Y. Wu, M.H. Pan, J.R. Chen, C.J. Chen, G.P. Chang-Chien, C.H. Hsu, C.S. Liu, and M.T. Wu. 2006. Sperm DNA damage correlates with polycyclic aromatic hydrocarbons biomarker in coke-oven workers. *International Archives of Occupational and Environmental Health* 79(5):349–356.

Hu, H., S. Ha, B.H. Henderson, T.D. Warner, J. Roth, H. Kan, and X. Xu. 2015. Association of atmospheric particulate matter and ozone with gestational diabetes mellitus. *Environmental Health Perspectives* 123(9):853–859.

Huang, C.C., H.J. Wen, P.C. Chen, T.L. Chiang, S.J. Lin, and Y.L. Guo. 2015. Prenatal air pollutant exposure and occurrence of atopic dermatitis. *British Journal of Dermatology* 173(4):981–988.

Huang, J.V., G.M. Leung, and C.M. Schooling. 2017. The association of air pollution with pubertal development: Evidence from Hong Kong's "Children of 1997" birth cohort. *American Journal of Epidemiology* 185(10):914–923.

Hui, L.L., H.S. Lam, E.Y. Lau, E.A. Nelson, T.W. Wong, and R. Fielding. 2016. Prenatal dioxin exposure and neurocognitive development in Hong Kong 11-year-old children. *Environmental Research* 150:205–212.

Huppe, V., Y. Kestens, N. Auger, M. Daniel, and A. Smargiassi. 2013. Residential proximity to gasoline service stations and preterm birth. *Environmental Science and Pollution Research* 20(10):7186–7193.

Hwang, B.F., Y.L. Lee, and J.J.K. Jaakkola. 2011. Air pollution and stillbirth: A population-based case-control study in Taiwan. *Environmental Health Perspectives* 119(9):1345–1349.

Hwang, B.F., Y.L. Lee, and J.J. Jaakkola. 2015. Air pollution and the risk of cardiac defects: A population-based case-control study. *Medicine* 94(44):e1883.

Ibrahimou, B., A.N. Albatineh, H.M. Salihu, and J. Gasana. 2017. Ambient $PM_{2.5}$ aluminum and elemental carbon and placental abruption morbidity. *Journal of Occupational and Environmental Medicine* 59(2):148–153.

IOM (Institute of Medicine). 2005. *Gulf War and health, volume 3: Fuels, combustion products, and propellants*. Washington, DC: The National Academies Press.

IOM. 2011. *Long-term health consequences of exposure to burn pits in Iraq and Afghanistan*. Washington, DC: The National Academies Press.

IOM. 2014. *Veterans and Agent Orange: Update 2012*. Washington, DC: The National Academies Press.

Iszatt, N., H. Stigum, E. Govarts, L.P. Murinova, G. Schoeters, T. Trnovec, J. Legler, C. Thomsen, G. Koppen, and M. Eggesbo. 2016. Perinatal exposure to dioxins and dioxin-like compounds and infant growth and body mass index at seven years: A pooled analysis of three European birth cohorts. *Environment International* 94:399–407.

Jacobs, M., G. Zhang, S. Chen, B. Mullins, M. Bell, L. Jin, Y. Guo, R. Huxley, and G. Pereira. 2017. The association between ambient air pollution and selected adverse pregnancy outcomes in China: A systematic review. *Science of the Total Environment* 579:1179–1192.

Janssen, B.G., E. Munters, N. Pieters, K. Smeets, B. Cox, A. Cuypers, F. Fierens, J. Penders, J. Vangronsveld, W. Gyselaers, and T.S. Nawrot. 2012. Placental mitochondrial DNA content and particulate air pollution during in utero life. *Environmental Health Perspectives* 120(9):1346–1352.

Janssen, B.G., L. Godderis, N. Pieters, K. Poels, M. Kicinski, A. Cuypers, F. Fierens, J. Penders, M. Plusquin, W. Gyselaers, and T.S. Nawrot. 2013. Placental DNA hypomethylation in association with particulate air pollution in early life. *Particle and Fibre Toxicology* 10:22.

Janssen, B.G., H.M. Byun, W. Gyselaers, W. Lefebvre, A.A. Baccarelli, and T.S. Nawrot. 2015. Placental mitochondrial methylation and exposure to airborne particulate matter in the early life environment: An ENVIRONAGE birth cohort study. *Epigenetics* 10(6):536–544.

Janssen, B.G., N.D. Saenen, H.A. Roels, N. Madhloum, W. Gyselaers, W. Lefebvre, J. Penders, C. Vanpoucke, K. Vrijens, and T.S. Nawrot. 2017. Fetal thyroid function, birth weight, and in utero exposure to fine particle air pollution: A birth cohort study. *Environmental Health Perspectives* 125(4):699–705.

Jedrychowski, W., A. Galas, A. Pac, E. Flak, D. Camman, V. Rauh, and F. Perera. 2005. Prenatal ambient air exposure to polycyclic aromatic hydrocarbons and the occurrence of respiratory symptoms over the first year of life. *European Journal of Epidemiology* 20(9):775–782.

Jedrychowski, W.A., F.P. Perera, U. Maugeri, E. Mroz, M. Klimaszewska-Rembiasz, E. Flak, S. Edwards, and J.D. Spengler. 2010a. Effect of prenatal exposure to fine particulate matter on ventilatory lung function of preschool children of non-smoking mothers. *Paediatric and Perinatal Epidemiology* 24(5):492–501.

Jedrychowski, W.A., F.P. Perera, U. Maugeri, D. Mrozek-Budzyn, E. Mroz, M. Klimaszewska-Rembiasz, E. Flak, S. Edwards, J. Spengler, R. Jacek, and A. Sowa. 2010b. Intrauterine exposure to polycyclic aromatic hydrocarbons, fine particulate matter and early wheeze: Prospective birth cohort study in 4-year olds. *Pediatric Allergy and Immunology* 21(4 Pt 2):e723–e732.

Jedrychowski, W., F. Perera, U. Maugeri, D. Mrozek-Budzyn, R.L. Miller, E. Flak, E. Mroz, R. Jacek, and J.D. Spengler. 2011a. Effects of prenatal and perinatal exposure to fine air pollutants and maternal fish consumption on the occurrence of infantile eczema. *International Archives of Allergy and Immunology* 155(3):275–281.

Jedrychowski, W., J.D. Spengler, U. Maugeri, R.L. Miller, D. Budzyn-Mrozek, M. Perzanowski, E. Flak, E. Mroz, R. Majewska, I. Kaim, and F. Perera. 2011b. Effect of prenatal exposure to fine particulate matter and intake of paracetamol (acetaminophen) in pregnancy on eczema occurrence in early childhood. *Science of the Total Environment* 409(24):5205–5209.

Jedrychowski, W., U. Maugeri, E. Mroz, E. Flak, M. Rembiasz, R. Jacek, and A. Sowa. 2012. Fractional exhaled nitric oxide in healthy non-asthmatic 7-year olds and prenatal exposure to polycyclic aromatic hydrocarbons: Nested regression analysis. *Pediatric Pulmonology* 47(11):1131–1139.

Jedrychowski, W.A., F.P. Perera, J.D. Spengler, E. Mroz, L. Stigter, E. Flak, R. Majewska, M. Klimaszewska-Rembiasz, and R. Jacek. 2013. Intrauterine exposure to fine particulate matter as a risk factor for increased susceptibility to acute broncho-pulmonary infections in early childhood. *International Journal of Hygiene and Environmental Health* 216(4):395–401.

Jedrychowski, W.A., F.P. Perera, R. Majewska, D. Camman, J.D. Spengler, E. Mroz, L. Stigter, E. Flak, and R. Jacek. 2014. Separate and joint effects of transplacental and postnatal inhalatory exposure to polycyclic aromatic hydrocarbons: Prospective birth cohort study on wheezing events. *Pediatric Pulmonology* 49(2):162–172.

Jedrychowski, W.A., F.P. Perera, D. Camann, J. Spengler, M. Butscher, E. Mroz, R. Majewska, E. Flak, R. Jacek, and A. Sowa. 2015a. Prenatal exposure to polycyclic aromatic hydrocarbons and cognitive dysfunction in children. *Environmental Science and Pollution Research International* 22(5):3631–3639.

Jedrychowski, W.A., F.P. Perera, R. Majewska, D. Mrozek-Budzyn, E. Mroz, E.L. Roen, A. Sowa, and R. Jacek. 2015b. Depressed height gain of children associated with intrauterine exposure to polycyclic aromatic hydrocarbons (PAH) and heavy metals: The cohort prospective study. *Environmental Research* 136:141–147.

Jedrychowski, W.A., F.P. Perera, U. Maugeri, R. Majewska, E. Mroz, E. Flak, D. Camann, A. Sowa, and R. Jacek. 2015c. Long term effects of prenatal and postnatal airborne PAH exposures on ventilatory lung function of non-asthmatic preadolescent children: Prospective birth cohort study in Krakow. *Science of the Total Environment* 502:502–509.

Jedrychowski, W.A., R. Majewska, J.D. Spengler, D. Camann, E.L. Roen, and F.P. Perera. 2017. Prenatal exposure to fine particles and polycyclic aromatic hydrocarbons and birth outcomes: A two-pollutant approach. *International Archives of Occupational and Environmental Health* 90(3):255–264.

Jeng, H.A., C.H. Pan, and M.R. Chao. 2013a. 1-Hydroxypyrene as a biomarker for assessing the effects of exposure to polycyclic aromatic hydrocarbons on semen quality and sperm DNA integrity. *Journal of Environmental Science and Health* 48(2):152–158.

Jeng, H.A., C.H. Pan, W.Y. Lin, M.T. Wu, S. Taylor, G.P. Chang-Chien, G. Zhou, and N. Diawara. 2013b. Biomonitoring of polycyclic aromatic hydrocarbons from coke oven emissions and reproductive toxicity in nonsmoking workers. *Journal of Hazardous Materials* 244–245:436–443.

Jeng, H.A., D. Yordt, S. Davis, and J.R. Swanson. 2015. Assessment of alteration of reproductive system in vivo induced by subchronic exposure to benzo(a)pyrene via oral administration. *Environmental Toxicology* 30(1):1–8.

Jenkins, T.G., E.R. James, D.F. Alonso, J.R. Hoidal, P.J. Murphy, J.M. Hotaling, B.R. Cairns, D.T. Carrell, and K.I. Aston. 2017. Cigarette smoking significantly alters sperm DNA methylation patterns. *Andrology* 5(6):1089–1099.

Jurewicz, J., K. Polanska, and W. Hanke. 2013a. Exposure to widespread environmental toxicants and children's cognitive development and behavioral problems. *International Journal of Occupational Medicine and Environmental Health* 26(2):185–204.

Jurewicz, J., M. Radwan, W. Sobala, S. Brzeznicki, D. Ligocka, P. Radwan, M. Bochenek, and W. Hanke. 2013b. Association between a biomarker of exposure to polycyclic aromatic hydrocarbons and semen quality. *International Journal of Occupational Medicine and Environmental Health* 26(5):790–801.

Jurewicz, J., M. Radwan, W. Sobala, K. Polanska, P. Radwan, L. Jakubowski, A. Ulanska, and W. Hanke. 2015. The relationship between exposure to air pollution and sperm disomy. *Environmental and Molecular Mutagenesis* 56(1):50–59.

Kakeyama, M., T. Endo, Y. Zhang, W. Miyazaki, and C. Tohyama. 2014. Disruption of paired-associate learning in rat offspring perinatally exposed to dioxins. *Archives of Toxicology* 88(3):789–798.

Kalkbrenner, A.E., G.C. Windham, M.L. Serre, Y. Akita, X. Wang, K. Hoffman, B.P. Thayer, and J.L. Daniels. 2015. Particulate matter exposure, prenatal and postnatal windows of susceptibility, and autism spectrum disorders. *Epidemiology* 26(1):30–42.

Kamelia, L., J. Louisse, L. de Haan, I.M.C.M. Rietjens, and P.J. Boogaard. 2017. Prenatal developmental toxicity testing of petroleum substances: Application of the mouse embryonic stem cell test (EST) to compare in vitro potencies with potencies observed in vivo. *Toxicology in Vitro* 44:303–312.

Kerin, T., H. Volk, W. Li, F. Lurmann, S. Eckel, R. McConnell, and I. Hertz-Picciotto. 2018. Association between air pollution exposure, cognitive and adaptive function, and ASD severity among children with autism spectrum disorder. *Journal of Autism and Developmental Disorders* 48(1):137–150.

Kim, A., M. Park, T.K. Yoon, W.S. Lee, J.-J. Ko, K. Lee, and J. Bae. 2011. Maternal exposure to benzo[b]fluoranthene disturbs reproductive performance in male offspring mice. *Toxicology Letters* 203(1):54–61.

Kim, E., H. Park, Y.C. Hong, M. Ha, B.N. Kim, Y. Kim, Y.M. Roh, B.E. Lee, J.M. Ryu, B.M. Kim, and E.H. Ha. 2014. Prenatal exposure to $PM_{2.5}$ and NO_2 and children's neurodevelopment from birth to 24 months of age: Mothers and Children's Environmental Health (MOCEH) study. *Science of the Total Environment* 481(1):439–445.

Kim, E., H. Park, E.A. Park, Y.C. Hong, M. Ha, H.C. Kim, and E.H. Ha. 2016. Particulate matter and early childhood body weight. *Environment International* 94:591–599.

Kisin, E.R., N. Yanamala, M.T. Farcas, D.W. Gutkin, M.R. Shurin, V.E. Kagan, A.D. Bugarski, and A.A. Shvedova. 2015. Abnormalities in the male reproductive system after exposure to diesel and biodiesel blend. *Environmental and Molecular Mutagenesis* 56(2):265–276.

Knopik, V.S., M.A. Maccani, S. Francazio, and J.E. McGeary. 2012. The epigenetics of maternal cigarette smoking during pregnancy and effects on child development. *Developmental Psychopathology* 24(4):1377–1390.

Kobayashi, Y., T. Hirano, T. Omotehara, R. Hashimoto, Y. Umemura, H. Yuasa, N. Masuda, N. Kubota, K. Minami, S. Yanai, M. Ishihara-Sugano, Y. Mantani, T. Yokoyama, H. Kitagawa, and N. Hoshi. 2015. Immunohistochemical analysis of 2,3,7,8-tetrachlorodibenzo-*p*-dioxin (TCDD) toxicity on the developmental dentate gyrus and hippocampal fimbria in fetal mice. *Journal of Veterinary Medical Science* 77(11):1355–1361.

Kobayashi, S., F. Sata, C. Miyashita, S. Sasaki, S. Ban, A. Araki, H. Goudarzi, J. Kajiwara, T. Todaka, and R. Kishi. 2017. Dioxin-metabolizing genes in relation to effects of prenatal dioxin levels and reduced birth size: The Hokkaido study. *Reproductive Toxicology* 67:111–116.

Lafuente, R., N. Garcia-Blaquez, B. Jacquemin, and M.A. Checa. 2016. Outdoor air pollution and sperm quality. *Fertility and Sterility* 106(4):880–896.

Lai, H.K., H. Tsang, and C.M. Wong. 2013. Meta-analysis of adverse health effects due to air pollution in Chinese populations. *BMC Public Health* 13:360.

Laiosa, M.D., E.R. Tate, L.S. Ahrenhoerster, Y. Chen, and D. Wang. 2016. Effects of developmental activation of the aryl hydrocarbon receptor by 2,3,7,8-tetrachlorodibenzo-*p*-dioxin on long-term self renewal of murine hematopoietic stem cells. *Environmental Health Perspectives* 124(7):957–965.

Lamichhane, D.K., J.-H. Leem, J.-Y. Lee, and H.-C. Kim. 2015. A meta-analysis of exposure to particulate matter and adverse birth outcomes. *Environmental Health and Toxicology* 30(0):e2015011.

Langlois, P.H., A.T. Hoyt, P.J. Lupo, C.C. Lawson, M.A. Waters, T.A. Desrosiers, G.M. Shaw, P.A. Romitti, and E.J. Lammer. 2012. Maternal occupational exposure to polycyclic aromatic hydrocarbons and risk of neural tube defect-affected pregnancies. *Birth Defects Research, Part A—Clinical and Molecular Teratology* 94(9):693–700.

Langlois, P.H., A.T. Hoyt, P.J. Lupo, C.C. Lawson, M.A. Waters, T.A. Desrosiers, G.M. Shaw, P.A. Romitti, and E.J. Lammer. 2013. Maternal occupational exposure to polycyclic aromatic hydrocarbons and risk of oral cleft-affected pregnancies. *Cleft Palate–Craniofacial Journal* 50(3):337–346.

Langlois, P.H., A.T. Hoyt, T.A. Desrosiers, P.J. Lupo, C.C. Lawson, M.A. Waters, C.M. Rocheleau, G.M. Shaw, P.A. Romitti, S.M. Gilboa, and S. Malik. 2014. Maternal occupational exposure to polycyclic aromatic hydrocarbons and small for gestational age offspring. *Occupational and Environmental Medicine* 71(8):529–535.

Latzin, P., M. Roosli, A. Huss, C.E. Kuehni, and U. Frey. 2009. Air pollution during pregnancy and lung function in newborns: A birth cohort study. *European Respiratory Journal* 33(3):594–603.

Lavigne, E., J. Ashley-Martin, L. Dodds, T.E. Arbuckle, P. Hystad, M. Johnson, D.L. Crouse, A.S. Ettinger, G.D. Shapiro, M. Fisher, A.S. Morisset, S. Taback, M.F. Bouchard, L. Sun, P. Monnier, R. Dallaire, and W.D. Fraser. 2016. Air pollution exposure during pregnancy and fetal markers of metabolic function. *American Journal of Epidemiology* 183(9):842–851.

Lavigne, E., M.A. Belair, M.T. Do, D.M. Stieb, P. Hystad, A. van Donkelaar, R.V. Martin, D.L. Crouse, E. Crighton, H. Chen, J.R. Brook, R.T. Burnett, S. Weichenthal, P.J. Villeneuve, T. To, S. Cakmak, M. Johnson, A.S. Yasseen, K.C. Johnson, M. Ofner, L. Xie, and M. Walker. 2017. Maternal exposure to ambient air pollution and risk of early childhood cancers: A population-based study in Ontario, Canada. *Environment International* 14:139–147.

Lee, P.C., E.O. Talbott, J.M. Roberts, J.M. Catov, R.K. Sharma, and B. Ritz. 2011. Particulate air pollution exposure and C-reactive protein during early pregnancy. [Erratum appears in *Epidemiology* 2011, 22(5):752]. *Epidemiology* 22(4):524–531.

Lee, P.C., E.O. Talbott, J.M. Roberts, J.M. Catov, R.A. Bilonick, R.A. Stone, R.K. Sharma, and B. Ritz. 2012. Ambient air pollution exposure and blood pressure changes during pregnancy. *Environmental Research* 117:46–53.

Lee, P.C., J.M. Roberts, J.M. Catov, E.O. Talbott, and B. Ritz. 2013. First trimester exposure to ambient air pollution, pregnancy complications and adverse birth outcomes in Allegheny County, PA. *Maternal and Child Health Journal* 17(3):545–555.

Lertxundi, A., M. Baccini, N. Lertxundi, E. Fano, A. Aranbarri, M.D. Martinez, M. Ayerdi, J. Alvarez, L. Santa-Marina, M. Dorronsoro, and J. Ibarluzea. 2015. Exposure to fine particle matter, nitrogen dioxide and benzene during pregnancy and cognitive and psychomotor developments in children at 15 months of age. *Environment International* 80:33–40.

Li, X., C. Shen, X. Liu, J. He, Y. Ding, R. Gao, X. Mu, Y. Geng, Y. Wang, and X. Chen. 2017. Exposure to benzo[a]pyrene impairs decidualization and decidual angiogenesis in mice during early pregnancy. *Environmental Pollution* 222:523–531.

Li, Y., K. Wang, Q.Y. Zou, R.R. Magness, and J. Zheng. 2015. 2,3,7,8-Tetrachlorodibenzo-*p*-dioxin differentially suppresses angiogenic responses in human placental vein and artery endothelial cells. *Toxicology* 336:70–78.

Liang, Z., L. Wu, L. Fan, and Q. Zhao. 2014. Ambient air pollution and birth defects in Haikou city, Hainan province. *BMC Pediatrics* 14:283.

Lin, C.C., S.K. Yang, K.C. Lin, W.C. Ho, W.S. Hsieh, B.C. Shu, and P.C. Chen. 2014. Multilevel analysis of air pollution and early childhood neurobehavioral development. *International Journal of Environmental Research and Public Health* 11(7):6827–6841.

Lin, H.L., Z.J. Liang, T. Liu, Q. Di, Z.M. Qian, W.L. Zeng, J.P. Xiao, X. Li, L.C. Guo, W.J. Ma, and Q.G. Zhao. 2015. Association between exposure to ambient air pollution before conception date and likelihood of giving birth to girls in Guangzhou, China. *Atmospheric Environment* 122:622–627.

Liu, L., Y. Wang, C. Shen, J. He, X. Liu, Y. Ding, R. Gao, and X. Chen. 2016a. Benzo(a)pyrene inhibits migration and invasion of extravillous trophoblast HTR-8/SVneo cells via activation of the ERK and JNK pathway. *Journal of Applied Toxicology* 36(7):946–955.

Liu, W., C. Huang, Y. Hu, Q. Fu, Z. Zou, C. Sun, L. Shen, X. Wang, J. Cai, J. Pan, Y. Huang, J. Chang, Y. Sun, and J. Sundell. 2016b. Associations of gestational and early life exposures to ambient air pollution with childhood respiratory diseases in Shanghai, China: A retrospective cohort study. *Environment International* 92–93:284–293.

Liu, X., X. Jin, R. Su, and Z. Li. 2017a. The reproductive toxicology of male SD rats after $PM_{2.5}$ exposure mediated by the stimulation of endoplasmic reticulum stress. *Chemosphere* 189:547–555.

Liu, C.B., X.R. Hong, M. Shi, X.Q. Chen, H.J. Huang, J.H. Chen, K. Yang, S.Q. Chen, H.Q. Chen, H.D. Kan, and Q.H. Sun. 2017b. Effects of prenatal PM_{10} exposure on fetal cardiovascular malformations in Fuzhou, China: A retrospective case-control study. *Environmental Health Perspectives* 125(5):057001-1– 057001-8.

Lu, C., L. Deng, C. Ou, H. Yuan, X. Chen, and Q. Deng. 2017. Preconceptional and perinatal exposure to traffic-related air pollution and eczema in preschool children. *Journal of Dermatological Science* 85(2):85–95.

Luderer, U., F. Christensen, W.O. Johnson, J. She, H.S.S. Ip, J. Zhou, J. Alvaran, E.F. Krieg, Jr, and J.S. Kesner. 2017a. Associations between urinary biomarkers of polycyclic aromatic hydrocarbon exposure and reproductive function during menstrual cycles in women. *Environment International* 100:110–120.

Luderer, U., M.B. Myers, M. Banda, K.L. McKim, L. Ortiz, and B.L. Parsons. 2017b. Ovarian effects of prenatal exposure to benzo[a]pyrene: Roles of embryonic and maternal glutathione status. *Reproductive Toxicology* 69:187–195.

Lupo, P.J., P.H. Langlois, J. Reefhuis, C.C. Lawson, E. Symanski, T.A. Desrosiers, Z.G. Khodr, A.J. Agopian, M.A. Waters, K.N. Duwe, R.H. Finnell, L.E. Mitchell, C.A. Moore, P.A. Romitti, and G.M. Shaw. 2012a. Maternal occupational exposure to polycyclic aromatic hydrocarbons: Effects on gastroschisis among offspring in the National Birth Defects Prevention Study. *Environmental Health Perspectives* 120(6):910–915.

Lupo, P.J., E. Symanski, P.H. Langlois, C.C. Lawson, S. Malik, S.M. Gilboa, L.J. Lee, A.J. Agopian, T.A. Desrosiers, M.A. Waters, P.A. Romitti, A. Correa, G.M. Shaw, and L.E. Mitchell. 2012b. Maternal occupational exposure to polycyclic aromatic hydrocarbons and congenital heart defects among offspring in the National Birth Defects Prevention Study. *Birth Defects Research, Part A—Clinical and Molecular Teratology* 94(11):875–881.

Ma, J., X. Chen, Y. Liu, Q. Xie, Y. Sun, J. Chen, L. Leng, H. Yan, B. Zhao, and N. Tang. 2015. Ancestral TCDD exposure promotes epigenetic transgenerational inheritance of imprinted gene *IGF2*: Methylation status and DNMTs. *Toxicology and Applied Pharmacology* 289(2):193–202.

MacIntyre, E.A., U. Gehring, A. Molter, E. Fuertes, C. Klumper, U. Kramer, U. Quass, B. Hoffmann, M. Gascon, B. Brunekreef, G.H. Koppelman, R. Beelen, G. Hoek, M. Birk, J.C. de Jongste, H.A. Smit, J. Cyrys, O. Gruzieva, M. Korek, A. Bergstrom, R.M. Agius, F. de Vocht, A. Simpson, D. Porta, F. Forastiere, C. Badaloni, G. Cesaroni, A. Esplugues, A. Fernandez-Somoano, A. Lerxundi, J. Sunyer, M. Cirach, M.J. Nieuwenhuijsen, G. Pershagen, and J. Heinrich. 2014. Air pollution and respiratory infections during early childhood: An analysis of 10 European birth cohorts within the ESCAPE Project. *Environmental Health Perspectives* 122(1):107–113.

Mahalingaiah, S., J.E. Hart, F. Laden, A. Aschengrau, and S.A. Missmer. 2014. Air pollution exposures during adulthood and risk of endometriosis in the Nurses' Health Study II. *Environmental Health Perspectives* 122(1):58–64.

Mahalingaiah, S., J.E. Hart, F. Laden, L.V. Farland, M.M. Hewlett, J. Chavarro, A. Aschengrau, and S.A. Missmer. 2016. Adult air pollution exposure and risk of infertility in the Nurses' Health Study II. *Human Reproduction* 31(3):638–647.

Manikkam, M., C. Guerrero-Bosagna, R. Tracey, M.M. Haque, and M.K. Skinner. 2012a. Transgenerational actions of environmental compounds on reproductive disease and identification of epigenetic biomarkers of ancestral exposures. *PLOS ONE* 7:e31901.

Manikkam, M., R. Tracey, C. Guerrero-Bosagna, and M.K. Skinner. 2012b. Dioxin (TCDD) induces epigenetic transgenerational inheritance of adult onset disease and sperm epimutations. *PLOS ONE* 7:e46249.

Manikkam, M., R. Tracey, C. Guerrero-Bosagna, and M.K. Skinner. 2012c. Pesticide and insect repellent mixture (permethrin and DEET) induces epigenetic transgenerational inheritance of disease and sperm epimutations. *Reproductive Toxicology* 34:708–719.

Mannetje, A., A. Eng, C. Walls, E. Dryson, M. Kogevinas, C. Brooks, D. McLean, S. Cheng, A.H. Smith, and N. Pearce. 2016. Sex ratio of the offspring of New Zealand phenoxy herbicide producers exposed to 2,3,7,8- tetrachlorodibenzo-*p*-dioxin. *Occupational and Environmental Medicine* 31(1):24–29.

Mao, G., R.M. Nachman, Q. Sun, X. Zhang, K. Koehler, Z. Chen, X. Hong, G. Wang, D. Caruso, G. Zong, C. Pearson, H. Ji, S. Biswal, B. Zuckerman, M. Wills-Karp, and X. Wang. 2017. Individual and joint effects of early-life ambient exposure and maternal prepregnancy obesity on childhood overweight or obesity. *Environmental Health Perspectives* 125(6):067005-2– 067005-10.

Marshall, E.G., G. Harris, and D. Wartenberg. 2010. Oral cleft defects and maternal exposure to ambient air pollutants in New Jersey. *Birth Defects Research* 88(4):205–215.

Martens, D.S., S. Gouveia, N. Madhloum, B.G. Janssen, M. Plusquin, C. Vanpoucke, W. Lefebvre, B. Forsberg, M. Nording, and T.S. Nawrot. 2017a. Neonatal cord blood oxylipins and exposure to particulate matter in the early-life environment: An ENVIRONAGE birth cohort study. *Environmental Health Perspectives* 125(4):691–698.

Martens, D.S., B. Cox, B.G. Janssen, D.B.P. Clemente, A. Gasparrini, C. Vanpoucke, W. Lefebvre, H.A. Roels, M. Plusquin, and T.S. Nawrot. 2017b. Prenatal air pollution and newborns' predisposition to accelerated biological aging. *JAMA Pediatrics* 171(12):1160–1167.

Martinez-Zamora, M.A., L. Mattioli, J. Parera, E. Abad, J.L. Coloma, B. van Babel, M.T. Galceran, J. Balasch, and F. Carmona. 2015. Increased levels of dioxin-like substances in adipose tissue in patients with deep infiltrating endometriosis. *Human Reproduction* 30(5):1059–1068.

Masiol, M., T. Mallon, K.M. Haines, M.J. Utell, and P.K. Hopke. 2016a. Airborne dioxins, furans and polycyclic aromatic hydrocarbons exposure to military personnel in Iraq. *Journal of Occupational and Environmental Medicine* 58(8):S22–S30.

Masiol, M., T. Mallon, K.M. Haines, M.J. Utell, and P.K. Hopke. 2016b. Source apportionment of airborne dioxins, furans and polycyclic aromatic hydrocarbons at a U.S. forward operating air base during the Iraq war. *Journal of Occupational and Environmental Medicine* 58(8):S31–S37.

Mattie, D.R., G.B. Merit, J.R. Cooper, T.R. Sterner, and C.D. Fleming. 2000. *Reproductive effects of JP-8 jet fuel on male and female Sprague-Dawley rats after exposure by oral gavage*. AFRL-HE-WP-TR-2000-0067. Wright-Patterson AFB, OH: Air Force Research Laboratory.

Mattison, D.R., N.B. White, and M.R. Nightingale. 1980. The effect of benzo(a)pyrene on fertility, primordial oocyte number, and ovarian response to pregnant mare's serum gonadotropin. *Pediatric Pharmacology (New York)* 1(2):143–151.

Mayo Clinic. 2018a. *Placenta accreta*. https://www.mayoclinic.org/diseases-conditions/placenta-accreta/symptoms-causes/syc-20376431 (accessed July 21, 2018).

Mayo Clinic. 2018b. *Placenta previa*. https://www.mayoclinic.org/diseases-conditions/placenta-previa/symptoms-causes/syc-20352768 (accessed July 21, 2018).

Mayo Clinic. 2018c. *Placental abruption*. https://www.mayoclinic.org/diseases-conditions/placental-abruption/symptoms-causes/syc-20376458 (accessed July 21, 2018).

Mayo Clinic. 2018d. *Preeclampsia*. https://www.mayoclinic.org/diseases-conditions/preeclampsia/symptoms-causes/syc-20355745 (accessed July 21, 2018).

McCallister, M.M., Z. Li, T. Zhang, A. Ramesh, R.S. Clark, M. Maguire, B. Hutsell, M.C. Newland, and D.B. Hood. 2016. Revealing behavioral learning deficit phenotypes subsequent to in utero exposure to benzo(a)pyrene. *Toxicological Sciences* 149(1):42–54.

Meier, M.J., J.M. O'Brien, M.A. Beal, B. Allan, C.L. Yauk, and F. Marchetti. 2017. In utero exposure to benzo[a]pyrene increases mutation burden in the soma and sperm of adult mice. *Environmental Health Perspectives* 125(1):82–88.

Mendola, P., M. Wallace, B.S. Hwang, D. Liu, C. Robledo, T. Mannisto, R. Sundaram, S. Sherman, Q. Ying, and K.L. Grantz. 2016. Preterm birth and air pollution: Critical windows of exposure for women with asthma. *Journal of Allergy and Clinical Immunology* 138(2):432–440.

Merklinger-Gruchala, A., G. Jasienska, and M. Kapiszewska. 2017. Effect of air pollution on menstrual cycle length: A prognostic factor of women's reproductive health. *International Journal of Environmental Research and Public Health* 14(7):20.

Miao, Y., C. Zhou, Q. Bai, Z. Cui, X. ShiYang, Y. Lu, M. Zhang, X. Dai, and B. Xiong. 2018. The protective role of melatonin in porcine oocyte meiotic failure caused by the exposure to benzo(a)pyrene. *Human Reproduction* 33(1):116–127.

Michikawa, T., S. Morokuma, S. Yamazaki, K. Fukushima, K. Kato, and H. Nitta. 2016. Exposure to air pollutants during the early weeks of pregnancy, and placenta praevia and placenta accreta in the western part of Japan. *Environment International* 92–93:464–470.

Miyashita, C., Y.A. Bamai, A. Araki, S. Itoh, M. Minatoya, S. Kobayashi, J. Kajiwara, T. Hori, and R. Kishi. 2018. Prenatal exposure to dioxin-like compounds is associated with decreased cord blood IgE and increased risk of wheezing in children aged up to 7 years: The Hokkaido study. *Science of the Total Environment* 610–611:191–199.

Mobasher, Z., M.T. Salam, T.M. Goodwin, F. Lurmann, S.A. Ingles, and M.L. Wilson. 2013. Associations between ambient air pollution and hypertensive disorders of pregnancy. *Environmental Research* 123:9–16.

Mocarelli, P., P.M. Gerthoux, L.L. Needham, D.G. Patterson, G. Limonta, R. Falbo, and P. Brambilla. 2011. Perinatal exposure to low doses of dioxin can permanently impair human semen quality. *Environmental Health Perspectives* 119(5):713–718.

Morales, E., R. Garcia-Esteban, O.A. De La Cruz, M. Basterrechea, A. Lertxundi, M.D. Martinez Lopez de Dicastillo, C. Zabaleta, and J. Sunyer. 2015. Intrauterine and early postnatal exposure to outdoor air pollution and lung function at preschool age. *Thorax* 70(1):64–73.

Moridi, M., S. Ziaei, and A. Kazemnejad. 2014. Exposure to ambient air pollutants and spontaneous abortion. *Journal of Obstetrics and Gynaecology Research* 40(3):743–748.

Mortimer, K., R. Neugebauer, F. Lurmann, S. Alcorn, J. Balmes, and I. Tager. 2008. Air pollution and pulmonary function in asthmatic children: Effects of prenatal and lifetime exposures. *Epidemiology* 19(4):550–557; discussion 561–562.

Muenyi, C.S., S.L. Carrion, L.A. Jones, L.H. Kennedy, A.T. Slominski, C.H. Sutter, and T.R. Sutter. 2014. Effects of in utero exposure of C57BL/6J mice to 2,3,7,8-tetrachlorodibenzo-*p*-dioxin on epidermal permeability barrier development and function. *Environmental Health Perspectives* 122(10):1052–1058.

Nachman, R.M., G. Mao, X. Zhang, X. Hong, Z. Chen, C.S. Soria, H. He, G. Wang, D. Caruso, C. Pearson, S. Biswal, B. Zuckerman, M. Wills-Karp, and X. Wang. 2016. Intrauterine inflammation and maternal exposure to ambient $PM_{2.5}$ during preconception and specific periods of pregnancy: The Boston birth cohort. *Environmental Health Perspectives* 124(10):1608–1615.

NASEM (National Academies of Sciences, Engineering, and Medicine). 2016. *Veterans and Agent Orange: Update 2014*. Washington, DC: The National Academies Press.

Neugebauer, J., J. Wittsiepe, M. Kasper-Sonnenberg, N. Schoneck, A. Scholmerich, and M. Wilhelm. 2015. The influence of low level pre- and perinatal exposure to PCDD/Fs, PCBs, and lead on attention performance and attention-related behavior among German school-aged children: Results from the Duisburg Birth Cohort Study. *International Journal of Hygiene and Environmental Health* 218(1):153–162.

Nieuwenhuijsen, M.J., X. Basagana, P. Dadvand, D. Martinez, M. Cirach, R. Beelen, and B. Jacquemin. 2014. Air pollution and human fertility rates. *Environment International* 70:9–14.

Nilsson, E., G. Larsen, M. Manikkam, C. Guerrero-Bosagna, M.I. Savenkova, and M.K. Skinner. 2012. Environmentally induced epigenetic transgenerational inheritance of ovarian disease. *PLOS ONE* 7:e36129.

Nishijo, M., T.T. Pham, A.T. Nguyen, N.N. Tran, H. Nakagawa, L.V. Hoang, A.H. Tran, Y. Morikawa, M.D. Ho, T. Kido, M.N. Nguyen, H.M. Nguyen, and H. Nishijo. 2014. 2,3,7,8-Tetrachlorodibenzo-*p*-dioxin in breast milk increases autistic traits of 3-year-old children in Vietnam. *Molecular Psychiatry* 19(11):1220–1226.

Nishijo, M., P.T. Tai, N.T.N. Anh, T.N. Nghi, H. Nakagawa, H. Van Luong, T.H. Anh, Y. Morikawa, T. Waseda, T. Kido, and H. Nishijo. 2015. Urinary amino acid alterations in 3-year-old children with neurodevelopmental effects due to perinatal dioxin exposure in Vietnam: A nested case-control study for neurobiomarker discovery. *PLOS ONE* 10(1):e0116778.

Nobles, C.J., E.F. Schisterman, S. Ha, G.M. Buck Louis, S. Sherman, and P. Mendola. 2018. Time-varying cycle average and daily variation in ambient air pollution and fecundability. *Human Reproduction* 33(1):166–176.

Noel, J.K., S. Namazi, and R.L. Haddock. 2015. Disparities in infant mortality due to congenital anomalies on Guam. *Hawaii Journal of Medicine and Public Health* 74(12):397–402.

Nowack, N., J. Wittsiepe, M. Kasper-Sonnenberg, M. Wilhelm, and A. Scholmerich. 2015. Influence of low-level prenatal exposure to PCDD/Fs and PCBs on empathizing, systemizing and autistic traits: Results from the Duisburg Birth Cohort Study. *PLOS ONE* 10(6):e0129906.

NRC (National Research Council). 2010. *Review of the Department of Defense Enhanced Particulate Matter Surveillance Program Report*. Washington, DC: The National Academies Press.

O'Brien, J.L., P.H. Langlois, C.C. Lawson, A. Scheuerle, C.M. Rocheleau, M.A. Waters, E. Symanski, P.A. Romitti, A.J. Agopian, and P.J. Lupo. 2016. Maternal occupational exposure to polycyclic aromatic hydrocarbons and craniosynostosis among offspring in the National Birth Defects Prevention Study. *Birth Defects Research, Part A—Clinical and Molecular Teratology* 106(1):55–60.

Ogliari, K.S., A.J. Lichtenfels, M.R. de Marchi, A.T. Ferreira, M. Dolhnikoff, and P.H. Saldiva. 2013. Intrauterine exposure to diesel exhaust diminishes adult ovarian reserve. *Fertility and Sterility* 99(6):1681–1688.

Omidakhsh, N., G.R. Bunin, A, Ganguly, B. Ritz, N. Kennedy, O.S. von Ehrenstein, N. Krause, and J.E. Heck. 2018. Parental occupational exposures and the risk of childhood sporadic retinoblastoma: A report from the Children's Oncology Group. *Occupational and Environmental Medicine* 75(3):205–211.

Orione, M.A.M., C.A. Silva, A.M.E. Sallum, L.M.A. Campos, C.H. Omori, A.L.F. Braga, and S.C.L. Farhat. 2014. Risk factors for juvenile dermatomyositis: Exposure to tobacco and air pollutants during pregnancy. *Arthritis Care and Research* 66(10):1571–1575.

Oshiro, W.M., T.E. Beasley, K.L. McDaniel, P.A. Evansky, S.A. Martin, V.C. Moser, M.E. Gilbert, and P.J. Bushnell. 2015. Prenatal exposure to vapors of gasoline-ethanol blends causes few cognitive deficits in adult rats. *Neurotoxicology and Teratology* 49:59–73.

Owagboriaye, F.O., G.A. Dedeke, J.S. Ashidi, A.A. Aladesida, and W.E. Olooto. 2017. Effect of gasoline fumes on reproductive function in male albino rats. *Environmental Science and Pollution Research* 1–11.

Padula, A.M., I.B. Tager, S.L. Carmichael, S.K. Hammond, F. Lurmann, and G.M. Shaw. 2013a. The association of ambient air pollution and traffic exposures with selected congenital anomalies in the San Joaquin Valley of California. *American Journal of Epidemiology* 177(10):1074–1085.

Padula, A.M., I.B. Tager, S.L. Carmichael, S.K. Hammond, W. Yang, F. Lurmann, and G.M. Shaw. 2013b. Ambient air pollution and traffic exposures and congenital heart defects in the San Joaquin Valley of California. *Paediatric and Perinatal Epidemiology* 27(4):329–339.

Padula, A.M., I.B. Tager, S.L. Carmichael, S.K. Hammond, W. Yang, F.W. Lurmann, and G.M. Shaw. 2013c. Traffic-related air pollution and selected birth defects in the San Joaquin Valley of California. *Birth Defects Research* 97(11):730–735.

Padula, A.M., E.M. Noth, S.K. Hammond, F.W. Lurmann, W. Yang, I.B. Tager, and G.M. Shaw. 2014. Exposure to airborne polycyclic aromatic hydrocarbons during pregnancy and risk of preterm birth. *Environmental Research* 135:221–226.

Padula, A.M., W. Yang, S.L. Carmichael, I.B. Tager, F. Lurmann, S.K. Hammond, and G.M. Shaw. 2015. Air pollution, neighbourhood socioeconomic factors, and neural tube defects in the San Joaquin Valley of California. *Paediatric and Perinatal Epidemiology* 29(6):536–545.

Pan, X., X. Liu, X. Li, N. Niu, X. Yin, N. Li, and Z. Yu. 2015. Association between environmental dioxin-related toxicants exposure and adverse pregnancy outcome: Systematic review and meta-analysis. *International Journal of Fertility & Sterility* 8(4):351–366.

Pearce, M.S., S.V. Glinianaia, J. Rankin, S. Rushton, M. Charlton, L. Parker, and T. Pless-Mulloli. 2010. No association between ambient particulate matter exposure during pregnancy and stillbirth risk in the north of England, 1962–1992. *Environmental Research* 110(1):118–122.

Pedersen, M., L. Stayner, R. Slama, M. Sorensen, F. Figueras, M.J. Nieuwenhuijsen, O. Raaschou-Nielsen, and P. Dadvand. 2014. Ambient air pollution and pregnancy-induced hypertensive disorders: A systematic review and meta-analysis. *Hypertension* 64(3):494–500.

Pedersen, M., M.A. Mendez, B. Schoket, R.W. Godschalk, A. Espinosa, A. Landstrom, C.M. Villanueva, D.F. Merlo, E. Fthenou, E. Gracia-Lavedan, F.J. van Schooten, G. Hoek, G. Brunborg, H.M. Meltzer, J. Alexander, J.K. Nielsen, J. Sunyer, J. Wright, K. Kovacs, K. de Hoogh, K.B. Gutzkow, L.J. Hardie, L. Chatzi, L.E. Knudsen, L. Anna, M. Ketzel, M. Haugen, M. Botsivali, M.J. Nieuwenhuijsen, M. Cirach, M.B. Toledano, R.B. Smith, S. Fleming, S. Agramunt, S.A. Kyrtopoulos, V. Lukacs, J.C. Kleinjans, D. Segerback, and M. Kogevinas. 2015. Environmental, dietary, maternal, and fetal predictors of bulky DNA adducts in cord blood: A European mother–child study (NewGeneris). [Erratum appears in *Environmental Health Perspectives* 2016, 124(1):A12]. *Environmental Health Perspectives* 123(4):374–380.

Perera, F., D. Tang, R. Whyatt, S.A. Lederman, and W. Jedrychowski. 2005a. DNA damage from polycyclic aromatic hydrocarbons measured by benzo[a]pyrene–DNA adducts in mothers and newborns from Northern Manhattan, the World Trade Center Area, Poland, and China. *Cancer Epidemiology, Biomarkers & Prevention* 14(3):709–714.

Perera, F.P., D. Tang, V. Rauh, K. Lester, W.Y. Tsai, Y.H. Tu, L. Weiss, L. Hoepner, J. King, G. Del Priore, and S.A. Lederman. 2005b. Relationships among polycyclic aromatic hydrocarbon–DNA adducts, proximity to the World Trade Center, and effects on fetal growth. *Environmental Health Perspectives* 113(8):1062–1067.

Perera, F.P., D. Tang, V. Rauh, Y.H. Tu, W.Y. Tsai, M. Becker, J.L. Stein, J. King, G. Del Priore, and S.A. Lederman. 2007. Relationship between polycyclic aromatic hydrocarbon–DNA adducts, environmental tobacco smoke, and child development in the World Trade Center Cohort. *Environmental Health Perspectives* 115(10):1497–1502.

Perera, F., W.Y. Tang, J. Herbstman, D. Tang, L. Levin, R. Miller, and S.M. Ho. 2009a. Relation of DNA methylation of 5'-CpG island of ACSL3 to transplacental exposure to airborne polycyclic aromatic hydrocarbons and childhood asthma. *PLOS ONE* 4(2):e4488.

Perera, F.P., Z. Li, R. Whyatt, L. Hoepner, S. Wang, D. Camann, and V. Rauh. 2009b. Prenatal airborne polycyclic aromatic hydrocarbon exposure and child IQ at age 5 years. *Pediatrics* 124(2):e195–e202.

Perera, F.P., S. Wang, J. Vishnevetsky, B. Zhang, K.J. Cole, D. Tang, V. Rauh, and D.H. Phillips. 2011. Polycyclic aromatic hydrocarbons-aromatic DNA adducts in cord blood and behavior scores in New York City children. *Environmental Health Perspectives* 119(8):1176–1181.

Perera, F.P., D. Tang, S. Wang, J. Vishnevetsky, B. Zhang, D. Diaz, D. Camann, and V. Rauh. 2012. Prenatal polycyclic aromatic hydrocarbon (PAH) exposure and child behavior at age 6–7 years. *Environmental Health Perspectives* 120(6):921–926.

Perera, F.P., H.W. Chang, D. Tang, E.L. Roen, J. Herbstman, A. Margolis, T.J. Huang, R.L. Miller, S. Wang, and V. Rauh. 2014. Early-life exposure to polycyclic aromatic hydrocarbons and ADHD behavior problems. *PLOS ONE* 9(11):e111670.

Perera, F., D.H. Phillips, Y. Wang, E. Roen, J. Herbstman, V. Rauh, S. Wang, and D. Tang. 2015. Prenatal exposure to polycyclic aromatic hydrocarbons/aromatics, BDNF and child development. *Environmental Research* 142:602–608.

Peterson, B.S., V.A. Rauh, R. Bansal, X. Hao, Z. Toth, G. Nati, K. Walsh, R. Miller, F. Arias, D. Semanek, and F. Perera. 2015. Effects of prenatal exposure to air pollutants (polycyclic aromatic hydrocarbons) on the development of brain white matter, cognition, and behavior in later childhood. *JAMA Psychiatry* 72(6):531–540.

Pham, T.T., M. Nishijo, A.T.N. Nguyen, N.N. Tran, L.V. Hoang, A.H. Tran, T.V. Nguyen, and H. Nishijo. 2015. Perinatal dioxin exposure and the neurodevelopment of Vietnamese toddlers at 1 year of age. *Science of the Total Environment* 536:575–581.

Pirkle, J.L., E.J. Sampson, L.L. Needham, D.G. Pattterson, and D.L. Ashley. 1995. Using biological monitoring to assess human exposure to priority toxicants. *Environmental Health Perspectives* 103(Suppl 3):45–48.

Poirier, M.C., A. Weston, B. Schoket, H. Shamkhani, C.F. Pan, M.A. McDiarmid, B.G. Scott, D.P. Deeter, J.M. Heller, D. Jacobson-Kram, and N. Rothman. 1998. Biomonitoring of United States Army soldiers serving in Kuwait in 1991. *Cancer Epidemiology, Biomarkers & Prevention* 7(6):545–551.

Polanska, K., W. Hanke, W. Sobala, S. Brzeznicki, and D. Ligocka. 2010. Exposure to polycyclic aromatic hydrocarbons and newborn biometric indicators. *International Journal of Occupational Medicine and Environmental Health* 23(4):339–346.

Polanska, K., J. Jurewicz, and W. Hanke. 2012. Exposure to environmental and lifestyle factors and attention-deficit/hyperactivity disorder in children: A review of epidemiological studies. *International Journal of Occupational Medicine and Environmental Health* 25(4):330–355.

Polanska, K., W. Hanke, W. Sobala, M. Trzcinka-Ochocka, D. Ligocka, S. Brzeznicki, H. Strugala-Stawik, and P. Magnus. 2013. Developmental effects of exposures to environmental factors: The Polish Mother and Child Cohort Study. *Biomedical Research International* 2013:629716.

Polanska, K., G. Dettbarn, J. Jurewicz, W. Sobala, P. Magnus, A. Seidel, and W. Hanke. 2014. Effect of prenatal polycyclic aromatic hydrocarbons exposure on birth outcomes: The Polish Mother and Child Cohort Study. *Biomedical Research International* 2014:408939.

Poursafa, P., S. Baradaran-Mahdavi, B. Moradi, S. Haghjooy Javanmard, M. Tajadini, F. Mehrabian, and R. Kelishadi. 2016. The relationship of exposure to air pollutants in pregnancy with surrogate markers of endothelial dysfunction in umbilical cord. *Environmental Research* 146:154–160.

Radwan, M., J. Jurewicz, W. Sobala, S. Brzeznicki, P. Radwan, L. Jakubowski, W. Hawula, A. Ulanska, and W. Hanke. 2016. Human sperm aneuploidy after exposure to polycyclic aromatic hydrocarbons. *Reproduction, Fertility and Development* 28(9):1376–1381.

Rankin, J., T. Chadwick, M. Natarajan, D. Howel, M.S. Pearce, and T. Pless-Mulloli. 2009. Maternal exposure to ambient air pollutants and risk of congenital anomalies. *Environmental Research* 109(2):181–187.

Raz, R., A.L. Roberts, K. Lyall, J.E. Hart, A.C. Just, F. Laden, and M.G. Weisskopf. 2015. Autism spectrum disorder and particulate matter air pollution before, during, and after pregnancy: A nested case-control analysis within the Nurses' Health Study II cohort. *Environmental Health Perspectives* 123(3):264–270.

Reutman, S.R., G.K. LeMasters, E.A. Knecht, R. Shukla, J.E. Lockey, G.E. Burroughs, and J.S. Kesner. 2002. Evidence of reproductive endocrine effects in women with occupational fuel and solvent exposures. *Environmental Health Perspectives* 110(8):805–811.

Ricke, W.A., C.W. Lee, T.R. Clapper, A.J. Schneider, R.W. Moore, K.P. Keil, L.L. Abler, J.L. Wynder, A. Lopez Alvarado, I. Beaubrun, J. Vo, T.M. Bauman, E.A. Ricke, R.E. Peterson, and C.M. Vezina. 2016. In utero and lactational TCDD exposure increases susceptibility to lower urinary tract dysfunction in adulthood. *Toxicological Sciences* 150(2):429–440.

Roberts, L.G., T.M. Gray, M.C. Marr, R.W. Tyl, G.W. Trimmer, G.M. Hoffman, F.J. Murray, C.R. Clark, and C.A. Schreiner. 2014a. Health assessment of gasoline and fuel oxygenate vapors: Developmental toxicity in mice. *Regulatory Toxicology and Pharmacology* 70(2 Suppl):S58–S68.

Roberts, L.G., T.M. Gray, G.W. Trimmer, R.M. Parker, F.J. Murray, C.A. Schreiner, and C.R. Clark. 2014b. Health assessment of gasoline and fuel oxygenate vapors: Developmental toxicity in rats. *Regulatory Toxicology and Pharmacology* 70(2 Suppl):S69–S79.

Robledo, C.A., P. Mendola, E. Yeung, T. Mannisto, R. Sundaram, D. Liu, Q. Ying, S. Sherman, and K. L. Grantz. 2015. Preconception and early pregnancy air pollution exposures and risk of gestational diabetes mellitus. *Environmental Research* 137:316–322.

Rosa, M.J., A.C. Just, I. Kloog, I. Pantic, L. Schnaas, A. Lee, S. Bose, Y.M. Chiu, H.L. Hsu, B. Coull, J. Schwartz, S. Cohen, M.M. Tellez Rojo, R.O. Wright, and R.J. Wright. 2017a. Prenatal particulate matter exposure and wheeze in Mexican children: Effect modification by prenatal psychosocial stress. *Annals of Allergy, Asthma, & Immunology* 119(3):232–237.

Rosa, M.J., A.C. Just, M.S. Guerra, I. Kloog, H.L. Hsu, K.J. Brennan, A.M. Garcia, B. Coull, R.J. Wright, M.M. Tellez Rojo, A.A. Baccarelli, and R.O. Wright. 2017b. Identifying sensitive windows for prenatal particulate air pollution exposure and mitochondrial DNA content in cord blood. *Environment International* 98:198–203.

Rowan-Carroll, A., M.A. Beal, A. Williams, F. Marchetti, and C.L. Yauk. 2017. Dose-response mutation and spectrum analyses reveal similar responses at two microsatellite loci in benzo(a)pyrene-exposed mouse spermatogonia. *Mutagenesis* 32(4):463–470.

Rubes, J., S.G. Selevan, D.P. Evenson, D. Zudova, M. Vozdova, Z. Zudova, W.A. Robbins, and S.D. Perreault. 2005. Episodic air pollution is associated with increased DNA fragmentation in human sperm without other changes in semen quality. *Human Reproduction* 20(10):2776–2783.

Rudra, C.B., M.A. Williams, L. Sheppard, J.Q. Koenig, and M.A. Schiff. 2011. Ambient carbon monoxide and fine particulate matter in relation to preeclampsia and preterm delivery in western Washington State. *Environmental Health Perspectives* 119(6):886–892.

Rundle, A., L. Hoepner, A. Hassoun, S. Oberfield, G. Freyer, D. Holmes, M. Reyes, J. Quinn, D. Camann, F. Perera, and R. Whyatt. 2012. Association of childhood obesity with maternal exposure to ambient air polycyclic aromatic hydrocarbons during pregnancy. *American Journal of Epidemiology* 175(11):1163–1172.

Saadat, M., and N. Monzavi. 2008. Genetic polymorphisms of glutathione S-transferase T1 (GSTT1) and alterations of sex hormones in filling-station workers. *Fertility and Sterility* 89(6):1777–1780.

Saadat, M., S. Bahaoddini, and I. Saadat. 2013. Alteration of serum sex hormonal profile in male gasoline filling station workers in respect to their polymorphism of glutathione S-transferase M1. *Environmental Toxicology and Pharmacology* 35(2):265–269.

Saenen, N.D., M. Plusquin, E. Bijnens, B.G. Janssen, W. Gyselaers, B. Cox, F. Fierens, G. Molenberghs, J. Penders, K. Vrijens, P. De Boever, and T.S. Nawrot. 2015. In utero fine particle air pollution and placental expression of genes in the brain-derived neurotrophic factor signaling pathway: An ENVIRONAGE birth cohort study. *Environmental Health Perspectives* 123(8):834–840.

Saenen, N.D., K. Vrijens, B.G. Janssen, N. Madhloum, M. Peusens, W. Gyselaers, C. Vanpoucke, W. Lefebvre, H.A. Roels, and T.S. Nawrot. 2016. Placental nitrosative stress and exposure to ambient air pollution during gestation: A population study. *American Journal of Epidemiology* 184(6):442–449.

Saenen, N.D., K. Vrijens, B.G. Janssen, H.A. Roels, K.Y. Neven, W. Vanden Berghe, W. Gyselaers, C. Vanpoucke, W. Lefebvre, P. De Boever, and T.S. Nawrot. 2017. Lower placental leptin promoter methylation in association with fine particulate matter air pollution during pregnancy and placental nitrosative stress at birth in the ENVIRONAGE cohort. *Environmental Health Perspectives* 125(2):262–268.

Safe, T.M., and A.E. Luebke. 2016. Prenatal low dosage dioxin (TCDD) exposure impairs cochlear function resulting in auditory neuropathy. *Hearing Research* 331:7–12.

Saigal, S., and L.W. Doyle. 2008. An overview of mortality and sequelae of preterm birth from infancy to adulthood. *The Lancet* 371(9608):261–269.

Salam, M.T., H.M. Byun, F. Lurmann, C.V. Breton, X. Wang, S.P. Eckel, and F.D. Gilliland. 2012. Genetic and epigenetic variations in inducible nitric oxide synthase promoter, particulate pollution, and exhaled nitric oxide levels in children. *Journal of Allergy and Clinical Immunology* 129(1):232–239.

Sanabria, M., M.S. Cucielo, M.T. Guerra, C. Dos Santos Borges, T.P. Banzato, J.E. Perobelli, G.A. Leite, J.A. Anselmo-Franci, and W. De Grava Kempinas. 2016. Sperm quality and fertility in rats after prenatal exposure to low doses of TCDD: A three-generation study. *Reproductive Toxicology* 65:29–38.

Sapkota, A., A.P. Chelikowsky, K.E. Nachman, A.J. Cohen, and B. Ritz. 2012. Exposure to particulate matter and adverse birth outcomes: A comprehensive review and meta-analysis. *Air Quality, Atmosphere and Health* 5(4):369–381.

Savitz, D.A., B. Elston, J.F. Bobb, J.E. Clougherty, F. Dominici, K. Ito, S. Johnson, T. McAlexander, Z. Ross, J.L.C. Shmool, T.D. Matte, and G.A. Wellenius. 2015. Ambient fine particulate matter, nitrogen dioxide, and hypertensive disorders of pregnancy in New York City. *Epidemiology* 26(5):748–757.

Schembari, A., M.J. Nieuwenhuijsen, J. Salvador, A. de Nazelle, M. Cirach, P. Dadvand, R. Beelen, G. Hoek, X. Basagana, and M. Vrijheid. 2014. Traffic-related air pollution and congenital anomalies in Barcelona. *Environmental Health Perspectives* 122(3):317–323.

Schneider, A.J., R.W. Moore, A.M. Branam, L.L. Abler, K.P. Keil, V. Mehta, C.M. Vezina, and R.E. Peterson. 2014. In utero exposure to TCDD alters Wnt signaling during mouse prostate development: Linking ventral prostate agenesis to downregulated beta-catenin signaling. *Toxicological Sciences* 141(1):176–187.

Shah, P.S., T. Balkhair, and Knowledge Synthesis Group on Determinants of Preterm/LBW Births. 2011. Air pollution and birth outcomes: A systematic review. *Environment International* 37(2):498–516.

Sholts, S.B., M. Korkalainen, U. Simanainen, H.M. Miettinen, H. Hakansson, and M. Viluksela. 2015. In utero/lactational and adult exposures to 2,3,7,8-tetrachlorodibenzo-*p*-dioxin (TCDD) show differential effects on craniofacial development and growth in rats. *Toxicology* 337:30–38.

Shrestha, A., B. Ritz, M. Wilhelm, J. Qiu, M. Cockburn, and J.E. Heck. 2014. Prenatal exposure to air toxics and risk of Wilms' tumor in 0- to 5-year-old children. *Journal of Occupational and Environmental Medicine* 56(6):573–578.

Silva da Silva, C., J.M. Rossato, J.A. Vaz Rocha, and V.M. Vargas. 2015. Characterization of an area of reference for inhalable particulate matter ($PM_{2.5}$) associated with genetic biomonitoring in children. *Mutation Research Genetic Toxicology and Environmental Mutagenesis* 778:44–55.

Singh, V.K., J. Singh, M. Anand, P. Kumar, D.K. Patel, M.M. Krishna Reddy, and M.K. Javed Siddiqui. 2008. Comparison of polycyclic aromatic hydrocarbon levels in placental tissues of Indian women with full- and preterm deliveries. *International Journal of Hygiene and Environmental Health* 211(5–6):639–647.

Slama, R., S. Bottagisi, I. Solansky, J. Lepeule, L. Giorgis-Allemand, and R. Sram. 2013. Short-term impact of atmospheric pollution on fecundability. *Epidemiology* 24(6):871–879.

Slotkin, T.A., S. Skavicus, J. Card, R.T.D. Giulio, and F.J. Seidler. 2017. In vitro models reveal differences in the developmental neurotoxicity of an environmental polycylic aromatic hydrocarbon mixture compared to benzo[a]pyrene: Neuronotypic PC12 cells and embryonic neural stem cells. *Toxicology* 377:49–56.

Snijder C.A., N. Roeleveld, E. Te Velde, E.A. Steegers, H. Raat, A. Hofman, V.W. Jaddoe, and A. Burdorf. 2012. Occupational exposure to chemicals and fetal growth: The Generation R Study. *Human Reproduction* 27(3):910–920.

Son, J.Y., H.J. Lee, P. Koutrakis, and M.L. Bell. 2017. Pregnancy and lifetime exposure to fine particulate matter and infant mortality in Massachusetts, 2001–2007. *American Journal of Epidemiology* 186(11):1268–1276.

Song, X.F., Z.Y. Chen, Z.J. Zang, Y.N. Zhang, F. Zeng, Y.P. Peng, and C. Yang. 2013. Investigation of polycyclic aromatic hydrocarbon level in blood and semen quality for residents in Pearl River Delta Region in China. *Environment International* 60:97–105.

Soto-Martinez, M., and P.D. Sly. 2010. Relationship between environmental exposures in children and adult lung disease: The case for outdoor exposures. *Chronic Respiratory Disease* 7(3):173–186.

Spektor, D.M., 1998. A review of the scientific literature as it pertains to Gulf War illnesses. Volume 6: Oil well fires. Santa Monica, CA: RAND.

Stingone, J.A., T.J. Luben, J.L. Daniels, M. Fuentes, D.B. Richardson, A.S. Aylsworth, A.H. Herring, M. Anderka, L. Botto, A. Correa, S.M. Gilboa, P.H. Langlois, B. Mosley, G.M. Shaw, C. Siffel, A.F. Olshan, and the National Birth Defects Prevention Study. 2014. Maternal exposure to criteria air pollutants and congenital heart defects in offspring: Results from the National Birth Defects Prevention Study. *Environmental Health Perspectives* 122(8):863–872.

Stingone, J.A., K.H. McVeigh, and L. Claudio. 2016. Association between prenatal exposure to ambient diesel particulate matter and perchloroethylene with children's 3rd grade standardized test scores. *Environmental Research* 148:144–153.

Suades-Gonzalez, E., M. Gascon, M. Guxens, and J. Sunyer. 2015. Air pollution and neuropsychological development: A review of the latest evidence. *Endocrinology* 156(10):3473–3482.

Sugai, E., W. Yoshioka, M. Kakeyama, S. Ohsako, and C. Tohyama. 2014. In utero and lactational exposure to 2,3,7,8-tetrachlorodibenzo-*p*-dioxin modulates dysregulation of the lipid metabolism in mouse offspring fed a high-calorie diet. *Journal of Applied Toxicology* 34(3):296–306.

Sun, X., X. Luo, C. Zhao, R.W. Chung Ng, C.E. Lim, B. Zhang, and T. Liu. 2015. The association between fine particulate matter exposure during pregnancy and preterm birth: A meta-analysis. *BMC Pregnancy and Childbirth* 15(300):300.

Sun, X., X. Luo, C. Zhao, B. Zhang, J. Tao, Z. Yang, W. Ma, and T. Liu. 2016. The associations between birth weight and exposure to fine particulate matter $PM_{2.5}$ and its chemical constituents during pregnancy: A meta-analysis. *Environmental Pollution* 211:38–47.

Suzuki, Y., M. Niwa, J. Yoshinaga, Y. Mizumoto, S. Serizawa, and H. Shiraishi. 2010. Prenatal exposure to phthalate esters and PAHs and birth outcomes. *Environment International* 36(7):699–704.

Tai, P.T., M. Nishijo, T.N. Nghi, H. Nakagawa, H. Van Luong, T.H. Anh, and H. Nishijo. 2016. Effects of perinatal dioxin exposure on development of children during the first 3 years of life. *Journal of Pediatrics* 175:159–166.e152.

Takeda, T., M. Fujii, Y. Hattori, M. Yamamoto, T. Shimazoe, Y. Ishii, M. Himeno, and H. Yamada. 2014a. Maternal exposure to dioxin imprints sexual immaturity of the pups through fixing the status of the reduced expression of hypothalamic gonadotropin-releasing hormone. *Molecular Pharmacology* 85(1):74–82.

Takeda, T., J. Taura, Y. Hattori, Y. Ishii, and H. Yamada. 2014b. Dioxin-induced retardation of development through a reduction in the expression of pituitary hormones and possible involvement of an aryl hydrocarbon receptor in this defect: A comparative study using two strains of mice with different sensitivities to dioxin. *Toxicology and Applied Pharmacology* 278(3):220–229.

Takeda, T., Y. Matsuo, K. Nishida, A. Fujiki, Y. Hattori, T. Koga, Y. Ishii, and H. Yamada. 2017. α-Lipoic acid potentially targets AMP-activated protein kinase and energy production in the fetal brain to ameliorate dioxin-produced attenuation in fetal steroidogenesis. *Journal of Toxicological Sciences* 42(1):13–23.

Talbott, E.O., V.C. Arena, J.R. Rager, J.E. Clougherty, D.R. Michanowicz, R.K. Sharma, and S.L. Stacy. 2015. Fine particulate matter and the risk of autism spectrum disorder. *Environmental Research* 140:414–420.

Tang, D., T.Y. Li, J.J. Liu, Y.H. Chen, L. Qu, and F. Perera. 2006. PAH–DNA adducts in cord blood and fetal and child development in a Chinese cohort. *Environmental Health Perspectives* 114(8):1297–1300.

Tang, W.Y., L. Levin, G. Talaska, Y.Y. Cheung, J. Herbstman, D. Tang, R.L. Miller, F. Perera, and S.M. Ho. 2012. Maternal exposure to polycyclic aromatic hydrocarbons and 5′-CpG methylation of interferon-gamma in cord white blood cells. *Environmental Health Perspectives* 120(8):1195–1200.

Tang, D., J. Lee, L. Muirhead, T.Y. Li, L. Qu, J. Yu, and F. Perera. 2014a. Molecular and neurodevelopmental benefits to children of closure of a coal burning power plant in China. *PLOS ONE* 9(3):e91966.

Tang, D., T.Y. Li, J.C. Chow, S.U. Kulkarni, J.G. Watson, S.S.H. Ho, Z.Y. Quan, L.R. Qu, and F. Perera. 2014b. Air pollution effects on fetal and child development: A cohort comparison in China. *Environmental Pollution* 185:90–96.

Tang, W., L. Du, W. Sun, Z. Yu, F. He, J. Chen, X. Li, X. Li, L. Yu, and D. Chen. 2017. Maternal exposure to fine particulate air pollution induces epithelial-to-mesenchymal transition resulting in postnatal pulmonary dysfunction mediated by transforming growth factor-β/Smad3 signaling. *Toxicology Letters* 267:11–20.

Tanwar, V., J.M. Adelstein, J.A. Grimmer, D.J. Youtz, B.P. Sugar, and L.E. Wold. 2017a. $PM_{2.5}$ exposure in utero contributes to neonatal cardiac dysfunction in mice. *Environmental Pollution* 230:116–124.

Tanwar, V., M.W. Gorr, M. Velten, C.M. Eichenseer, V.P. Long, 3rd, I.M. Bonilla, V. Shettigar, M.T. Ziolo, J.P. Davis, S.H. Baine, C.A. Carnes, and L.E. Wold. 2017b. In utero particulate matter exposure produces heart failure, electrical remodeling, and epigenetic changes at adulthood. *Journal of the American Heart Association* 6(4):e005796.

Teng, C., Z. Wang, and B. Yan. 2016. Fine particle-induced birth defects: Impacts of size, payload, and beyond. *Birth Defects Research, Part C: Embryo Today* 108(3):196–206.

Tetreault, L.F., M. Doucet, P. Gamache, M. Fournier, A. Brand, T. Kosatsky, and A. Smargiassi. 2016. Childhood exposure to ambient air pollutants and the onset of asthma: An administrative cohort study in Quebec. *Environmental Health Perspectives* 124(8):1276–1282.

Thiering, E., J. Cyrys, J. Kratzsch, C. Meisinger, B. Hoffmann, D. Berdel, A. Von Berg, S. Koletzko, C. P. Bauer, and J. Heinrich. 2013. Long-term exposure to traffic-related air pollution and insulin resistance in children: Results from the GINIplus and LISAplus birth cohorts. *Diabetologia* 56(8):1696–1704.

Thirtamara Rajamani, K., S. Doherty-Lyons, C. Bolden, D. Willis, C. Hoffman, J. Zelikoff, L.C. Chen, and H. Gu. 2013. Prenatal and early-life exposure to high-level diesel exhaust particles leads to increased locomotor activity and repetitive behaviors in mice. *Autism Research* 6(4):248–257.

Thomson, E.M., D. Vladisavljevic, S. Mohottalage, P. Kumarathasan, and R. Vincent. 2013. Mapping acute systemic effects of inhaled particulate matter and ozone: Multiorgan gene expression and glucocorticoid activity. *Toxicological Sciences* 135(1):169–181.

Tracey, R., M. Manikkam, C. Guerrero-Bosagna, and M.K. Skinner. 2013. Hydrocarbons (jet fuel JP-8) induce epigenetic transgenerational inheritance of obesity, reproductive disease and sperm epimutations. *Reproductive Toxicology* 36:104–116.

Tran, N.N., T.T. Pham, K. Ozawa, M. Nishijo, A.T. Nguyen, T.Q. Tran, L.V. Hoang, A.H. Tran, V.H. Phan, A. Nakai, Y. Nishino, and H. Nishijo. 2016. Impacts of perinatal dioxin exposure on motor coordination and higher cognitive development in Vietnamese preschool children: A five-year follow-up. *PLOS ONE* 11(1):e0147655.

U.S. Army. 2001. *Female reproductive effects of exposure to jet fuel at U.S. Air Force bases*. Fort Detrick, MD: U.S. Army Medical Research and Material Command.

van den Hooven, E.H., Y. De Kluizenaar, F.H. Pierik, A. Hofman, S.W. Van Ratingen, P.Y.J. Zandveld, J.P. MacKenbach, E.A.P. Steegers, H.M.E. Miedema, and V.W.V. Jaddoe. 2011. Air pollution, blood pressure, and the risk of hypertensive complications during pregnancy: The Generation R Study. *Hypertension* 57(3):406–412.

van den Hooven, E.H., Y. de Kluizenaar, F.H. Pierik, A. Hofman, S.W. van Ratingen, P.Y.J. Zandveld, J. Lindemans, H. Russcher, E.A.P. Steegers, H.M.E. Miedema, and V.W.V. Jaddoe. 2012a. Chronic air pollution exposure during pregnancy and maternal and fetal C-reactive protein levels: The Generation R Study. *Environmental Health Perspectives* 120(5):746–751.

van den Hooven, E.H., F.H. Pierik, Y. de Kluizenaar, A. Hofman, S.W. van Ratingen, P.Y. Zandveld, H. Russcher, J. Lindemans, H.M. Miedema, E.A. Steegers, and V.W. Jaddoe. 2012b. Air pollution exposure and markers of placental growth and function: The Generation R Study. *Environmental Health Perspectives* 120(12):1753–1759.

van Drooge, B.L., A. Marqueno, J.O. Grimalt, P. Fernandez, and C. Porte. 2017. Comparative toxicity and endocrine disruption potential of urban and rural atmospheric organic PM_1 in JEG-3 human placental cells. *Environmental Pollution* 230:378–386.

van Esterik, J.C., H.W. Verharen, H.M. Hodemaekers, E.R. Gremmer, B. Nagarajah, J.H. Kamstra, M.E. Dolle, J. Legler, and L.T. van der Ven. 2015. Compound- and sex-specific effects on programming of energy and immune homeostasis in adult C57BL/6JxFVB mice after perinatal TCDD and PCB 153. *Toxicology and Applied Pharmacology* 289(2):262–275.

van Rossem, L., S.L. Rifas-Shiman, S.J. Melly, I. Kloog, H. Luttmann-Gibson, A. Zanobetti, B.A. Coull, J.D. Schwartz, M.A. Mittleman, E. Oken, M.W. Gillman, P. Koutrakis, and D.R. Gold. 2015. Prenatal air pollution exposure and newborn blood pressure. *Environmental Health Perspectives* 123(4):353–359.

Van Tung, D., T. Kido, S. Honma, H.D. Manh, D.D. Nhu, R. Okamoto, S. Maruzeni, M. Nishijo, H. Nakagawa, P.T. Ngoc, N. Van Toan, N.N. Hung, N.H. Minh, and L.K. Son. 2016. Low birth weight of Vietnamese infants is related to their mother's dioxin and glucocorticoid levels. *Environmental Science and Pollution Research International* 23(11):10922–10929.

Velali, E., E. Papachristou, A. Pantazaki, T. Choli-Papadopoulou, N. Argyrou, T. Tsourouktsoglou, S. Lialiaris, A. Constantinidis, D. Lykidis, T.S. Lialiaris, A. Besis, D. Voutsa, and C. Samara. 2016. Cytotoxicity and genotoxicity induced in vitro by solvent-extractable organic matter of size-segregated urban particulate matter. *Environmental Pollution* 218:1350–1362.

Vinikoor-Imler, L.C., S.C. Gray, S.E. Edwards, and M.L. Miranda. 2012. The effects of exposure to particulate matter and neighbourhood deprivation on gestational hypertension. *Paediatric and Perinatal Epidemiology* 26(2):91–100.

Vinikoor-Imler, L.C., J.A. Davis, R.E. Meyer, and T.J. Luben. 2013. Early prenatal exposure to air pollution and its associations with birth defects in a state-wide birth cohort from North Carolina. *Birth Defects Research* 97(10):696–701.

Vinikoor-Imler, L.C., T.G. Stewart, T.J. Luben, J.A. Davis, and P.H. Langlois. 2015. An exploratory analysis of the relationship between ambient ozone and particulate matter concentrations during early pregnancy and selected birth defects in Texas. *Environmental Pollution* 202:1–6.

Vishnevetsky, J., D. Tang, H.W. Chang, E.L. Roen, Y. Wang, V. Rauh, S. Wang, R.L. Miller, J. Herbstman, and F.P. Perera. 2015. Combined effects of prenatal polycyclic aromatic hydrocarbons and material hardship on child IQ. *Neurotoxicology and Teratology* 49:74–80.

Volk, H.E., F. Lurmann, B. Penfold, I. Hertz-Picciotto, and R. McConnell. 2013. Traffic-related air pollution, particulate matter, and autism. *JAMA Psychiatry* 70(1):71–77.

von Ehrenstein, O.S., J.E. Heck, A.S. Park, M. Cockburn, L. Escobedo, and B. Ritz. 2016. In utero and early-life exposure to ambient air toxics and childhood brain tumors: A population-based case-control study in California, USA. *Environmental Health Perspectives* 124(7):1093–1099.

Voynow, J.A., and R. Auten. 2015. Environmental pollution and the developing lung. *Clinical Pulmonary Medicine* 22(4):177–184.

Vrijheid, M., D. Martinez, S. Manzanares, P. Dadvand, A. Schembari, J. Rankin, and M. Nieuwenhuijsen. 2011. Ambient air pollution and risk of congenital anomalies: A systematic review and meta-analysis. *Environmental Health Perspectives* 119(5):598–606.

Wajda, A., J. Lapczuk, M. Grabowska, E. Pius-Sadowska, M. Slojewski, M. Laszczynska, E. Urasinska, B. Machalinski, and M. Drozdzik. 2017. Cell and region specificity of aryl hydrocarbon receptor (AhR) system in the testis and the epididymis. *Reproductive Toxicology* 69:286–296.

Wakx, A., A. Regazzetti, D. Dargere, N. Auzeil, S. Gil, D. Evain-Brion, O. Laprevote, and P. Rat. 2016. New in vitro biomarkers to detect toxicity in human placental cells: The example of benzo[A]pyrene. *Toxicology in Vitro* 32:76–85.

Walker, V.R., A.L. Boyles, K.E. Pelch, S.D. Holmgren, A.J. Shapiro, C.R. Blystone, M.J. Devito, R.R. Newbold, R. Blain, P. Hartman, K.A. Thayer, and A.A. Rooney. 2018. Human and animal evidence of potential transgenerational inheritance of health effects: An evidence map and state-of-the-science evaluation. *Environment International* 115:48–69.

Wang, L., and H. Choi. 2014. Using semiparametric-mixed model and functional linear model to detect vulnerable prenatal window to carcinogenic polycyclic aromatic hydrocarbons on fetal growth. *Biometrical Journal* 56(2):243–255.

Wang, C., X.G. Yuan, C.P. Liu, S.N. Zhai, D.W. Zhang, and Y.X. Fu. 2017a. Preliminary research on DNA methylation changes during murine palatogenesis induced by TCDD. *Journal of Cranio-Maxillofacial Surgery* 45(5):678–684.

Wang, H., X. Peng, F. Cao, Y. Wang, H. Shi, S. Lin, W. Zhong, and J. Sun. 2017b. Cardiotoxicity and mechanism of particulate matter 2.5 ($PM_{2.5}$) exposure in offspring rats during pregnancy. *Medical Science Monitor* 23:3890–3896.

Wang, L., S. Lin, J. Zhang, T. Tian, L. Jin, and A. Ren. 2017c. Fetal DNA hypermethylation in tight junction pathway is associated with neural tube defects: A genome-wide DNA methylation analysis. *Epigenetics* 12(2):157–165.

Wang, R., W.P. Wang, L. Ao, Z. Wang, X.L. Hao, and H.D. Zhang. 2017d. Benzo a pyrene-7,8-diol-9,10-epoxide suppresses the migration and invasion of human extravillous trophoblast HTR-8/SVneo cells by down-regulating MMP2 through inhibition of FAK/SRC/PI3K/AKT pathway. *Toxicology* 386:72–83.

Wang, W., R. Wang, Q. Zhang, G. Mor, and H. Zhang. 2018. Benzo(a)pyren-7,8-dihydrodiol-9,10-epoxide induces human trophoblast Swan 71 cell dysfunctions due to cell apoptosis through disorder of mitochondrial fission/fusion. *Environmental Pollution* 233:820–832.

Warren, J.L., J.A. Stingone, A.H. Herring, T.J. Luben, M. Fuentes, A.S. Aylsworth, P.H. Langlois, L.D. Botto, A. Correa, and A.F. Olshan. 2016. Bayesian multinomial probit modeling of daily windows of susceptibility for maternal $PM_{2.5}$ exposure and congenital heart defects. *Statistics in Medicine* 35(16):2786–2801.

Weldy, C.S., Y. Liu, Y.C. Chang, I.O. Medvedev, J.R. Fox, T.V. Larson, W.M. Chien, and M.T. Chin. 2013. In utero and early life exposure to diesel exhaust air pollution increases adult susceptibility to heart failure in mice. *Particle and Fibre Toxicology* 10(1):59.

Weldy, C.S., Y. Liu, H.D. Liggitt, and M.T. Chin. 2014. In utero exposure to diesel exhaust air pollution promotes adverse intrauterine conditions, resulting in weight gain, altered blood pressure, and increased susceptibility to heart failure in adult mice. *PLOS ONE* 9(2):e88582.

Wesselink, A., M. Warner, S. Samuels, A. Parigi, P. Brambilla, P. Mocarelli, and B. Eskenazi. 2014. Maternal dioxin exposure and pregnancy outcomes over 30 years of follow-up in Seveso. *Environment Internationa*l 63:143–148.

Winckelmans, E., K. Vrijens, M. Tsamou, B.G. Janssen, N.D. Saenen, H.A. Roels, J. Kleinjans, W. Lefebvre, C. Vanpoucke, T.M. de Kok, and T.S. Nawrot. 2017. Newborn sex-specific transcriptome signatures and gestational exposure to fine particles: Findings from the ENVIRONAGE birth cohort. *Environmental Health* 16(1):52.

Wu, J., H. Hou, B. Ritz, and Y. Chen. 2010. Exposure to polycyclic aromatic hydrocarbons and missed abortion in early pregnancy in a Chinese population. *Science of the Total Environment* 408(11):2312–2318.

Wu, J., M. Wilhelm, J. Chung, and B. Ritz. 2011. Comparing exposure assessment methods for traffic-related air pollution in an adverse pregnancy outcome study. *Environmental Research* 111(5):685–692.

Wu, L., L. Jin, T. Shi, B. Zhang, Y. Zhou, T. Zhou, W. Bao, H. Xiang, Y. Zuo, G. Li, C. Wang, Y. Duan, Z. Peng, X. Huang, H. Zhang, T. Xu, Y. Li, X. Pan, Y. Xia, X. Gong, W. Chen, and Y. Liu. 2017. Association between ambient particulate matter exposure and semen quality in Wuhan, China. *Environment International* 98:219–228.

Wu, Y., X. Chen, Q. Zhou, Q. He, J. Kang, J. Zheng, K. Wang, and T. Duan. 2014. ITE and TCDD differentially regulate the vascular remodeling of rat placenta via the activation of AhR. *PLOS ONE* 9(1):e86549.

Xia, X., A. Carroll-Haddad, N. Brown, M.J. Utell, C.T. Mallon, and P.K. Hopke. 2016. Polycyclic aromatic hydrocarbons and polychlorinated dibenzo-*p*-dioxins/dibenzofurans in microliter samples of human serum as exposure indicators. *Journal of Occupational and Environmental Medicine* 58(8 Suppl 1):S72–S79.

Xia, Y., P. Zhu, Y. Han, C. Lu, S. Wang, A. Gu, G. Fu, R. Zhao, L. Song, and X. Wang. 2009. Urinary metabolites of polycyclic aromatic hydrocarbons in relation to idiopathic male infertility. *Human Reproduction* 24(5):1067–1074.

Xu, X., H. Hu, S. Ha, and J. Roth. 2014. Ambient air pollution and hypertensive disorder of pregnancy. *Journal of Epidemiology and Community Health* 68(1):13–20.
Yan, Z., H. Zhang, C. Maher, E. Arteaga-Solis, F.A. Champagne, L. Wu, J.D. McDonald, B. Yan, G.J. Schwartz, and R.L. Miller. 2014. Prenatal polycyclic aromatic hydrocarbon, adiposity, peroxisome proliferator-activated receptor (PPAR) γ methylation in offspring, grand-offspring mice. *PLOS ONE* 9(10):e110706.
Yang, A., N.A. Janssen, B. Brunekreef, F.R. Cassee, G. Hoek, and U. Gehring. 2016. Children's respiratory health and oxidative potential of $PM_{2.5}$: The PIAMA birth cohort study. *Occupational and Environmental Medicine* 73(3):154–160.
Yang, P., Y.X. Wang, Y.J. Chen, L. Sun, J. Li, C. Liu, Z. Huang, W.Q. Lu, and Q. Zeng. 2017a. Urinary polycyclic aromatic hydrocarbon metabolites and human semen quality in China. *Environmental Science and Technology* 51(2):958–967.
Yang, P., Y.X. Wang, L. Sun, Y.J. Chen, C. Liu, L.L. Huang, W.Q. Lu, and Q. Zeng. 2017b. Urinary metabolites of polycyclic aromatic hydrocarbons, sperm DNA damage and spermatozoa apoptosis. *Journal of Hazardous Materials* 329:241–248.
Yang, P., Y.J. Gong, W.C. Cao, R.X. Wang, Y.X. Wang, C. Liu, Y.J. Chen, L.L. Huang, S.H. Ai, W.Q. Lu, and Q. Zeng. 2018. Prenatal urinary polycyclic aromatic hydrocarbon metabolites, global DNA methylation in cord blood, and birth outcomes: A cohort study in China. *Environmental Pollution* 234:396–405.
Yang, Q., Y. Zhao, X. Qiu, C. Zhang, R. Li, and J. Qiao. 2015. Association of serum levels of typical organic pollutants with polycystic ovary syndrome (PCOS): A case-control study. *Human Reproduction* 30(8):1964–1973.
Yao, C., Y. Chen, X. Zhu, Y. Liu, J. Zhang, L. Hou, Y. Xu, C. Zhang, and J. Cao. 2016. Air pollution and the risk of birth defects in Anqing City, China. *Journal of Occupational and Environmental Medicine* 58(4):e124–e127.
Ye, M., M. Warner, P. Mocarelli, P. Brambilla, and B. Eskenazi. 2018. Prenatal exposure to TCDD and atopic conditions in the Seveso second generation: A prospective cohort study. *Environmental Health* 17(1):22.
Yi, D., Y. Yuan, L. Jin, G. Zhou, H. Zhu, R. H. Finnell, and A. Ren. 2015. Levels of PAH–DNA adducts in cord blood and cord tissue and the risk of fetal neural tube defects in a Chinese population. *NeuroToxicology* 46:73–78.
Yin, S., M. Tang, F. Chen, T. Li, and W. Liu. 2017. Environmental exposure to polycyclic aromatic hydrocarbons (PAHs): The correlation with and impact on reproductive hormones in umbilical cord serum. *Environmental Pollution* 220(Pt B):1429–1437.
Yorifuji, T., S. Kashima, M. Higa Diez, Y. Kado, S. Sanada, and H. Doi. 2016. Prenatal exposure to traffic-related air pollution and child behavioral development milestone delays in Japan. *Epidemiology* 27(1):57–65.
Yuan, Y., L. Jin, L. Wang, Z. Li, L. Zhang, H. Zhu, R.H. Finnell, G. Zhou, and A. Ren. 2013. Levels of PAH–DNA adducts in placental tissue and the risk of fetal neural tube defects in a Chinese population. *Reproductive Toxicology* 37:70–75.
Zhan, S., X. Zhang, S. Cao, and J. Huang. 2015. Benzo(a)pyrene disrupts mouse preimplantation embryo development. *Fertility and Sterility* 103(3):815–825.
Zhou, N., Z. Cui, S. Yang, X. Han, G. Chen, Z. Zhou, C. Zhai, M. Ma, L. Li, M. Cai, Y. Li, L. Ao, W. Shu, J. Liu, and J. Cao. 2014. Air pollution and decreased semen quality: A comparative study of Chongqing urban and rural areas. *Environmental Pollution* 187:145–152.
Zhou, Y., S. M. Gilboa, M. L. Herdt, P. J. Lupo, W. D. Flanders, Y. Liu, M. Shin, M. A. Canfield, and R. S. Kirby. 2017. Maternal exposure to ozone and $PM_{2.5}$ and the prevalence of orofacial clefts in four U.S. states. *Environmental Research* 153:35–40.
Zhu, X., Y. Liu, Y. Chen, C. Yao, Z. Che, and J. Cao. 2015a. Maternal exposure to fine particulate matter ($PM_{2.5}$) and pregnancy outcomes: A meta-analysis. [Erratum appears in *Environmental Science and Pollution Research International* 22(5):3397–3399]. *Environmental Science and Pollution Research International* 22(5):3383–3396.
Zhu, Y., C. Zhang, D. Liu, K.L. Grantz, M. Wallace, and P. Mendola. 2015b. Maternal ambient air pollution exposure preconception and during early gestation and offspring congenital orofacial defects. *Environmental Research* 140:714–720.

7

Solvents

Solvents have a variety of uses in the military, and many of them were shipped in large quantities to the Persian Gulf. Some of the known uses for the military's various solvents include the maintenance of vehicles and equipment, cleaning, and degreasing. However, there is little information on which solvents were used in the Gulf War and the Post-9/11 conflicts, for what purposes, and in what quantity.

Although Congress identified several of the insecticides and other toxicants for study in the legislation on Gulf War exposures, it did not identify the specific solvents that should be examined by the committees of the *Gulf War and Health* series. The Volume 2 committee identified a large number of solvents sent to the Gulf War (see Appendix D in *Volume 2*), many of which have been extensively studied. To identify the solvents used in the Gulf War, the committee gathered information from several sources, including veterans' testimony and reports from the Office of the Special Assistant for Gulf War Illnesses (OSAGWI, 2000) and the Department of Defense (DoD) Defense Logistics Agency. Through its research the committee ultimately identified 53 solvents for review (see Table 7-1, adapted from Appendix D in *Volume 2*).

As the Volume 11 committee had a defined period in which to complete its review, the decision was made to update the toxicological and epidemiological information on the solvents discussed in *Volume 2* and to add any solvents that were sent to the Gulf in large quantities (more than 1,000 liters) and that had a threshold limit value[1] (TLV) of less than or equal to 100 ppm. However, solvents for which little or no information was available on the reproductive or developmental effects of the chemical (e.g., amyl acetate) were not given further consideration by the Volume 11 committee. The committee found no specific information on the exposures of Post-9/11 service members to solvents during deployment. The solvents considered by the Volume 11 committee are listed in Table 7-1.

[1] *Threshold limit values* (TLVs®) refer to airborne concentrations of chemical substances and represent conditions under which it is believed that nearly all workers may be repeatedly exposed, day after day, over a working lifetime, without adverse effects. TLVs are not regulatory standards, but rather recommendations developed and maintained by the American Conference of Governmental Industrial Hygienists.

TABLE 7-1 Solvents Sent to the 1990–1991 Gulf War

Solvents of Interest (as in Volume 2, Appendix D)	Health Effects in Vol. 2[a]	R/D tox data in Vol. 2[b]	Listed in OSAGWI[c]	>1kL sent to Gulf War[d]	TLV ≤100 ppm[e]	R/D Tox[f]	Health Effects in Vol. 11
Acetic acid**					X		
Acetone	X	X		X			
Amyl acetate				X	X		
Benzene	X	X			X		X
Ethylene glycol monobutyl ether (2-butoxyethanol)	X			X	X		X
Butyl acetate	X	X	X				
Butyl alcohol**					X		
Camphor**					X		
Chloroform	X				X		
Cresol**					X		
Cresylic acid**							
Cyclohexanol	X	X		X	X		
Cyclohexanone**					X		
Dichlorodifluoro-methane**							
Diethylene glycol	X	X		X			X
Diethylene glycol monobutyl ether				X			X
Diethylene triamine**					X		
Dipropylene glycol**							X
Ethanol**	X			X			
Ethyl acetate**							
2-ethyl butanol**							X
Ethylene glycol	X			X		R (A)	X
Ethylene glycol monoethyl ether	X	X			X	R (E)	X
Ethylene glycol monomethyl ether	X	X			X		X
Ethyl ether**							
Glycerol**							
n-heptane**							
Hexyl alcohol**							
Hexylene glycol	X			X	X		
Isoamyl acetate					X		
Isopentyl alcohol**							
Isopropyl alcohol**	X			X			

TABLE 7-1 Continued

Solvents of Interest (as in Volume 2, Appendix D)	Health Effects in Vol. 2[a]	R/D tox data in Vol. 2[b]	Listed in OSAGWI[c]	>1kL sent to Gulf War[d]	TLV ≤100 ppm[e]	R/D Tox[f]	Health Effects in Vol. 11
Methanol	X			X		D (E)	
1-methoxy-2-propanol acetate	X	X	X				
Methylene chloride	X	X		X	X		
Methyl ethyl ketone	X	X	X	X		D (E)	
Methyl isoamyl ketone			X		X		
Methyl isobutyl ketone	X		X	X	X	D (E)	
Methyl propyl ketone			X				
Morpholine**					X		
Naphtha	X	X		X	X		
Phenol**					X		
Polyalkylene glycol**							
Potassium hydroxide**				X			
Propylene glycol	X			X			X
Stoddard solvent	X			X	X		
Tetrachloroethylene	X	X		X	X	D (A)	X
Toluene	X	X	X	X	X		X
1,1,1-trichloroethane (methylchloroform)**				X			
1,1,2-trichloro-1,2,2-trifluoroethane**				X			
Trichloroethylene	X	X		X	X	D (A/E)	X
Tricresyl phosphate**							
Xylenes	X	X	X	X	X	D (A)	X
Propylene glycol monoethyl ether	X						X
Propylene glycol monomethyl ether	X	X					X

NOTES: kL=kiloliter; OSAGWI=Office of the Special Assistant for Gulf War Illnesses.

[a] These solvents were reviewed by the Volume 2 committee (IOM, 2003).

[b] Reproductive and/or developmental toxicity data regarding the effects of these solvents were reported by the Volume 2 committee (IOM, 2003).

[c] These solvents were present during Gulf War deployment according to reports from veterans (OSAGWI, 2000).

[d] Solvents sent to the theater of operations as indicated by DoD Defense Logistics Agency (OSAGWI, 2000).

[e] Threshold limit value (TLV) is an occupational exposure limit set by the American Conference of Governmental Industrial Hygienists to represent the upper limit of exposure considered safe for humans over a lifetime. Lower values represent more toxic substances (ACGIH, 2018).

[f] Reproductive (R) or developmental (D) toxicity data available from either an Agency for Toxic Substances and Disease Registry toxicological profile (A) or from a U.S. Environmental Protection Agency (E) document such as a support document for the Integrated Risk Integration System database or a human health assessment.

** Not discussed in Volume 11.

The most thoroughly documented solvent exposure involved the spray painting of military vehicles with chemical-agent-resistant coating (CARC) (IOM, 2003). Thousands of military vehicles deployed to the Gulf War were painted with tan CARC to provide camouflage protection for the desert environment as well as to provide a surface that could be easily decontaminated. Not all military personnel involved in CARC painting were trained in spray painting operations, and some might not have had or used all the necessary personal protective equipment, thus increasing their potential exposure to the cleaning solvents and paints (IOM, 2003). Personnel who participated in CARC painting were likely exposed to solvents in the CARC formulations, paint thinners, and cleaning products. As noted in a report by the Office of the Special Assistant for Gulf War Illnesses (OSAGWI), some of the solvents used to clean painting equipment might have been purchased locally and therefore not identified (OSAGWI, 2000).

In addition to the solvents sent to the Gulf War or Post-9/11 conflicts in large quantities or of great toxicity, in some cases exposure to volatile organic compounds (VOCs) and to the solvents themselves in ambient air were the result of incomplete combustion from diesel exhaust and burn pits. There is overlap between the two sources. For example, trichloroethylene (TCE) and tetrachloroethylene (PCE) were sent to the Gulf as solvents but were detected in air monitoring samples collected at Joint Base Balad (JBB), one of the largest U.S. military bases in Iraq, as the result of the operation of a large burn pit there. Several VOCs were detected only in air samples from JBB and were not sent to the Middle East as solvents (e.g., hexane); these VOCs are not discussed in depth in this volume, but more information on their health impacts may be found in the Institute of Medicine report *Long-Term Health Consequences of Exposure to Burn Pits in Iraq and Afghanistan* (IOM, 2011).

It is important to note that many of the epidemiologic studies that examine the potential reproductive and developmental effects of solvents—particularly in occupational settings or during the course of environmental exposures—involve a mixture of solvents, although investigators generally attempt either to measure levels of specific solvents or to use job matrices to estimate exposures. Because of the variety of uses for these solvents in the Gulf War and Post-9/11 conflicts, there were a number of possible routes of exposure for service members, including—in descending order of likelihood based on the described uses—inhalation, dermal, and oral pathways. These routes of exposure are associated with differing rates of systemic exposure, metabolism, and elimination from the body. The lack of precise exposure information for each solvent is a significant weakness for many of the studies considered in this section, and it adds uncertainty in extrapolating from occupational and environmental exposures, such as working in a dry cleaning facility or automotive repair facility, to the exposures that may have been experienced by veterans during deployment. Furthermore, many of the occupational studies report on exposure to several or many toxicants. Where there are studies of reproductive or developmental effects as a result of exposure to several of the committee's toxicants of concern, the Volume 11 committee cites the study for each relevant solvent.

The Volume 11 committee began its consideration of the reproductive and developmental effects of solvents by reviewing the findings of the 2003 Volume 2 committee. Although the Volume 2 committee reached conclusions on the category of association for specific solvents and most reproductive and developmental health outcomes (e.g., that there was evidence of a causal association between benzene exposure and acute leukemia in adults), it was unable to reach a consensus on the category of association for parental preconception exposure to solvents and the developmental health effect of childhood leukemia. The Volume 2 committee did reach a consensus that there was inadequate/insufficient evidence to determine whether an association existed for:

- Solvents and male or female infertility after the cessation of exposure;
- Parental preconception exposure to solvents and neuroblastoma and childhood brain cancers;

- Parental preconception exposure to solvents and spontaneous abortion or other adverse pregnancy outcomes; and
- Parental preconception exposure to solvents and congenital malformations.

In the following sections, the Volume 11 committee considers the epidemiologic and toxicologic information available on benzene, toluene, xylene, TCE, PCE, and glycols and glycol ethers derived from reports by authoritative bodies such as the Environmental Protection Agency (EPA) and the Agency for Toxic Substances and Disease Registry (ATSDR) and from literature searches for scientific studies published since *Volume 2*. It is important to note that the committee did not consider human or animal studies where the exposures attempted to mimic those of abuse scenarios such as solvent sniffing or "huffing." This exposure scenario was considered to be nonrepresentative of those that might be encountered by male or female veterans while on deployment.

BENZENE

Benzene is an aromatic hydrocarbon. It was widely used as a solvent in the past, and it was reported to be among the solvents used by Gulf War veterans (IOM, 2003); the Volume 11 committee was unable to identify any information on its use in the Post-9/11 conflicts. This hydrocarbon is also considered to be a VOC due to its physicochemical properties. Benzene is a known human carcinogen and causes leukemia (IARC, 2012). Although no longer used as a general purpose solvent because of concerns regarding its toxicity, benzene continues to be used in the synthesis of other chemicals, and it is a component of gasoline, diesel fuel, and JP-8 jet fuel. The Occupational Safety and Health Administration's permissible exposure level for benzene in workplace air is 1 ppm (time-weighted average) (OSHA, 2018).

Benzene was also one of the 12 most frequently measured pollutants in air samples taken at JBB in 2007 and 2009 (IOM, 2011). The base was home to a large airstrip and a large burn pit for waste. Air sampling, conducted by the U.S. Army to determine if service members on base were exposed to hazardous substances as a result of the burning of waste in the large burn pit, showed average benzene concentrations of 2.7 to 9.1 $\mu g/m^3$ (0.85 to 2.85 ppb), depending on the year (2007 or 2009) of sampling and sampling location.

These data show that both Gulf War and Post-9/11 service members may have been exposed, voluntarily and involuntarily, to benzene from several sources during their deployment, whether from its use as a solvent, as a component of jet and vehicle fuels, or as a byproduct of waste disposal in burn pits. Benzene is also a component of tobacco smoke. Environmental tobacco smoke is the single greatest source of indoor benzene concentrations, with emissions from cigarette smoking ranging from 430 to 590 μg per cigarette (Singer et al., 2003; WHO, 2010).

The epidemiologic studies reviewed below are summarized in Table 7-2 at the end of the section.

Reproductive Effects

Reproductive Effects in Men and Women

The Volume 2 committee reviewed several studies that assessed the risk of spontaneous abortions in the partners of men who were occupationally exposed to benzene in Finland (Lindbohm et al., 1991), France (Stucker et al., 1994), and China (Xu et al., 1998). The risk of spontaneous abortion was not significantly increased with low-level benzene exposures (concentrations not measured) for the Finnish workers exposed prior to conception (odds ratio [OR]=1.0, 95% confidence interval [CI] 0.7–1.3) or for the French workers exposed to 5 ppm (relative risk [RR]=1.1, 95% CI 0.6–2.0). However, female workers in the Chinese petrochemical industry exposed to undefined levels of benzene had a significantly increased risk of spontaneous abortion (RR=2.5, 95% CI 1.7–3.7) (Xu et al., 1998).

The 2007 *ATSDR Toxicological Profile for Benzene* and the 2015 *Addendum to the Toxicological Profile for Benzene* (ATSDR, 2007a, 2015a) reviewed numerous studies on the reproductive effects of benzene in humans. In one study, male workers with occupational exposure to benzene showed no statistically significant changes in the volume, appearance, pH, viscosity, or liquefaction of their semen compared with unexposed workers. However, when the men were stratified according to their duration of exposure, there were significant effects which included decreases in total sperm count and sperm motility, increased percentages of morphologically abnormal sperm, and increased sperm comet tail length (a measure of deoxyribonucleic acid [DNA] integrity) across all exposure groups (0–5 years, 5–10 years, and 10–15 years) compared with unexposed controls. The study did not include an evaluation of reproductive success in these workers (Katukam et al., 2012). ATSDR (2015a) reported that occupational exposure to benzene was also associated with genotoxic effects in sperm, including increased rates of chromosomal aberrations (e.g., breaks, deletions, translocations, and aneuploidy) for a number of sperm chromosomes (Ji et al., 2012; Kim et al., 2010; Marchetti et al., 2012; Schmid et al., 2006; Xing et al., 2010).

The Volume 11 committee considered three new studies in its assessment of possible reproductive effects that may be associated with benzene exposure. The three studies (Ji et al., 2012; Marchetti et al., 2012; Xing et al., 2010) reported on results of the China Benzene and Sperm Study, a cross-sectional study of chromosomal aberrations in 33 male workers who used benzene-containing glues in manufacturing, compared with 33 unexposed workers (from a meat packing plant) in Tianjin, China; all the men had worked in the plants for at least 1 year. Personal passive air sampling was conducted, and urine, blood, and sperm samples were collected from the subjects. Benzene concentrations in the workplace air ranged from below a detection limit of 0.2 ppm to 24 ppm (median, 2.9 ppm), with 27% of the men (n=9) being exposed to concentrations of ≤1 ppm. Xing et al. (2010) found, when compared with the unexposed workers, there was an increased frequency of aneuploid sperm in the low-exposed (1 ppm mean concentration) and high-exposed (7.7 ppm mean concentration) groups for disomy X, with an incidence rate ratio (IRR) of 2.0 (95% CI 1.1–3.4) and 2.8 (95% CI 1.5–4.9), respectively; there was also an increased risk for overall hyperhaploidy for chromosomes X, Y, and 21 (IRR=1.6, 95% CI 1.0–2.4 for low exposure, and IRR=2.3, 95% CI 1.5–3.6 for high exposure). The frequencies of disomy 21 were also significantly increased in the low-exposure men (IRR=2.1, 95% CI 1.0–4.7), and the frequency of disomy Y was increased in the high-exposure men (IRR=2.6, 95% CI 1.4–4.8). Ji et al. (2012) found that the sperm of these workers showed an increase in sex chromosome disomy but not chromosome 21. A significant correlation in frequency of sex chromosome disomy was observed between blood lymphocytes and sperm for the unexposed workers but not for exposed workers. Structural but not numerical chromosomal aberrations were increased in 30 of the exposed men (low exposure IRR=1.42, 95% CI 1.10–1.83; moderate exposure IRR=1.44, 95% CI 1.12–1.85; and high exposure IRR=1.75, 95% CI 1.36–2.24) compared with 11 unexposed men (Marchetti et al., 2012).

Adverse Pregnancy Outcomes

The Volume 2 committee (IOM, 2003) identified one study that reported an association between low birth weight and benzene exposure during pregnancy in female workers at a petrochemical facility in China. The effect was increased when benzene exposure was combined with work stress (Chen et al., 2000).

The 2015 ATSDR review *Addendum to the Toxicological Profile for Benzene* reported on one study (Zahran et al., 2012) that found a significantly increased risk of low birth weight with increasing benzene levels in ambient air in a study of resident births in the United States. No other relevant studies were discussed (ATSDR, 2015a).

The Volume 11 committee evaluated six studies that reported on fetal outcomes for women with prenatal exposures to benzene, four of which assessed benzene as a component of ambient air pollution (Estarlich et al., 2011; Ghosh et al., 2013; Llop et al., 2010; Zahran et al., 2012). In an assessment of 785 pregnant women with residential exposure to benzene in ambient outdoor air in Valencia, Spain, Llop et al. (2010) found an increased risk of preterm birth for women exposed throughout their entire pregnancies to estimated benzene levels of >2.7 μg/m^3 (OR=6.46, 95% CI 1.58–26.35). In a further study of a larger cohort of 2,337 pregnant women in four regions of Spain, Estarlich et al. (2011) found that exposure to ambient benzene (mean=1.6 μg/m^3), as estimated for the residence of each woman for each trimester and for the entire pregnancy, was not associated with reduced birth weight (OR=16.2, 95% CI –24.6–56.9), birth length (OR=0.16, 95% CI –0.03–0.35), or head circumference (OR=0.04, 95% CI –0.09–0.17) for any trimester or across the entire pregnancy. Ghosh et al. (2013) assessed the effects of air pollution, including benzene concentrations (mean=1.1 ppb), on the risk of having an infant with term low-birth weight. For third-trimester exposures, there was a slight but significant increase in the risk of a term low-birth weight infant (OR=1.03, 95% CI 1.00–1.05) among births to women living within 5 miles (8 km) of an air toxics monitoring station in Los Angeles, California, in 1995–2006.

Zahran et al. (2012), also cited in ATSDR (2015a), conducted a study of birth weights in 1.6 million singleton births in 422 U.S. counties across the nation. The researchers assessed maternal exposure to benzene on the basis of county-level ambient concentrations in 1996 and 1999, during which period benzene levels in gasoline dropped from 5% to 1%. A decrease in birth weight of 16.5 g (95% CI –17.6– –15.4 g) was found for each unit increase in benzene concentration. Furthermore, a 1 mg/m^3 increase in exposure significantly increased the risk of a low-birth-weight infant (OR=1.07, 95% CI 1.06–1.08).

In 2005–2006, Slama et al. (2009) recruited 271 nonsmoking pregnant French women to participate in the EDEN mother–infant cohort. Women wore a passive air sampler for a week during the 27th gestational week to measure ambient benzene levels. The median benzene exposure was 1.8 μg/m^3 (5th percentile=0.5 μg/m^3 and 95th percentile=7.5 μg/m^3). Benzene exposure was associated with a 68 g mean decrease in birth weight and a 1.9 mm decrease in mean head circumference at birth (95% CI –3.8–0.0 mm), and there was an estimated 1.5 mm decrease in fetal head circumference (95% CI –3.1–0 mm) at the end of the second trimester.

Ruckart et al. (2014) conducted a cross-sectional study of 11,896 births at the U.S. Marine Corps base Camp Lejeune, North Carolina, during 1968–1985. During this period the groundwater on the base was contaminated with benzene and other solvents. The authors used birth certificate information to identify mothers at delivery and groundwater modeling to estimate solvent concentrations. The researchers found no association between residential prenatal exposure to any concentration of benzene during the entire pregnancy and the risk of a small for gestational age infant, preterm birth, reduced mean birth weight, or full-term low birth weight. A nonsignificant monotonic exposure–response relationship was also observed for benzene exposure throughout pregnancy and term low birth weight (highest exposure level OR=1.5, 85% CI 0.9–2.3). However, a significant association was shown between benzene and adjusted mean birth weight difference compared with unexposed births (mean difference= –36.2 g, 95% CI –72.3– –0.1).

Animal Studies

Animal studies have been conducted to evaluate the reproductive effects of both inhalation and oral exposures of benzene in male animals. Although *Volume 2* did not include any animal studies on benzene, ATSDR thoroughly reviewed the animal literature concerning the reproductive effects of benzene via inhalation or oral exposure (ATSDR, 2007a, 2015a). ATSDR reported that although benzene does not appear to be teratogenic in animal studies, it may be fetotoxic (able to cause harm to the fetus) at concentrations that also cause maternal toxicity. ATSDR concluded that there was limited evidence from animal studies that oral exposure to benzene affects reproductive organs and that there was no information on the reproductive effects from inhalation exposure.

The Volume 11 committee identified one new animal study on the reproductive effects of benzene exposure that had not been reviewed by the IOM or ATSDR. Singh and Bansode (2011) fed male rats 0.5 mL or 1 mL benzene/kg (440 or 880 mg/kg) for 14 and 9 days, respectively. At autopsy, 1 day after exposure ended, the high-dose group exhibited a significantly decreased mean seminal vesicle weight (approximately 40% less than that of controls), with degenerative changes in the testes, such as giant cell formation, cytoplasmic vacuolization, pyknosis, chromatolysis, and the desquamation and dissolution of germ cells in the tubular lumen. The low-dose group (440 mg/kg) also had significantly decreased numbers of non-pachytene and pachytene spermatocytes, round and elongated spermatids, and decreased diameters of seminiferous tubules and Leydig cell nuclei. There was no loss in other reproductive organ weights; all animals given the high dose died.

Developmental Effects

The Volume 2 committee did not consider any studies of benzene exposure and developmental effects in humans or animals, but ATSDR did review numerous studies on the developmental effects of benzene in humans (ATSDR, 2007a, 2015a). The resulting review concluded that the epidemiological studies focused on developmental endpoints had considerable limitations, and ATSDR drew no conclusions on the possible effects of benzene in humans. The 2015 addendum reported on several epidemiological studies published since the toxicological profile that provided more information on potential developmental effects resulting from maternal inhalation exposure to benzene in ambient air. In a population-based study in Texas, Lupo et al. (2011) assessed the risk for neural tube defects, expressed in the form of spina bifida or anencephaly, as a result of prenatal exposure to ambient air pollutants. The estimated benzene levels were categorized as low (0.12–0.45 μg/m^3; referent), medium-low (>0.45–0.98 μg/m^3), medium (>0.98–1.52 μg/m^3), medium-high (>1.52–2.86 μg/m^3), and high (>2.86–7.44 μg/m^3). There were increased risks of spina bifida at ambient benzene concentrations compared to low levels (medium-low OR=1.77, 95% CI 1.04–3.00; medium OR=1.90, 95% CI 1.11–3.24; medium high OR=1.40, 95% CI 0.82–2.38; and high concentration OR=2.30, 95% CI 1.22–4.33). Anencephaly was not significantly associated with any benzene concentration. Ramakrishnan et al. (2013) estimated ambient air benzene levels near mothers' residences in Texas and compared those with the risk of having an oral cleft among offspring born between 1999 and 2008. No significant associations were found between benzene exposure and a cleft lip with and without cleft palate (OR=0.95, 95% CI 0.81–1.12) or between benzene exposure and a cleft palate without a cleft lip (OR=0.85, 95% CI 0.67–1.09).

The Volume 11 committee considered three meta-analyses that looked at the relationship between prenatal exposure to benzene and the risk of childhood leukemia: Zhou et al. (2014), Carlos-Wallace et al. (2016), and Filippini et al. (2015). In the Zhou et al. (2014) meta-analysis exposure to benzene was categorized for solvents (n=7), petroleum (n=7), or paint (n=7). For those three exposures, derived from 28 case-control studies and a cohort study, the pooled ORs for acute lymphoblastic leukemia (ALL) were

1.25 (95% CI 1.09–1.45) for solvents, 1.23 (95% CI 1.02–1.47) for paint, and 1.42 (95% CI 1.10–1.84) for petroleum; there was significant heterogeneity across the studies for paint, but not for solvents or petroleum. The authors concluded that childhood ALL was associated with maternal benzene exposure during pregnancy.

Carlos-Wallace et al. (2016) reviewed 20 studies of the association between occupational (n=17) or household product exposure (n=3) and childhood leukemia. The summary relative risk (sRR) for any childhood leukemia for the 20 studies combined was 1.96 (95% CI 1.60–2.41). Six of the studies provided data on acute myeloid leukemia (AML), giving a sRR of 2.34 (95% CI 1.72–3.18), and 14 studies reported on ALL for a sRR of 1.57 (95% CI 1.30–1.90). The risk of childhood leukemia was greater when the mother had been exposed to benzene (sRR=1.96, 95% CI 1.52–2.55; 13 studies) than when the father had been exposed (sRR=1.23, 95% CI 1.08–1.39; 14 studies). Maternal and paternal occupational exposure to benzene were both significantly associated with an increased risk (sRR=1.71, 95% CI 1.14–2.58; 7 studies, and sRR=1.18, 95% CI 1.00–1.41; 6 studies, respectively), as was household product use (sRR=1.67, 95% CI 1.24–2.26; 6 studies). Maternal exposure during gestation posed the greatest risk of childhood leukemia (sRR=2.06, 95% CI 1.51–2.81; 9 studies). Preconception (≥2 years before birth) exposure to benzene did not increase the risk when it was the mothers who were exposed (sRR=1.32, 95% CI 0.92–1.89; 6 studies), but it did when fathers were exposed (sRR=1.31, 95% CI 1.11–1.54; 8 studies), whereas neither maternal nor paternal periconception (approximately 1 year before birth) exposure was significantly associated with an increase in risk of childhood leukemia (sRR=1.29, 95% CI 0.97–1.71; 3 studies, and sRR=1.13, 95% CI 0.94–1.37; 4 studies, respectively). The authors concluded that there were associations between childhood leukemia and some benzene exposures.

Filippini et al. (2015) conducted a meta-analysis of 6 ecologic and 20 case-control studies to evaluate the association between traffic-related air pollution and the risk of childhood leukemia, with an emphasis on the effects of maternal residential exposures to nitrogen dioxide (NO_2) and benzene during pregnancy. On the basis of four studies (one of which reported on both ALL and AML), benzene was found to have an OR of 1.64 (95% CI 0.91–2.95) for any childhood leukemia. When stratified by leukemia type, the two relevant studies resulted in an OR of 1.09 (95% CI 0.67–1.77) for ALL and 2.28 (95% CI 1.09–4.75) for AML. The authors concluded that their results "support a link between ambient exposure to traffic pollution and childhood leukemia risk, particularly due to benzene."

In one of the few studies that conducted a trimester-by-trimester assessment of the risk of childhood leukemia from maternal exposure to air toxics, including benzene, Heck et al. (2014) used the California Cancer Registry to identify children under 6 years of age who had been diagnosed with either ALL (n=69) or AML (n=46) between 1990 and 2007. Both the cases and the 19,209 controls lived within either 2 km (for ALL) or 6 km (for AML) of an air toxics monitoring station. For each trimester of pregnancy, the averages of about seven air toxic measurements were used to calculate individual exposures. A single interquartile increase in benzene concentrations did not significantly increase the risk for ALL in the first trimester (OR=0.85, 95% CI 0.58–1.26) or the second trimester (OR=1.16, 95% CI 0.80–1.67), but it did increase the risk significantly in the third trimester (OR=1.50, 95% CI 1.08–2.09). Similar results were seen for the risk of AML for each trimester (ORs=1.13 [95% CI 0.64–2.01], 1.30 [95% CI 0.74–2.28], and 1.75 [95% CI 1.04–2.93], respectively). The authors concluded that ambient exposures to benzene during pregnancy may increase leukemia risk in children.

Senkayi et al. (2014) assessed the association between air pollution from airports and road traffic and childhood leukemia in Texas. They included all the airports in the state of Texas and 2,134 incidences of childhood leukemia (children age 9 and under) statewide over a 10-year period in their model. Benzene emissions from the airports were found to be a statistically significant predictor variable for the incidence of childhood leukemia (β=0.23, 95% CI 0.15–0.31).

The association between ALL in 416 Australian children under the age of 15 and parental exposure to a variety of chemical toxicants was examined by Reid et al. (2011). Parents reported relevant information about their potential exposures, including their occupations, and an expert reviewed the likelihood of their exposure to exhausts, solvents (including benzene specifically), glues, and paints up to 2 years prior to the birth of the child and 1 year afterward. Neither maternal nor paternal exposure to low or moderate/substantial levels of benzene at any time prior to or during pregnancy was associated with a significant increase in the risk of childhood ALL.

Childhood brain cancers and their association with ambient air toxics were studied by von Ehrenstein et al. (2016) for children under 6 years of age diagnosed in 1990–2007. Exposure was based on measurements of ambient air toxics within a 5-mile radius of a monitor. The study included 43 cases of central nervous system (CNS) primitive neuroectodermal tumor (PNET), 34 cases of medulloblastoma, and 106 cases of astrocytoma from the California Cancer Registry along with 30,569 controls, all of them living within 5 miles of a monitor. PNETs were positively associated with interquartile range (1.216) increases in prenatal exposure to benzene (OR=2.14, 95% CI 1.12–4.06), although medulloblastomas and astrocytomas were not (OR=0.82, 95% CI 0.36–1.87 and OR=0.83, 95% CI 0.53–1.29, respectively).

In the large registry-based case-control NORD-TEST study, the risk of testicular germ cell tumors was studied in men ages 14–49 years (n=8,112; controls=26,264) diagnosed in 1978–2012 in Finland, Norway, and Sweden (Le Cornet et al., 2017). Prenatal exposures were assessed on the basis of the men's parents' occupations prior to the men's birth. The parental occupations prior to the child's birth were based on national censuses and job codes. No significant associations were found between prenatal maternal exposure in the year prior to birth or paternal exposure and the risk of testicular germ cell tumors across all three countries (OR=1.24, 95% CI 0.83–1.85 and OR=0.99, 95% CI 0.86–1.15, respectively).

Two studies evaluated the association between birth defects and benzene exposure from ambient air during pregnancy. One was a retrospective cohort study of birth defects (critical congenital heart defects [n=2,028], orofacial clefts [n=1,299], and spina bifida [n=271]) in children born to mothers residing in Florida from 2000 to 2009 (Tanner et al., 2015). Estimates of maternal exposures to the ambient air levels of particulate matter $(PM)_{2.5}$ and benzene were derived by aggregating ambient measurement data from EPA. The mothers with the highest level of exposure to benzene were at the greatest risk of having a child with an isolated cleft palate (adjusted prevalence ratio [aPR] 4th quartile=1.52, 95% CI 1.13–2.04) or any orofacial cleft (aPR 4th quartile=1.29, 95% CI 1.08–1.56, compared with the lowest quartile). Furthermore, there was an inverse association between exposure to benzene and the heart defect described as non-isolated pulmonary atresia (aPR 4th quartile=0.19, 95% CI 0.04–0.84), but there was no such association for other heart defects. The authors found no significant associations between estimated benzene exposures and any other birth defects.

In a smaller study in Italy, Vinceti et al. (2016) compared the prenatal benzene exposures of 228 children born with birth defects and 228 children without birth defects. The ambient benzene levels from vehicle exhaust, which were estimated based on dispersion modeling, were 23.5 mg/km and 0.82 mg/km for light and heavy vehicles, respectively, in the urban areas, and 2.96 mg/km and 0.31 mg/km in the rural areas. There was no increased risk for any birth defect associated with the average or maximal levels of benzene.

Ruckart et al. (2013) conducted a case-control study to assess the frequency of birth defects and childhood cancers in children born to mothers at Camp Lejeune, North Carolina, between 1968 and 1985. Birth certificates were used to identify the 51 cases and 526 control parent–child pairs. Prenatal benzene exposure in the first trimester, dichotomized to exposed/unexposed, was not significantly associated with an increased risk of childhood leukemia or non-Hodgkin's lymphoma or oral cleft defects. However, first-trimester exposure to benzene was strongly associated with an increased risk of neural tube defects (OR=4.1, 95% CI 1.4–12.0).

The committee identified only two studies that assessed the association between a prenatal benzene exposure and cognitive and psychomotor development in children. Lertxundi et al. (2015) studied a population-based cohort of 438 mother–child pairs in Spain, recruited in 2006–2008 during each mother's first-trimester antenatal care visit. Air sampling was used to determine ambient levels of $PM_{2.5}$ and NO_2, and benzene concentrations were estimated using land use regression models. Children were assessed at about 15 months of age using the Bayley Scales of Infant Development. The authors concluded that there was no significant association between exposure to benzene in ambient air and development in children.

The Volume 11 committee identified one study that assessed the impact of exposure to residential benzene on the expression of microRNA (miR)-155 and miR-223 in maternal and cord blood as part of the German Lifestyle and Environmental Factors and Their Influence on Newborns Allergy Risk study in 2006–2008 (Herberth et al., 2014). miR-155 and miR-223 are known to be involved in regulatory T-cell formation or function. The median benzene concentration measured in the homes during weeks 34–36 of pregnancy was 1.01 $\mu g/m^3$. Higher concentrations of benzene was significantly associated increased levels of miR-223 in maternal blood (means ratio=1.18, 95% CI 1.07–1.30), but not miR-155. Benzene levels were not significantly associated with levels of miR-155 or miR-223 in cord blood (95% CIs included 1.0). High miR-223 expression was associated with lower regulatory T-cell numbers in maternal and cord blood. Toluene concentrations were also associated with miR-223 in maternal blood, but not the expression of either microribonucleic acid (miRNA) in cord blood, and xylenes were not associated with miRNA in either maternal or cord blood (see the following sections on toluene and xylenes).

Animal Studies

ATSDR (2007a) included numerous animal studies that reported that inhalation exposure to benzene produced fetotoxicity as evidenced by decreased body weight and by increased skeletal variants such as missing sternebrae and extra ribs, although ATSDR did not consider these to be malformations, but rather the result of maternal toxicity. Alterations in hematopoiesis was also observed in the fetuses and offspring of pregnant mice exposed via inhalation to low levels of benzene. The oral studies in animals cited by ATSDR did not show any developmental effects.

One animal study on the neurodevelopmental effects of benzene was identified by the Volume 11 committee. Lo Pumo et al. (2006) found that the exposure of pregnant rats to 0.1 mg/kg benzene resulted in impaired cognition and motor behavior in male offspring at 2 months of age; females were not assessed. No teratogenic effects were seen in the offspring of either sex.

The Volume 11 committee identified several studies that assessed the effects of benzene on fetal metabolism. Fetal transcription factor c-Myb gene levels were elevated 24 h after pregnant mice were given intraperitoneal injections of 800 mg/kg benzene on gestation days (GDs) 10 and 11. Benzene also caused oxidative stress, as evidenced by decreases in the ratio of reduced to oxidized glutathione in maternal and embryonic tissues at both 4 h and 24 h after exposure; however, the decreases were no longer evident at 48 hours after dosing (Wan and Winn, 2008). There was no embryo lethality.

The effect of benzene on oxidative stress was also examined by Badham and colleagues in a series of experiments with mice (Badham and Winn 2010a,b; Philbrook and Winn, 2015). Pregnant mice received intraperitoneal doses of 200 or 400 mg/kg benzene on GDs 8, 10, 12, and 14; animals were sacrificed on GD 15. Neither dose resulted in any maternal or fetal toxicity; however, at 200 mg/kg there was significantly altered erythroid and myeloid progenitor cell growth in the hematopoietic tissue of the fetuses; increases in the reactive oxygen species, but not oxidative stress markers in the fetal hematopoietic tissue; and significantly reduced fetal liver IκB-α protein levels in the fetuses (Badham and Winn, 2010a). Female offspring, but not male offspring, of dams treated with 200 mg/kg benzene had a significant increase in the number of erythroid-colony-forming units on GD 16 ($p<0.05$), although a significant decrease in the numbers of hematopoietic-colony-forming units was seen at postnatal day (PND) 2 ($p<0.05$); these effects were not seen in the offspring of dams receiving 400 mg/kg (Badham and Winn, 2010b). Philbrook and Winn (2015) explored the effects of prenatal exposures to benzene on epigenetic modifications. Pregnant CD-1 mice were dosed on GDs 8, 10, 12, and 14 with 200 mg/kg benzene and maternal bone marrow and fetal livers assessed for global DNA methylation, promoter-specific methylation of the tumor suppressor gene p15, and levels of acetylated histones H3, H4, and H3K56 and methylated histones H3K9 and H3K27. The authors found that although there was decreased global DNA methylation in maternal bone marrow, fetal livers showed no effect on global DNA methylation, p15 promoter methylation, or any measured histone modifications and recommended further investigation of the whole genome and epigenome.

The responses of mice to benzene may vary by strain. Badham et al. (2010) found that CD-1 mice, but not C57BL/6N mice, that had been prenatally exposed to 200 mg/kg benzene on GDs 8, 10, 12, and 14 had a significant increase in the incidence of hepatic and hematopoietic tumors at 1 year of age. Male CD-1 offspring had more hepatic tumors, while female mice had predominantly hematopoietic tumors. Female CD-1 offspring exposed transplacentally also had significantly suppressed bone marrow CD11b(+) cells at 1 year after birth.

Lau et al. (2009) administered daily intraperitoneal injections of benzene (200 or 400 mg/kg) to pregnant mice on GDs 7 to 15. On PND 9, the bone marrow micronucleus frequency was significantly elevated in the offspring of the high-dose group, although neither dose significantly altered the formation of γ-H2A.X fetal liver cells or in PND 9 bone marrow cells. No recombination events were detected in the fetal liver.

Synthesis and Conclusions

Given the ubiquity of benzene in ambient air and as a component of both fuels and exhaust from the combustion of fuels and other hydrocarbons, it is not surprising that benzene is relatively well studied. However, many of the studies of benzene have focused on its carcinogenicity, particularly as a causal agent for leukemia in adults. Benzene's potential to cause reproductive and developmental effects has been assessed in occupational studies of both male and female workers. Studies of the effects of prenatal exposure to benzene have generally been done by measuring its concentrations in ambient air—frequently by comparing maternal exposures at residences near roads versus residences further from obvious benzene sources.

Reproductive Effects

The effects of benzene exposure on male reproduction have been studied in occupational settings, primarily in China. The Volume 11 committee considered three new studies (Ji et al., 2012; Marchetti et al., 2012; Xing et al., 2010) from the cross-sectional China Benzene and Sperm Study. The researchers that found that occupational exposure to benzene even at the lowest concentration measured (1 ppm) was associated with genotoxic effects in sperm, including increases in aneuploidy, disomy, and hyperhaploidy. However, these studies reported on only one small cohort, with just 33 exposed and 33 unexposed workers. A larger study by Katukam et al. (2012) of 160 workers also with industrial exposure to benzene reported sperm DNA damage (an increase in comet tail length) in the workers and other adverse sperm effects were seen. One animal study also showed that benzene has adverse effects on sperm parameters (Singh and Bansode, 2011).

Studies from the 1990s of occupational exposure of Finnish, French, or Chinese men to benzene reported that the men's partners were not at increased risk of spontaneous abortion (IOM, 2003). The Volume 11 committee evaluated six studies that reported on fetal outcomes for women with prenatal exposures to benzene, four of which assessed benzene as a component of ambient air pollution (Estarlich et al., 2011; Ghosh et al., 2013; Llop et al., 2010; Zahran et al., 2012); the results were mixed. Llop et al. (2010) found an increased risk of preterm births with increasing benzene exposure in women in Spain, whereas Estarlich et al. (2011) found that benzene exposure was not associated with reduced birth weight or head circumference at any time during pregnancy. In two U.S. studies (Ghosh et al., 2013; Zahran et al., 2012) and one French study (Slama et al., 2009), benzene exposure was associated with a significantly increased risk of having a low-birth-weight infant and, in the French study, with decreased head circumference. A new study of infants born to women who lived at Camp Lejeune, North Carolina, during a period when the water was contaminated with benzene and other solvents found that benzene exposure during pregnancy was not associated with an increased risk for adverse birth outcomes. Thus, the results of the studies of prenatal benzene exposure on adverse birth outcomes were mixed.

The Volume 11 committee concludes that there is limited/suggestive evidence of an association exists between exposure to benzene and reproductive effects in men.

The Volume 11 committee also concludes that there is inadequate/insufficient evidence to determine whether an association exists between exposure to benzene and reproductive effects in women, or with adverse pregnancy outcomes.

Developmental Effects

Benzene is often singled out as an air toxic and traffic pollutant, with exposures at some point between conception and diagnosis reported to increase the risk of child leukemia (Heck et al., 2014; Senkayi et al., 2014). One challenge with these reports is that the windows of relevant exposure have not been defined. As noted earlier, benzene is a known carcinogen and causes leukemia in adults, but there is no evaluation that is specific for childhood leukemia (IARC, 2012). IARC notes that studies "support the idea that genotoxic and non-genotoxic events following exposure to benzene may be initiators of childhood leukemia in utero" (IARC, 2012). The 2015 *Addendum to the ATSDR Toxicological Profile*, after an evaluation of numerous epidemiological studies on developmental effects following maternal exposure to benzene in ambient air, found that there was a significant increase in the risk of spina bifida but not anencephaly or cleft lip with or without cleft palate (ATSDR, 2015a).

The Volume 11 committee reviewed three meta-analyses, all of which concluded that there is an association between prenatal exposure to benzene in ambient air and an increased risk of childhood leukemia. These findings were supported by Heck et al. (2014), who assessed benzene exposure by trimester and found that exposures in the third but not first or second trimester were associated with an increased risk of both ALL and AML in children. Living near an airport was found to increase the risk of childhood leukemia, and the risk was associated with benzene emissions (Senkayi et al., 2014). These results were contradicted, however, by an Australian study that found no increase in the risk of ALL in children whose parents had any exposure to benzene prior to or during the pregnancy.

One study of brain cancers in children in relation to ambient benzene concentrations in California found a strong positive increase in the presence of PNETs with increases in benzene, but there was no increase in the risk of medulloblastomas or astrocytomas (von Ehrenstein et al., 2014).

Studies on the association between exposure to benzene and birth defects have offered mixed results. Two studies (Ramakrishnan et al., 2013; Ruckart et al., 2013) found no association between prenatal maternal exposure to benzene in, respectively, ambient air or drinking water and cleft lips in offspring; however, a study by Tanner et al. (2015) found that mothers with the highest benzene exposure were at the greatest risk of having a child with a cleft palate or any orofacial cleft, although there were no associations with other birth defects, including heart defects. The study by Ruckart et al. (2013) of children born to mothers who had resided at Camp Lejeune, North Carolina, found that first-trimester exposure to drinking water contaminated with benzene significantly increased the risk of neural tube defects.

The committee considered only one study of prenatal benzene exposure and neurodevelopment in children, which was carried out in Spain. No association was found.

The Volume 11 committee concludes that there is sufficient evidence of an association between prenatal exposure to benzene and childhood leukemia.

The Volume 11 committee also concludes that there is inadequate/insufficient evidence to determine whether an association exists between prenatal exposure to benzene and other developmental effects in children.

TABLE 7-2 Summary of Reproductive and Developmental Effects of Benzene

Study	Design/Population	Exposure	Results
Reproductive Effects			
Reproductive Effects in Men			
Marchetti et al. (2012)	Cross-sectional 30 exposed and 11 nonexposed male workers in Tianjin, China.	Occupational exposures to benzene-containing glues versus working in a meat packing plant; personal passive air badges and urine samples were used to monitor benzene levels. Workers stratified to low-, moderate-, and high-exposure groups with median air benzene concentrations of 1.2, 3.7, and 8.4 ppm, respectively.	Sperm DNA damage. Exposure to benzene was associated with chromosomal structural aberrations in sperm, but not numerical abnormalities; adjusted IRRs for all structural aberrations combined were 1.42 (95% CI 1.10–1.83), 1.44 (95% CI 1.12–1.85), and 1.75 (95% CI 1.36–2.24) in the low-, moderate-, and high-exposed men compared with unexposed men.
Ji et al. (2012)	See Marchetti et al. (2012).	See Marchetti et al. (2012).	Sperm aneuploidy compared to aneuploidy in blood lymphocytes. Benzene exposure was positively associated with the gain of chromosome 21, but not sex chromosomes, in blood lymphocytes; significant increase in sex chromosomes in sperm, but not chromosome 21. Also a significant correlation between the gain of sex chromosomes in blood lymphocytes and sperm among unexposed subjects, but not among exposed workers.
Xing et al. (2010)	Cohort 33 exposed men (17 with low benzene exposures and 16 with high exposures) compared with 33 nonexposed male workers in Tianjin, China.	Occupational exposures to benzene-containing glues versus working in a meat packing plant; personal passive air badges were used for 2 days, and urine spot samples were used to monitor benzene levels. Benzene exposures lasted for at least 1 year. Air concentrations ranged from below the detection limit to 24 ppm (median, 2.9 ppm), with 9 men exposed to ≤1 ppm benzene.	Sperm DNA damage. Occupational exposures to benzene were associated with increased frequencies of aneuploid sperm for chromosomes X, Y, or 21; significant exposure-dependent increases in the frequencies of sperm with disomy X, disomy Y, and hyperhaploidy in exposed men ($p<0.05$).

continued

TABLE 7-2 Continued

Study	Design/Population	Exposure	Results
Adverse Birth Outcomes			
Slama et al. (2009)	Cohort—EDEN study 271 pregnant women in two French maternity hospitals in 2005–2006.	Median benzene concentration as measured by personal air samplers worn by the women for 1 week was 1.8 μg/m^3 (5th, 95th percentiles, 0.5, 7.5 μg/m^3, respectively).	Decrease in birth weight (–68 g) and mean head circumference (–1.9 mm).
Zahran et al. (2012)	Cohort 1.6 million births in 422 U.S. counties.	Maternal exposure based on median county-level ambient concentrations of benzene in 1999 compared with 1996 (benzene levels in gasoline dropped from 5% to 1% during this time).	Unit increase (mg/m^3) in benzene concentration decreased birth weight by 16.5 g (95% CI 17.6–15.4); a 1 mg/m^3 increase in benzene exposure increased the odds of a low-birth-weight outcome by a factor of 1.07 (95% CI 1.06–1.08).
Ruckart et al. (2014)	Cross-sectional 11,896 infants born to women who consumed contaminated drinking water at Marine Corps base Camp Lejeune during 1968–1985.	Benzene exposure stratified to no exposure, low exposure (>0–<1 ppb), and high exposure (≥1 ppb) for SGA, low birth weight, and birth weight; for preterm exposure stratified to below versus above 10 ppb based on modeled concentration for entire pregnancy.	SGA, low exposure OR=1.0 (95% CI 0.9–1.2), high exposure OR=1.2 (95% CI 0.9–1.5); PTB, low exposure OR=1.0 (95% CI 0.9–1.3), high exposure OR=0.8 (95% CI 0.6–1.1); term low birth weight low exposure OR=1.0 (95% CI 0.8–1.4), high exposure OR=1.5 (95% CI 0.9–2.3); birth weight low exposure md= –14.5 grams (p=1.8), high exposure md= –36.2 grams (p=0.05). Adjusted for prenatal care, sex of child, mother's race, parity, and rank of military member.
Developmental Effects			
Ramakrishnan et al. (2013)	Case-control 3,945 case of oral clefts versus 15,780 controls born in Texas in 1999–2008.	Estimates of average annual exposure to environmental concentrations of each BTEX compound for maternal census tract at birth based on 2005 EPA National-Scale Air Toxics Assessment Hazardous Air Pollutant Exposure Model; the mean level of benzene was 0.85 mg/m^3.	Birth defects: oral clefts. Mothers with high levels of estimated benzene exposure (≥1.38 mg/m^3) were not more likely to have offspring with cleft lip with or without cleft palate (OR=0.95; 95% CI 0.81–1.12) or isolated cleft palate (OR=0.85; 95% CI 0.67–1.09) compared with mothers who had low levels of exposure (≤0.58 mg/m^3); adjusted for birth year, infant sex, maternal race/ethnicity, education, age, smoking, and season of conception.

Study	Design/Population	Exposure	Results
Tanner et al. (2015)	Retrospective cohort 973,797 infants with congenital malformations (2,028 with critical congenital heart defects, 1,299 with orofacial clefts, and 271 with spina bifida) and 973,797 infants with no malformations, born in Florida from 2000 to 2009.	Birth defects, including critical congenital heart defects, orofacial clefts, and spina bifida, identified from the Florida Birth Defects Registry. Estimates of maternal exposures to $PM_{2.5}$ and benzene were derived by aggregation of ambient measurement data, from the EPA Air Quality System.	Birth defects: oral clefts. Mothers with the highest level of exposure to benzene were more likely to deliver an infant with an isolated cleft palate (aPR 4th quartile=1.52, 95% CI 1.13–2.04) or any orofacial cleft (aPR 4th quartile=1.29, 95% CI 1.08–1.56). There was a negative association between exposure to benzene and non-isolated pulmonary atresia (aPR 4th quartile=0.19, 95% CI 0.04–0.84). No other significant effects.
Ruckart et al. (2013)	Case-control 6 cases of neural tube defects, 3 cases of oral clefts, 2 cases of leukemia or non-Hodgkin's lymphoma versus health controls born during 1968–1985 to mothers who lived at the Marine Corps base Camp Lejeune.	Exposure to benzene in water at Camp Lejeune during first trimester of pregnancy (exposed versus unexposed; actual benzene levels in contaminated drinking water not given).	Birth defects: NTDs. NTD: OR=4.1, 95% CI 1.4–12.0; Oral cleft defect: OR=0.7, 95% CI 0.2–2.2; Childhood leukemia or non-Hodgkin's lymphoma: OR=0.8, 95% CI 0.2–3.8.
Vinceti et al. (2016)	Case-control 228 cases of birth defects versus 228 controls in Italy.	Modeling of benzene exposure as air pollution with some sampling to confirm maternal exposure during pregnancy.	Birth defects. No association between benzene and any birth defect or chromosomal abnormality.
Zhou et al. (2014)	Meta-analysis of maternal benzene exposures and risk of childhood ALL. Studies published before 9/1/2013. Twenty-eight case-control studies and one cohort study included in the analysis (16,695 cases and 1,472,786 controls).	Self-reported maternal solvent, paint, petroleum exposure, and smoking during pregnancy. No air modeling was done, nor were any measurements taken.	Childhood leukemia (ALL). Pooled ORs: solvents (n=7 studies) OR=1.25 (95% CI 1.09-1.45); paint (n=7 studies) OR=1.23 (95% CI 1.02–1.47); petroleum exposure (n=7 studies) OR=1.42 (95% CI 1.10–1.84); smoking during pregnancy (n=18 studies) OR=0.99 (95% CI 0.93–1.06).

continued

TABLE 7-2 Continued

Study	Design/Population	Exposure	Results
Filippini et al. (2015)	Meta-analysis of 6 ecologic and 20 case-control studies on traffic-related air pollution and risk of childhood leukemia; emphasis on effects of maternal residential exposures to NO_2 and benzene.	Exposure data not reported. Heterogeneity of how exposure was determined.	Childhood leukemia. On the basis of 4 studies, benzene showed an OR of 1.64 (95% CI 0.91–2.95) for any childhood leukemia. When stratified by leukemia type, the two relevant studies resulted in an OR of 1.09 (95% CI 0.67–1.77) for ALL and 2.28 (95% CI 1.09–4.75) for AML.
Carlos-Wallace et al. (2016)	Meta-analysis of occupational and household product exposures to benzene and risk of childhood leukemia completed during 1987–2014.	Exposure metrics included occupational and household use of benzene and solvents, traffic density, and traffic-related air pollution.	Childhood leukemia. Pooled estimate for all childhood leukemia and any benzene exposure RR=1.96 (95% CI 1.53–2.52; n=20 studies); AML RR=2.34 (95% CI 1.72–3.18; n=6 studies); ALL RR=1.57 (95% CI 1.21–2.05; n=14 studies). RR was higher for maternal than paternal exposure, in studies that assessed benzene versus all solvents, and in studies of gestational exposure. In studies of traffic density or traffic-related air pollution: pooled estimate for all leukemia RR=1.48 (95% CI 1.10–1.99; n=12 studies); AML RR=2.07 (95% CI 1.34–3.20); ALL RR=1.49 (95% CI 1.07–2.08). In studies that used detailed models of traffic pollution RR=1.70, 95% CI 1.16–2.49.
Slater et al. (2011)	Case-control 443 infants (<1 year) with leukemia versus 324 controls.	Maternal exposure to petroleum products in month before birth or during pregnancy; not benzene-specific.	Childhood leukemia. Exposure to petroleum products preconception or during prenatal period was significantly associated with infant leukemia: AML OR=2.33, 95% CI 1.30–4.18; and ALL OR=2.48, 95% CI 1.37–4.48; and during entire pregnancy AML OR=2.54, 95% CI 1.40–4.62.

Study	Design/Population	Exposure	Results
Heck et al. (2014)	Case-control—California Cancer Registry 69 cases of ALL and 46 cases of AML age <6 years, and 19,209 controls from California birth records. 1990–2007	Children lived within 2 km (ALL) and 6 km (AML) of an air toxics monitoring station. In the first trimester, average of 6.9 air toxic measurements used to calculate an individual's exposure; a similar number were used in the second (mean=6.9) and third (mean=7.3) trimesters.	Childhood leukemia. One interquartile increase in benzene concentrations did not significantly increase the risk for ALL in the first trimester (OR=0.85, 95% CI 0.58–1.26) or second trimester (OR=1.16, 95% CI 0.80–1.67), but the risk was significantly increased in the third trimester (OR=1.50, 95% CI 1.08–2.09). Similar results were seen for the risk of AML for each trimester: ORs=1.13 (95% CI 0.64–2.01), 1.30 (95% CI 0.74–2.28), and 1.75 (95% CI 1.04–2.93), respectively.
Senkayi et al. (2014)	Ecological Incidence of childhood leukemia in children ≤9 years old in Texas by census block and by county. 1995–2005	Benzene esposures modeled based on emissions from all airports in state of Texas. No actual measurements reported. Benzene was singled out as an emission of concern and was specifically modeled.	Childhood leukemia. Benzene emissions from the airports were found to be statistically significant predictor variable for the incidence of childhood leukemia (β=0.230, 95% CI 0.15–0.31).
Reid et al. (2011)	Case-control 416 cases of ALL <15 years old diagnosed 2003–2006 (including 379 mothers, 328 case fathers) versus parents of healthy children (854 mothers, 748 fathers) from the Australian population.	Exposure to benzene estimated based on occupation for before birth, after birth, 1 year before birth, and 2 years before birth (mother only). Exposure levels not defined.	Childhood leukemia. Paternal exposure to low levels of benzene at any time prior to birth was not associated with an increased risk of ALL (OR=1.07, 95% CI 0.43–2.63 for maternal exposure; OR=1.38, 95% CI 0.82–2.32 for paternal exposure), nor was moderate to high exposure (OR=0.93, 95% CI 0.42–2.09 for maternal exposure; OR=0.79, 95% CI 0.51–1.23 for paternal exposure).
von Ehrenstein et al. (2016)	Case-control—California Cancer Registry 43 CNS PNET, 34 medulloblastoma, and 106 astrocytoma cases and 30,569 controls ≤6 years of age diagnosed 1990–2007.	Exposure estimated based on air monitor.	Childhood cancer. PNETs associated with interquartile increases in prenatal exposure to benzene (OR=2.14, 95% CI 1.12–4.06), although medulloblastomas and astrocytomas were not associated with benzene exposure (OR=0.82, 95% CI 0.36–1.87; and OR=0.83, 95% CI 0.53–1.29, respectively).

continued

TABLE 7-2 Continued

Study	Design/Population	Exposure	Results
Lertxundi et al. (2015)	Cohort 438 children from Guipozcoa, Spain. 2006–2008	Prenatal benzene exposure estimated based on proximity to steel and iron industry and traffic, air monitors, and land use regression models.	Neurodevelopment assessed at 15 months of age. Benzene levels showed a negative, but non-significant associations with mental and motor development scores both under a model that did not account for distances and a model that accounted for them (i.e., distance from the closest pollution release and transfer-listed facility and for distance from the closest road with traffic density >20,000 vehicles/day). Analysis of prenatal benzene exposure combined with NO_2 exposure resulted in negative, nonsignificant associations with mental and motor scores.
Herberth et al. (2014)	441 children and 315 pregnant mothers in prospective mother–child study (Lifestyle and Environmental Factors and Their Influence on Newborns Allergy Risk).	Benzene concentrations measured in maternal residence with passive monitor; median concentration was 1.01 $\mu g/m^3$. Blood samples and urine samples taken from mother at 34th week of pregnancy and cord blood collected at birth. Urine analyzed for benzene metabolite S-phenylmercapturic acid.	Higher concentrations of benzene were significantly associated with increased levels of miR-223 in maternal blood (means ratio=1.18, 95% CI 1.07–1.30) but not miR-155. Benzene levels were not significantly associated with levels of miR-155 or miR-223 in cord blood (95% CIs included 1.0). High miR-223 expression was significantly associated with lower Treg numbers in maternal and cord blood (CIs did not include 1.0).

NOTE: ALL=acute lymphoblastic leukemia; AML=acute myeloid leukemia; aPR=adjusted prevalence ratio; BTEX=benzene, toluene, ethylbenzene, xylene; CI=confidence interval; CNS=central nervous system; DNA=deoxyribonucleic acid; EPA=U.S. Environmental Protection Agency; IRR=incidence rate ratio; md=mean difference; miR=micro-ribonucleic acid; NO_2=nitrogen dioxide; NTD=neural tube defect; OR=odds ratio; PM=particulate matter; PNET=primitive neuroectodermal tumor; PTB=preterm birth; RR=relative risk; SGA=small for gestational age; Treg=regulatory T cell.

TOLUENE

Toluene is a widely used aromatic hydrocarbon. Toluene is a component of gasoline and is also found as a combustion product of fuel. It was sent to the Gulf War as a solvent in quantities greater than 1 kiloliter. The Volume 2 committee reported that "toluene is also present in paints, thinners, cleaning agents, and glue and is widely abused as an inhalant" (IOM, 2003). It may replace benzene in some industrial applications.

Toluene is a monosubstituted benzene derivative sometimes known as methylbenzene. It is frequently considered in combination with benzene, ethylbenzene, and xylenes as a mixture called BTEX. ATSDR (2015b) reported on the toxicokinetics of toluene and stated, "In both humans and rats, up to about 75–80% of inhaled toluene that is absorbed can be accounted for as hippuric acid in the urine" (Lof et al., 1993; Ogata, 1984; Tardif et al., 1998). The report also said that most absorbed toluene is rapidly eliminated from the body.

Toluene was among the 12 most frequently detected VOCs at the three sampling locations at JBB in both 2007 and 2009 (IOM, 2011). It was detected in 63 of 66 air samples in 2007 and in 56 of 57 air samples in 2009. Air concentrations ranged from nondetectable to approximately 55, the highest concentration measured of any of the 12 VOCs, with an average concentration of 18.6 μg/m^3. The committee that wrote that report considered the likely major source of the toluene to be the combustion of petroleum-based fuel.

Toluene was also detected in the contaminated water supply at Camp Lejeune, North Carolina, possibly as a degradation product of PCE (NRC, 2009). Toluene was detected in a few water samples collected in 1984 and 1985, and the maximum concentration reported in any one well was 12 μg/L, but it was not detected in the vast majority of samples.

Epidemiologic studies on the reproductive and developmental effects of toluene reviewed below are summarized in Table 7-3 at the end of this section.

Reproductive Effects

Reproductive Effects in Men

The Volume 2 committee identified several studies that examined the effects of toluene exposure on male infertility. Plenge-Böenig and Karmaus (1999) examined male and female infertility in printing-industry workers using time to pregnancy (TTP) as the effect. Workers were interviewed about their occupational and reproductive histories, and their exposure to toluene was categorized according to job descriptions and previous measurements by industrial hygienists. Toluene exposure appeared to have no effect on TTP for exposed men, regardless of the extent of their exposure (fecund-ability ratio [FR]=1.05, 95% CI 0.93–1.19).

One report on a multitude of reproductive outcomes following male exposure to toluene was identified by the Volume 11 committee. Reproductive outcomes in 398 Dutch male painters following exposure to organic solvents, using toluene as the marker of exposure, were examined by Hooiveld et al. (2006); 302 carpenters were the unexposed referents. Toluene exposure at 3 months before pregnancy for painters was estimated to range from 0.17 to 4.66 mg/m^3, below the occupational exposure limit of 150 mg/m^3 in the Netherlands. Compared with carpenters, painters with occupational exposure in the 3 months before pregnancy were not at increased risk of prolonged TTP (OR=1.1, 95% CI 0.7–1.9) or decreased fecundability (FR=0.9, 95% CI 0.8–1.1).

There have been several small studies on the effects of toluene on male reproductive hormones. As reported in *Gulf War and Health, Volume 2*, Svensson et al. (1992a,b) found that exposure to toluene was associated with lower blood concentrations of follicle-stimulating hormone (FSH), luteinizing hormone (LH), prolactin, and testosterone in young male rotogravure printers as compared with factory workers. The authors stated that the effects may be transitory, as the decreases in LH and FSH levels were reversed in a subset of the printers after a 4-week exposure-free period. ATSDR's *Draft Toxicological Profile for Toluene* (2015b) reported on two small studies of reproductive hormones related to toluene exposure. One study in which 1,225 male printers in Germany were compared with unexposed workers found that the serum levels of FSH, LH, and testosterone were not significantly different between those exposed to median toluene concentrations of 24 ppm (printers) and those exposed to 4.5 ppm (nonprinters) for at least 20 years (Gericke et al., 2001). Luderer et al. (1999) exposed five men and five women in the follicular phase to 0 or 50 ppm toluene for 3 hours. There were no significant direct effects of exposure on LH, FSH, and testosterone levels, with the exception of a significant decline in LH in men during exposure compared with sham exposure; however, ATSDR stated that it was difficult to assess this result in terms of what it implied for reproductive function.

The Volume 11 committee identified one new study of the effects of toluene exposure on semen. A small study in China of 24 men with occupational exposure to high concentrations of benzene, toluene, and xylenes (mean concentrations in work air were 103.34, 42.73, and 8.21 mg/m^3, respectively) and 37 unexposed workers found a positive correlation between semen liquefaction and the toluene concentration in the semen (β=0.2571; significant T=0.047) (Xiao et al., 2001).

Reproductive Effects in Women

The Volume 2 committee reported on two studies that assessed reproductive effects in women who had been exposed to toluene. In one of them, Plenge-Böenig and Karmaus (1999) found, in contrast to their findings on men discussed earlier, that women who were exposed to toluene in a printing facility had an increased TTP (FR=0.52, 95% CI 0.28–0.99). ATSDR did not report on any studies of female reproductive effects in humans.

The Volume 11 committee did not identify any new studies on the effects of toluene on female reproduction.

Adverse Pregnancy Outcomes

The Volume 2 committee cited one case-control study by Taskinen et al. (1994) that found that women who worked in a laboratory with exposure to toluene were at an increased risk of spontaneous abortion (OR=4.7, 95% CI 1.4–15.9). A study in Finland that included biological monitoring of 120 male workers found consistent increases in the risk of spontaneous abortion in the partners of men with high or frequent exposure to toluene (OR=2.3, 95% CI 1.1–4.7) (Taskinen et al., 1989).

The ATSDR *Draft Toxicological Profile for Toluene* (2015b) reviewed three studies not included in *Gulf War and Health, Volume 2* on the occurrence of spontaneous abortion in women exposed to toluene (Lindbohm et al., 1991; Ng et al., 1992; Taskinen et al., 1989). All three studies found an increased risk, but the latter two studies had substantial limitations, such as a small number of cases. ATSDR concluded, "Current data do not provide convincing evidence that acute or repeated inhalation exposure to toluene may cause reproductive effects in humans."

The Hooiveld et al. (2006) study, whose results on male reproductive effects were described earlier, also found that, when compared with unexposed carpenters, the exposure of Dutch male painters to toluene did not significantly increase their partners' risks of spontaneous abortion (OR=1.1, 95% CI 0.4–2.7), preterm birth (OR=1.2, 95% CI 0.7–2.2), or low-birth-weight infants (OR=1.7, 95% CI 0.9–3.2). The Volume 11 did not identify any additional studies on the effects of maternal or paternal exposure to toluene and adverse pregnancy outcomes.

Animal Studies

There were no animal studies of possible reproductive effects of toluene cited in *Gulf War and Health, Volume 2* (IOM, 2003).

The ATSDR *Draft Toxicological Profile for Toluene* included inhalation studies in rats at toluene concentrations ≥2,000 ppm. In female animals exposed to 3,000 ppm, reproductive effects included abnormalities of the ovaries (Tap et al., 1996). In male rats, the effects included reduced sperm count, motility, and quality as well as altered reproductive organ weight and histology (Kanter, 2011; Ono et al., 1996, 1999). However, Ono et al. (1996) found that although there were changes in sperm count and epididymis weight, there was no corresponding change in reproductive performance (e.g., fertility). Studies in rats exposed repeatedly by inhalation to toluene, including a two-generation reproductive toxicity study, have shown no evidence of adverse effects on mating or fertility at concentrations as high as 1,200–2,000 ppm (API, 1981, 1985; Ono et al., 1996; Roberts et al., 2003; Thiel and Chahoud, 1997). Thus, ATSDR concluded that the majority of animal studies provided little evidence for toluene having reproductive toxicity.

The Volume 11 committee did not identify any additional animal studies on the possible reproductive effects of toluene in male or female animals.

Developmental Effects

Several developmental endpoints have been studied following parental exposure to toluene—specifically childhood cancers and several types of birth defects—and were reported in *Volume 2*, by ATSDR, and by the Volume 11 committee in this volume. In addition, the Volume 11 committee identified one paper that examined cancer in adult men whose parents had occupational exposure to toluene.

Volume 2 discussed only one study that examined developmental effects in children that may have resulted from maternal or paternal exposure to toluene. Shu et al. (1999) found that children born to women who had a history of exposure to toluene were not at increased risk of ALL (OR=1.5, 95% CI 0.6–3.8) and that there was also no increased risk for children whose fathers had preconception exposure to toluene.

The Volume 11 committee identified two new studies of cancer in the children of parents who had been exposed to toluene. Heck et al. (2014)—also discussed in the section on benzene—assessed the risk of childhood leukemia after maternal exposure to air toxics, including toluene, by trimester in children in California who had been diagnosed with either ALL (n=69) or AML (n=46) between 1990 and 2007. The cases, along with the 19,209 controls, lived within either 2 km (for ALL) or 6 km (for AML) of an air toxics monitoring station. For each trimester of pregnancy, averages of the measurements of about 7 air toxics were used to calculate individual exposures. A one-interquartile increase in toluene concentrations did not significantly increase the risk for ALL in the any trimester (first trimester OR=0.95, 95% CI 0.68–1.32; second trimester OR=1.02, 95% CI 0.73, 1.42; third trimester OR=1.22, 95% CI 0.90–1.65), or for the entire pregnancy (OR=1.11, 95% CI 0.71–1.74). Similar results were seen for the risk of AML for the first and second trimester (OR=1.25, 95% CI 0.83–1.88 and OR=1.31,

95% CI 0.88–1.94, respectively), but the risk of AML was significantly increased for the third trimester (OR=1.50, 95% CI 1.04–2.16) and for the entire pregnancy (OR=1.78, 95% CI 1.03–3.06).

In the large registry-based NORD-TEST study, the risk of testicular germ cell tumors was studied in men ages 14–49 years diagnosed between 1978 and 2012 in Finland, Norway, and Sweden, on the basis of the men's parents' occupations prior to the men's birth (Le Cornet et al., 2017). The parents' occupations prior to the child's birth were determined by examining national censuses and job codes. Although the authors found no association between prenatal maternal exposure to solvents and testicular germ cell tumors across all the countries combined, they did find an association with maternal exposure to toluene in the year before birth (OR=1.67, 95% CI 1.02–2.73), but not with paternal exposure.

ATSDR (2015b) reported on several studies of fetotoxicity following the intentional inhalation of large quantities of toluene or other organic solvents by women while pregnant; however, the Volume 11 committee does not find those exposure scenarios to be representative of those likely to be experienced by women during deployment. ATSDR identified one small study of low-level occupational exposure to toluene as well as other solvents and chemicals in Finland that suggested that there was an increased risk of CNS anomalies and neural tube closure defects in children of 14 exposed women (Holmberg, 1979).

The Volume 11 committee identified one paper that examined birth defects in children born to fathers with occupational exposure to toluene. In the Hooiveld et al. (2006) study cited earlier, which used toluene as a marker of exposure to solvents, 398 Dutch male painters were compared with 302 carpenters as the unexposed referents. Toluene exposure at 3 months before pregnancy for painters was predicted to range from 0.17 to 4.66 mg/m^3, which was below the occupational exposure limit of 150 mg/m^3 in the Netherlands. Compared with carpenters, painters with occupational exposure in the 3 months before pregnancy did have a significantly increased risk of birth defects in offspring (OR=2.4, 95% CI 1.2–4.9), particularly congenital malformations (OR=6.2, 95% CI 1.4–27.9).

The Volume 11 committee considered several papers on birth effects in children born to mothers with environmental exposure to toluene. Lupo et al. (2011) assessed the risk for neural tube defects, expressed in the form of spina bifida or anencephaly, as a result of prenatal exposure to ambient air pollutants in a population-based study in Texas. The estimated toluene levels, using the 1999 EPA ASPEN model, were categorized as low (0.01–0.31 μg/m^3 for spina bifida, 0.01–0.30 μg/m^3 for anencephaly), medium-low (>0.31–1.50 μg/m^3 for spina bifida, >0.30–1.53 μg/m^3 for anencephaly), medium (>1.50–2.84 μg/m^3 for spina bifida, >1.53–2.85 μg/m^3 for anencephaly), medium-high (>2.84–5.96 μg/m^3 for spina bifida, >2.85–5.90 μg/m^3 for anencephaly), and high (>5.96–14.3 μg/m^3 for spina bifida, >5.90–14.3 μg/m^3 for anencephaly). Although the risks were increased for both spina bifida and anencephaly at all toluene concentrations, none of the increases were significant. Ramakrishnan et al. (2013) assessed the risk for oral clefts in children whose mothers gave birth in Texas between 1999 and 2008 (estimated mean concentration of toluene in ambient air was 1.70 mg/m^3). Mothers with estimated high exposure to toluene were no more likely to have a child with cleft lip with or without cleft palate (OR=1.01, 95% CI 0.86–1.19) or a nonsyndromic isolated cleft palate (OR=0.91, 95% CI 0.72–1.17) than mothers with estimated low exposure.

The Volume 11 committee identified one study that assessed the impact of exposure to residential toluene on the expression of miR-155 and miR-223 in maternal and cord blood as part of the German Lifestyle and Environmental Factors and Their Influence on Newborns Allergy Risk study in 2006–2008 (Herberth et al., 2014). miR-155 and miR-223 are known to be involved in regulatory T-cell formation or function. The median toluene concentration measured in the homes during weeks 34–36 of pregnancy was 6.95 μg/m^3. Higher concentrations of toluene were significantly associated with increased levels of miR-223 in maternal blood (means ratio=1.10, 95% CI 1.02–1.18), but not miR-155 levels. Cord blood miR-155 expression was related to lower S-benzylmercapturic acid concentrations, a toluene metabolite, in maternal urine, but miR-233 was not; toluene concentrations did not affect expression of either miRNA in cord blood. miR155 expression was not associated with lower Treg numbers in maternal and cord blood. Benzene concentrations were also associated with miR-223 in maternal blood, but not the expression of either miRNA in cord blood, and xylenes were not associated with miRNA in either maternal or cord blood (see the earlier section on benzene and the next section on xylenes).

Animal Studies

There were no toxicological or animal studies of possible developmental effects of toluene exposure cited in *Gulf War and Health, Volume 2*.

ATSDR (2015b) reported on several developmental toxicity studies done with rats, mice, and rabbits exposed to toluene. The results of numerous studies indicate that toluene by inhalation does not cause either toxic effects in the mother or developmental effects in the offspring when animals are exposed at levels <1,000 ppm administered for 6–7 hours/day during gestation (API, 1978, 1991, 1992; Jones and Balster, 1997; Klimisch et al., 1992; Ono et al., 1995; Roberts et al., 2007; Saillenfait et al., 2007; Thiel and Chahoud, 1997; Tsukahara et al., 2009; Win-Shwe et al., 2012; Yamamoto et al., 2009). However, at doses exceeding 1,000 ppm, retarded fetal growth and skeletal development and also altered development of behavior have been observed in offspring, while maternal toxicity is also evident (API, 1991, 1992; Dalgaard et al., 2001; Hass et al., 1999; Hougaard et al., 2003; Jones and Balster, 1997; Ono et al., 1995; Roberts et al., 2007; Saillenfait et al., 2007; Thiel and Chahoud, 1997).

ATSDR also reported on two studies of the continuous exposure of rats, mice, and rabbits to 133–399 ppm toluene during gestation, which resulted in reduced maternal body weight and reduced body weight and delayed skeletal ossification in the fetuses (Hudak and Ungvary, 1978; Ungvary and Tatrai, 1985).

The Volume 11 committee considered three additional studies on potential developmental effects from prenatal exposure to toluene. Hougaard et al. (2005) assessed whether prenatal exposure to 1,500 ppm toluene, 6 h/day, on GDs 7–20 resulted in increased effects in the female offspring of pregnant rats when combined with maternal exposure to chronic mild stress on GDs 9–20. Toluene exposure resulted in a greater decrease in plasma corticosterone in the offspring after acute stress on PND 27 as compared with the unexposed control or the chronic mild-stress animals. Maternal exposure to stress combined with toluene did not appear to exacerbate any neurotoxic effects. In a similar study, Soberanes-Chavez et al. (2013) exposed pregnant mice to restraint stress, to toluene (8,000 ppm whole body, 30 minutes, twice per day from GD 7 to parturition), or to a combination of the two. Only male pups were assessed postnatally. Exposure to toluene alone or with stress did not affect the length of gestation, the number of live pups, or the sex ratio. However, exposure to toluene significantly increased the risk of neonatal death (RR=4.2, 95% CI 1.2–14.8), with an even greater increase when toluene was combined with stress (RR=7.8, 95% CI 2.4–25.3). Toluene exposure also resulted in a significantly lower body weight at weaning. The committee notes that, given the large confidence intervals, these data should be interpreted with caution.

In a study to assess whether prenatal exposure to abusive levels of toluene impaired the neurodevelopment of offspring, Callan et al. (2017) exposed pregnant rats to 8,000 or 12,000 ppm toluene for 15 minutes twice daily from GD 8 through GD 20. Male and female offspring exposed to the lower dose exhibited no differences from controls in initial acquisition in the Morris water maze on PND 28 or on PND 44; however, rats exposed to 12,000 ppm displayed performance deficits during a probe trial and in reversal learning on PND 44.

Synthesis and Conclusions

The Volume 2 committee did not reach any conclusions on the category of association between exposure to toluene and any health outcomes, including reproductive or developmental effects.

Reproductive Effects

ATSDR (2015b) found that the data did not provide convincing evidence that acute or repeated inhalation exposure to toluene caused reproductive effects in humans. ATSDR presented limited evidence in humans to indicate that occupational exposure to toluene may lead to an increased incidence of spontaneous abortion (Lindbohm et al., 1991; Ng et al., 1992; Taskinen et al., 1989) or to decreased fecundity in female workers (Plenge-Böenig and Karmaus, 1999).

The Volume 11 committee found some evidence that exposure to toluene may adversely affect the reproductive health of women, such as fertility and the risk of spontaneous abortion (Taskinen et al., 1989). There were few studies of the reproductive effects of toluene in men, and the results showed few adverse effects on reproductive hormones or time to pregnancy (Hooiveld et al., 2006), although one study in Finland did find a significant increase in the risk of spontaneous abortion with high or frequent toluene exposure (Taskinen et al., 1989). The subjects in these studies were typically exposed to other solvents in addition to toluene. The animal studies provide little evidence on the reproductive toxicity of toluene.

The Volume 11 committee notes there are many unanswered questions regarding the reproductive effects of toluene since most studies predate the development of epigenetic biomarkers, which might help identify subclinical risk, and nearly all human studies are likely underpowered and have substantial confounders since most subjects were exposed to mixtures of chemicals. There are no data on the role of toluene exposure in the transgenerational transmission of adverse health effects or in epigenetic effects in either humans or animals.

The Volume 11 committee concludes that there is inadequate/insufficient evidence to determine whether an association exists between exposure to toluene and reproductive effects in men or women, or with adverse pregnancy outcomes.

Developmental Effects

Although there are a few studies that show that addictive inhalation of solvents by mothers during pregnancy can affect the fetal brain (ATSDR, 2015b), the Volume 11 committee did not find addiction to be a relevant exposure scenario for deployed women. Studies of prenatal exposure to low levels of toluene in ambient air did not support an increased risk of birth defects (Ramakrishnan et al., 2013) or of childhood cancer (Heck et al., 2014). Again, the maternal exposures in these studies were to mixtures that contained toluene. Animal studies did not show developmental effects with exposure to low levels of toluene, although two studies showed that toluene exposure in combination with chronic mild stress did result in adverse effects on pups.

The Volume 11 committee concludes that there is inadequate/insufficient evidence to determine whether an association exists between prenatal exposure to toluene and developmental effects.

TABLE 7-3 Summary of Reproductive and Developmental Effects of Toluene

Study	Design/Population	Exposure	Results
Reproductive Effects			
Xiao et al. (2001)	Case-control 24 men occupationally exposed for at least 1 year to benzene, toluene, and xylene versus 37 unexposed controls in Zhejiang, China.	Mean concentrations (range) of benzene, toluene, xylene in work air were 103.34 (0~7070.3), 42.73 (0~435.8), 8.21 (0~133.1) mg/m^3, respectively. Concentrations also measured in blood and semen.	Semen parameters. Mean sperm vitality, sperm activity, and acrosin activity reduced in the exposed workers ($p<0.01$); γ-glutamyltransferase activity and lactate dehydrogenase-C4 relative activity in exposed men were lower than those in the control workers. Benzene, toluene, and xylene were detected in blood and semen of exposed workers only.
Hooiveld et al. (2006)	Case-control 1,578 male painters versus 1,537 male carpenters in the Netherlands born 1950–1975.	Toluene was a marker of exposure to any solvents. Among painters, modeled toluene exposure at 3 months before pregnancy ranged from 0.17 to 4.66 mg/m^3. These values were all well below the Dutch occupational exposure limit for toluene (150 mg/m^3). Exposure categorized by tertiles (0.17–0.38, 0.38–1.02, and 1.03–4.66 mg/m^3).	Male fertility and adverse pregnancy outcomes. TTP: OR=1.1, 95% CI 0.7–1.9, ORs for prolonged TTP were similar in all exposed categories. Fecundability: FR=0.9, 95% CI 0.8–1.1. Spontaneous abortion: OR=1.1, 95% CI 0.4–2.7. PTB: OR=1.2, 95% CI 0.7–2.2, no differences in PTB among the exposure groups. LBW: OR=1.7, 95% CI 0.9–3.2, risk of LBW increased with increasing exposure (low exposure OR=1.5, 95% CI 0.5–4.3, high exposure OR=1.9, 95% CI 0.8–4.7; p-trend=0.05). Birth defects (OR=2.4, 95% CI 1.2–4.9), mainly due to a higher risk of congenital malformations (OR=6.2, 95% CI 1.4–27.9). Malformations reported by painters were: cardiovascular (n=4), gastrointestinal (n=2), central nervous system (n=1), eye (n=1), urogenital malformations (n=1), oro-facial clefts (n=3), Down's syndrome (n=1), and other syndromes (n=3). Nonexposed workers reported one urogenital defect and one hip dysplasia. A dose–response relationship (p-trend=0.03) was observed for all birth defects (low OR=2.1, 95% CI 0.7–5.9; intermediate OR=3.0, 95% CI 1.3–7.0; high OR=2.2, 95% CI 0.8–6.0). In both occupational groups, about 50% of the reported cases of functional developmental disorders had a diagnosis of ADHD, metabolome disease, or hyperactivity.

continued

TABLE 7-3 Continued

Study	Design/Population	Exposure	Results
Developmental Effects			
Ramakrishnan et al., 2013	Case-control 3,945 cases of oral clefts from the Texas Birth Defects Registry versus 15,780 controls in Texas. 1999–2008	Estimates of average annual exposure to each BTEX component based on mother's residence at birth by census-tract in Texas based on 2005 EPA National-Scale Air Toxics Assessment Hazardous Air Pollutant Exposure Model; estimated mean toluene concentration=1.70 μg/m³ (SD 0.97).	Birth defects: oral clefts. Mothers with high exposure to toluene were no more likely to have a child with cleft lip with or without cleft palate (OR=1.01, 95% CI 0.86–1.19) or nonsyndromic isolated cleft palate (OR=0.91, 95% CI 0.72–1.17) than mothers with estimated low exposure. Results were similar for benzene, ethylbenzene, and xylenes.
Heck et al. (2014)	Case-control 69 cases of ALL and 46 cases of AML from California Cancer Registry records of children age <6 years, and 19,209 controls from California birth records. 1990–2007	Exposure estimated based on residence distance to air toxics monitoring station (within 2 km for ALL, and 6 km for AML).	Childhood leukemia. Toluene exposure (per interquartile increase) did not significantly increase the risk for ALL in any trimester (OR=0.95, 95% CI 0.68–1.32), for the first trimester (OR=1.22, 95% CI 0.90–1.65), or for the entire pregnancy (OR=1.11, 95% CI 0.71–1.74). Similar results were seen for the risk of AML for the first and second trimester (OR=1.25, 95% CI 0.83–1.88 and OR=1.31, 95% CI 0.88–1.94, respectively), but the risk of AML was significantly increased for the third trimester (OR=1.50, 95% CI 1.04–2.16) and for the entire pregnancy (OR=1.78, 95% CI 1.03–3.06).
Herberth et al. (2014)	441 children and 315 pregnant mothers in prospective mother–child study (Lifestyle and Environmental Factors and Their Influence on Newborns Allergy Risk).	Toluene concentrations measured in maternal residence with passive monitor; median concentration was 6.95μg/m³. Blood samples and urine samples taken from mother at 34th week of pregnancy and cord blood collected at birth. Urine analyzed for toluene metabolite S-benzylmercapturic acid.	Higher concentrations of toluene were significantly associated with increased levels of miR-223 in maternal blood (means ratio=1.10, 95% CI 1.02–1.18), but not miR-155 levels. Cord blood miR-155 expression was related to lower S-benzylmercapturic acid concentrations in maternal urine, but miR-233 was not; toluene concentrations did not affect expression of either miRNA in cord blood. miR-155 expression was not associated with lower Treg numbers in maternal and cord blood.

NOTE: ADHD=attention deficit hyperactivity disorder; ALL=acute lymphoblastic leukemia; AML=acute myeloid leukemia; BTEX=benzene, toluene, ethylbenzene and xylene; CI=confidence interval; EPA=U.S. Environmental Protection Agency; FR=fecundability ratio; LBW=low birth weight; miR=micro-ribonucleic acid; miRNA=micro-ribonucleic acid; OR=odds ratio; PTB=preterm birth; SD=standard deviation; Treg=regulatory T cell; TTP=time to pregnancy.

XYLENES

Xylenes, like toluene, are components of gasoline and are also found as combustion products of fuel. Xylenes are thought to have been sent to the Gulf War in quantities greater than 1 kiloliter.

Xylenes were among the 12 most frequently detected VOCs at the three sampling locations at JBB in both 2007 and 2009 (IOM, 2011), although the concentrations varied considerably depending on where the sampling was conducted on the base and the time of year. The air concentrations of total xylenes ranged from levels below the detection limit to greater than 50 $\mu g/m^3$ (second only to toluene). The authoring committee considered the likely major source of the xylenes to be unspecified combustion.

Xylene, or dimethyl benzene, is an organic aromatic hydrocarbon widely used in the production of ethyl benzene, polyester, and plastic. Like benzene and toluene, xylenes are commonly used industrial solvents and are frequently considered as part of the benzene-toluene-ethylbenzene-xylene (BTEX) complex. Also, like toluene, they are methylated forms of benzene with two methyl groups; there are three isomeric forms of xylene: *ortho-*, *meta-*, and *para-*.

Epidemiologic studies on the reproductive and developmental effects of xylenes reviewed below are summarized in Table 7-4 at the end of this section.

Reproductive Effects

Reproductive Effects in Men and Women

The Volume 2 committee (IOM, 2003) did not discuss any studies of male or female reproductive effects following exposure to xylene. Similarly, EPA and ATSDR did not present any human studies on reproductive effects following xylene exposure in their reviews (ATSDR, 2007b; EPA, 2003).

The Volume 11 committee identified only one small study, also discussed in the sections on benzene and toluene, of the effects of xylene exposure. This was the study of 24 men in China with occupational exposure to a mixture of high concentrations of benzene, toluene, and xylenes along with 37 unexposed workers who served as controls (Xiao et al., 2001). Multiple-regression results showed that decreased seminal γ-glutamyltransferase activity (which reflects the function of the prostate) was associated with increased xylene levels in the blood of exposed men.

Among 1,408 newly wed female petrochemical workers in China, exposure to xylene—as part of a mixture that also included benzene, toluene, and styrene—was correlated with an increased risk of oligomenorrhea (menstrual cycle length >35 days) (OR=1.63, 95% CI 1.04–2.53) (Cho et al., 2001).

Adverse Pregnancy Outcomes

The Volume 2 committee (IOM, 2003) identified one case-control study by Taskinen et al. (1994) that examined the risk of spontaneous abortion among female laboratory workers potentially exposed to solvents (206 cases and 329 controls). The authors reported that exposure to xylene was associated with an increased risk of spontaneous abortion (OR=3.1, 95% CI 1.3–7.5).

EPA (2003) did not identify any studies on adverse birth outcomes in children exposed prenatally to xylenes. ATSDR (2007b) reported on two studies of birth outcomes associated with parental exposure to xylenes, one of which was Taskinen et al. (1994), which was also discussed by the Volume 2 committee. The other study—by Lindbohm et al. (1990)—found no significant increase in the risk of spontaneous abortion among Finnish workers for whom there were biomonitoring data on xylene levels. ATSDR (2007b) concluded that "the available studies of reproductive toxicity from occupational exposure to xylenes were not definitive because of the small number of subjects and/or concurrent exposure to other chemicals."

EPA reached similar conclusions on the potential association between spontaneous abortion and exposure to xylenes, but it also noted the lack of specificity in the exposures (EPA, 2000). Ambient solvents modelled by land use regression in a large California study were associated with an increased risk of low birth weight for gestational age with higher exposure to several solvents including xylene, however, the effect estimate was small (OR=1.03, 95% CI 1.01–1.06) (Ghosh et al., 2013).

The Volume 11 committee did not identify any new studies on birth outcomes in humans following maternal or paternal exposure to xylenes.

Animal Studies

ATSDR (2007b) found no reproductive effects in rats exposed via inhalation to 500 ppm xylene before mating and during gestation and lactation. No histopathological changes in the reproductive organs were seen in rats and mice in intermediate and chronic oral bioassays at mixed xylene concentrations of, respectively, 800 and 1,000 mg/kg/day, given 5 days/week.

The Volume 11 committee did not identify any new relevant animal studies on the reproductive effects of xylene.

Developmental Effects

The Volume 2 (IOM, 2003) committee considered several studies that looked at solvents in general and that reported results for xylenes specifically. Olshan and colleagues (1999) found an increased risk of neuroblastoma in children whose fathers were painters (OR=2.1, 95% CI 0.9–4.8); this was the most relevant of the 73 paternal occupations listed for solvent exposure. In a follow-up study, a job-exposure matrix was used to evaluate maternal and paternal occupational exposure to 65 chemical compounds or broad categories of substances (De Roos et al., 2001). Using this approach, the authors found no significant increase in the risk of neuroblastoma in children born to mothers or fathers with occupational exposure to xylene (OR for paternal exposure=1.4, 95% CI 0.5–4.3). In a study of occupational exposures among parents in the Children's Cancer Group, there was no association found between self-reported paternal preconception exposure to xylenes and ALL in their children (OR=1.2, 95% CI 0.8–1.8) (Shu et al., 1999). Results were not reported for maternal exposure for any time prior to or during pregnancy.

EPA and ATSDR reported few data on developmental outcomes associated with prenatal xylene exposure (ATSDR, 2007b; EPA, 2003). EPA's *Toxicological Review of Xylenes* (2003) did not identify any studies on the possible developmental toxicity of inhaled xylenes in humans. ATSDR (2007b) concluded that the "data are limited for assessing the relationship between inhalation of xylene and developmental effects because the available studies involved concurrent exposure to other solvents in addition to xylene in the workplace (Holmberg and Nurminen, 1980; Kucera, 1968; Taskinen et al., 1989; Windham et al., 1991), and because of the small number of subjects, ranging from 9 to 61 (Taskinen et al., 1989; Windham et al., 1991)."

The Volume 11 committee identified three new studies that reported on developmental effects in children following maternal exposure to xylenes. In a study discussed earlier in the sections on benzene and toluene, Ramakrishnan et al. (2013) estimated ambient air levels of numerous air pollutants, including xylenes, near mothers' residences in Texas and used the Texas Birth Defects registry to examine the occurrence of oral cleft among these mothers' children between 1999 and 2008. No significant associations were found between a mother's exposure to xylene (high versus low exposure) and the likelihood of having a child with cleft lip with or without cleft palate (aOR=0.93, 95% CI 0.80–1.10) or isolated cleft palate (aOR=0.85, 95% CI 0.66–1.08). In a second study—also discussed in the sections on benzene and toluene—Lupo et al. (2011) assessed the risk for neural tube defects, expressed in the form of spina bifida or anencephaly, as a result of prenatal exposure to ambient air pollutants in a population-based study in Texas. Estimated xylene levels (ranging from 0–8.84 μg/m^3) were associated with increased, but not significant, risks for both spina bifida and anencephaly.

Heck et al. (2014)—also discussed earlier in the sections on benzene and toluene—used the California Cancer Registry to identify children under 6 years of age who had been diagnosed with either ALL (n=69) or AML (n=46) between 1990 and 2007. The authors then looked for a relationship between xylene exposure and leukemia in those cases along with 19,209 controls, all of whom lived within either 2 km (for ALL) or 6 km (for AML) of an air toxics monitoring station. In the each trimester of pregnancy, an average of about seven air toxic measurements were used to calculate individual exposures. A one-interquartile increase in o-xylene or m/p-xylenes concentration did not significantly increase the risk for ALL or AML at any time during pregnancy. However, when the authors assessed the relationships as a function of trimester only, they found that during the third trimester exposure to m/p-xylenes significantly increased the risk of ALL (OR=1.37, 95% CI 1.01–1.85) and exposure to o-xylene significantly increased the risk of AML (OR=1.33, 95% CI 1.05–1.69).

The Volume 11 committee identified one study that assessed the impact of exposure to residential xylenes on the expression of miR-155 and miR-223 in maternal and cord blood as part of the German Lifestyle and Environmental Factors and Their Influence on Newborns Allergy Risk study in 2006–2008 (Herberth et al., 2014). miR-155 and miR-223 are known to be involved in regulatory T-cell formation or function. The median xylenes concentrations for the m/p-isomers was 1.55 μg/m^3 and for o-isomer was 0.49 μg/m^3. Higher concentrations of any xylenes were not significantly associated increased levels of miR-223 or miR-155 in either maternal or cord blood (all CIs included 1.0). Benzene and toluene concentrations were both associated with miRNA-223 in maternal blood, but not the expression of either miRNA in cord blood (see earlier sections on benzene and toluene).

Animal Studies

The Volume 2 committee did not include any animal studies of the developmental toxicity of xylenes.

In its *Toxicological Review of Xylenes*, EPA reported on several animal studies that examined the developmental effects in offspring following maternal inhalation exposure (EPA, 2003). In one study by Hass et al. (1995), neurodevelopmental impairments (rotarod performance) were observed in the female but not male offspring of pregnant rats exposed to 500 ppm, although the impairments did not reach statistical significance. Animal studies that looked at standard developmental endpoints in rats and mice reported decreased body weights in dams at doses of 700 ppm xylene or greater as well as fetal skeletal and visceral malformations; doses as low as 230 ppm resulted in increased abortions in rabbits, and decreased fetal body weight and fetal survival were observed in rats at 350 ppm. However, EPA noted that these effects were seen at concentrations greater than those associated with neurobehavioral effects in adults.

ATSDR (2007b) reviewed the studies cited by EPA as well as new studies and found that "in general, developmental studies in animals reported adverse fetal effects only at concentrations that caused maternal toxicity." Inhalation studies in animals exposed prenatally to ≥350 ppm xylenes resulted in a delayed ossification of the skeleton and reduced fetal body weight, but the concentrations also caused maternal toxicity. In rats, prenatal inhalation exposure to 500 ppm m-xylene has been associated with postnatal neurobehavioral deficits (decreased rotarod performance); oral exposure to 2,060 mg/kg/day of mixed xylenes has been associated with cleft plate and decreased fetal weight; and dermal exposure to xylene has been associated with biochemical changes in fetal and maternal brain tissue.

The Volume 11 committee did not identify any relevant new animal studies on the developmental effects of xylene.

Synthesis and Conclusions

Reproductive Effects

The data on the reproductive effects of xylenes are scant. Most studies have investigated the effects of the mixture BTEX, not xylenes specifically, and nearly all occur in the context of mixed exposures. Single studies suggested that occupational exposures to xylene may be associated with oligomenorrhea in women and reduced seminal γ-glutamyltransferase activity in men, although both studies were small.

Only two studies of the effects of prenatal occupational exposure to xylenes on the risk of spontaneous abortion were identified by ATSDR (2007b), and the results were contradictory. The Volume 11 committee did not identify any new literature on the reproductive effects of xylenes.

The Volume 11 committee concludes that there is inadequate/insufficient evidence to determine whether an association exists between exposure to xylenes and reproductive effects in men or women, or with adverse pregnancy outcomes.

Developmental Effects

One study suggested that BTEX exposure may increase the risk of low birth weight for gestational age, although the effect size was small. Some data suggest that xylenes exhibit developmental neurotoxicity but primarily at very high doses, and there is some suggestive evidence of an increased risk of AML in children if mothers are exposed in the third trimester, but the results overall are not conclusive.

EPA and ATSDR reviewed several animal studies that showed various developmental effects, including skeletal malformations, decreased fetal weight and viability, and, in one study, neurologic effects associated with gestational exposure to xylenes. ATSDR cautioned that the developmental effects were generally seen at doses that caused maternal toxicity.

Therefore, the Volume 11 committee concludes that there is inadequate/insufficient evidence to determine whether an association exists between prenatal exposure to xylenes and developmental effects.

TABLE 7-4 Summary of Reproductive and Developmental Effects of Xylenes

Study	Design/Population	Exposure	Results
Xiao et al. (2001)	Case-control 24 men occupationally exposed for at least 1 year. to benzene, toluene, and xylene in Zhejiang, China; 37 unexposed controls. Blood and sperm were collected from all subjects.	Concentrations of xylene measured by monitors; mean=8.21 (range=0~133.1) mg/m^3.	Semen parameters. Xylene detected in blood and semen of exposed workers only. Decreased seminal γ-glutamyltransferase activity was associated with xylene levels in the blood of exposed men (β=30.28, B=7.58, p=0.0002) but not related to other parameters; exposures measured in air and semen were not related to any outcomes.
Ramakrishnan et al. (2013)	Case-control 3,945 cases of oral clefts from the Texas Birth Defects Registry versus 15,780 population controls, born 1999–2008.	Estimates of average annual exposure based on maternal residence at delivery modeled at the census tract level using 2005 EPA National-Scale Air Toxics Assessment Hazardous Air Pollutant Exposure Model; mean xylene concentration=0.70 µg/m^3.	Birth defects: oral clefts. Cleft lip with or without cleft palate: High versus low exposure OR=0.93, 95% CI 0.80–1.10. Cleft palate only: high versus low exposure OR=0.85, 95% CI 0.66–1.08). Adjusted for birth year, infant sex, maternal race/ethnicity, education, age, smoking, and season of conception; findings were similar for benzene, ethyl benzene, and toluene.
Heck et al. (2014)	Case-control 69 cases of ALL and 46 cases of AML from California Cancer Registry records of children age <6 years versus 19,209 controls from California birth records in 1990–2007.	Exposure estimated based on maternal residence at birth's distance to an air monitoring station (2 km for ALL, and 6 km for AML).	Childhood leukemia. Per interquartile increase in xylene: o-xylene and ALL: 1st trimester OR=0.84, 95% CI 0.60–1.17); 2nd trimester OR=0.99, 95% CI 0.72–1.35; 3rd trimester OR=1.29, 95% CI 0.99–1.68; entire pregnancy OR=1.07, 95% CI 0.70–1.62. o-xylene and AML: 1st trimester OR=1.15, 95% CI 0.78–1.71; 2nd trimester OR=1.20, 95% CI 0.81–1.77; 3rd trimester OR=1.38, 95% CI 0.95–1.99; entire pregnancy OR=1.48, 95% CI 0.88–2.47. m/p-xylenes and ALL: 1st trimester OR=1.07, 95% CI 0.84–1.37; 2nd trimester OR=1.04, 95% CI 0.75–1.43; 3rd trimester OR=1.33, 95% CI 1.05–1.69; entire pregnancy OR=1.38, 95% CI 0.92–2.08. m/p-xylenes and AML: 1st trimester OR=1.03, 95% CI 0.71–1.51; 2nd trimester OR=1.20, 95% CI 0.86–1.68; 3rd trimester OR=1.37, 95% CI 1.01–1.85; entire pregnancy OR=1.51, 95% CI 0.93–2.44.

continued

TABLE 7-4 Continued

Study	Design/Population	Exposure	Results
Herberth et al. (2014)	441 children and 315 pregnant mothers in prospective mother–child study in Germany (Lifestyle and Environmental Factors and Their Influence on Newborns Allergy Risk).	Xylene concentrations measured in maternal residence with passive monitor; median concentrations for the m-+p-isomers was 1.55 μg/m^3 and the o-isomer was 0.49 μg/m^3. Blood samples and urine samples taken from mother at 34th week of pregnancy and cord blood collected at birth.	Higher concentrations of toluene were not significantly associated with increased levels of miR-223 or miR-155 in maternal blood or cord blood.

NOTE: ALL=acute lymphoblastic leukemia; AML=acute myeloid leukemia; CI=confidence interval; EPA=U.S. Environmental Protection Agency; miR=microribonucleic acid; OR=odds ratio.

TRICHLOROETHYLENE (TCE)

TCE is a commonly used solvent and is relatively well studied with regard to its toxicity in both humans and animals. EPA considers TCE to be carcinogenic to humans by all routes of exposure and, furthermore, has identified it as a potential threat to human health through noncancer toxicity to the CNS, kidney, liver, immune system, male reproductive system, and developing embryos/fetuses (Chiu et al., 2013).

TCE was sent to the 1990–1991 Gulf War in quantities greater than 1 kiloliter (see Table 7-1). The Volume 11 committee was unable to identify any information on the amount of TCE that was sent to the Post-9/11 conflicts. However, TCE was one of 47 chemicals detected in at least 5% of the air monitoring samples collected at JBB in 2007 and 2009 (IOM, 2011).

DoD and the Department of Veterans Affairs are also concerned about TCE because it was a major contaminant of the water supply system at the U.S. Marine Corps base Camp Lejeune in North Carolina from 1957 until the contaminated wells were closed in 1985. Residents, including children and pregnant women, were exposed to TCE, PCE, benzene, toluene, and other halogenated hydrocarbons, many of them degradation products of PCE, the most commonly detected contaminant (NRC, 2009). TCE concentrations in the well water varied greatly depending on the well and date of sampling, but they ranged from undetectable to 18,900 μg/L in 1980–1985 (NRC, 2009).

TCE metabolism in humans and animals occurs by cytochrome P450 and glutathione conjugation pathways. The major urinary metabolites of TCE in humans are the oxidative metabolites trichloroacetic acid, trichloroethanol, trichloroethanol-glucuronide (ATSDR, 2014), and dichloroacetic acid (IOM, 2003). The metabolism of TCE is relatively rapid, with a renal elimination half-life of about 10 hours following inhalation exposure (ATSDR, 2014).

For its assessment of the reproductive and developmental effects of TCE, the Volume 11 committee considered four earlier, comprehensive reports—*Gulf War and Health, Volume 2* (IOM, 2003), the 2009 NRC report on contaminated water at Camp Lejeune, EPA's *Toxicological Review of Trichloroethylene* (EPA, 2011), and the 2014 ATSDR publication *Draft Toxicological Profile for Trichloroethylene*—as well as any new studies published in the years since 2014. The committee notes that many of the key studies on TCE were reviewed by more than one of those organizations. The epidemiologic studies on the reproductive and developmental effects of TCE reviewed below are summarized in Table 7-5 at the end of this section.

Reproductive Effects

The potential reproductive effects of TCE have been studied by numerous researchers and have been evaluated by several organizations, including the NRC, EPA, and ATSDR. The 2009 NRC report on PCE- and TCE-contaminated drinking water at Camp Lejeune found limited suggestive evidence of an association between TCE, PCE, or solvent mixtures and female infertility; however, there was inadequate/insufficient evidence to determine whether an association existed between exposure to TCE, PCE, or solvent mixtures and female infertility after the exposure ceased; between maternal or paternal preconception exposure and miscarriage, preterm birth, or fetal growth restriction; or between prenatal exposure and preterm birth or fetal growth restriction (NRC, 2009).

Reproductive Effects in Men and Women

The Volume 2 committee reported on only one study of male reproductive effects (Sallmén et al., 1998). In this Finnish study of self-reported paternal exposure (with biological measurements of exposure in 69% of men) to a variety of solvents, including TCE, exposure to any level of TCE did not have an impact on TTP. Studies of exposure to TCE among 85 male workers found moderate decreases in FSH and testosterone and stronger increases in dehydroepiandrosterone sulfate with increasing duration of exposure, but these hormonal changes were not linked to reproductive effects (Chia et al., 1997; Goh et al., 1998).

In its 2006 review, NRC found no data on the effects of TCE on human male reproduction; however, animal studies suggested that TCE "is toxic to spermatogenesis and sperm fertilizing ability." In 2009, NRC did not find any epidemiologic studies on the possible effects of TCE exposure, whether occupational or environmental, on semen quality or male fertility.

EPA (2011) reported that of the 10 studies on male reproductive effects it considered (7 populations, 1 case study; all but 1 study looked at fewer than 100 men), all but 1 found significant associations between TCE exposure and increased sperm concentration and decreased sperm quality parameters, altered sexual drive or function, or altered serum hormone levels; however, the effects on male fertility were not reported for most of the studies or were unchanged. EPA concluded that the "database as a whole suggests that TCE does induce male reproductive toxicity independent of systemic effects."

In 2014, ATSDR cited several studies (Bardodej and Vyskocil, 1956; El Ghawabi et al., 1973) that reported reproductive effects in men occupationally exposed to TCE, such as decreased potency or sexual disturbances and changes in sperm morphology; other studies cited by ATSDR, however, found that TCE had no effect on male reproduction (Rasmussen et al., 1988; Sallmén et al., 1998). ATSDR stated, "Evidence of trichloroethylene-induced effects in occupationally-exposed men includes reports of decreased potency, altered sex drive or function, decreased sperm quality, and decreased serum levels of reproductive hormones" (ATSDR, 2014).

Regarding female reproductive effects, the Volume 2 committee identified two studies that looked at maternal exposure to TCE and reproductive effects (IOM, 2003). Sallmén et al. (1995) found that among Finnish women occupationally exposed to high levels of TCE in the 12 months before pregnancy, fecundability was reduced, but not significantly (incidence density ratio [IDR]=0.61, 95% CI 0.28–1.33).

The EPA (2011) toxicologic review of TCE included only two studies on the effects of TCE on female reproduction. One was a study in Finland (Sallmén et al., 1995; cited in IOM, 2003), and the other was carried out at Rocky Mountain Arsenal in Colorado (ATSDR, 2001), neither of which showed a significant effect on fertility.

The Volume 11 committee did not identify any new studies on possible reproductive effects in men or women following environmental or occupational exposure to TCE.

Adverse Pregnancy Outcomes

Volume 2 included a study of Finnish women with occupational exposures to TCE that showed an increased risk of spontaneous abortion (OR=2.2, 95% CI 1.2–4.1) (Lindbohm et al., 1990).

The 2006 NRC report found that women in three states (eastern North Carolina, western New York State, and New Jersey) who were exposed to TCE-contaminated drinking water while pregnant gave birth to babies with reduced birth weights. For the Camp Lejeune population in eastern North Carolina, the longer the exposure to TCE, the greater the decrease in birth weight. In 2009, an NRC committee that reviewed health effects at Camp Lejeune found some indication that solvent exposure during, but not before, pregnancy was associated with an increased risk of miscarriage, although it was not associated with preterm birth or reduced birth weight, and there was no direct evidence on perinatal mortality (NRC, 2009).

The EPA reviewed the evidence for adverse fetal outcomes from prenatal exposure to TCE, and the resulting report included many studies that were discussed in the 2006 and 2009 NRC reports (EPA,

2011). In general, the epidemiologic studies reported associations between parental exposure to TCE, both occupational and environmental, and spontaneous abortion or perinatal death and also decreased birth weight or small for gestational age, although other studies reported mixed or null findings. EPA noted that many of these studies were small in size and a number of them reported on exposures to mixtures of solvents, not TCE alone. EPA concluded on the basis of the epidemiologic and animal data that "TCE exposure poses a potential hazard for prenatal loses and decreased growth or birth weight of offspring" (EPA, 2011).

ATSDR (2014) cited several studies that reported adverse fetal outcomes following residential or occupational exposure to TCE. The results were mixed for an increased risk of spontaneous abortion, and some studies found that prenatal maternal exposures to TCE were associated with lower birth weights.

The Volume 11 committee considered two additional studies. The first study was on fetal outcomes for women exposed to TCE present in indoor air via soil-vapor intrusion in Endicott, New York (Forand et al., 2012). Among the 1,090 births to women who were exposed to TCE levels ranging from 0.18 to 140 $\mu g/m^3$, the adjusted rate ratios (aRRs) versus births to unexposed women were significantly higher for low birth weight (<2,500 g; aRR=1.36; 95% CI 1.07–1.73), small for gestational age (aRR=1.23, 95% CI 1.03–1.48), and full-term low birth weight (aRR=1.68, 95% CI 1.20–2.34). RRs for other endpoints—preterm birth (<37 weeks), very preterm birth (<32 weeks), and very low birth weight (<1,500 g)—were also elevated, but not significantly. The authors noted, however, that socioeconomic factors, particularly maternal smoking, may have led to some confounding of results.

In the second study, Ruckart et al. (2014) conducted a cross-sectional study of 11,896 births at Camp Lejeune, North Carolina, during 1968–1985, the period of groundwater contamination with TCE and other solvents (including benzene, as discussed earlier), using birth certificate information and groundwater modeling. Term low birth weight was defined as full-term babies (≥37 weeks gestation) weighing <2,500 grams at birth. For small for gestation age births, three categories were evaluated: newborns weighing <5th and <10th percentiles based on sex- and race-specific weight by gestational week norms from New Jersey, and newborns weighing less <10th percentile based on sex-specific growth curves for California. Exposure to any concentration of TCE during the entire pregnancy was associated with a significantly reduced mean birth weight (β= –78.3g, 95% CI –115.0– –41.7). It was also associated with an increased risk of a small-for-gestational-age infant at any concentration during pregnancy, including at the lowest tertile of exposure (OR=1.2, 95% CI 1.1–1.5). It was not associated with preterm births or term low birth weight.

Animal Studies

Volume 2 reported that inhalation of TCE in male rats results in dose-related increases in Leydig cell tumors (IOM, 2003). NRC (2006) reported that multiple rodent studies indicate that TCE affects spermatogenesis and the fertilizing capability of sperm in males. The second NRC review (2009) reported on a few animal studies, including some with inhalation exposure that showed a potential association with male infertility, particularly decreased sperm count and motility and increased numbers of abnormal sperm.

The EPA toxicological review (2011) also found that some, but not all, animal studies reported adverse effects of TCE on male reproduction, including sperm measures, libido/copulatory behaviors, and serum hormone levels as well as histopathological lesions in the testes or epididymides and altered in vitro sperm–oocyte binding or in vivo fertilization due to TCE or metabolites.

The animal studies cited by ATSDR (2014) in the TCE profile supported the epidemiologic studies on the effects of TCE on male and female reproduction. Exposure to TCE via inhalation was a reproductive toxicant in male rats and mice, resulting in testicular atrophy, decreased sperm count and motility, and increased abnormal sperm morphology. In one study, male rats administered TCE by gavage at 1,000 mg/kg/day, 5 days/week for 6 weeks had impaired copulatory behavior (Zenick et al., 1984).

Regarding female fertility and pregnancy outcomes, NRC (2006) found animal studies that indicate that TCE leads to decreased fertilizability of oocytes in females. The 2006 NRC committee found that animal studies also suggested that TCE may be a reproductive toxicant in rats and that its effect requires metabolic activation by cytochrome P450 2E1 (CYP2E1), but the relevance of these studies to human reproduction was not clear. In studies on female rats described in the 2009 NRC report on Camp Lejeune, exposure before mating and during pregnancy was correlated with reduced offspring survival at high concentrations that also produced maternal toxicity. Studies of mating pairs of rats or mice exposed during mating and throughout one or more pregnancies also showed reduced numbers of litters and increased perinatal mortality. NRC (2006) reported that multiple animal studies have found decreased fetal growth after maternal exposure to TCE. In animal studies, decreased intrauterine growth has been found consistently after maternal exposure to TCE (Fisher et al., 2001; Johnson et al., 1998a,b; Smith et al., 1989, 1992).

EPA (2011) found that animal studies supported the human data: decreased fetal weight, decreased live birth weights, and decreased postnatal growth were found in rats and mice, although there were species differences in the outcomes reported for Fischer 344 or Wistar rats (increased risk of adverse outcomes) versus Sprague Dawley rats (no increase in risk). It further reported that although one study in rats showed reduced in vitro oocyte fertilizability, other laboratory animal studies of oral exposure did not report adverse effects on female reproductive function.

In the 2014 ATSDR review, animal studies supported the epidemiologic findings of reduced fertility and adverse birth outcomes, although only when the animals received repeated high doses of TCE. The only study of female rats found no reproductive effects following preconception exposure. In a continuous breeding study, oral administration of 300 mg/kg/day of TCE from 7 days before mating through the birth of the F2 generation resulted in no reproductive effects in rats. A similar study in mice treated with up to 750 mg/kg/day found no treatment-related effects on mating, fertility, or reproductive performance in either the F0 or F1 mice, but sperm motility was reduced by 45% in F0 males and by 18% in F1 males, and F1 males exhibited significantly increased mean relative weights of the left testis/epididymis and right epididymis; the effects in the F2 generation were not reported by ATSDR. No treatment-related effects on fertility were seen in studies of female rats receiving TCE from the drinking water during premating or gestation at estimated doses as high as 129 mg/kg/day.

The Volume 11 committee identified only one new animal study on the effects of TCE exposure on reproduction. Wu and Berger (2007) exposed female rats to TCE in drinking water on days 1 to 5, days 6 to 10, or days 11 to 14 of the 2-week interval preceding ovulation (oocytes collected the morning of day 15). TCE-treated oocytes had a greater incidence of protein carbonyls (an indicator of oxidative damage) and were less fertilizable than controls.

Developmental Effects

Several developmental effects have been assessed in children who were exposed to TCE either via the mother during gestation or via the father prior to conception. The health outcomes that have been examined include childhood cancer, specifically leukemia, and cardiac birth defects.

The Volume 2 committee reported on three studies that evaluated the association between prenatal exposure to TCE and childhood leukemia. Paternal preconception exposure to TCE was not significantly associated with childhood leukemia (De Roos et al., 2001; Lowengart et al., 1987; Shu et al.,

1999). However, maternal prenatal exposure to any solvent was associated with an increased risk of acute lymphocytic leukemia in children, although exposure to TCE specifically was not (De Roos et al., 2001; Shu et al., 1999).

The 2006 NRC report found that prenatal exposure to TCE via drinking contaminated water was associated in several epidemiological studies with a two- to threefold increase in the risk of congenital heart defects of the interventricular septae and heart valves. The biological plausibility of this correlation was enhanced by similar defects being reported in animal studies, although the NRC committee found the animal studies to be inconsistent and noted that there were species differences in response, with avian studies being the most convincing.

The 2009 NRC report on contaminated water at Camp Lejeune concluded that although the epidemiologic evidence of an association between chronic exposure to TCE or PCE and congenital malformations was judged to be inadequate to support conclusions, the toxicologic data from several studies reviewed by the committee, particularly the inhalation exposure study conducted in rats on GDs 6–20 by Carney et al. (2006), provided strong evidence that neither solvent was associated with congenital cardiovascular malformations in rats at concentrations up to those that have minimal maternal toxicity. Many of the developmental animal studies considered by the committee exposed the dams to TCE not only during gestation but also during lactation, which is not a relevant window of exposure for this report. The 2009 NRC committee noted that there was no evidence of second-generation effects from continuous breeding experiments in rats and mice.

Epidemiologic studies on postnatal developmental effects following prenatal exposure was assessed by EPA in its extensive 2011 toxicological review of TCE (EPA, 2011). EPA found that both human and animal studies indicated that a number of congenital malformations were associated with prenatal maternal environmental and occupational exposure to TCE; these exposures were via inhalation and consumption of contaminated drinking water. Some—but not all—epidemiologic studies found increases in total birth defects, oral cleft defects, eye/ear defects, kidney/urinary tract disorders, musculoskeletal birth anomalies, lung/respiratory tract disorders, skeletal defects, and cardiac defects. For some of these outcomes, such as eye/ear defects and kidney/urinary tract disorders, there was only one positive study (e.g., Lagakos et al., 1986). Prenatal exposure to TCE in humans was also associated with neuroanatomical changes such as neural tube defects (ATSDR, 2014; Bove, 1996; Bove et al., 1995; Lagakos et al., 1986) and encephalopathy (White et al., 1997) and also with clinical neurological changes such as impaired cognition (White et al., 1997) and speech and hearing impairment (Burg and Gist, 1999; White et al., 1997). In animal studies, the administration of TCE, whether by the inhalation or oral route of exposure, was also associated with anatomical and developmental neurotoxicity.

The most studied birth defects were those of the cardiovascular system, particularly the heart. EPA (2011) found that the epidemiologic studies, when considered as a group, showed a significant increase in the incidence of cardiac defects in children with prenatal exposure to TCE, whether from maternal inhalation of contaminated air or maternal consumption of contaminated water (ATSDR, 2008; Bove et al., 1995; Goldberg et al., 1990; Yauck et al., 2004). The animal data on cardiac defects following prenatal exposure to TCE were inconsistent; several studies found cardiac defects in rat pups born to dams administered TCE in drinking water, but some well-conducted studies did not. EPA pointed out that although some animal and mechanistic studies may have had limitations, they provided a "plausible mechanistic basis for defects in septal and valvular morphogenesis observed in rodents, and consequently support the plausibility of cardiac defects induced by TCE in humans" (EPA, 2011).

Studies on the risk of childhood cancer as a result of prenatal exposure to TCE were inconclusive, and EPA cited an ongoing study by ATSDR of childhood cancer at Camp Lejeune as a potential future resource.

ATSDR (2014) reviewed two studies of maternal exposure to TCE via inhalation and several studies of maternal exposure to TCE via contaminated drinking water and concluded that it was not possible to determine on the basis of those studies if TCE caused developmental effects, including cardiac effects and hearing impairment, in prenatally exposed offspring.

The Volume 11 committee considered six studies (Brender et al., 2014; Cordier et al., 2012; Forand et al., 2012; Heck et al., 2014; Ruckart et al., 2013; Swartz et al., 2015) and one systematic review (Makris et al., 2016) that examined developmental effects in children born to women with gestational exposure to TCE; one additional study assessed both maternal and paternal exposures (Le Cornet et al., 2017). In the Forand et al. (2012) study, cited under Reproductive Effects, children born to women with inhalation exposure to TCE as a result of soil-vapor intrusion were found to be at a significantly increased risk of cardiac defects (RR=2.15, 95% CI 1.27–3.62) and conotruncal defects (RR=4.91, 95% CI 1.58–15.24); the risks were elevated for all reportable birth defects and for surveillance birth defects, but not significantly so.

The PELAGIE mother–child cohort in Brittany, France (Cordier et al., 2012), examined the association between solvent exposure (as determined by questionnaires and, in a subset, the presence of urinary metabolites of TCE) and congenital malformations in a subset of 3,421 women who returned the inclusion questionnaire before 19 weeks of gestation; pregnancy outcomes were obtained from maternity hospital records for 3,399 pregnancies, including 79 cases and 580 controls. Levels of trichloracetic acid and trichloroethanol greater than or equal to 0.01 mg/L in urine were both associated with an increased risk of limb malformations (OR=8.0, 95% CI 2.5–25.9 and OR=5.8, 05% CI 1.4–23.6, respectively); trichloroethanol was also associated with an increased risk of any malformation (OR=3.3, 95% CI 1.3–8.3).

As discussed in the section on benzene, Ruckart et al. (2013) conducted a case-control study to assess the frequency of birth defects and childhood cancers in children born to mothers at Camp Lejeune, North Carolina, between 1968 and 1985, who may have consumed drinking water contaminated with solvents, including TCE. Birth certificates were used to identify the 51 cases and 526 control parent–child pairs. Prenatal TCE exposure in the first trimester was not associated with a significantly increased risk of childhood leukemia, non-Hodgkin's lymphoma, oral cleft defects, or neural tube defects.

Brender et al. (2014) examined the risk of birth defects in children born between 1996 and 2008 in Texas and maternal residential proximity to industrial releases of chlorinated solvents, including TCE. TCE was not significantly associated with any of the birth defects considered: any neural tube defect, anencephaly, spina bifida, conotruncal heart defects, obstructive heart defects, any oral clefts, cleft palate only, or cleft lip with or without cleft palate, or any type of limb deficit. A correlation between TCE exposure and septal heart defects was barely significant (OR=1.06, 95% CI 1.02–1.10) and showed a positive trend with TCE emissions (p-value for trend=0.002). When analyses were stratified by maternal age, infants born to exposed mothers who were 35 years of age or older had a significantly greater risk of several defects, whereas risks were less among children born to women less than 35 years of age: oral clefts (OR=1.39, 95% CI 1.06–1.83 versus OR=1.02, 95% CI 0.91–1.14) and any heart defect (OR=1.04, 95% CI 1.00–1.07 versus OR=1.13, 95% CI 1.04–1.22).

In a study of the risk of neural tube defects in children born in Texas between 1999 and 2004, Swartz et al. (2015) estimated the ambient levels of 32 hazardous air pollutants, including TCE, using the EPA 1999 Assessment System for Population Exposure Nationwide. The authors used hierarchical Bayesian modeling, which included stochastic search variable selection (SSVS). Among the 25 hazardous air pollutants used in the model, only quinolone and TCE had Bayes factors greater than 1. The OR for the medium level of TCE exposure and spina bifida was 2.00 (95% CI 1.14–3.61); the joint model without the SSVS found only the medium level of TCE to be associated with spina bifida (OR=5.72, 95% CI 1.44–24.16).

Heck et al. (2014)—also discussed in the section on benzene—assessed the risk of childhood leukemia following maternal exposure to air toxics, including TCE, by trimester, in children in California who had been diagnosed with either ALL (n=69) or AML (n=46) between 1990 and 2007. A one-interquartile increase in TCE concentrations did not increase the risk for ALL during the first, second, or third trimester or during the entire pregnancy, nor the risk of AML at any time during the pregnancy.

In the NORD-TEST study described in the benzene section, there was no increased risk of testicular germ cell tumors in men aged 14–49 years relative to their parents exposures to TCE in the year prior to their birth in Finland, Norway, and Sweden (OR=0.98, 95% CI 0.62–1.54 and OR=1.10, 95% CI 0.94–1.28, for maternal and paternal occupational exposures, respectively) (Le Cornet et al., 2017).

In a systematic review of the risk of cardiac defects following TCE exposure, Makris et al. (2016) examined seven epidemiologic studies. Most of the studies had been included in the EPA (2011) assessment cited earlier. The authors found that "TCE has the potential to cause cardiac defects in humans when exposure occurs at sufficient doses during a sensitive window of fetal development" (Makris et al., 2016).

Animal Studies

The 2006 NRC committee identified multiple mammalian and avian studies that suggested that TCE or one or more of its metabolites (trichloroacetic acid and dichloroacetic acid) can cause cardiac teratogenesis, although the committee noted that the avian studies were the most convincing, as the rodent studies had mixed results, suggesting either methodological or strain differences. The committee noted that the "low-dose studies showing a positive correlation in TCE-induced cardiac teratogenesis showed unusually flat dose–response curves and came from a single laboratory" (NRC, 2006).

The NRC committee that examined the effects of TCE and PCE in drinking water at Camp Lejeune (NRC, 2009) concluded that the toxicologic data provide strong evidence that neither solvent is associated with congenital malformations in rats, based on the then-recent studies by Carney et al. (2006) that showed no effects on the development of the heart or other organs in the rat at concentrations up to a minimal maternally toxic concentration. The committee discussed four studies in rats that suggested the existence of neurologic effects in offspring following gestational exposure via drinking water.

The EPA (2011) toxicological review of TCE concluded, based on multiple well-conducted studies in rats and mice, that exposure to TCE poses a risk for prenatal losses and decreased growth or birth weight in offspring. EPA found mixed evidence concerning the connection between TCE and cardiac defects; it reported that numerous studies had found that the oral administration of TCE in maternal drinking water during gestation induces cardiac malformations in rat fetuses, while several other well-conducted studies had not found induction of cardiac defects in rats, mice, or rabbits when TCE was administered by inhalation or gavage.

The animal studies cited by ATSDR suggest that TCE not only can cause cardiac malformations via oral exposure but also can damage the immune system in developing fetuses and produce neurologic defects (ATSDR, 2014).

The Volume 11 committee identified several new animal studies that examined the effects of TCE on fetal development. Warren et al. (2006) assessed whether the prenatal exposure of rats to TCE and its oxidative metabolites, trichloroacetate (TCA) and dichloroacetate (DCA), affects eye development. Pregnant rats received oral doses of either TCE (500 mg/kg/day), TCA (300 mg/kg/day), or DCA (300 mg/kg/day) on GDs 6–15. On GD 21, fetal eyes were measured for lens area, globe area, medial canthus distance, and interocular distance. No gross ocular malformations were seen for the TCE, TCA, and DCA treatment groups. All four ocular measures were reduced after exposure to TCA or to DCA, but the reductions were not significant for the TCA; TCE had no effect.

Palbykin et al. (2011) found that 10 ppb of TCE administered via drinking water to pregnant Sprague-Dawley rats beginning on GD 0 induced DNA hypermethylation in the reduced *Serca2* promotor region of rat embryonic cardiac tissue examined on GD 10, which corresponds to the first phase of heart development. Gilbert et al. (2014) sought to determine if the timing of TCE exposure during development resulted in different immunotoxic responses. Pregnant MRL+/+ mice received oral doses of 0, 0.01, or 0.1 mg/mL TCE from GDs 0 to birth. Peripheral CD4+ T cells from the offspring of both groups had alterations in retrotransposon (intracisternal A particle and murine endogenous retrovirus) expression indicative of epigenetic alterations. Some effects, such as alterations in thymus cellularity, were found only in offspring exposed to TCE during gestation.

Synthesis and Conclusions

TCE has been studied by several governmental and other organizations. It has been identified as a contaminant in drinking water or air at several locations. It has numerous industrial applications that may result in occupational exposures.

Reproductive Effects

NRC, EPA, and ATSDR have all reviewed multiple studies that assessed the effect of occupational exposure to TCE on male reproduction. EPA reviewed 10 studies, 9 of which included fewer than 100 men and which found significant adverse effects on semen quality. However, what impact these effects had on fertility was not reported in the studies. ATSDR cited other studies which did not find any effect of TCE on male reproduction. The Volume 11 committee did not identify any new studies of TCE exposure and male reproduction. Many, but not all, of the animal studies considered by EPA indicated that TCE may have adverse effects on male reproduction, including altered hormone levels and lesions in the testes. Together these data suggest that TCE may affect semen parameters, but the studies are limited by the small numbers of subjects and need confirmation.

There is little information on the effects of occupational or environmental TCE exposure on female reproduction. Animal studies on the subject have mixed results.

Most of the studies reviewed by NRC, EPA, and ATSDR have found prenatal exposure to TCE to be associated with a number of adverse pregnancy outcomes, particularly an increased risk of spontaneous abortion and decreased birth weight. Most of the studies were small in size, and the exposures were usually to a mixture of solvents, although some studies did make efforts to isolate exposure to specific solvents, including TCE. One study reviewed by the Volume 11 committee (Forand et al., 2012) found that environmental exposure to TCE was significantly associated with several birth outcomes, such as low birth weight and small for gestational age, but not with others (e.g., preterm birth). The animal studies cited by NRC, EPA and ATSDR supported the epidemiologic studies with findings of reduced fertility and fetal loss, although two continuous breeding studies did not find any substantial reproductive effects in the F0 or F1 generations.

The Volume 11 committee concludes that there is limited/suggestive evidence of an association between exposure to TCE and reproductive effects in men.

The Volume 11 committee also concludes that there is inadequate/insufficient evidence to determine whether an association exists between exposure to TCE and reproductive effects in women.

The Volume 11 committee also concludes that there is limited/suggestive evidence of an association between exposure to TCE and adverse pregnancy outcomes.

Developmental Effects

There have been a number of studies examining possible developmental effects, particularly birth defects, following mothers' occupational or environmental exposures to TCE. These studies have produced mixed results. Some, but not all, of the epidemiologic studies have found that prenatal exposure to TCE may result in numerous birth defects, including oral clefts, eye/ear defects, neural tube defects, and other neurological changes. However, the study of TCE-contaminated drinking water at Camp Lejeune did not find any increased risk for neural tube or oral cleft defects.

The most studied birth defects are those of the cardiovascular system. EPA (2011) concluded that the epidemiologic and animal data together supported the "plausibility of cardiac defects induced by TCE in humans." ATSDR (2014) found that TCE caused developmental effects, including cardiac defects, in offspring following prenatal exposure to TCE. The five studies considered by the Volume 11 committee also assessed the risk of congenital malformations or cancer in children born to mothers with exposure to TCE during pregnancy. Three of the studies—Forand et al. (2012), Cordier et al. (2012), and Swartz et al. (2015)—each found increased risks of defects in children prenatally exposed to TCE via maternal inhalation, although the types of defects varied among the studies: respectively, cardiac and conotruncal defects, limb malformation, and spina bifida. On the other hand, Brender et al. (2014) found no significant associations between maternal exposures to TCE in ambient air and any birth defects, and Heck et al. (2014) found no associations between maternal exposures to TCE in ambient air and childhood leukemia. EPA was unable to explain the disparity in results among the five studies.

Animal studies were also somewhat equivocal with regard to the effects of prenatal exposure to TCE on offspring. Although EPA (2011) concluded that the animal studies supported its contention that TCE causes cardiac malformations in rat fetuses as well as other adverse birth outcomes, it acknowledged that several other well-conducted studies did not support that conclusion, and it stated that the dissection techniques used in those studies may have precluded any finding of the malformations. ATSDR (2014) stated that the epidemiological studies it reviewed indicated that exposure to TCE via air and drinking water may be associated with developmental effects, but this was not the finding of the NRC (2009) committee. The Volume 11 committee reviewed one new animal study that showed no effect of prenatal exposure to TCE on fetal eye development (Warren et al., 2006). Gilbert et al. (2014) found that prenatal TCE exposure may cause epigenetic alterations in immunologic responses in fetal mice.

Thus, several human studies indicate that some birth defects, particularly cardiac defects, might be associated with maternal inhalation exposure to TCE during pregnancy, although some studies did not find any such associations. The animal data also provide support the association between prenatal exposure to TCE and developmental effects, particularly cardiac malformation. Although both EPA and ATSDR found that prenatal TCE exposure may result in developmental effects, a 2009 NRC committee did not. Further research on the potential for developmental effects following prenatal exposure to TCE in both animals and humans is warranted.

The Volume 11 committee concludes that there is limited/suggestive evidence of an association between prenatal exposure to TCE and developmental effects.

TABLE 7-5 Summary of Reproductive and Developmental Effects of TCE

Study	Design/Population	Exposure	Results
Reproductive Effects			
Forand et al. (2012)	Cohort 1,090 TCE exposed births in Endicott, NY, versus 3.6 million births in NY state (excluding New York City) based on birth records from 1978–2002. There was an industrial spill of trichloroethane in 1979 in Endicott.	Estimated for maternal residence at birth based on census block-level exposure.	Adverse birth outcomes. LBW: RR=1.36, 95% CI 1.07–1.73; very LBW: RR=1.61, 95% CI 0.94–2.78; PTB: RR=1.02, 95% CI 0.82–1.27; very PTB: RR=1.37, 95% CI 0.87–2.14; SGA: RR=1.23, 95% CI 1.03–1.48; term LBW: RR=1.68, 95% CI 1.20–2.34. Adjusted for mother's age, education, race, number of previous births, infant's sex, adequate prenatal care.
Ruckart et al. (2014)	Cohort 11,896 infants born to women who consumed contaminated drinking water at the Marine Corps base Camp Lejeune, NC, during 1968–1985.	TCE exposure for entire pregnancy estimated based on residence and fate and transport models. Stratified to 5 exposure levels: no exposure, low (>0–<1.7 ppb), medium (≥1.7–<3.1 ppb), medium-high (≥3.1–9.8), and high exposure (≥9.8 ppb).	Adverse birth outcomes. SGA: low OR=1.2, 95% CI 1.1–1.5; medium OR=1.3, 95% CI 1.1–1.5; medium-high OR=1.1, 95% CI 1.0–1.4; high OR=1.5, 95% CI 1.2–1.9. PTB: low OR=1.1, 95% CI 0.9–1.3; medium OR=1.0, 95% CI 0.8–1.3; medium-high OR=1.3, 95% CI 1.0–1.6; high OR=1.1, 95% CI 0.6–1.1. LBW not associated with any level of TCE exposure. Mean birth weight difference: low md= –42.2, 95% CI –66.7– –17.7; medium md= –48.8, 95% CI –77.4– –20.3; medium-high md= –40.5, 95% CI –72.3– –8.7; high md= –78.3, 95% CI –115.0– –41.7. Birth weight adjusted for sex of child, mother's race, parity.
Developmental Effects			
Forand et al. (2012)	Cohort 1,090 TCE exposed births in Endicott, NY, versus 3.6 million births in NY state (excluding New York City) based on birth records from 1978–2002. There was an industrial spill of trichloroethane in 1979 in Endicott.	Estimated for maternal residence at birth based on census block-level exposure.	Birth defects. 44 birth defects diagnosed during 1983–2000. All birth defects: RR=1.07, 95% CI 0.78–1.47; All cardiac defects: RR=2.15, 95% CI 1.27–3.62, n=15; Major cardiac defects: RR=2.40, 95% CI 1.00–5.77, n=6; Conotruncal defects: RR=4.91, 95% CI 1.58–15.24, n=3. Adjusted for mother's age, education, race, number of previous births, infant's sex, adequate prenatal care.

Study	Design/Population	Exposure	Results
Cordier et al. (2012)	Cohort—PELAGIE study of 3,399 pregnant women in Brittany, France in 2002–2006. Nested case-control study: 79 cases of nonchromosomal, nongenetic major malformations versus 580 controls.	Self-reported residential and occupational exposure to solvents (29% reported occupational exposure). Nested case-control study: exposure was based on 10 urinary metabolites collected in early pregnancy.	Birth defects. In the whole cohort, risk of any major malformation based on self-reported exposure frequency: occasional exposure OR=2.1 (95% CI 1.0–4.4), regular exposure OR=2.7 (95% CI 1.5–5.0), p-value for trend=0.001; and based on job exposure matrix–defined exposure: medium OR=1.5 (95% CI 0.8-2.8), high OR=3.2 (95% CI 1.2-8.7), p-value for trend=0.02. Hobby exposure not associated with malformations. Adjusted for maternal age group, tobacco use, alcohol use, folic acid supplementation, and years of schooling. Nested case-control study. Levels of trichloracetic acid and trichloroethanol ≥ 0.01 mg/L in urine were both associated with an increased risk of limb malformations (OR=8.0, 95% CI 2.5–25.9 and OR=5.8, 05% CI 1.4–23.6, respectively); trichlorethanol was associated with an increased risk of any malformation (OR=3.3, 95% CI 1.3–8.3). Ethoxyacetic acid was associated with oral clefts (OR=10.9, 95% CI 2.4–50.0) and limb malformations (OR=3.1, 95% CI 1.1–8.2). Other metabolites not associated with malformations.
Ruckart et al. (2013)	Case-control 15 cases of NTD, 24 cases of oral clefts, and 13 cases of childhood hematopoietic cancer, versus 524 controls born during 1968–1985 to mothers who lived at the Marine Corps base Camp Lejeune.	Exposure during the 1st trimester of pregnancy categorized as unexposed, low (>0–≤ 2ppb), high (>2 ppb), below MCL (>0–≤5 ppb), above MCL (>5 ppb), or unexposed/exposed; estimates modeled using fate and transport models.	Birth defects (neural tube or oral cleft defects) and childhood cancers. ORs for NTDs, oral cleft defects, or childhood leukemia or non-Hodgkin's lymphoma were not significantly increased for any TCE exposure level.

continued

TABLE 7-5 Continued

Study	Design/Population	Exposure	Results
Brender et al. (2014)	Case-control 3,245 cases of NTD, 2,406 cases of limb deficiencies, 7,416 cases of oral clefts, and 60,154 cases of heart defects identified from the Texas Birth Defects Registry and 280,764 controls randomly selected from birth certificate data, frequency matched to cases by year of delivery and mother's residence in 1996–2008.	Maternal residential distance to industrial sources of emissions. Data for air emissions of TCE from Texas industrial facilities were obtained from EPA Toxic Release Inventory program. TCE emissions (lbs. released by facilities/year) categorized as 0.01–56.69, 56.70–284.39, and >284.39 lbs/year.	Birth defects. TCE was not associated with NTDs OR=0.95 (95% CI 0.83–1.09); anencephaly OR=0.99 (95% CI 0.76–1.29); spina bifida OR=0.94 (95% CI 0.79–1.12); conotruncal heart defects OR=0.98 (95% CI 0.87–1.10), obstructive heart defects OR=1.03 (95% CI 0.92–1.15); any oral clefts OR=1.02 (95% CI 0.92–1.13); any type of limb deficit (OR=1.01, 95% CI 0.88–1.17). Septal heart defects were associated with TCE exposure (OR=1.06, 95% CI 1.02–1.10, p-value for trend=0.002). Other solvents were more strongly associated with septal heart defects. Adjusted for birth year, maternal age, education, race/ethnicity, and public health region of residence.
Swartz et al. (2015)	Case-control 533 cases of spina bifida from the Texas Birth Defects Registry versus 3,695 controls selected from birth certificates, matched to cases by year of birth. 1999–2004	Exposure estimated based on maternal residence at birth and census tract-level estimates of air pollutants obtained from the EPA 1999 Assessment System for Population Exposure Nationwide Inhalation exposure. TCE exposure classified as high exposure (>95th percentile; 0.16 μg/m^3), medium exposure (5th–95th percentile, 0.05–0.11 μg/m^3), and low exposure (<5th percentile, reference).	Birth defects (spina bifida). Medium exposure level OR=2.00, 95% CI 1.14–3.61, Bayes factor=3.79; high exposure level OR=1.32, 95% CI 0.61–2.80, Bayes factor=0.60. Analysis used hierarchical Bayesian logistic regression models with stochastic search variable selection.
Heck et al. (2014)	Case-control 69 cases of ALL and 46 cases of AML from California Cancer Registry records of children diagnosed <age 6 years, and 19,209 controls from California birth records. 1990–2007	Prenatal exposure to air pollutants estimated based on data from air monitoring stations. Children lived within 2 km (ALL) and 6 km (AML) of an air toxics monitoring station.	Childhood leukemia. TCE was not associated with ALL during the 1st, 2nd, or 3rd trimesters or during the entire pregnancy (OR=1.01, 95% CI 0.90–1.14; OR=0.92, 95% CI 0.72–1.19; OR=1.01, 95% CI 0.81–1.26; OR=0.98, 95% CI 0.79–1.23, respectively, per IQR increase), nor the risk of AML during the 1st, 2nd, or 3rd trimesters or during the entire pregnancy (OR=0.95, 95% CI 0.77–1.17; OR=0.89, 95% CI 0.67–1.18; OR=0.98, 95% CI 0.80–1.21; OR=0.92, 95% CI 0.71–1.20, respectively, per IQR increase).

NOTE: ALL=acute lymphoblastic leukemia; AML=acute myeloid leukemia; CI=confidence interval; EPA=U.S. Environmental Protection Agency; IQR=interquartile range; LBW=low birth weight; MCL=maximum contaminant level; md=mean difference; NTD=neural tube defect; OR=odds ratio; PTB=preterm birth; RR=relative risk; SGA=small for gestational age; TCE=trichloroethylene.

TETRACHLOROETHYLENE

Tetrachloroethylene (also called perchloroethylene, PCE, or perc) is a widely used industrial solvent. PCE has been the major solvent used in dry cleaning and is used in metal degreasing as well as in numerous industrial applications.

PCE has been detected in ambient air, where it results both from industrial emissions and from the combustion of organic materials; it has also been detected in drinking water contaminated by industrial leaks into groundwater. In 2007 and 2009 PCE was measured in air samples of emissions from a large-scale burn pit at JBB in Iraq (IOM, 2011). PCE was also a major contaminant of the drinking water at Camp Lejeune, North Carolina. PCE entered the base's drinking water through the groundwater as a result of spills and improper disposal from an off-site dry cleaner. It was estimated that the PCE contamination there began in 1957 and continued until the groundwater wells were closed in 1985. The levels of PCE in the Camp Lejeune drinking water exceeded the EPA maximum contaminant level of 5 μg/L; for example, levels of 76–104 μg/L were found in samples taken from Tawara Terrace in August 1982 (Faye and Green, 2007a,b; NRC, 2009). Groundwater contamination from PCE has also been found at other sites in the United States, including areas around Woburn, Massachusetts, and Endicott, New York.

PCE and its metabolites can be measured in humans, although the half-life of PCE is relatively short, with the chemical being mostly metabolized within days of exposure. The urinary metabolites of PCE are trichloroacetic acid and dichloroacetic acid (ATSDR, 2014).

In its assessment of the reproductive and developmental effects of PCE, the Volume 11 committee considered four earlier, comprehensive reports—*Gulf War and Health, Volume 2* (IOM, 2003), the 2009 NRC report on contaminated water at Camp Lejeune, the 2012 EPA *Toxicological Review of Tetrachloroethylene (Perchloroethylene)*, and the 2014 ATSDR *Draft Toxicological Profile for Tetrachloroethylene*—as well as any new studies it found that had been published in recent years. The committee notes that many of the studies on PCE have been reviewed by more than one of the above organizations. The epidemiologic studies on the reproductive and developmental effects of PCE reviewed below are summarized in Table 7-6 at the end of this section.

Reproductive Effects

Reproductive Effects in Men and Women

The Volume 2 committee (IOM, 2003) did not identify any studies of occupational or environmental exposure of men or women to PCE and its effect on semen quality or male fertility or on female reproduction.

The 2009 NRC review found only one study of men occupationally exposed to solvents (painters and millwrights), although not to PCE specifically, that found an association between the levels of exposure to chlorinated solvents and increasing levels of FSH, but not concentrations of LH or TTP (Luderer et al., 2004). The NRC committee concluded that there continued to be inadequate/insufficient evidence to determine whether an association exists between chronic exposure to TCE or PCE and male infertility.

In 2012, EPA summarized studies of PCE effects on semen quality (Eskenazi et al., 1991b) and male fertility (Eskenazi et al., 1991b; Rachootin and Olsen, 1983) as well as TTP (Sallmén et al., 1998). Most of these studies assessed effects in men who worked in dry cleaning facilities. EPA found that although there was one study (Eskenazi et al., 1991b) reporting that PCE had effects on some sperm parameters, those results, when considered against other studies finding no such adverse outcomes, were not sufficient to conclude that PCE was associated with adverse effects on male reproduction.

ATSDR (2014) reviewed many of the same studies as those cited by EPA. It included the Eskenazi et al. (1991a,b) and the Sallmén et al. (1998) studies of male reproductive effects following inhalation exposure to PCE. ATSDR also reported on the study by Sallmén et al. (1995) that examined women who had been biologically monitored for exposure to organic solvents at the Finnish Institute of Occupational Health and asked about possible solvent exposure in the 12 months before pregnancy. Using a fecundability measure termed the IDR, Sallmén et al. reported that women with exposure to PCE had reduced fecundity (IDR=0.69, 95% CI 0.31–1.52).

The Volume 11 committee did not identify any new literature on the effects of exposure to PCE on male or female reproduction.

Adverse Pregnancy Outcomes

The Volume 2 committee identified several studies, mostly of Scandinavian women or men who worked in dry cleaning facilities, of the effects of PCE exposure on fetal outcomes, particularly the occurrence of spontaneous abortion. The results of the studies were inconsistent, as noted earlier.

Olsen et al. (1990) combined data from Sweden, Denmark, and Finland and found a slight increase in the risk of spontaneous abortion for women who worked in dry cleaning with potential low exposure (OR=1.17, 95% CI 0.74–1.85), and the increase was greater for women with high exposure (OR=2.88, 95% CI 0.98–8.44). Lindbohm and colleagues studied Finnish women and men who had been occupationally exposed to organic solvents. For women who were exposed during the first trimester of their pregnancy, there was a significant association between solvent exposure and spontaneous abortion (OR=2.2, 95% CI 1.2–4.1) (Lindbohm et al., 1990); however, there was no significant association between paternal occupational exposure to PCE and spontaneous abortion (PCE=0.7, 95% CI 0.2–2.4) (Lindbohm et al., 1991). The study used the time of spermatogenesis (80 days before conception) as the relevant window of exposure.

A study of dry cleaners in the United Kingdom who were exposed to PCE (Doyle et al., 1997) found no association with spontaneous abortion (OR=1.03, 95% CI 0.48–2.21). Ahlborg (1990) found a nonsignificant increased risk of spontaneous abortion (OR=1.1, 95% CI 0.6–2.0) in a study of women working in laundry or dry cleaning facilities in Sweden who had exposures during the first trimester. By contrast, Kyyronen et al. (1989) found a significant increase in spontaneous abortion among women in Finland who reported high exposures to PCE in dry cleaning facilities (OR=3.6, 95% CI 1.3–11.2).

The 2012 EPA review included many of the same studies of the effects of PCE and other solvents on female reproduction as reviewed by the Volume 2 committee or the NRC committee on Camp Lejeune (NRC, 2009). New studies published after the 2009 NRC report included findings of associations between PCE exposure and various adverse pregnancy outcomes, including spontaneous abortion (Aschengrau et al., 2009), low birth weight, and shortened gestational duration (Aschengrau et al., 2008).

EPA (2012) found three studies of paternal occupational exposure to PCE prior to conception that did not find increases in the risk of spontaneous abortion (Eskenazi et al., 1991a; Lindbohm et al., 1991; Taskinen et al., 1989), although the exposures in the latter two studies were to a multitude of solvents. The EPA report also included new studies of two populations living in Massachusetts that had been exposed to PCE-contaminated drinking water (Aschengrau et al., 2008, 2009; Lagakos et al., 1986). No associations were found between exposure to PCE in drinking water and the incidence of spontaneous abortion in either population. EPA noted that the studies of drinking water contamination evaluated populations with much lower exposures than those experienced by the occupational cohorts.

EPA (2012) also assessed the effect of PCE exposure on other birth outcomes. Several studies suggested that prenatal PCE exposure in drinking water was associated with low birth weight (Bove et al., 1995; Lagakos et al., 1986; Sonnenfeld et al., 2001). However, in the Cape Cod population studies done by Aschengrau et al. (2008), individuals were exposed to a wide range of PCE in drinking water, and the authors did not find an association between exposure and birth weight or gestational duration.

EPA found that "Overall, no associations were noted in several studies that assessed maternal or paternal occupational exposure to PCE and increased incidence of stillbirths, congenital anomalies, or decreased birth weight (Lindbohm, 1995; Windham et al., 1991; Olsen et al., 1990; Kyyronen et al., 1989; Taskinen et al., 1989; Bosco et al., 1987)."

The 2014 ATSDR *Draft Toxicological Profile for Tetrachloroethylene* also assessed many of the studies reviewed by the IOM, NRC, and EPA. It was not possible to draw any conclusions concerning the association between maternal or paternal exposure to PCE and adverse reproductive effects in men, women, or fetuses because of the limitations of the epidemiologic studies, such as confounding from multiple exposures and small numbers of study participants.

The Volume 11 committee considered two new studies that examined reproductive effects in humans following prenatal PCE exposure. In a further study of eight towns in Cape Cod, Massachusetts, that had PCE contamination in the water system between 1969 and 1990, Carwile et al. (2014) found that PCE exposure during pregnancy for 1,091 women was not significantly associated with overall ischemic placental disease, preeclampsia, placental abruption, or small-for-gestational-age infants among women with cumulative exposure levels below the median (<28 g PCE). However, women with PCE exposures greater than the sample median (>28.9 g PCE) were at a significantly increased risk for stillbirth ≥27 weeks gestation (RR=2.38, 95% CI 1.01–5.59).

Ruckart et al. (2014) conducted a cross-sectional study of 11,896 births at Camp Lejeune, North Carolina, during 1968–1985, the period of groundwater contamination with PCE and other solvents (including, as discussed earlier, benzene and TCE), using birth certificate information and groundwater modeling. There was no association found between residential prenatal exposure to any concentration of PCE (≥81.4 ppb) during the entire pregnancy and the risk of a full-term low birth weight or reduced mean birth weight. However, there was a slight but significant increase in the risk of a small-for-gestational-age infant at a PCE concentration of ≥35.8–<52.7 ppb (OR=1.2, 95% CI 1.0–1.4), although not at other concentrations, and PCE at a concentration of ≥81.4 ppb was associated with a significantly increased risk of preterm birth (OR=1.3, 95% CI 1.0–1.6).

Animal Studies

There were no animal studies of PCE's reproductive or developmental effects discussed by the Volume 2 committee (IOM, 2003). The 2006 NRC report examined a study by Berger and Horner (2003) that found that exposure to 0.9% PCE in drinking water reduced the percentage of females ovulating ($p<0.05$); however, there were no effects on oocyte fertilizability or on the number of penetrated sperm per oocyte. Females who were exposed to 1,700 ppm PCE via inhalation for two 1-hour periods per day for 2 weeks experienced a slight reduction in the fertilizability of their oocytes ($p<0.05$), and the number of penetrated sperm per oocyte was also reduced; there were no clinical signs of toxicity.

The 2009 NRC report found that maternal exposure to PCE led to reduced fetal weight in rats and that maternal exposure to high levels of PCE via inhalation reduced intrauterine growth.

The 2012 EPA review of animal studies reported a decrease in mean testes weight in F1 males in a two-generation inhalation study of PCE (Tinston, 1994), although there were no effects on male or female fertility or other evidence of alterations in reproductive function. Beliles et al. (1980) also found no sperm abnormalities in rats following up to 10 weeks of PCE inhalation exposures at 100 or 500 ppm, although they did find an increase in abnormal sperm heads in mice after 4 weeks of exposure to 500 ppm only.

ATSDR (2014) reported that inhalation exposures of female rats and rabbits at concentrations between 300 and 1,254 ppm during gestation resulted in increased pre- and post-implantation losses, decreased litter sizes, and decreased survival during lactation; these results were not seen in mice. Decreased fetal and maternal weight were observed in rats and mice exposed to concentrations of 300–664 ppm during gestation.

The Volume 11 committee did not identify any new animal studies on the reproductive effects of PCE.

Developmental Effects

The authoritative reviews of PCE conducted by NRC, ATSDR, and EPA cited in the preceding section also examined the developmental effects of exposure to PCE on infants and children. These findings are summarized below.

The Volume 2 committee (IOM, 2003) considered a number of studies that examined maternal and paternal solvent exposure before or during pregnancy and did not find a pattern of association with any congenital malformations. However, the four key studies cited by the committee for neural tube defects, including spina bifida (Blatter et al., 1996, 1997; Shaw et al., 1999a) and gastroschisis (Torfs et al., 1996), did not show increased risks of congenital malformations that were associated specifically with paternal or prenatal maternal PCE exposure.

The Volume 2 committee identified two studies that reported on the risk of childhood cancers and prenatal PCE exposure. Shu et al. (1999), in an extensive study of ALL in children, found a nonsignificant association with the mothers' self-reports of prenatal exposure to PCE (OR=1.4, 95% CI 0.2–8.6) but not with the fathers' preconception exposures (OR=0.8, 95% CI 0.5–1.5). De Roos et al. (2001) found no association between the risk of childhood neuroblastoma in children and their fathers' preconception occupational exposure to PCE (OR=0.5, 95% CI 0.1–1.7). Thus, the Volume 2 committee concluded that there was inadequate/insufficient evidence to determine whether an association exists between chronic exposure to solvents and congenital malformations or childhood cancer.

The 2009 NRC review identified three new studies that assessed the relationship between parental exposure to PCE and childhood leukemia—one cohort study with incidence data (Morgan and Cassady, 2002) and two case-control studies (Costas et al., 2002; Infante-Rivard, 2005). No significant increase in the incidence of childhood leukemia was found for residents of a California community exposed to PCE- and TCE-contaminated drinking water (standardized incidence ratio=1.09, 99% CI 0.38–2.31) (Morgan and Cassady, 2002), nor was there an association between maternal preconception and prenatal occupational exposure to PCE and leukemia in offspring (OR=0.96, 95% CI 0.41–2.25) (Infante-Rivard, 2005). The third study cited by the NRC committee, a case-control study by Costas et al.(2002), also found no significant association. Thus, the NRC committee concluded that there was inadequate/insufficient evidence to determine whether an association exists between PCE and childhood leukemia.

The NRC committee also considered a study by Janulewicz et al. (2008) that assessed prenatal exposure to PCE in contaminated water in a Cape Cod community. The researchers found that mothers' prenatal PCE exposure was not associated with disorders of attention, learning, and behavior in their children at 5 years of age, as determined by an examination of school records.

The 2012 EPA review evaluated the epidemiologic and animal literature on PCE exposure and adverse developmental outcomes in offspring. Epidemiologic studies of PCE assessed birth anomalies, postnatal development learning and behavior, and schizophrenia in children with prenatal exposure to PCE (Aschengrau et al., 2009; Bosco et al., 1987; Janulewicz et al., 2008; Lagakos et al., 1986; McDonald et al., 1987; Olsen et al., 1990; Perrin et al., 2007). Lagakos et al. (1986), in a study of drinking water contaminated with PCE, TCE, and other chlorinated organics in Woburn, Massachusetts, found that exposure to PCE was associated with a significantly increased risk of eye/ear anomalies (OR=14.9, p<0.0001) and CNS, chromosomal, or oral cleft abnormalities (OR=4.5, p=0.01); no other abnormalities reached significance. Aschengrau et al. (2009) reported similar results for infants born in eight towns in Cape Cod that had PCE-contaminated water, although the number of anomalies was low. PCE levels in residential areas in Falmouth, Massachusetts, ranged from undetectable to 80 μg/L in water pipes along main streets with high water flow and from 1,600 to 7,750 μg/L in water pipes along dead end streets with low water flow. The OR for all anomalies combined for children in the uppermost quartile of PCE exposure was 1.5 (95% CI 0.9–2.5); among offspring with any prenatal exposure, the OR for neural tube defects was 3.5 (95% CI 0.8–14.0) and for oral clefts was 3.2 (95% CI 0.7–15.0). The researchers reported that diagnoses of attention deficit disorder, hyperactive disorder, or educational problems, as reported by the mothers about their children, were not associated with PCE (Janulewicz et al., 2008). However, Perrin et al. (2007) reported that prenatal exposure to PCE at a dry cleaning facility was associated with a diagnosis of schizophrenia when the offspring were ages 21–33 years. EPA concluded that "the literature is insufficient to draw conclusions regarding effects of PCE exposure on development in infants and children" (EPA, 2012).

ATSDR (2014) reviewed much of the same information as EPA (2012) did and noted that in many of the epidemiologic studies subjects had multiple exposures, which made it difficult to make any conclusions as to the reproductive and developmental effects associated with PCE specifically. In a study focusing on risky behaviors, Aschengrau et al. (2011) found that at the highest tertile of prenatal PCE exposure there was a slight but significant increase in adolescent smoking (RR=1.6, 95% CI 1.1–2.3) and alcohol use (RR=1.3, 95% CI 1.0–1.7); the increase was not seen for all exposure categories or for lower exposures. For drug use, the risks were greater for teens in the highest tertile of exposure (OR=1.6, 95% CI 1.2–2.2) and for adults (OR=1.5, 95% CI 1.2–1.9). Aschengrau et al. (2012) also found a non-significant risk for bipolar disorder, post-traumatic stress disorder, and schizophrenia, but not for depression, among exposed subjects. In a follow-up study in the Cape Cod population, Janulewicz et al. (2012) performed neuropsychological testing in the original cohort, although only 35 prenatally exposed and 28 unexposed adults agreed to participate. No evidence was found of an association between prenatal exposure and the results of neuropsychological tests for omnibus intelligence, academic achievement, or language endpoints; however, there were suggestive, but not significant, associations between prenatal exposure and decrements in visuospatial functioning, learning and memory, motor speed, attention, and mood in the adults. The authors attributed the equivocal findings to the small sample size.

The Volume 11 committee considered eight new publications that examined developmental outcomes in children exposed prenatally to PCE. Four of the publications reported further assessments of the Cape Cod cohort described earlier, which was exposed to PCE from contaminated drinking water from 1969 to 1983 (Aschengrau et al., 2015; Gallagher et al., 2017; Janulewicz et al., 2013; Mahalingaiah et al., 2016). PCE measurements taken in 1980 from Cape Cod public drinking water supplies ranged from 1.5 μg/L to 7,750 μg/L (Janulewicz et al., 2012). Janulewicz et al. (2013) reported findings on 26 PCE-exposed and 16 unexposed adults who were examined with structural magnetic resonance imaging of the brain. No significant differences were found between the exposed and unexposed groups on most measures (e.g., white matter hypointensities, total cerebral and cerebellum white or gray matter volumes), but the parahippocampal gyrus was larger, on average, in exposed subjects (p=0.03), as was the thalamus (p=0.05). In a larger follow-up study of 831 participants with prenatal and postnatal (to 5 years of age) exposure to PCE and 547 unexposed participants, Aschengrau et al. (2015) found no associations between PCE exposure and the occurrence of obesity, diabetes, cardiovascular disease, hypertension, color blindness, near- and farsightedness, and dry eyes. However, there was an increased risk of cancer among those with early life exposure versus the unexposed (OR=1.8, 95% CI 0.8–4.0) and an increased risk of epilepsy (OR=1.5, 95% CI 0.6–3.6), although neither increase was significant. The committee notes that interpretation is difficult because of the small number of cases and the use of self-reported outcomes that were not confirmed by medical records. Gallagher et al. (2017) assessed whether the children with prenatal exposure to PCE in the Cape Code drinking water were more likely to engage in risky behaviors, alcohol consumption, and illicit drug use as adolescents and whether alcohol use by the mother affected the child's risk-taking behaviors. Compared with unexposed controls (n=242), adolescents with maternal exposure to only PCE (n=361) were at an increased risk of using two or more major drugs (RR=1.6, 95% CI 1.0–2.4) and of having more than five drinks of alcohol in 4 days (RR=1.3, 95% CI 1.0–1.6), and adolescents with early life exposure to both PCE and alcohol (n=302) were at even greater risk for major drug use (RR=1.9, 95% CI 1.2–3.0) and heavy alcohol consumption (RR=1.4, 95% CI 1.1–1.47). The authors note, however, that there are difficulties in conducting such a retrospective study, including poor response rate and recall bias among both adolescents and mothers. Finally, Mahalingaiah et al. (2016) looked at the reproductive health of female offspring born to women born 1969–1983 who were exposed during pregnancy to PCE in the Cape Cod drinking water. The female children were between 23 and 39 years old at the time of the survey in 2006–2008. Of the four reproductive health outcomes assessed—adult-onset polycystic ovary syndrome, endometriosis, difficulty conceiving, and miscarriage—there was no association between PCE exposure and an increased risk of any of the outcomes.

In a study of children who attended third grade in public schools in New York City, Stingone et al. (2016) found that those with higher prenatal exposure to diesel PM and PCE (average concentration=0.68 mg/m^3) had a greater risk of failing to meet math, but not English language arts, test standards (OR=1.1, 95% CI 1.07–1.12) than children with lower levels of exposure. This risk associated with the combined exposure was greater than for children with exposure to greater levels of diesel PM only (RR= 1.03, 95% CI 0.99–1.06) or to PCE only (RR=1.03, 95% CI 1.00–1.06). The exposure estimates were based on EPA's 1996 National Air Toxics Assessment for residential census tracts.

Heck et al. (2014), which was also discussed in the section on benzene, assessed the risk of childhood leukemia following maternal exposure to air toxics, including PCE, by trimester, in children in California who had been diagnosed with either ALL (n=69) or AML (n=46) between 1990 and 2007. A one-interquartile increase in PCE concentrations at any time during pregnancy did not significantly increase the risk for ALL or AML.

In the only new study to examine birth defects as well as childhood cancers, Ruckart et al. (2013) conducted a case-control study of children born to mothers at Camp Lejeune between 1968 and 1985 who may have consumed drinking water contaminated with solvents, including PCE. Birth certificates were used to identify the 51 cases and 526 control parent–child pairs. Prenatal PCE exposure in the first trimester at concentrations below the maximum contaminant level of 5 ppb was significantly associated with an increased risk of neural tube defects (OR=3.7, 95% CI 1.0–14.1); however, when the exposures were dichotomized to exposed/unexposed, there was no increased risk. Exposure to PCE at any level was not associated with a significantly increased risk of oral cleft defects or childhood leukemia or non-Hodgkin's lymphoma.

In the NORD-TEST study—also described in the benzene section—there were no significant associations between prenatal maternal exposure or paternal exposure to TCE in the year prior to birth and the risk of testicular germ cell tumors in men ages 14–49 years in Finland, Norway, and Sweden combined. However, there was an increased risk of testicular germ cell tumors for Finnish men with prenatal paternal exposure to PCE (OR=2.42, 95% CI 1.32–4.41) (Le Cornet et al., 2017).

Animal Studies

The Volume 2 committee did not report on any studies of developmental effects in animals following prenatal exposure to PCE.

NRC (2009) concluded that animal studies supported the epidemiologic findings for the most part. The NRC committee stated that "the toxicologic data provide strong evidence that neither solvent is associated with congenital malformations in rats"; however, it continued, other animal studies in rats "exposed to PCE prenatally or postnatally suggest that there may be sensitive windows for neurobehavioral impairment during development" (NRC, 2009).

EPA (2012) reported on a two-generation inhalation study in rats conducted by Tinston (1994). Decreased pup weights and reduced postnatal survival were seen in both generations, and behavioral alterations were observed in the F1 pups. One of the indications that in utero exposure has effects on prenatal survival was an increased degree of pre- and post-implantation loss that was seen in rats, mice, and rabbits (Schwetz et al., 1975; Szakmáry et al., 1997). In rats the oral administration of 900 mg/kg/day of PCE on GDs 6–13 resulted in an increased risk of micro/anophthalmia in the offspring. Rats exposed prenatally to PCE via inhalation also exhibited altered neurological function (Nelson et al., 1980; Szakmáry et al., 1997; Tinston, 1994) and reductions in brain acetylcholine and dopamine (Nelson et al., 1980). Several of the animal studies of reproductive and developmental effects cited by EPA had substantial limitations, including a lack of a dose response because of the use of only one treatment level and also a lack of reporting details. Nevertheless, EPA found that the PCE "database included assessments of the various potential manifestations of developmental toxicity, i.e., alterations in survival, growth, morphology, and functional development" (EPA, 2012).

The animals studies cited by ATSDR (2014) had several developmental toxicity endpoints such as alterations in fetal survival, growth, morphology (skeletal ossification in mice), and functional development, which were also described in the EPA review. ATSDR reported that delayed skeletal development was observed in rats and mice exposed to concentrations of 300–664 ppm PCE during gestation. Gestational exposure to 900 ppm PCE was associated with behavioral and neurochemical alterations in some rat offspring.

The Volume 11 committee did not find any new animal studies on the developmental effects of PCE.

Synthesis and Conclusions

The reproductive and development effects of PCE, like those of TCE, have been reviewed by several governmental and other organizations, including NRC, EPA, and ATSDR. Although PCE is a widely used solvent, particularly for dry cleaning, there is a dearth of information on its reproductive and developmental effects.

Reproductive Effects

The reproductive effects of PCE on males are unclear, and there are relatively few studies on which to base conclusions, although Eskenazi et al. (1991b) found that PCE had adverse effects on sperm quality. Studies of the effects of PCE exposure on female reproduction are also scarce. The adverse pregnancy outcomes reported in several occupational studies are not consistent. Although some studies in Scandinavian populations suggest that maternal occupational exposure to PCE may increase the risk of spontaneous abortion, studies in a Massachusetts residential population found no association between PCE in drinking water and spontaneous abortion, birth weight, or gestational age. NRC and ATSDR found that the data were insufficient to draw any conclusions on the effects of PCE on reproductive endpoints, and EPA found that there were no associations between maternal or paternal occupational exposure to PCE and an increased incidence of adverse pregnancy outcomes.

The new studies reviewed by the Volume 11 committee found no increase in adverse pregnancy outcomes, although a study of the Massachusetts population (discussed above) reported that exposures higher than the cumulative median concentration (28.9 g) increased the risk of stillbirth and placental abruption (Carwile et al., 2014). Animal studies were inconsistent concerning the effects of PCE that they reported on sperm, male or female fertility, and birth outcomes, and there were species differences.

The Volume 11 committee finds that there is inadequate/insufficient evidence to determine whether an association exists between exposure to PCE and reproductive effects in men or women, or with adverse pregnancy outcomes.

Developmental Effects

Numerous researchers have assessed the effects of prenatal exposure, primarily maternal, on developmental effects, including childhood cancers, birth defects, and neurodevelopmental deficits. Several studies looking for a link between childhood leukemia and prenatal exposure to PCE, usually from the maternal consumption of contaminated drinking water, did not find a significantly increased risk of the disease among children who had been prenatally exposed. However, prenatal exposure to PCE was associated with other developmental outcomes in children, including the risks of eye/ear anomalies and CNS/chromosomal/oral cleft abnormalities. Several studies of the Cape Cod, Massachusetts, population that consumed PCE-contaminated drinking water found that mothers' consumption of contaminated water was associated with a slight but significant increase in risky behaviors (e.g., smoking, alcohol use) in their children. Although prenatal exposure was associated with increases in neurobehavioral outcomes, none of the associations reached significance (Aschengrau et al., 2012; Janulewicz et al., 2012), nor was there an effect on brain morphology in the exposed children (Janulewicz et al., 2013). Animal studies generally support the findings in humans of birth defects and altered neurological function in offspring who were exposed, or whose parents were exposed, to PCE.

The Volume 11 committee concludes that there is limited/suggestive evidence of an association between prenatal exposure to PCE and developmental effects.

TABLE 7-6 Summary of Reproductive and Developmental Effects of Tetrachloroethylene

Study	Design/Population	Exposure	Results
Reproductive Effects			
Carwile et al. (2014)	Cohort—Cape Cod, MA. 1,766 pregnancies in Cape Cod. 834 PCE-exposed and 932 unexposed. 1969–1983 (See Aschengrau et al., 2015)	PCE-contaminated drinking water in Cape Cod, MA, 1969–1990. Exposure status based on maps of the pipe distribution network surrounding the birth residence with a leaching and transport model to determine final PCE exposure delivered to each residence. Average monthly PCE exposure during the last menstrual period year ranged from 0–89.2 g (median=0.9 g) and cumulative PCE exposure before the last menstrual period month and year ranged from 0–3,600 g (median=28.9 g) among exposed pregnancies. Analyses did not differentiate between prenatal and early childhood exposure.	Adverse pregnancy outcomes (ischemic placental diseases: birth weight and gestational age determined from birth certificates; placental abruption or separation, preeclampsia, vaginal bleeding were self-reported). Average monthly PCE exposure during the last menstrual period year was not associated with overall ischemic placental disease: for PCE ≥sample median (0.57 g–132 g) versus no exposure, RR=0.90, 95% CI 0.65–1.24; placental abruption RR=1.35, 95% CI 0.68–2.67; preeclampsia RR=0.36, 95% CI 0.12–1.07; SGA RR=0.98, 95% CI 0.66–1.45; stillbirth RR=2.38, 95% CI 1.01–5.59. Adjusted for hypertension before or during pregnancy, smoking, parity, and previous ischemic placental disease, maternal age, year pregnancy ended, gestational weight gain (varied by outcomes).
Ruckart et al. (2014)	Cohort—11,896 infants born to women who consumed contaminated drinking water at the Marine Corps base Camp Lejeune, NC. 1968–1985	PCE-contaminated drinking water at Camp Lejeune. Exposure estimates based on place of residence and fate and transport models. Exposure for entire pregnancy was stratified to 5 levels: no exposure, low (>0–<35.8 ppb), medium (≥35.8–<52.7 ppb), medium-high (≥52.7–81.4), and high exposure (≥81.4 ppb) for SGA and PTBs; levels for term LBW and birth weight were no exposure, low (>0–<35.9 ppb), medium (≥35.9–<52.6 ppb), medium-high (≥52.6–80.7 ppb), and high (≥81.4 ppb).	Adverse pregnancy outcomes (PTB, SGA, LBW, mean birth weight deficit from birth certificates). PCE exposure over entire pregnancy not associated with LBW. SGA low OR=1.0, 95% CI 0.9–1.2; medium OR=1.2, 95% CI 1.0–1.4; medium-high OR=1.0, 95% CI 0.8–1.2; high RR=1.0, 95% CI 0.8–1.2. PTB low OR=1.0, 95% CI 0.9–1.2; medium OR=0.9, 95% CI 0.7–1.1; medium-high OR=0.8, 95% CI 0.6–1.0; high OR=1.3, 95% CI 1.0–1.6. Mean birth weight difference (grams) low md=4.4, 95% CI 17.4–26.1; medium md= –28.5, 95% CI –55.1– –1.9; medium-high md=3.8, 95% CI –28.3–36.0; high md=8.2, 95% CI –29.5–46.0. Adjusted for prenatal care, sex of child, mother's race, mother's age, mothers' education, parity, mother had a previous fetal death, father's age, and rank of military member.

continued

TABLE 7-6 Continued

Study	Design/Population	Exposure	Results
Developmental Effects			
Janulewicz et al. (2013)	Cohort—Cape Cod, MA. 42 subjects who were exposed to PCE prenatally and underwent structural MRI (26 exposed and 16 unexposed); average age 30 years. (See Aschengrau et al., 2015)	PCE-contaminated drinking water in Cape Cod, MA, 1969–1983. Exposure status based on maps of the pipe distribution network surrounding the birth residence with a leaching and transport model to determine final PCE exposure delivered to each residence. Among exposed individuals, PCE levels ranged 0.4–1,255 g during the prenatal exposure period and 0.7–3,413 g during the postnatal exposure period.	Brain structure. No statistically significant differences between the exposed and unexposed groups on measures of white matter hypointensities, total cerebral white matter volume, total cerebellum white matter volume, total cerebral gray matter volume, total cerebellum gray matter volume; or on measures of cingulate, entorhinal cortex, caudate, putamen, pallidum, hippocampal, amygdala, or accumbens volumes (all $p>0.05$). The parahippocampal gyrus was larger in exposed subjects ($\beta=473.6\ mm^3$, 95% CI 37.5–909.7, $p=0.03$) and the thalamus proper was also larger ($\beta=929.4\ mm^3$, 95% CI –14.7–1873.5, $p=0.05$).
Aschengrau et al. (2015)	Cohort—Cape Cod, MA. 1,512 children born in Cape Cod, 1968–1983 (831 participants with prenatal and early childhood exposure to PCE versus 547 participants with no exposure). (See Janulewicz et al., 2013; Carwile et al., 2014; Mahalingaiah et al., 2016)	PCE-contaminated drinking water in Cape Cod, MA, 1969–1983. Exposure status based on maps of the pipe distribution network surrounding the birth residence with a leaching and transport model to determine final PCE exposure delivered to each residence. Exposure estimated for prenatal period through age 5. Cumulative mean (SD) exposures were estimated to be 32.6 (88.6) and 109.0 (283.3) g, respectively, for prenatal (9 months) and early childhood (5 years). Analyses did not differentiate between prenatal and early childhood exposure.	Adult health assessed by questionnaire. No significant associations between any early life PCE exposure or exposure above the median and cancer, diabetes, hypertension, cardiovascular disease, epilepsy, obesity, color blindness, near-sightedness, or dry eyes (all $p>0.05$).

Study	Design/Population	Exposure	Results
Mahalingaiah et al. (2016)	Cohort—Cape Cod, MA. 500 PCE exposed and 331 unexposed female children born 1969–1983 to mothers from Cape Cod. Enrollment 2006–2008. (See Aschengrau et al., 2015)	PCE-contaminated drinking water in Cape Cod, MA, 1969–1983. Exposure status based on maps of the pipe distribution network surrounding the birth residence with a leaching and transport model to determine final PCE exposure delivered to each residence. Exposure estimated for prenatal period through age 5. Cumulative prenatal and early childhood exposure: mean=121.7 g, SD=268.4, median=32.6 g. Analyses did not differentiate between prenatal and early childhood exposure.	Female reproductive disorders in adult women assessed by questionnaire. For any PCE exposure: polycystic ovary syndrome RR=0.9, 95% CI 0.5–1.6); endometriosis RR=1.0, 95% CI 0.5–1.8); trouble getting pregnant RR=1.0, 95% CI 0.6–1.6; and miscarriage RR=0.9, 95% CI 0.6–1.4. Adjusted for child's age.
Stingone et al. (2016)	Cohort 201,559 children born between 1994 and 1998 who attended New York City public schools in third grade.	Average annual ambient PCE estimated from census tract for residence at birth and EPA's 1996 National Air Toxics Assessment. Categorized into low (range=0.84–9.2 $\mu g/m^3$) and high exposure (range=0.28–0.84 $\mu g/m^3$). The average PCE concentration was 0.68 mg/m^3 in the study area. Sensitivity analyses were conducted to assess impact on children who did not move from the census tract after birth. Analyses did not differentiate between prenatal and early childhood exposure.	Standardized test scores in third grade. Children with high exposures to both diesel PM and PCE had greater risk of failing to meet test-based standards for mathematics than children with lower levels of exposure to both pollutants (RR=1.1, 95% CI 1.07–1.12) and for children with greater exposure to PCE only (RR=1.03, 95% CI 1.00–1.06). Children with high exposure to PCE and diesel PM had greater risk of failing to meet test-based standards for English language arts than children with lower levels of exposure to both pollutants (RR=1.03, 95% CI 1.01–1.04); and for high PCE exposure only (RR=1.02, 95% CI 1.00–1.04). Sensivity analyses limited to students that did not move from the census tract after birth found no significant associations. Adjusted for maternal race, age, marital status, nativity, educational attainment, use of tobacco and/or alcohol during pregnancy, and primary payor for delivery; eligibility for school lunch program, days absent from third grade, blood lead level, neighborhood deprivation score.

continued

TABLE 7-6 Continued

Study	Design/Population	Exposure	Results
Heck et al. (2014)	Case-control—Air Pollution and Childhood Cancer Study of 69 cases of ALL and 46 cases of AML from California Cancer Registry versus 19,209 controls from California birth records, age <6 years and born from 1990–2007.	Children lived within 2 km (ALL) and 6 km (AML) of an air toxics monitoring station. PCE exposure estimated for each trimester and first year of life based on maternal residence at birth and air monitoring data.	Childhood leukemia. Analyses reported risks per IQR increase in PCE. ALL: 1st trimester OR=0.97, 95% CI 0.69–1.37; 2nd trimester OR=1.06, 95% CI 0.76–1.48; 3rd trimester OR=1.13, 95% CI 0.84–1.52; entire pregnancy OR=1.08, 95% CI 0.72–1.61; 1st year of life OR=1.21, 95% CI 0.75–1.96. AML: 1st trimester OR=1.02, 95% CI 0.73–1.41; 2nd trimester OR=1.06, 95% CI 0.82–1.38; 3rd trimester OR=1.11, 95% CI 0.90–1.36; entire pregnancy OR=1.16, 95% CI 0.75–1.80; 1st year of life OR=1.17, 95% CI 0.79–2.16. Adjusted for maternal race/ethnicity, birth year, parity, maternal birthplace, and neighborhood socioeconomic index.
Ruckart et al. (2013)	Nested case-control 12,493 births at Camp Lejeune, NC, 1968–1985. 15 NTDs, 23 oral clefts, 13 childhood hematopoietic cancers.	PCE-contaminated drinking water at Camp Lejeune, 1968–1985. Exposure estimates based on place of residence and fate and transport models. Maternal exposure to PCE during the first trimester of pregnancy was categorized as unexposed (ref); low (0–<44 ppb), high (≥44 ppb); above or below MCL (5 ppb); or any exposure.	Birth defects and childhood cancers with medical confirmation. NTDs: <MCL OR=3.7, 95% CI 1.0–14.1; >MCL OR=0.4, 95% CI 0.1–1.8; any exposure OR=0.8, 95% CI 0.3–2.5. Oral clefts: low OR=0.6, 95% CI 0.2–2.0; high OR=0.5, 95% CI 0.1–1.7; <MCL OR=1.0, 95% CI 0.2–4.4; >MCL OR=0.5, 95% CI 0.2–1.3; any exposure OR=0.6, 95% CI 0.2–1.4. Hematopoietic cancers: low OR=1.8, 95% CI 0.5–6.6; high OR=1.4, 95% CI 0.3–5.6; any exposure OR=1.6, 95% CI 0.5–4.8. Unadjusted results reported.

NOTE: ALL=acute lymphoblastic leukemia; AML=acute myeloid leukemia; CI=confidence interval; EPA=U.S. Environmental Protection Agency; IQR=interquartile ratio; LBW=low birth weight; MCL=maximum contaminant level; md=mean difference; MRI=magnetic resonance imaging; NTD=neural tube defect; OR=odds ratio; PCE=tetrachloroethylene; PM=particulate matter; PTB=preterm birth; RR=relative risk; SD=standard deviation; SGA=small for gestational age.

GLYCOLS AND GLYCOL ETHERS

The glycol ethers are a group of solvents classified on the basis of the alkyl ethers of one of two parent alcohols: the 2-carbon chain ethylene glycol or the 3-carbon chain propylene glycol. The glycol ethers include the following: glycol ethers (unspecified), ethylene glycol ethers, diethylene glycol, propylene glycol, ethylene glycol monomethyl ether (EGME, 2-methoxyethanol), ethylene glycol monoethyl ether (EGEE, 2-ethoxythanol), ethylene glycol monobutyl ether (EGBE, 2-butoxyethanol), and propylene glycol monomethyl ether (PGME). Glycol ethers are commonly used industrially in paints and cleaners as well as in the manufacture of semiconductors; the latter source of exposure has been examined in several epidemiologic studies. Ethylene glycol monobutyl ether (EGBE, 2-butoxyethanol) is widely used as a solvent in protective surface coatings; as an ingredient in paint thinners and strippers, silicon caulks, cutting oils, hydraulic fluids; and as a degreaser (ATSDR, 1998). Propylene glycol is a colorless, odorless, water-soluble liquid used in commercial formulations of foods, drugs, and cosmetics and to generate artificial smoke. Propylene glycol is designated as a generally recognized as safe additive by the Food and Drug Administration (ATSDR, 1997). Ethylene glycol is a toxic chemical that is a component of antifreeze and hydraulic fluids (ATSDR, 2010).

Ethylene glycol monobutyl ether, diethylene glycol, diethylene glycol monobutyl ether, ethylene glycol, and propylene glycol were all sent to the Persian Gulf in quantities of greater than 1 kiloliter (see Table 7-1). The glycols and glycol ethers discussed in this chapter are listed in Table 7-7. The Volume 11 committee did not identify any information on the use of or quantities of glycols or glycol ethers that may have been sent to the Post-9/11 conflicts. The epidemiologic studies on the reproductive and developmental effects of glycols and glycol ethers reviewed below are summarized in Table 7-8 at the end of this section.

Toxic metabolites of glycols and glycol ethers are excreted in the urine (see Table 7-7). The metabolites include 2-methosxyacetic acid (2-MMA), a metabolite of EGME; ethoxyacetic acid (EAA), glycolic acid, and oxalic acid, which are metabolites of ethylene glycol; and 2-butoxyacetic acid, a metabolite of 2-butoxyethanol. Propylene glycol may be detected in serum and urine with an elimination half-life following oral exposure of about 4 hours; it degrades in the body in about 48 hours (ATSDR, 1997). The differing toxicity of the glycols and glycol ethers is thought to be due to their metabolites (IOM, 2003).

TABLE 7-7 Glycols and Glycol Ethers Discussed in the Chapter

Chemical Name	Abbreviation	Urinary Metabolites
Ethylene glycol		Glycolic acid Oxalic acid Ethoxyacetic acid (EAA)
Propylene glycol		
Diethylene glycol	DEG	
Ethylene glycol monomethyl ether (2-methoxyethanol)	EGME	2-methoxyacetic acid (2-MMA)
Ethylene glycol monoethyl ether (2-ethoxyethanol)	EGEE	
Ethylene glycol monobutyl ether (2-butoxyethanol)	EGBE	
Propylene glycol monomethyl ether	PGME	
Diethylene glycol monobutyl ether	DEGBE	

Reproductive Effects

Reproductive Effects in Men and Women

The Volume 2 committee reported on the effects that glycols and glycol ethers had on reproduction in exposed men and women, including semen characteristics and fertility. Most of the studies of these effects were small, and the participants had concurrent exposures to other chemicals. Veulemans et al. (1993) examined semen characteristics in 1,019 men occupationally exposed to ethylene glycol ethers who had been clinically diagnosed as infertile or subfertile, with 475 male patients of the same clinic who were diagnosed as fertile serving as controls. The authors found no association between urinary EAA and abnormal semen characteristics; they suggested that the results might be due to a latent period between exposure and the time when observable effects are seen. In another occupational case-control study, Ratcliffe et al. (1989) found decreases in mean sperm count in workers exposed to EGME at a metal-casting company, but no marked changes in sperm motility, structure, or velocity or in testicular volume after adjustments had been made for many potential confounders; the study had low statistical power. Welch et al. (1988) examined exposure to the ethylene glycol ethers—EGME and EGEE—among shipyard painters and found a higher prevalence of oligospermia and azoospermia and a higher, but nonsignificant, risk of decreased sperm count per ejaculate in the exposed group (OR=1.85, 95% CI 0.6–5.6); again, no important differences were found in sperm structure, motility, or viability.

The Volume 11 committee identified two new studies on the effects of glycol ethers on male reproductive function. The committee notes that in both studies there was concurrent occupational exposure to other chemicals, thus making interpretation of the results difficult.

In a study of 109 men in Paris, France, 48 of whom had occupational exposure to glycol ethers, Multigner et al. (2007) assessed the urinary levels of glycol metabolites. The men provided semen samples 2 to 3 months after they had provided urine samples. Compared with controls, sperm concentration, total sperm count, the percentage of rapid progressive sperm, and the percentage of morphologically normal sperm were significantly lower in the exposed group ($p<0.001$), although there were no differences in semen pH or sperm viability. Serum testosterone, LH, and inhibin B concentrations were similar in the two groups. FSH concentration was not significantly increased in the exposed group. Exposure to high levels of glycol ethers was associated with a significantly increased risk of a low percentage of rapid progressive sperm motility (OR=10.2, 95% CI 1.3–82.5), whereas no significant associations were observed for low sperm concentration, a low percentage of morphologically normal sperm, low seminal volume, or low total progressive sperm motility.

Cherry et al. (2008) reported a case-referent study of 2,118 men attending fertility clinics in the United Kingdom. Self-reports of exposure were reviewed by an industrial hygienist who estimated the men's level of exposure to solvents, particularly glycol ethers, in the 3 months prior to their clinic visits. Exposure to higher levels of glycol ethers was associated with an increased risk of low motile sperm concentration: low exposure (OR=0.93 95% CI 0.74–1.17); moderate exposure (OR=1.65 95% CI 1.06–2.54); and high exposure (OR=2.54 95% CI 1.23–5.27). Exposure to low or high levels of other VOCs was not significantly associated with low motile sperm concentrations, although moderate exposure was (OR=1.55, 95% CI 1.10–2.18).

Male and female workers in the semiconductor industry are known to be exposed to ethylene glycol ethers. The Volume 2 committee examined several studies of reproductive effects, primarily TTP, in these workers. Solvent-exposed male workers at an Italian mint (Figa-Talamanca et al., 2000) did not have a significantly elevated risk of a conception delay of more than 6 months (OR=1.69, 95% CI 0.62–4.62). Samuels et al. (1995) found no increases in TTP in a subset of workers (FR=1.03, 95% CI 0.70–1.51) in whom exposure to ethylene glycol ethers was of particular concern.

Correa et al. (1996) examined the extent of subfertility (defined as taking more than 1 year to conceive) in six female workers and for 561 pregnancies of wives of male workers. In the female employees, there was a significantly increased risk of subfertility (OR=4.6, 95% CI 1.6–13.3), but not in the wives of male workers (OR=1.7, 95% CI 0.7–4.3).

ATSDR (2010) did not identify any studies on reproductive effects in humans after the inhalation of or oral exposure to ethylene glycol. The ATSDR *Toxicological Profile for Propylene Glycol* (1997) was included in the Volume 2 deliberations, although that committee concluded that any reproductive effects reported in that profile were inconclusive. The profile did not include any human studies of reproductive effects following exposure to propylene glycol. In the 1998 report *Toxicological Profile for 2-Butoxyethanol and 2-Butoxyethanol Acetate*, ATSDR reported that there were no data on whether 2-butoxyethanol (EGBE) or 2-butoxyethanol acetate caused reproductive effects in humans.

The Volume 11 committee identified one new study on the association between women's exposure to glycol ethers (primarily from cosmetics use) and TTP (Garlantezec et al., 2013). In a study on the PELAGIE cohort in France, the researchers measured glycol ether metabolites in the urine of 519 pregnant women; the samples were collected before 19 weeks of pregnancy. TTP information was collected at the beginning of the pregnancy. Both butoxyacetic and phenoxyacetic acids, which are both glycol ether metabolites, were detected in 93% of the urine samples; however, only the fourth-quartile concentration of phenoxyacetic acid (≥1.38 mg/L) was significantly associated with an increased TTP (OR=0.70, 95% CI 0.52–0.95).

Adverse Pregnancy Outcomes

The Volume 2 committee (IOM, 2003) considered two epidemiologic studies on pregnancy and birth outcomes performed with a cohort of female semiconductor workers exposed to ethylene glycol ethers (particularly in the fabrication process) and other chemicals. A study of 152 fabrication and 251 non-fabrication female workers at two semiconductor manufacturing plants found nonsignificantly reduced fecundability (longer TTP) in a subset of those with exposure to ethylene glycol ethers (FR=0.37, 95% CI 0.11–1.19) (Eskenazi et al., 1995). Women were followed for an average of five menstrual cycles, and daily urine samples were analyzed to confirm clinical spontaneous abortions and early fetal losses. In a large study by Swan et al. (1995; cited but not discussed in *Volume 2*), 891 women who worked in semiconductor fabrication were asked whether they had experienced a spontaneous abortion. Exposure to glycol ethers and other chemicals during the first trimester of pregnancy was assessed on the basis of job descriptions. The risk of spontaneous abortion was significantly increased for fabrication workers with the greatest predicted exposure to ethylene glycol ether (RR=2.67, 95% CI 1.33–5.36), and there was no increase associated with exposure to propylene glycol ether. Correa et al. (1996), discussed in the previous section, noted a trend for an increased risk of spontaneous abortion with higher exposures to glycol ethers.

The Volume 11 committee did not identify any new studies on adverse pregnancy outcomes in association with exposure to glycol ethers.

Animal Studies

The Volume 2 committee (IOM, 2003) noted that the evidence from animal studies indicated that exposure to ethylene glycol ethers was associated with testicular atrophy, decreased sperm motility, and abnormal sperm structure in rats, mice, and rabbits (Bruckner and Warren, 2001). It also reviewed studies of the oral toxicity of three ethylene glycol ethers—EGME, EGEE, EGBE—in rats and mice in 2-week and 13-week drinking water studies conducted by the National Toxicology Program (Dieter, 1993). The rats were estimated to have consumed 100–400 mg/kg of EGME, 200–1,600 mg/kg of EGEE, and 70–300 mg/kg of EGBE; mice consumed 200–1,300 mg/kg of EGME, 400–2,800 mg/kg of EGEE, and 90–1,400 mg/kg of EGBE. There was testicular atrophy in the males of both species for both EGME and EGEE; no other effects on reproductive organs in either species at any dose were reported for the three solvents. In the 13-week studies, rats received 750–6,000 ppm EGME, 1,250–20,000 ppm EGEE, or 750–6,000 ppm EGBE, and mice received 2,000–10,000 ppm EGME, 2,500–40,000 ppm EGEE, or 750–6,000 ppm EGBE. Rats and mice receiving EGME or EGEE—but not EGBE—had histopathologic changes in the testes; a more severe degeneration of the germinal epithelium in the seminiferous tubules of the testes was observed with EGME exposure in both species. Some ovarian and uterine atrophy was observed in both rats and mice administered EGEE and EGME, but almost entirely at the highest dose levels tested (Dieter, 1993).

ATSDR (1998) reported on several animal studies with EGBE, none of which showed reproductive effects in male or female animals following inhalation exposure. ATSDR (2010) discussed several animal studies of reproductive effects and exposure to ethylene glycol. Testis and uterine weights and histopathology were not affected in mice treated with ethylene glycol for 4 consecutive days and evaluated 1 day later (Hong et al., 1988). However, intermediate-duration oral exposure to ethylene glycol in three multigenerational studies (one in rats and two in mice) and several shorter exposure studies (15–20 days in rats and mice) resulted in effects on fertility, fetal viability, and male reproductive organs in mice, although not in rats.

ATSDR (1997) included one long-term inhalation study of propylene glycol in rats that showed no adverse effects on the ability to produce live young or on the survival of the offspring.

The Volume 11 committee considered 13 animal studies on the male reproductive effects of a variety of ethylene glycols and glycol ethers, particularly EGME. In 2- and 13-week repeat-dose oral toxicity studies in rats, Johnson et al. (2005) found that diethylene glycol monobutyl ether (DEGBE) administered in drinking water at 0, 50, 250, or 1,000 mg/kg/day had no effect on sperm parameters or testis histopathology.

As part of an in vitro fertilization assay, Berger et al. (2000) found that 50–100 mg EGME/kg reduced the sperm fertilizing capacity for zone-free oocytes in male rats but that sperm motility was not affected. In another study of the male reproductive toxicity, Watanabe et al. (2000) administered EGME daily at 100 and 200 mg/kg/day for 2 weeks or 100 mg/kg/day for 4 weeks to 6- and 8-week-old male rats. In the 2-week, 200 mg/kg and 4-week, 100 mg/kg groups, testis and epididymis weights were decreased, and a histopathological examination showed severe degenerative changes in the testis, such as an atrophy of the seminiferous tubules and multinucleated giant cell formation in all the rats in the 2-week, 200 mg/kg group, while at 100 mg/kg/days both the 2-week and 4-week groups had a degeneration of pachytene spermatocytes which underwent apoptotic death, with a resulting decrease in the number of germ cells. EGME (200 mg/kg) administered orally to male rats for 3, 6, or 14 days resulted in the degeneration of spermatocytes in late-stage tubules and spermatocyte depletion at day 4, with the severity of effects increasing with prolonged exposure (Enright et al., 2013).

Yoon et al. (2003) found that EGEE, administered via gavage to male rats at 0, 100, 200, 400, and 800 mg/kg body weight/day for 4 weeks, was associated with decreases in the weight of the testis and epididymis and in the number of testicular cells as well as an exfoliation of germ cells into the tubular lumen at doses of ≥200 mg/kg, and with testicular degeneration at a dose of 400 mg/kg. EGEE also reduced sperm motility in both the cauda epididymis and the "spermaduct" when given to rats at 600 mg/kg for 5 weeks (Wang et al., 2006). Doses of 0, 100, 200, and 400 mg/kg EGEE administered orally by gavage to male rats for 14 consecutive days caused significant alterations in glutathione levels, superoxide dismutase catalase activities, malondialdehyde levels, glutathione-S-transferase and lactate dehydrogenase activities in the testes and spermatozoa with severe degeneration of the testes, and a significant decrease in daily sperm production and in the number of epididymal and testicular spermatozoa and sperm. EGEE also significantly increased the total spermatozoa abnormalities without affecting the spermatozoa live-dead ratio at all dose levels when compared with the control group (Adedara and Farombi, 2010).

Mechanistic studies of EGME in male rats that were exposed to 30 or 100 mg/kg/day for 1, 4, and 14 days found that the higher dose produced testicular damage at 14 days. An analysis of the metabolites in serum, urine, liver, and testis suggested that EGME may induce toxicity via the inhibition of flavoprotein dehydrogenase-catalyzed reactions (Takei et al., 2010).

Several studies examined the effect of EGME or its metabolite 2-MMA on gene expression. Bagchi et al. (2010) assessed the effect of 2-MMA on cultured mouse testicular TM3 Leydig cells after 3, 8, and 24 hours of treatment. Progressive changes in gene expression were seen as consistent with a reproductive system disease. In another study, 6 hours after male rats received single oral doses of 50 or 2,000 mg/kg EGME, a slight degeneration of the spermatocytes was observed in rats given the high, but not the low, dose. Significant increases in three spermatogenesis-related genes—*heat shock protein 70-2*, *insulin growth factor binding protein 3*, and *glutathione S transferase*—were detected prior to the appearance of obvious pathological changes in the testis at the 2,000 mg/kg dose (Fukushima et al., 2005). Fukushima et al. (2011) found similar results when male rats were treated with 50 or 2,000 mg/kg EGME for 6 or 24 hours. Again, no changes in the testis were observed at 50 mg, but at 2,000 mg/kg there was a slight decrease of phacytene spermatocytes at 6 hr and a severe decrease at 24 hr. After 24 hr, significant changes in marker genes involved in spermatogenesis were observed: miR-449a and miR-92a decreased, and miR-320, miR-134 and miR-188 increased, while only miR-760-5p increased after 6 hr. Matsuyama et al. (2018) gave male rats single doses of 200, 600, or 2,000 mg/kg EGME and studied the resulting changes in the transcript levels of genes, including spermatocyte-specific genes. The two higher doses of EGME caused dose-dependent testicular toxicity, including the degeneration and necrosis of spermatocytes, and this injury correlated with decreased spermatocyte-specific gene expression. Specific gene expression changes were for *Pbk* (0.11- and 0.05-fold changes at 600 and 2,000 mg/kg, respectively); *Phf2* (0.11- and 0.09-fold changes at 600 and 2,000 mg/kg, respectively); *Prok2* (0.13- and 0.09-fold changes at 600 and 2,000 mg/kg, respectively); and *Mllt*10 (0.18- and 0.12-fold changes at 600 and 2,000 mg/kg, respectively). An analysis of upstream regulators suggested that oxidative stress, protein kinase activation, and histone acetylation, but not decreased testicular testosterone, were involved in the EGME-induced spermatocyte toxicity.

Sakurai et al. (2015) studied gene expression changes in the testis of cynomolgus monkeys following oral administration of EGME at 0 or 300 mg/kg for 4 days. All the monkeys given the 300 mg/kg dose had testicular toxicity, as demonstrated by decreases in pachytene spermatocytes and round spermatids. Sixteen down-regulated and 347 up-regulated miRNAs were detected in the testis. Levels of miR-1228 and miR-2861 increased in the testis of EGME-treated animals, which the authors state reflects recovery from EGME-induced testicular damages via the stimulation of cell proliferation and the differentiation of sperm.

For female reproduction, ATSDR (1997) reported that in rats exposed to propylene glycol in drinking water there were no adverse effects on any measure of reproduction, including the number of litters, litter size, pup weight, or sex ratio, even at the highest dose, nor was there any effect on the reproductive capacity of the offspring from the high-dose group. Some female rats and rabbits that breathed in large amounts of EGBE while they were pregnant delivered fewer offspring than pregnant rats or rabbits that were not exposed; the doses also produced maternal toxicity. The live offspring of these exposed mothers did not exhibit any adverse effects. EGMBE did not produce other developmental effects in the offspring of animals exposed via inhalation at doses that did not produce maternal toxicity (ATSDR, 1998). ATSDR (2010) reported that inhaled ethylene glycol in mice and rats resulted in effects on implant viability and live fetal weight, although no dose–response relationships were provided. Nose-only studies also showed reduced live fetal body weight, although ATSDR considered the results to be inconclusive for inhalation exposure because of the confounding caused by concomitant oral exposure. ATSDR also reported that intermediate-duration oral exposure to ethylene glycol included decreased the body weights of pups.

The Volume 11 committee identified several new studies on the effects of glycol ethers or ethylene glycols on female reproduction in animal models. The reproductive toxicity of diethylene glycol (DEG) was studied in a continuous breeding study in CD-1 mice (Williams et al., 1990). The animals were administered 0, 0.35, 1.75, and 3.5% w/v DEG for 14 weeks in drinking water; the doses were such that the highest dose was estimated to reduce body weight by 10%, the middle dose would produce no or minimal toxicity, and the lowest dose was the estimated no-observed effect level. At 3.5% DEG, breeding pairs of animals had significantly decreased numbers of litters per pair, live pups per litter, the proportion of pups born alive, live pup weight, and the numbers of pairs producing third, fourth, and fifth litters; this dose also resulted in a significant increase in the cumulative days to litter.

The toxicity of EGME to the ovary was studied by Dodo et al. (2009) in rats that received 0, 30, 100, or 300 mg/kg for 2 or 4 weeks (repeated-dose toxicity studies) or the same doses for 2 weeks prior to mating, during mating, and until day 6 of pregnancy (fertility study). Continuous diestrus and alterations of ovarian morphology were observed for doses ≥100 mg/kg at both 2 and 4 weeks regardless of period of administration. In the fertility study, doses ≥100 mg/kg resulted in irregular estrous cycles, prolonged mating periods, lower pregnancy rates, and decreased corpora lutea of pregnancy.

Weng et al. (2010) administered via gavage approximately 0 mg/kg/day, 80 mg/kg/day, 118 mg/kg/day, or 310 mg/kg/day of EGME to 6-week-old female Swiss CD-1 mice for 7 days. The mice were then induced to ovulate and mated with nonexposed males. There were no significant differences among the dose groups in terms of the number of pups per litter, oocyte apoptosis ratios, or the number of retrieved oocytes following the induction of ovulation, although there was greater variance in the number of pups per litter in the highest-dose group. The cumulus-oocyte complex apoptosis ratios were significantly different across the groups ($p \leq 0.001$), although the response was not dose-dependent. Berger et al. (2000) reported that EGME (0.15–0.25% in drinking water) administered to female rats for 14 days reduced the number of ovulated oocytes in an in vitro fertilization study.

Ballantyne and Snellings (2005) studied the reproductive toxicity of DEG in CD-1 mice and CD rats. Pregnant mice received 0 (distilled water), 559, 2,795, or 11,180 mg/kg/day, and pregnant rats received 0, 1,118, 4,472, and 8,944 mg/kg/day on GDs 6–15. At the highest doses in both species there was no effect on implantations, although there was maternal toxicity and reduced fetal body weights.

Developmental Effects

The Volume 2 committee also reviewed studies on parental exposure to glycols and the risk of childhood cancer. Feingold et al. (1992) found that paternal exposure to DEG in the year before birth was associated with a nonsignificant increase in the risk of ALL (OR=1.4, 95% CI 0.4–4.5) and of childhood brain cancer (OR=1.3, 95% CI 0.3–5.2).

Volume 2 (IOM, 2003) included a study of the occupational and hobby-related exposures experienced from 3 months before to 3 months after conception (periconception) by mothers of children with neural tube defects and controls in selected California counties (Shaw et al., 1999b). Periconceptional maternal exposure, based on mothers' reports of activities, to glycol ethers was associated with a nonsignificant

OR of 0.93 (95% CI 0.66–1.3). Other congenital malformations were studied by Cordier et al. (1997) and Lorente et al. (2000). Cordier et al. (1997) examined maternal exposure to glycol ethers during the first trimester of pregnancy using a job-exposure matrix. There was a significantly increased risk for congenital malformations (OR=1.44, 95% CI 1.10–1.90), particularly for first-trimester exposures and neural tube defects (OR=1.94, 95% CI 1.16–3.24), spina bifida (OR=2.37, 95% CI 1.22–4.62), cleft lip (OR=2.03, 95% CI 1.11–3.73), and multiple anomalies (OR=2.00, 95% CI 1.24–3.23). Similarly increased risks were seen in a study of first-trimester maternal occupational exposure to glycol ethers and cleft lip with or without cleft palate (OR=2.10, 95% CI 1.14–3.88), although the risk for cleft palate alone was not significant (OR=1.82, 95% CI 0.82–4.03) (Lorente et al., 2000).

ATSDR (2010) found that there were no additional studies on the developmental toxicity of ethylene glycol in humans.

The Volume 11 committee found one new study of the PELAGIE mother–child cohort in Brittany, France (Cordier et al., 2012). The association between solvent exposure (as determined by the presence of urinary metabolites of glycol ethers) and congenital malformations was assessed among a subset of 3,421 women who returned the inclusion questionnaire before 19 weeks of gestation; pregnancy outcomes were obtained from the maternity hospital records for 3,399 pregnancies (n=79 cases, 580 controls). Although several of the metabolites were associated with an increased risk of some form of congenital malformation, none of the increases were significant except for the metabolite EAA, which was associated with an increased risk of oral clefts (OR=10.9, 95% CI 2.4–50) and major limb malformation (OR=3.1, 95% CI 1.1–8.2), and 2-methoxypropionic acid, which was associated with a significantly increased risk of any malformation (OR=2.9, 95% CI 1.2–6.8) and of urinary tract malformations (OR=5.3, 95% CI 1.0–27.2). The committee notes that the number of cases for many of the malformations was small, making it difficult to generalize to a larger population.

In another analysis of the PELAGIE cohort, Béranger et al. (2017) measured urinary concentrations of glycol ethers metabolites in 204 women in the first 19 weeks of pregnancy and assessed neurocognitive abilities in their children at 6 years of age using the Wechsler Intelligence Scale for Children (WISC) Verbal Comprehension Index and Developmental Neuropsychological Assessment (NEPSY) battery (Design Copying and Arrows). Of the five glycol ether metabolites measured in maternal urine (2-butoxyacetic acid, EAA, EEAA, MAA, and phenoxyacetic acid), only two of them were associated with any differences in WISC or NEPSY scores: children of mothers in the highest tertile of urinary phenoxyacetic acid scored significantly lower on the WISC Verbal Comprehension test (β [third versus first tertile]= –6.53, 95% CI –11.44– –1.62) and children of mothers with higher concentrations of EAA scored lower on the NEPSY Design Copying subtest (β [third versus first tertile]= –0.11, 95% CI –0.21– –0.00).

Animal Studies

The Volume 2 committee did not report on animal studies of glycol ethers and ethylene glycols.

ATSDR (2010) reviewed several animal studies on the developmental toxicity of ethylene glycol via inhalation, oral, and dermal exposures in acute-duration studies and by oral exposure in intermediate-duration studies. The acute oral studies indicated that developmental effects—skeletal variation and total malformations—may occur in mice and rats. Ethylene glycol did not appear to be teratogenic in rabbits at maternally lethal doses or to be a developmental toxicant via dermal exposure. ATSDR reported that inhaled ethylene glycol in mice and rats produced effects similar to those seen with oral dosing but noted that all the studies were confounded by the concurrent ingestion of ethylene glycol deposited on the fur. Whole-body inhalation studies resulted in visceral and skeletal malformations in both rats and mice, although dose–response relationships were lacking. Nose-only studies also showed a significant increase in fused ribs, but confounding factors rendered the studies inconclusive. ATSDR found that the developmental effects of intermediate-duration oral exposure to ethylene glycol included kidney effects in offspring.

The Volume 11 committee reviewed the findings of developmental toxicity studies of several ethylene glycols and glycol ethers not cited by ATSDR. The exposure of pregnant rats and rabbits to EGEE, but not to PGME, caused fetal cardiovascular and skeletal abnormalities in both species at levels that did not result in maternal toxicity (Bruckner and Warren, 2001).

Ballantyne and Snellings (2005) studied the developmental toxicity of DEG in CD-1 mice and CD rats to determine the no-observed effect level. Pregnant mice received 0 (distilled water), 559, 2,795, and 11,180 mg/kg/day, and pregnant rats received 0, 1,118, 4,472, and 8,944 mg/kg/day on GDs 6–15. There was maternal toxicity at the highest doses in both species. There were no increases in fetal variations or malformations at any dose in mice. The highest dose in rats results in reduced fetal body weights. DEG did not affect fetal external or visceral variations; however, at the two highest doses there were significantly increased skeletal variations. There were no indications of embryotoxicity or teratogenic effects at any dose in either species.

In the Weng et al. (2010) study of the generational effects of EGME, 4- to 6-week-old female Swiss CD-1 mice were administered via gavage approximately 0 mg/kg/day, 80 mg/kg/day, 118 mg/kg/day, and 310 mg/kg/day of EGME for 7 days. Mice were induced to ovulate and then mated with nonexposed males. Female F1 offspring were induced to ovulate, and their oocytes were evaluated. EGME has no effect on the number of retrieved oocytes following the induction of ovulation effects or on the oocyte apoptosis ratio, but there was a dose-dependent increase in the cumulus-oocyte complex apoptosis ratios in the female offspring who were not directly exposed to EGME. In an in vitro study, Dayan and Hales (2012) compared the teratogenic effects of EGME (3, 10, or 30 mM) and its metabolite 2-MMA on limb development in embryos on GD 12. Only the highest dose of EGME significantly decreased limb development (14% at 30mM), whereas all the concentrations of 2-MMA significantly decreased limb development in a dose-dependent manner (12% at 3 mM; 40% at 10 mM; 64% at 30 mM).

The reproductive effects of ethylene glycol were assessed in a three-generation study in rats. Dietary doses of 1.0, 0.2, and 0.04 g/kg/day were given over three generations of reproduction. Each generation was bred once, and the F2 males from the reproduction study were bred to three consecutive lots of untreated females at weekly intervals. Doses of up to 1.0 mg/kg/day did not produce any reproductive or dominant lethal effects (DePass et al., 1986). Carney et al. (2008) reported that although ethylene glycol is teratogenic in rats, it is not teratogenic in rabbits, possibly due to rabbits' slower metabolism of ethylene glycol to its teratogenic metabolite, glycolic acid.

Synthesis and Conclusions

Several glycols and glycol ethers were sent to the Persian Gulf, although neither the Volume 2 nor the Volume 11 committee had information on their specific uses in theater. Although there have been studies examining the reproductive and developmental effects of many of these chemicals, they tend to have limitations. In the case of epidemiologic studies, for example, the fact that occupational exposures were rarely to a single glycol or glycol ether makes it difficult to attribute any observed effects to a specific chemical. For many of the glycol ethers, there may be only a single study for any given agent, which makes it difficult to generalize effects to the class of chemicals.

Reproductive Effects

The Volume 11 committee considered two new studies of the effects of exposure to glycol ethers on sperm quality (Cherry et al., 2008; Multigner et al., 2007). These two studies, along with earlier studies cited in *Volume 2*, indicated that exposure to glycol ethers is associated with the impairment of at least one sperm parameter. Exposure to ethylene glycol was found not to affect sperm quality, although this was attributed to the lag between exposure and measurement. A number of animal studies have shown that oral and inhalation exposure of male animals to glycol ethers adversely affects semen quality and increases testicular atrophy.

Other studies of occupational exposure to glycol ethers reported that exposure to glycol ethers was not associated with increased TTP in male workers (Correa et al., 1996; Figa-Talamanca et al., 2000; Samuels et al., 1995) but was in female workers (Correa et al., 1996). One study in France of the effects in women also found an increased TTP, although only at the highest concentrations (Garlantezec et al., 2013). Animal studies indicated that exposure to glycol ethers could result in uterine and ovarian atrophy.

Studies of female workers in the semiconductor industry (Eskenazi et al., 1995; Swan et al., 1995) have indicated that exposure to ethylene glycol ethers may increase the risk of spontaneous abortion. ATSDR reported on several studies in both rats and mice that showed adverse pregnancy outcomes, such as reduced pup body weight, after exposure to ethylene glycol via inhalation. The animal studies identified by the Volume 11 committee also show that high exposure to glycol ethers may have adverse effects on several pregnancy outcomes, particularly birth weights.

The Volume 11 committee concludes that there is limited/suggestive evidence of an association between exposure to glycols and glycol ethers and reproductive effects in men.

The Volume 11 committee also concludes that there is inadequate/insufficient evidence to determine whether an association exists between exposure to glycols and glycol ethers and reproductive effects in women, or with adverse pregnancy outcomes.

Developmental Effects

The Volume 11 committee considered four studies that evaluated congenital malformations associated with preconception or periconception exposure to glycol ethers, with inconsistent results. Two studies found that maternal exposure to glycol ethers in the first trimester of pregnancy significantly increased the risk of having a child with a neural tube defect, spina bifida, or other birth defects such as cleft palate (Cordier et al., 1997; Lorente et al., 2000). However, Shaw et al. (1999b) did not find an increased risk of neural tube defects when mothers were exposed for 3 months before or 3 months after conception. The fourth study, by Cordier et al. (2012), examined a different cohort of mother–infant pairs and found no significant associations between exposure to glycol ethers in early pregnancy and congenital malformations, with the exception of exposure to two metabolites: exposure to EAA at the highest level was significantly associated with oral clefts and major limb malformations, and any level of exposure to 2-methoxypropionic acid was associated with all malformations and urinary tract malformations specifically. Women in the last study also had exposure to other solvents, such as TCE and PCE. A study of children in this French cohort at 6 years of age indicated that prenatal exposure to some glycol ether metabolites (e.g., EAA) may affect neurodevelopment (Béranger et al., 2017). These studies indicated that glycol ethers may be associated with birth defects, but further study is needed.

Animal studies have not supported an association between ethylene glycols and developmental effects, and they suggest that prenatal exposure to glycol ethers does not cause malformations in offspring except at very high doses. The studies were inconsistent with regard to the developmental toxicity of ethylene glycol in animals, and propylene glycol had no adverse effects on development in animal studies. A review of the toxicity of ethylene glycols indicated that they are unlikely to be reproductive toxicants or to be embryotoxic in humans at "environmentally relevant doses" and that they do not cause developmental effects at doses that do not cause significant maternal toxicity (Fowles et al., 2017).

The Volume 11 committee concludes that there is limited/suggestive evidence of an association between prenatal exposure to glycols or glycol ethers and birth defects.

The Volume 11 committee also concludes that there is inadequate/insufficient evidence to determine whether an association exists between prenatal exposure to glycols or glycol ethers and any other developmental effects.

TABLE 7-8 Summary of Reproductive and Developmental Effects of Ethylene Glycols and Glycol Ethers

Study	Design/Population	Exposure	Results
Reproductive Effects			
Multigner et al. (2007)	Cross-sectional 98 men employed at the Paris Municipality during 2000–2001 and ages 20–55 years. 48 men were exposed to GEs and 50 were unexposed.	Occupational exposure assessed by self-report about occupational exposure to glycol ethers for the past 10 years and urinary metabolites, collected 1 month apart, at the end of 2 working weeks; semen and blood samples were collected 2–3 months later. Workplace materials were assessed for GE content by investigators. Urine samples analyzed for GE metabolites: methoxyacetic acid, ethoxyacetic acid, butoxyacetic acid, n-propoxyacetic acid, phenoxyacetic acid, and methoxypropionic acid. Participants were assigned exposure indexes based on the reported frequency of use of GE-containing products. Categorized as currently nonexposed (reference group) versus currently exposed. Analyses limited to BAA and 2-MPA.	Semen quality. BAA and 2-MPA not correlated with any semen parameters or hormone levels. No differences between mean volume, pH, multiple anomaly index, viability, or hormones (testosterone, FSH, LH, inhibin B). Exposed men had greater decrements in sperm concentration (md=45.0, 95% CI 21.0–69.1), sperm count (md=138.8, 95% CI 37.7–240.0), and % normal morphology (md=7.1, 95% CI 0.8–13.4). Past high exposure associated with semen parameters based on World Health Organization reference values: seminal volume OR=1.0, 95% CI 1.0–1.1; sperm concentration OR=3.0, 95% CI 0.6–14.6; rapid progressive motility OR=10.2, 95% CI 1.3–82.5; total progressive motility OR=4.3, 95% CI 0.9–20.9; morphology OR=3.2, 95% CI 0.9–11.8. Not significant for all parameters and past moderate exposure.
Cherry et al. (2008)	Case-control 2,118 employed men were recruited from 14 fertility clinics across the United Kingdom, 1999–2002. 874 cases with low motile sperm concentrations versus 1,244 controls with normal sperm.	GE exposure assessed by self-report in questionnaires and interviews with review by an industrial hygienist. Exposure for the 3 months prior to providing the semen sample was designated as no (reference value), low, moderate, or high.	Male infertility. Exposure to increasing levels of GE was associated with increasing risk of low motile sperm concentration: low exposure OR=0.93 (95% CI 0.74–1.17); moderate exposure OR=1.65 (1.06–2.54); high exposure OR=2.54 (1.23–5.27). Adjusted for surgery to the testes, previous conception, use of alcohol, wearing boxer shorts, and center.
Garlantezec et al. (2013)	Cohort—PELAGIE study 519 pregnant women in Brittany, France in 2002–2006. (see Cordier et al., 2012)	Exposure assessed by urinary metabolites, collected at 19 weeks of gestation (MAA, EAA, BAA, PAA, PhAA, MEAA, EEAA, and 2-MPA). Categorized by above or below the limit of detection (0.05 mg/L), quartiles, or continuous.	TTP. PhAA detected in 93% of samples; it was associated with TTP (OR=0.95, 95% CI 0.90–1.00, p-trend=0.02). BAA detected in 93% of urine samples; it was not associated with an increased TTP (OR=0.96, 95% CI 0.70–1.34, p-trend=0.86). Other metabolites not significant.

continued

TABLE 7-8 Continued

Study	Design/Population	Exposure	Results
Developmental Effects			
Cordier et al. (2012)	Cohort— PELAGIE study 3,399 pregnant women in Brittany, France. 2002–2006. Nested case-control study: 79 cases of non-chromosomal, nongenetic major malformations versus 580 controls. (see Garlantezec et al., 2013)	Exposure assessed by self-reported residential and occupational exposure to solvents (29% reported occupational exposure) and job-exposure matrix. Nested case-control study: Exposure was based on urinary metabolites of glycol ethers collected around 19 weeks gestation (MAA, EAA, BAA, PAA, PhAA, MEAA, EEAA, and 2-MPA). Categorized by above or below the limit of detection (0.05 mg/L).	Birth defects (any malformation, oral clefts, urinary tract defects, limb defects, or male genital defects). MAA, MEAA, EAA, PAA, BAA, and PhAA not associated with any defects. EEAA: oral cleft OR=10.9, 95% CI 2.4–50; major limb malformation (OR=3.1, 95% CI 1.1–8.2); not significant for other defects. 2-MPA: any malformation OR=2.9, 95% CI 1.2–6.8; urinary tract malformations OR=5.3, 95% CI 1.0–27.2; not significant for other defects.
El-Zein et al. (2007)	Nested case-control 41 children of female Mexican factory workers exposed. 6 children exposed to EGME in utero versus 12 children born to mothers not exposed during pregnancy (children were born 1–10 years after mothers left the factory).	Women were exposed to EGME while working at a factory in 1970–1977. Exposure was in utero or preconception.	Telomere length in peripheral blood lymphocutes in children ages 10–28 years old. In utero exposed offspring had reduced telomeres compared with unexposed offspring (mean=43.6 pixels, SE=7.6 versus mean=74.1 pixels, SE=1.9, $p<0.05$).

NOTE: BAA=butoxyacetic acid; CI=confidence interval; EAA=ethoxyacetic acid; EEAA=ethoxy ethoxyacetic acid; EGME=ethylene glycol monomethyl ether (2-methoxyethanol); FSH=follicle-stimulating hormone; GE=glycol ether; FSH=follicle-stimulating hormone; LH=luteninizing hormone; MAA=methoxyacetic acid; md=mean difference; MEAA=methoxy ethoxyacetic acid; 2-MPA=2-methoxypropionic acid; OR=odds ratio; PAA=n-propoxyacetic acid; PhAA=phenoxyacetic acid; SE=standard error; TTP=time to pregnancy.

REFERENCES

ACGIH (American Conference of Governmental Industrial Hygienists). 2018. Threshold limit values for chemical substances in the work environment. https://www.osha.gov/dsg/annotated-pels/tablez-1.html (accessed July 5, 2018).

Adedara, I.A., and E.O. Farombi. 2010. Induction of oxidative damage in the testes and spermatozoa and hematotoxicity in rats exposed to multiple doses of ethylene glycol monoethyl ether. *Human & Experimental Toxicology* 29(10):801–812.

Ahlborg, G., Jr. 1990. Pregnancy outcome among women working in laundries and dry-cleaning shops using tetrachloroethylene. *American Journal of Industrial Medicine* 17(5):567–575.

API (American Petroleum Institute). 1978. *Teratology study in rats: Toluene. Final report*. Washington, DC: American Petroleum Institute.

API. 1981. *Mutagenicity evaluation of toluene in the mouse dominant lethal assay*. Washington, DC: American Petroleum Institute.

API. 1985. *Two-generation reproduction/fertility study on a petroleum-derived hydrocarbon (toluene)*. Washington, DC: American Petroleum Institute.

API. 1991. *Toluene: Effect on pregnancy of the rat by inhalation (status report) with cover letter dated 02-21-91*. Washington, DC: American Petroleum Institute.

API. 1992. *A preliminary study of the effect of toluene on pregnancy of the rat (inhalation exposure)*. Washington, DC: American Petroleum Institute.

Aschengrau, A., J. Weinberg, S. Rogers, L. Gallagher, M. Winter, V. Vieira, T. Webster, and D. Ozonoff. 2008. Prenatal exposure to tetrachloroethylene-contamination drinking water and the risk of adverse birth outcomes. *Environmental Health Perspectives* 116(6):814–820.

Aschengrau, A., J.M. Weinberg, P.A. Janulewicz, L.G. Gallagher, M.R. Winter, V.M. Vieira, T.F. Webster, and D.M. Ozonoff. 2009. Prenatal exposure to tetrachloroethylene-contaminated drinking water and the risk of congenital anomalies: A retrospective cohort study. *Environmental Health: A Global Access Science Source* 8:44.

Aschengrau, A., J.M. Weinberg, P.A. Janulewicz, M.E. Romano, L.G. Gallagher, M.R. Winter, B.R. Martin, V.M. Vieira, T.F. Webster, R.F. White, and D.M. Ozonoff. 2011. Affinity for risky behaviors following prenatal and early childhood exposure to tetrachloroethylene (PCE)-contaminated drinking water: A retrospective cohort study. *Environmental Health* 10:102.

Aschengrau, A., J.M. Weinberg, P.A. Janulewicz, M.E. Romano, L.G. Gallagher, M.R. Winter, B.R. Martin, V.M. Vieira, T.F. Webster, R.F. White, and D.M. Ozonoff. 2012. Occurrence of mental illness following prenatal and early childhood exposure to tetrachloroethylene (PCE)-contaminated drinking water: A retrospective cohort study. *Environmental Health* 11:2.

Aschengrau, A., M.R. Winter, V.M. Vieira, T.F. Webster, P.A. Janulewicz, L.G. Gallagher, J. Weinberg, and D.M. Ozonoff. 2015. Long-term health effects of early life exposure to tetrachloroethylene (PCE)-contaminated drinking water: A retrospective cohort study. *Environmental Health* 14:36.

ATSDR (Agency for Toxic Substances and Disease Registry). 1997. *Toxicological profile for propylene glycol*. Atlanta, GA: U.S. Department of Health and Human Services.

ATSDR. 1998. *Toxicological profile for 2-butoxyethanol and 2-butoxyethanol acetate*. Atlanta, GA: U.S. Department of Health and Human Services.

ATSDR. 2001. *Final Report: Evaluation of priority health conditions in a community with historical contamination by trichloroethylene*. Atlanta, GA: U.S. Department of Health and Human Services.

ATSDR. 2007a. *Toxicological profile for benzene*. Atlanta, GA: U.S. Department of Health and Human Services.

ATSDR. 2007b. *Toxicological profile for xylene*. Atlanta, GA: U.S. Department of Health and Human Services.

ATSDR. 2008. *Toxicological profile for diazinon*. Atlanta, GA: U.S. Department of Health and Human Services.

ATSDR. 2010. *Toxicological profile for ethylene glycol*. Atlanta, GA: U.S. Department of Health and Human Services.

ATSDR. 2014. *Draft toxicological profile for trichloroethylene*. Atlanta, GA: U.S. Department of Health and Human Services.

ATSDR. 2015a. *Addendum to the toxicological profile for benzene*. Atlanta, GA: U.S. Department of Health and Human Services.

ATSDR. 2015b. *Draft toxicological profile for toluene*. Atlanta, GA: U.S. Department of Health and Human Services.

Badham, H.J., and L.M. Winn. 2010a. In utero exposure to benzene disrupts fetal hematopoietic progenitor cell growth via reactive oxygen species. *Toxicological Sciences* 113(1):207–215.

Badham, H.J., and L.M. Winn. 2010b. In utero and in vitro effects of benzene and its metabolites on erythroid differentiation and the role of reactive oxygen species. *Toxicology and Applied Pharmacology* 244(3):273–279.

Badham, H.J., D.P. LeBrun, A. Rutter, and L.M. Winn. 2010. Transplacental benzene exposure increases tumor incidence in mouse offspring: Possible role of fetal benzene metabolism. *Carcinogenesis* 31(6):1142–1148.

Bagchi, G., Y. Zhang, and D.J. Waxman. 2010. Impact of methoxyacetic acid on mouse Leydig cell gene expression. *Reproductive Biology and Endocrinology* 8:65.

Ballantyne, B., and W.M. Snellings. 2005. Developmental toxicity study with diethylene glycol dosed by gavage to CD rats and CD-1 mice. *Food and Chemical Toxicology* 43(11):1637–1646.

Bardodej, Z., and J. Vyskocil. 1956. The problem of trichloroethylene in occupational medicine: Trichloroethylene metabolism and its effect on the nervous system evaluated as a means of hygienic control. *Archives of Industrial Health* 56:581–592.

Beliles, R.P., D.J. Brusick, and F.J. Mecler. 1980. *Teratogenic–mutagenic risk of workplace contaminants: Trichloroethylene, perchloroethylene, and carbon disulfide*. Cincinnati, OH: National Institute for Occupation Safety and Health.

Béranger, R., R. Garlantézec, G.L. Maner-Idrissi, A. Lacroix, F. Rouget, J. Trowbridge, C. Warembourg, C. Monfort, F.L. Gléau, M. Jourdin, L. Multigner, S. Cordier, and C. Chevrier. 2017. Prenatal exposure to glycol ethers and neurocognitive abilities in 6-year-old children: The PELAGIE cohort study. *Environmental Health Perspectives* 125(4):684–690.

Berger, T., and C.M. Horner. 2003. In vivo exposure of female rats to toxicants may affect oocyte quality. [Erratum appears in *Reproductive Toxicology* 2004; 18(3):447]. *Reproductive Toxicology* 17(3):273–281.

Berger, T., M.G. Miller, and C.M. Horner. 2000. In vitro fertilization after in vivo treatment of rats with three reproductive toxicants. *Reproductive Toxicology* 14(1):45–53.

Blatter, B., N. Roeleveld, G. Zielhuis, F. Gabreels, and A. Verbeek. 1996. Maternal occupational exposure during pregnancy and the risk of spina bifida. *Occupational and Environmental Medicine* 53(2):80–86.

Blatter, B., R. Hermens, M. Bakker, N. Roeleveld, A.L. Verbeek, and G.A. Zielhuis. 1997. Paternal occupational exposure around conception and spina bifida in offspring. *American Journal of Industrial Medicine* 32(3):283–291.

Bosco, M.G., I. Figa-Talamanca, and S. Salerno. 1987. Health and reproductive status of female workers in dry cleaning shops. *International Archives of Occupational and Environmental Health* 59:295–301.

Bove, F.J. 1996. Public drinking water contamination and birthweight, prematurity, fetal deaths, and birth defects. *Toxicology and Industrial Health* 12:255–266.

Bove, F.J., M.C. Fulcomer, J.B. Klotz, J. Esmart, E.M. Dufficy, and J.E. Savrin. 1995. Public drinking water contamination and birth outcomes. *American Journal of Epidemiology* 141:850–862.

Brender, J.D., M.U. Shinde, F. Benjamin Zhan, X. Gong, and P.H. Langlois. 2014. Maternal residential proximity to chlorinated solvent emissions and birth defects in offspring: A case-control study. *Environmental Health* 13(1):96.

Bruckner, J., and D. Warren. 2001. Toxic effects of solvents and vapors. In C. Klaassen (ed.). *Casarett and Doull's toxicology: The basic science of poisons, 6th ed*. New York: McGraw-Hill.

Burg, J., and G. Gist. 1999. Health effects of environmental contaminant exposure: An intrafile comparison of the trichloroethylene subregistry. *Archives of Environmental & Occupational Health* 54:231–241.

Callan, S.P., A.K. Apawu, T.A. Mathews, and S.E. Bowen. 2017. Toluene's effects on activity and extracellular dopamine in the mouse are altered by $GABA_A$ antagonism. *Neuroscience Letters* 647:67–71.

Carlos-Wallace, F.M., L. Zhang, M.T. Smith, G. Rader, and C. Steinmaus. 2016. Parental, in utero, and early-life exposure to benzene and the risk of childhood leukemia: A meta-analysis. *American Journal of Epidemiology* 183(1):1–14.

Carney, E.W., B.A. Thorsrud, P.H. Dugard, and C.L. Zablotny. 2006. Developmental toxicity studies in Crl:CD (SD) rats following inhalation exposure to trichloroethylene and perchloroethylene. *Birth Defects Research, Part B—Developmental and Reproductive Toxicology* 77(5):405–412.

Carney, E.W., B. Tornesi, D.A. Markham, R.J. Rasoulpour, and N. Moore. 2008. Species-specificity of ethylene glycol–induced developmental toxicity: Toxicokinetic and whole embryo culture studies in the rabbit. *Birth Defects Research, Part B—Developmental and Reproductive Toxicology* 83(6):573–581.

Carwile, J.L., S. Mahalingaiah, M.R. Winter, and A. Aschengrau. 2014. Prenatal drinking-water exposure to tetrachloroethylene and ischemic placental disease: A retrospective cohort study. *Environmental Health* 13:72.

Chen, D., S.I. Cho, C. Chen, X. Wang, A.I. Damokosh, L. Ryan, T.J. Smith, D.C. Christiani, and X. Xu. 2000. Exposure to benzene, occupational stress, and reduced birth weight. *Occupational and Environmental Medicine* 57(10):661–667.

Cherry, N., H. Moore, R. McNamee, A. Pacey, G. Burgess, J.A. Clyma, M. Dippnall, H. Baillie, and A. Povey. 2008. Occupation and male infertility: Glycol ethers and other exposures. *Occupational and Environmental Medicine* 65(10):708–714.

Chia, S.E., V.H. Goh, and C.N. Ong. 1997. Endocrine profiles of male workers with exposure to trichloroethylene. *American Journal of Industrial Medicine* 32(3):217–222.

Chiu, W. A., J. Jinot, C.S. Scott, S.L. Makris, G.S. Cooper, R.C. Dzubow, A.S. Bale, M.V. Evans, K.Z. Guyton, N. Keshava, J.C. Lipscomb, S. Barone, Jr., J.F. Fox, M.R. Gwinn, J. Schaum, and J.C. Caldwell. 2013. Human health effects of trichloroethylene: Key findings and scientific issues. *Environmental Health Perspectives* 121(3):303–311.

Cho, S.I., A.I. Damokosh, and L.M. Ryan. 2001. Effects of exposure to organic solvents on menstrual cycle length. *Journal of Occupational and Environmental Medicine* 43(6):565–575.

Cordier, S., A. Bergeret, J. Goujard, M.C. Ha, S. Ayme, F. Bianchi, E. Calzolari, H.E.K. De Walle, R. Knill-Jones, S. Candela, I. Dale, B. Dananche, C. De Vigan, J. Fevotte, G. Kiel, L. Mandereau, J. Pompili, A. Nielsen, M.C. Cornel, E.Y. Haayer, M.Y.M.C. Smeets, T.M. Pal, V. Vodovar, O. Boiron, A. Seniori-Constantini, and A. Scarpelli. 1997. Congenital malformations and maternal occupational exposure to glycol ethers. *Epidemiology* 8(4):355–363.

Cordier, S., R. Garlantezec, L. Labat, F. Rouget, C. Monfort, N. Bonvallot, B. Roig, J. Pulkkinen, C. Chevrier, and L. Multigner. 2012. Exposure during pregnancy to glycol ethers and chlorinated solvents and the risk of congenital malformations. *Epidemiology* 23(6):806–812.

Correa, A., R. Gray, R. Cohen, N. Rothman, F. Shah, H. Seacat, and M. Corn. 1996. Ethylene glycol ethers and risks of spontaneous abortion and subfertility. *American Journal of Epidemiology* 143(7):707–717.

Costas, K., R.S. Knorr, and S.K. Condon. 2002. A case-control study of childhood leukemia in Woburn, Massachusetts: The relationship between leukemia incidence and exposure to public drinking water. *Science of the Total Environment* 300(1–3):23–35.

Dalgaard, M., A. Hossaini, K. S. Hougaard, U. Hass, and O. Ladefoged. 2001. Developmental toxicity of toluene in male rats: Effects on semen quality, testis morphology, and apoptotic neurodegeneration. *Archives of Toxicology* 75(2):103–109.

Dayan, C., and B.F. Hales. 2012. A model teratogen, 2-methoxyacetic acid, disrupts epigenetic programming leading to apoptosis during limb development in vitro. *Birth Defects Research, Part A—Clinical and Molecular Teratology* 94 (5):316.

De Roos, A.J., A.F. Olshan, K. Teschke, C. Poole, D.A. Savitz, J. Blatt, M. L. Bondy, and B.H. Pollock. 2001. Parental occupational exposures to chemicals and incidence of neuroblastoma in offspring. *American Journal of Epidemiology* 154(2):106–114.

DePass, L.R., M.D. Woodside, R.R. Maronpot, and C.S. Weil. 1986. Three-generation reproduction and dominant lethal mutagenesis studies of ethylene glycol in the rat. *Fundamental and Applied Toxicology* 7(4):566–572.

Dieter, M.P. 1993. *NTP Technical Report on toxicity studies of ethylene glycol ethers: 2-methoxyehtanol, 2-ethoxyethanol, 2-butoxyethanol (Cas Nos. 109-86-4, 110-80-5, 111-76-2) administered in drinking water to F344/N rats and B6C3F$_1$ mice*. Toxicity report series number 26. Research Triangle Park, NC: National Toxicology Program.

Dodo, T., Y. Taketa, M. Sugiyama, A. Inomata, J. Sonoda, Y. Okuda, H. Mineshima, S. Hosokawa, and T. Aoki. 2009. Collaborative work on evaluation of ovarian toxicity. 11) Two- or four-week repeated-dose studies and fertility study of ethylene glycol monomethyl ether in female rats. *Journal of Toxicological Sciences* 34(Suppl 1):SP121–SP128.

Doyle, P., E. Roman, V. Beral, and S.M. Brooke. 1997. Spontaneous abortion in dry cleaning workers potentially exposed to perchloroethylene. *Occupational and Environmental Medicine* 54(12):848–853.

El Ghawabi, S.M., M.B. Mansoor, and E. Gamel. 1973. Chronic trichloroethylene exposure. *Journal of the Egyptian Medical Association* 56:715–724.

El-Zein, R., T. Albrecht, E. Knutson, M.S. Legator, and S.Z. Abdel-Rahman. 2007. Reductions in telomere length in individuals exposed in utero to glycol ethers. *Archives of Environmental and Occupational Health* 62(3):161–163.

Enright, B.P., B. Tornesi, H. Lorenz, and K. Whitney. 2013. The inhibin B response to testicular toxicants ethylene glycol monomethyl ether or dibromoacetic acid in male rats. *Birth Defects Research, Part B—Developmental and Reproductive Toxicology* 98(1):35–40.

EPA (U.S. Environmental Protection Agency). 2000. *Xylenes (Mixed Isomers)*. https://www.epa.gov/sites/production/files/2016-09/documents/xylenes.pdf (accessed August 27, 2018).

EPA. 2003. *Toxicological review of xylenes*. Washington, DC: Environmental Protection Agency.

EPA. 2011. *Toxicological review of trichloroethylene*. Washington, DC: Environmental Protection Agency.

EPA. 2012. *Toxicological review of tetrachloroethylene (perchloroethylene)*. Washington, DC: Environmental Protection Agency.

Eskenazi, B., A.J. Wyrobek, L. Fenster, D. F. Katz, M. Sadler, J. Lee, M. Hudes, and D.M. Rempel. 1991a. A study of the effect of perchloroethylene exposure on semen quality in dry cleaning workers. *American Journal of Industrial Medicine* 20(5):575–591.

Eskenazi, B., L. Fenster, M. Hudes, A.J. Wyrobek, D. F. Katz, J. Gerson, and D.M. Rempel. 1991b. A study of the effect of perchloroethylene exposure on the reproductive outcomes of wives of dry-cleaning workers. *American Journal of Industrial Medicine* 20(5):593–600.

Eskenazi, B., E. Gold, S. Samuels, S. Wight, B. Lasley, S. Hammond, M. Rasor, and M. Schenker. 1995. Prospective assessment of fecundability of female semiconductor workers. *American Journal of Industrial Medicine* 28(6):817–831.

Estarlich, M., F. Ballester, I. Aguilera, A. Fernandez-Somoano, A. Lertxundi, S. Llop, C. Freire, A. Tardon, M. Basterrechea, J. Sunyer, and C. Iniguez. 2011. Residential exposure to outdoor air pollution during pregnancy and anthropometric measures at birth in a multicenter cohort in Spain. *Environmental Health Perspectives* 119(9):1333–1338.

Faye, R.E., and J.W. Green, Jr. 2007a. Analyses of groundwater flow, contaminant fate and transport, and distribution of drinking water at Tarawa Terrace and vicinity, U.S. Marine Corps Base Camp Lejeune, North Carolina: Historical reconstruction and present-day conditions—Chapter B: Geohydrologic framework of the Castle Hayne aquifer system. Atlanta, GA: Agency for Toxic Substances and Disease Registry. http://www.atsdr.cdc.gov/SITES/LEJEUNE/docs/ChapterB_TarawaTerrace.pdf (accessed December 12, 2008).

Faye, R.E., and J.W. Green, Jr. 2007b. Analyses of groundwater flow, contaminant fate and transport, and distribution of drinking water at Tarawa Terrace and vicinity, U.S. Marine Corps Base Camp Lejeune, North Carolina: Historical reconstruction and present-day conditions—Chapter E: Occurrence of contaminants in groundwater. Atlanta, GA: Agency for Toxic Substances and Disease Registry. http://www.atsdr.cdc.gov/SITES/LEJEUNE/docs/ChapterE_TarawaTerrace_revised0108.pdf (accessed December 12, 2008).

Feingold, L., D. Savitz, and E. John. 1992. Use of a job–exposure matrix to evaluate parental occupation and childhood cancer. *Cancer Causes and Control* 3(2):161–169.

Figa-Talamanca, I., G. Petrelli, R. Tropeano, G. Papa, and G. Boccia. 2000. Fertility of male workers of the Italian mint. *Reproductive Toxicology* 14:325–330.

Filippini, T., J.E. Heck, C. Malagoli, C. Del Giovane, and M. Vinceti. 2015. A review and meta-analysis of outdoor air pollution and risk of childhood leukemia. *Journal of Environmental Science and Health, Part C—Environmental Carcinogenesis and Ecotoxicology Reviews* 33(1):36–66.

Fisher, J.W., S.R. Channel, J. S. Eggers, P.D. Johnson, K.L. MacMahon, C.D. Goodyear, G.L. Sudberry, D.A. Warren, J.R. Latendresse, and L.J. Graeter. 2001. Trichloroethylene, trichloroacetic acid, and dichloroacetic acid: Do they affect fetal rat heart development? *International Journal of Toxicology* 20(5):257–267.

Forand, S.P., E.L. Lewis-Michl, and M.I. Gomez. 2012. Adverse birth outcomes and maternal exposure to trichloroethylene and tetrachloroethylene through soil vapor intrusion in New York State. *Environmental Health Perspectives* 120(4):616–621.

Fowles, J., M. Banton, J. Klapacz, and H. Shen. 2017. A toxicological review of the ethylene glycol series: Commonalities and differences in toxicity and modes of action. *Toxicology Letters* 278:66–83.

Fukushima, T., T. Yamamoto, R. Kikkawa, Y. Hamada, M. Komiyama, C. Mori, and I. Horii. 2005. Effects of male reproductive toxicants on gene expression in rat testes. *Journal of Toxicological Sciences* 30(3):195–206.

Fukushima, T., K. Taki, R. Ise, I. Horii, and T. Yoshida. 2011. MicroRNAs expression in the ethylene glycol monomethyl ether-induced testicular lesion. *Journal of Toxicological Sciences* 36(5):601–611.

Gallagher, L., T. Webster, and A. Aschengrau. 2017. Exploring associations between prenatal solvent exposures and teenage drug and alcohol use: A retrospective cohort study. *Environmental Health* 16(26):1–10.

Garlantezec, R., C. Warembourg, C. Monfort, L. Labat, J. Pulkkinen, N. Bonvallot, L. Multigner, C. Chevrier, and S. Cordier. 2013. Urinary glycol ether metabolites in women and time to pregnancy: The PELAGIE cohort. *Environmental Health Perspectives* 121(10):1167–1173.

Gericke, C., B. Hanke, and G. Beckmann. 2001. Multicenter field trial on possible health effects of toluene. III. Evaluation of effects after long-term exposure. *Toxicology* 168(2):185–209.

Ghosh, J.K. C., J.E. Heck, M. Cockburn, J. Su, M. Jerrett, and B. Ritz. 2013. Prenatal exposure to traffic-related air pollution and risk of early childhood cancers. *American Journal of Epidemiology* 178(8):1233–1239.

Gilbert, K.M., W. Woodruff, and S.J. Blossom. 2014. Differential immunotoxicity induced by two different windows of developmental trichloroethylene exposure. *Autoimmune Diseases* 2014:982073.

Goh, V.H., S.E. Chia, and C.N. Ong. 1998. Effects of chronic exposure to low doses of trichloroethylene on steroid hormone and insulin levels in normal men. *Environmental Health Perspectives* 106(1):41–44.

Goldberg, S.J., M.D. Lebowitz, E.J. Graver, and S. Hicks. 1990. An association of human congenital cardiac malformations and drinking water contaminants. *Journal of the American College of Cardiology* 16(1):155–164.

Hass, U., S.P. Lund, and L. Simonsen. 1995. Effects of prenatal exposure to xylene on postnatal development and behavior in rats. *Neurotoxicology and Teratology* 17:547–551.

Hass, U., S. Lund, and K. Hougaard. 1999. Developmental neurotoxicity after toluene inhalation exposure in rats. *Neurotoxicology and Teratology* 21(4):349–357.

Heck, J.E., A.S. Park, J. Qiu, M. Cockburn, and B. Ritz. 2014. Risk of leukemia in relation to exposure to ambient air toxics in pregnancy and early childhood. *International Journal of Hygiene and Environmental Health* 217(6):662–668.

Herberth, G., M. Bauer, M. Gasch, D. Ninz, S. Röder, S. Olek, T. Kohajda, U. Rolle-Kampczyk, M. von Bergen, U. Sack, M. Borte, and I. Lehmann. 2014. Maternal and cord blood miR-223 expression associates with prenatal tobacco smoke exposure and low regulatory T-cell numbers. *Journal of Allergy and Clinical Immunology* 133:543–550.

Holmberg, P.C. 1979. Central-nervous-system defects in children born to mothers exposed to organic solvents during pregnancy. *Lancet* 2:177–179.

Holmberg, P.C., and M. Nurminen. 1980. Congenital defects of the central nervous system and occupational factors during pregnancy. A case–referent study. *American Journal of Industrial Medicine* 1(2):167–176.
Hong, H., J. Canipe, and C. Jameson. 1988. Comparative effects of ethylene glycol and ethylene glycol monomethyl ether exposure on hematopoiesis and histopathology in B6C3Ff1 mice. *Journal of Environmental Pathology, Toxicology and Oncology* 8(7):27–38.
Hooiveld, M., W. Haveman, K. Roskes, R. Bretveld, I. Burstyn, and N. Roeleveld. 2006. Adverse reproductive outcomes among male painters with occupational exposure to organic solvents. *Occupational and Environmental Medicine* 63(8):538–544.
Hougaard, K.S., A.M. Hansen, U. Hass, and S.P. Lund. 2003. Toluene depresses plasma corticosterone in pregnant rats. *Pharmacology and Toxicology* 92(3):148–152.
Hougaard, K.S., M.B. Andersen, A.M. Hansen, U. Hass, T. Werge, and S. P. Lund. 2005. Effects of prenatal exposure to chronic mild stress and toluene in rats. *Neurotoxicology and Teratology* 27(1):153–167.
Hudak, A., and G. Ungvary. 1978. Embryotoxic effects of benzene and its methyl derivatives: Toluene, xylene. *Toxicology* 11:55–63.
IARC (International Agency for Research on Cancer). 2012. Benzene. In *Chemical agents and related occupations, volume 100F: A review of human carcinogens*. IARC monographs.
Infante-Rivard, C., J. Siemiatycki, R. Lakhani, and L. Nadon. 2005. Maternal exposure to occupational solvents and childhood leukemia. *Environmental Health Perspectives* 113(6):787–792.
IOM (Institute of Medicine). 2003. *Gulf War and health, volume 2: Insecticides and solvents*. Washington, DC: The National Academies Press.
IOM. 2011. *Long-term health consequences of exposure to burn pits in Iraq and Afghanistan*. Washington, DC: The National Academies Press.
Janulewicz, P.A., R.F. White, M.R. Winter, J.M. Weinberg, L.E. Gallagher, V. Vieira, T.F. Webster, and A. Aschengrau. 2008. Risk of learning and behavioral disorders following prenatal and early postnatal exposure to tetrachloroethylene (PCE)-contaminated drinking water. *Neurotoxicology and Teratology* 30(3):175–185.
Janulewicz, P.A., R.F. White, B.M. Martin, M.R. Winter, J.M. Weinberg, V. Vieira, and A. Aschengrau. 2012. Adult neuropsychological performance following prenatal and early postnatal exposure to tetrachloroethylene (PCE)-contaminated drinking water. *Neurotoxicology and Teratology* 34(3):350–359.
Janulewicz, P.A., R.J. Killiany, R.F. White, B.M. Martin, M.R. Winter, J.M. Weinberg, and A. Aschengrau. 2013. Structural magnetic resonance imaging in an adult cohort following prenatal and early postnatal exposure to tetrachloroethylene (PCE)-contaminated drinking water. *Neurotoxicology and Teratology* 38:13–20.
Ji, Z., R.H. Weldon, F. Marchetti, H. Chen, G. Li, C. Xing, E. Kurtovich, S. Young, T.E. Schmid, S. Waidyanatha, S. Rappaport, L. Zhang, and B. Eskenazi. 2012. Comparison of aneuploidies of chromosomes 21, X, and Y in the blood, lymphocytes, and sperm of workers exposed to benzene. *Environmental and Molecular Mutagenesis* 53(3):218–226.
Johnson, K., P.C. Baker, H.L. Kan, J.P. Maurissen, P.J. Spencer, and M.S. Marty. 2005. Diethylene glycol monobutyl ether (DGBE): Two- and thirteen-week oral toxicity studies in Fischer 344 rats. *Food and Chemical Toxicology* 43(3):467–481.
Johnson, P.D., B.V. Dawson, and S.J. Goldberg. 1998a. Cardiac teratogenicity of trichloroethylene metabolites. *Journal of the American College of Cardiology* 32(2):540–545.
Johnson, P.D., B.V. Dawson, and S.J. Goldberg. 1998b. A review: Trichloroethylene metabolites: Potential cardiac teratogens. B. *Environmental Health Perspectives* 104(Suppl 4):995–999.
Jones, H.E., and R.L. Balster. 1997. Neurobehavioral consequences of intermittent prenatal exposure to high concentrations of toluene. *Neurotoxicology and Teratology* 19(4):305–313.
Kanter, M. 2011. Thymoquinone reestablishes spermatogenesis after testicular injury caused by chronic toluene exposure in rats. *Toxicology and Industrial Health* 27(2):155–166.
Katukam, V., M. Kulakarni, R. Syed, K. Alharbi, and J. Naik. 2012. Effect of benzene exposure on fertility of male workers employed in bulk drug industries. *Genetic Testing and Molecular Biomarkers* 16(6):592–597.
Kim, Y.J., J.Y. Choi, Y.H., Cho, H.D. Woo, H.W. Chung. 2010. Micronucleus-centromere assay in workers occupationally exposed to low level of benzene. *Human & Experimental Toxicology* 29(5):343–350.
Klimisch, H.J., J. Hellwig, and A. Hofmann. 1992. Studies on the prenatal toxicity of toluene in rabbits following inhalation exposure and proposal of a pregnancy guidance value. *Archives of Toxicology* 66:373–381.
Kucera, J. 1968. Exposure to fat solvents: A possible cause for sacral agenesis in man. *Journal of Pediatrics* 72:857–859.
Kyyronen, P., H. Taskinen, M. Lindbohm, K. Hemminki, and O. Heinonen. 1989. Spontaneous abortions and congenital malformations among women exposed to tetrachloroethylene in dry cleaning. *Journal of Epidemiology and Community Health* 43(4):346–351.
Lagakos, S.W., B.J. Wessen, and M. Zelen. 1986. An analysis of contaminated well water and 32 health effects in Woburn, Massachusetts. *Journal of the American Statistical Association* 81:583–596.

Lau, A., C.L. Belanger, and L.M. Winn. 2009. In utero and acute exposure to benzene: Investigation of DNA double-strand breaks and DNA recombination in mice. *Mutation Research* 676(1–2):74–82.

Le Cornet, C., B. Fervers, E. Pukkala, T. Tynes, M. Feychting, J. Hansen, K. Togawa, K. C. Nordby, S. O. Dalton, S. Uuksulainen, P. Wiebert, T. Woldbæk, N.E. Skakkebæk, A. Olsson, and J. Schüz. 2017. Parental occupational exposure to organic solvents and testicular germ cell tumors in their offspring: NORD-TEST study. *Environmental Health Perspectives* 125(6):067023.

Lertxundi, A., M. Baccini, N. Lertxundi, E. Fano, A. Aranbarri, M.D. Martinez, M. Ayerdi, J. Alvarez, L. Santa-Marina, M. Dorronsoro, and J. Ibarluzea. 2015. Exposure to fine particle matter, nitrogen dioxide and benzene during pregnancy and cognitive and psychomotor developments in children at 15 months of age. *Environment International* 80:33–40.

Lindbohm, M.L. 1995. Effects of parental exposure to solvents on pregnancy outcome. *Journal of Occupational and Environmental Medicine* 37:908–914.

Lindbohm, M.L., H. Taskinen, and M. Sallmén. 1990. Spontaneous abortions among women exposed to organic solvents. *American Journal of Industrial Medicine* 17:449–463.

Lindbohm, M.L., K. Hemminki, M. G. Bonhomme, A. Anttila, K. Rantala, P. Heikkila, and M.J. Rosenberg. 1991. Effects of paternal occupational exposure on spontaneous abortions. *American Journal of Public Health* 81(8):1029–1033.

Llop, S., F. Ballester, M. Estarlich, A. Esplugues, M. Rebagliato, and C. Iniguez. 2010. Preterm birth and exposure to air pollutants during pregnancy. *Environmental Research* 110(8):778–785.

Lo Pumo, R., M. Bellia, A. Nicosia, V. Micale, and F. Drago. 2006. Long-lasting neurotoxicity of prenatal benzene acute exposure in rats. *Toxicology* 223(3):227–234.

Lof, A., E.W. Hjelm, A. Colmsjo, B.O. Lundmark, A. Norström, and A. Sato. 1993. Toxicokinetics of toluene and urinary excretion of hippuric acid after human exposure to 2H8-toluene. *British Journal of Industrial Medicine* 50:55–59.

Lorente, C., S. Cordier, A. Bergeret, H. De Walle, J. Goujard, S. Ayme, R. Knill-Jones, E. Calzolari, and F. Bianchi. 2000. Maternal occupational risk factors for oral clefts. *Scandinavian Journal of Work, Environment & Health* 26(2):137–145.

Lowengart, R., J. Peters, C. Cicioni, J. Buckley, L. Bernstein, S. Preston-Martin, and E. Rappaport. 1987. Childhood leukemia and parents' occupational and home exposures. *Journal of the National Cancer Institute* 79(1):39–46.

Luderer, U., M.S. Morgan, and C.A. Brodkin. 1999. Reproductive endocrine effects of acute exposure to toluene in men and women. *Occupational and Environmental Medicine* 56(10):657–666.

Luderer, U., A. Bushley, B.D. Stover, W.J. Bremner, E.M. Faustman, T.K. Takaro, H. Checkoway, and C. A. Brodkin. 2004. Effects of occupational solvent exposure on reproductive hormone concentrations and fecundability in men. *American Journal of Industrial Medicine* 46(6):614–626.

Lupo, P. J., E. Symanski, D. K. Waller, W. Chan, P. H. Langlois, M. A. Canfield, and L. E. Mitchell. 2011. Maternal exposure to ambient levels of benzene and neural tube defects among offspring: Texas, 1999–2004. *Environmental Health Perspectives* 119(3):397–402.

Mahalingaiah, S., M.R. Winter, and A. Aschengrau. 2016. Association of prenatal and early life exposure to tetrachloroethylene (PCE) with polycystic ovary syndrome and other reproductive disorders in the Cape Cod Health Study: A retrospective cohort study. *Reproductive Toxicology* 65:87–94.

Makris, S.L., C.S. Scott, J. Fox, T.B. Knudsen, A.K. Hotchkiss, X. Arzuaga, S.Y. Euling, C.M. Powers, J. Jinot, K.A. Hogan, B.D. Abbott, E.S. Hunter, and M.G. Narotsky. 2016. A systematic evaluation of the potential effects of trichloroethylene exposure on cardiac development. *Reproductive Toxicology* 65:321–358.

Marchetti, F., B. Eskenazi, R.H. Weldon, G. Li, L. Zhang, S.M. Rappaport, T.E. Schmid, C. Xing, E. Kurtovich, and A.J. Wyrobek. 2012. Occupational exposure to benzene and chromosomal structural aberrations in the sperm of Chinese men. *Environmental Health Perspectives* 120(2):229–234.

Matsuyama, T., K. Yabe, C. Kuwata, K. Ito, Y. Ando, H. Iida, and K. Mori. 2018. Transcriptional profile of ethylene glycol monomethyl ether-induced testicular toxicity in rats. *Drug and Chemical Toxicology* 41(1):105–112.

McDonald, A.D., J.C. McDonald, B. Armstrong, N. Cherry, C. Delorme, A. Nolin, and D. Robert. 1987. Occupation and pregnancy outcome. *British Journal of Industrial Medicine* 44:521–526.

Morgan, J.W., and R.E. Cassady. 2002. Community cancer assessment in response to long-time exposure to perchlorate and trichloroethylene in drinking water. *Journal of Occupational and Environmental Medicine* 44(7):616–621.

Multigner, L., E. Ben Brik, I. Arnaud, J.M. Haguenoer, P. Jouannet, J. Auger, and F. Eustache. 2007. Glycol ethers and semen quality: A cross-sectional study among male workers in the Paris municipality. *Occupational and Environmental Medicine* 64(7):467–473.

Nelson, B.K., B.J. Taylor, J.V. Setzer, and R.W. Hornung. 1980. Behavioral teratology of perchloroethylene in rats. *Journal of Environmental Pathology, Toxicology, and Oncology* 3(1–2):233–250.

Ng, T.P., S.C. Foo, and T. Yoong. 1992. Risk of spontaneous abortion in workers exposed to toluene. *British Journal of Industrial Medicine* 49:804–808.

NRC (National Research Council). 2006. *Assessing the human health risks of trichloroethylene: Key scientific issues*. Washington, DC: The National Academies Press.

NRC. 2009. *Contaminated water supplies at Camp Lejeune: Assessing potential health effects*. Washington, DC: The National Academies Press.

Ogata, M. 1984. Estimation of solvent concentrations in ambient air from urinary metabolite levels of workers exposed to solvents. *Industrial Health* 22:319–324.

Olsen, J., K. Hemminki, G. Ahlborg, T. Bjerkedal, P. Kyyronen, H. Taskinen, M. Lindbohm, O. Heinonen, L. Brandt, H. Kolstad, B. Halvorsen, and J. Egenaes. 1990. Low birthweight, congenital malformations, and spontaneous abortions among dry-cleaning workers in Scandinavia. *Scandinavian Journal of Work, Environment & Health* 16(3):163–168.

Olshan, A., A.J. De Roos, K. Teschke, J. Neglia, D. Stram, B. Pollock, and B. Pollock. 1999. Neuroblastoma and parental occupation. *Cancer Causes and Control* 10(6):539–549.

Ono, A., K. Sekita, and K. Ohno. 1995. Reproductive and developmental toxicity studies of toluene: I. Teratogenicity study of inhalation exposure in pregnant rats. *Journal of Toxicological Sciences* 20(2):109–134.

Ono, A., K. Sekita, and Y. Ogawa. 1996. Reproductive and developmental toxicity studies of toluene: II. Effects of inhalation exposure on fertility in rats. *Journal of Environmental Pathology, Toxicology and Oncology* 15(1):9–20.

Ono, A., K. Kawashima, and K. Sekita. 1999. Toluene inhalation induced epididymal sperm dysfunction in rats. *Toxicology* 139(3):193–205.

OSAGWI (Office of the Special Assistant for Gulf War Illnesses). 2000. *Environmental exposure report: Chemical agent resistant coating. Final report*. Washington, DC: U.S. Department of Defense, OSAGWI.

OSHA (Occupational Safety and Health Administration). 2018. Permissibile exposure limits/OSHA annotated table Z-1. https://www.osha.gov/dsg/annotated-pels/tablez-1.html#notes (accessed July 5, 2018).

Palbykin, B., J. Borg, P.T. Caldwell, J. Rowles, A.J. Papoutsis, D.F. Romagnolo, and O.I. Selmin. 2011. Trichloroethylene induces methylation of the *Serca2* promoter in H9c2 cells and embryonic heart. *Cardiovascular Toxicology* 11(3):204–214.

Perrin, M.C., M.G. Opler, S. Harlap, J. Harkavy-Friedman, K. Kleinhaus, D. Nahon, S. Fennig, E.S. Susser, and D. Malaspina. 2007. Tetrachloroethylene exposure and risk of schizophrenia: Offspring of dry cleaners in a population birth cohort, preliminary findings. *Schizophrenic Research* 90(1–3):251–254.

Philbrook, N.A., and L.M. Winn. 2015. Investigating the effects of in utero benzene exposure on epigenetic modifications in maternal and fetal CD-1 mice. *Toxicology and Applied Pharmacology* 289(1):12–19.

Plenge-Böenig, A., and W. Karmaus. 1999. Exposure to toluene in the printing industry is associated with subfecundity in women but not in men. *Occupational and Environmental Medicine* 56(7):443–448.

Rachootin, P., and J. Olsen. 1983. The risk of infertility and delayed conception associated with exposures in the Danish workplace. *Journal of Occupational and Environmental Medicine* 25:394–402.

Ramakrishnan, A., P.J. Lupo, A.J. Agopian, S.H. Linder, T.H. Stock, P.H. Langlois, and E. Craft. 2013. Evaluating the effects of maternal exposure to benzene, toluene, ethyl benzene, and xylene on oral clefts among offspring in Texas: 1999–2008. *Birth Defects Research* 97(8):532–537.

Rasmussen, K., S. Sabroe, and M. Wohlert. 1988. A genotoxic study of metal workers exposed to trichloroethylene: Sperm parameters and chromosome aberrations in lymphocytes. *International Archives of Occupational & Environmental Health* 60:419–423.

Ratcliffe, J., S. Schrader, D. Clapp, W. Halperin, T. Turner, and R. Hornung. 1989. Semen quality in workers exposed to 2-ethoxyethanol. *British Journal of Industrial Medicine* 46(6):151–157.

Reid, A., D.C. Glass, H.D. Bailey, E. Milne, B.K. Armstrong, F. Alvaro, and L. Fritschi. 2011. Parental occupational exposure to exhausts, solvents, glues and paints, and risk of childhood leukemia. *Cancer Causes and Control* 22(11):1575–1585.

Roberts, L. G., A.C. Bevans, and C.A. Schreiner. 2003. Developmental and reproductive toxicity evaluation of toluene vapor in the rat. I. Reproductive toxicity. *Reproductive Toxicology* 17(6):649–658.

Roberts, L.G., M.J. Nicolich, and C.A. Schreiner. 2007. Developmental and reproductive toxicity evaluation of toluene vapor in the rat. II. Developmental toxicity. *Reproductive Toxicology* 23(4):521–531.

Ruckart, P.Z., F. Bove, and M. Maslia. 2013. Evaluation of exposure to contaminated drinking water and specific birth defects and childhood cancers at Marine Corps Base Camp Lejeune, North Carolina: A case-control study. *Environmental Health and Preventive Medicine* 12:104.

Ruckart, P. Z., F. J. Bove, and M. Maslia. 2014. Evaluation of contaminated drinking water and preterm birth, small for gestational age, and birth weight at Marine Corps Base Camp Lejeune, North Carolina: A cross-sectional study. *Environmental Health and Preventive Medicine* 13(99):1–10.

Saillenfait, A.M., F. Gallissot, J.P. Sabate, N. Bourges-Abella, and S. Muller. 2007. Developmental toxic effects of ethylbenzene or toluene alone and in combination with butyl acetate in rats after inhalation exposure. *Journal of Applied Toxicology* 27(1):32–42.

Sakurai, K., K. Mikamoto, M. Shirai, T. Iguchi, K. Ito, W. Takasaki, and K. Mori. 2015. MicroRNA profiling in ethylene glycol monomethyl ether–induced monkey testicular toxicity model. *Journal of Toxicological Sciences* 40(3):375–382.

Sallmén, M., M.L. Lindbohm, and P. Kyyronen. 1995. Reduced fertility among women exposed to organic solvents. *American Journal of Industrial Medicine* 27(5):699–713.

Sallmén, M., M.L. Lindbohm, A. Anttila, P. Kyyronen, H. Taskinen, E. Nykyri, and K. Hemminki. 1998. Time to pregnancy among the wives of men exposed to organic solvents. *Occupational and Environmental Medicine* 55(1):24–30.

Samuels, S., S. McCurdy, Y.D. Poceka, S. Hammond, L. Missell, and M. Schenker. 1995. Fertility history of currently employed male semiconductor workers. *American Journal of Industrial Medicine* 28(6):873–882.

Schmid, T.E., B. Eskenazi, F. Marchetti, R. Gopalan, G. Li, D. Anderson, S. Rappaport, E. Kurtovich, and A.J. Wyrobek. 2006. Increased human DNA strand damage is associated with occupational exposure to benzene. *Environmental & Molecular Mutagenesis* 47(6):418.

Schwetz, B.A., B.K. J. Leong, and P.J. Gehring. 1975. The effect of maternally inhaled 24 trichloroethylene, perchloroethylene, methyl chloroform, and methylene chloride on 25 embryonal and fetal development in mice and rats. *Toxicology and Applied Pharmacology* 32:84–96.

Senkayi, S.N., M.L. Sattler, N. Rowe, and V.C.P. Chen. 2014. Investigation of an association between childhood leukemia incidences and airports in Texas. *Atmospheric Pollution Research* 5(2):189–195.

Shaw, G., C. Wasserman, C. O'Malley, V. Nelson, and R. Jackson. 1999a. Maternal pesticide exposure from multiple sources and selected congenital anomalies. *Epidemiology* 10(1):60–66.

Shaw, G., E. Velie, E. Katz, K. Morland, D. Schaffer, and V. Nelson. 1999b. Maternal occupational and hobby chemical exposures as risk factors for neural tube defects. *Epidemiology* 10(2):124–129.

Shu, X., P. Stewart, W. Wen, D. Han, J. Potter, J. Buckley, E. Heineman, and L.L. Robison. 1999. Parental occupational exposure to hydrocarbons and risk of acute lymphocytic leukemia in offspring. *Cancer Epidemiology, Biomarkers & Prevention* 8(9):783–791.

Singer, B.C., A.T. Hodgson, and W.W. Nazaroff. 2003. Gas-phase organics in environmental tobacco smoke: 2. Exposure-relevant emission factors and indirect exposures from habitual smoking. *Atmospheric Environment* 37(39–40):5551–5561.

Singh, R.K., and F.W. Bansode. 2011. Benzene-induced histopathological changes and germ cell population dynamics in testes of Sprague Dawley rats. *Journal of Environmental Biology* 32(6):687–694.

Slama, R., O. Thiebaugeorges, V. Goua, L. Aussel, P. Sacco, A. Bohet, A. Forhan, B. Ducot, I. Annesi-Maesano, J. Heinrich, G. Magnin, M. Schweitzer, M. Kaminski, M.A. Charles, and Eden Mother–Child Cohort Study Group. Group. 2009. Maternal personal exposure to airborne benzene and intrauterine growth. *Environmental Health Perspectives* 117(8):1313–1321.

Slater, M.E., A.M. Linabery, L.G. Spector, K.J. Johnson, J.M. Hilden, N.A. Heerema, L.L. Robison, and J.A. Ross. 2011. Maternal exposure to household chemicals and risk of infant leukemia: A report from the Children's Oncology Group. *Cancer Causes Control* 22(8):1197–1204.

Smith, M.K., J.L. Randall, E.J. Read, and J.A. Stober. 1989. Teratogenic activity of trichloroacetic acid in the rat. *Teratology* 40(5):445–451.

Smith, M.K., J.L. Randall, E.J. Read, and J.A. Stober. 1992. Developmental toxicity of dichloroacetate in the rat. *Teratology* 46(3):217–223.

Soberanes-Chavez, P., C. Lopez-Rubalcava, P. de Gortari, and S. L. Cruz. 2013. Exposure to toluene and stress during pregnancy impairs pups' growth and dams' lactation. *Neurotoxicology and Teratology* 40:9–16.

Sonnenfeld, N., I. Herts-Picciotto, and W.E. Kaye. 2001. Tetrachloroethylene in drinking water and birth outcomes at the U.S. Marine Corps Base at Camp Lejeune, North Carolina. *American Journal of Epidemiology* 154:902–908.

Stingone, J.A., K.H. McVeigh, and L. Claudio. 2016. Association between prenatal exposure to ambient diesel particulate matter and perchloroethylene with children's 3rd grade standardized test scores. *Environmental Research* 148:144–153.

Stucker, I., L. Mandereaum, M.P. Aubert-Berleur, F. Deplan, A. Paris, A. Richard, and D. Hemon. 1994. Occupational paternal exposure to benzene and risk of spontaneous abortion. *Occupational and Environmental Medicine* 51(7):475–478.

Svensson, B.G., G. Nise, E.M. Erfurth, A. Nilsson, and S. Skerfving. 1992a. Hormone status in occupational toluene exposure. *American Journal of Industrial Medicine* 22(1):99–107.

Svensson, B.G., G. Nise, E.M. Erfurth, and H. Olsson. 1992b. Neuroendocrine effects in printing workers exposed to toluene. *British Journal of Industrial Medicine* 49(6):402–408.

Swan, S.H., J.J. Beaumont, S.K. Hammond, J. Von Behren, R.S. Green, M.F. Hallock, S.R. Woskie, C.J. Hines, and M.B. Schenker. 1995. Historical cohort study of spontaneous abortion among fabrication workers in the Semiconductor Health Study: Agent-level analysis. *American Journal of Industrial Medicine* 28(6):751–769.

Swartz, M.D., Y. Cai, W. Chan, E. Symanski, L.E. Mitchell, H.E. Danysh, P.H. Langlois, and P.J. Lupo. 2015. Air toxics and birth defects: A Bayesian hierarchical approach to evaluate multiple pollutants and spina bifida children's environmental health. *Environmental Health* 14(1):16.

Szakmáry, É., G. Gungváry, and E. Tátrai. 1997. The offspring-damaging effect of tetrachloroethylene in rats, mice, and rabbits. *Central European Journal of Occupational and Environmental Medicine* 3(1):31–39.

Takei, M., Y. Ando, W. Saitoh, T. Tanimoto, N. Kiyosawa, S. Manabe, A. Sanbuissho, O. Okazaki, H. Iwabuchi, T. Yamoto, K.P. Adam, J.E. Weiel, J.A. Ryals, M.V. Milburn, and L. Guo. 2010. Ethylene glycol monomethyl ether-induced toxicity is mediated through the inhibition of flavoprotein dehydrogenase enzyme family. *Toxicological Sciences* 118(2):643–652.

Tanner, J.P., J.L. Salemi, A.L. Stuart, H. Yu, M. M. Jordan, C. DuClos, P. Cavicchia, J.A. Correia, S.M. Watkins, and R.S. Kirby. 2015. Associations between exposure to ambient benzene and $PM_{2.5}$ during pregnancy and the risk of selected birth defects in offspring. *Environmental Research* 142:345–353.

Tap, O., S. Solmaz, and S. Polat. 1996. The effect of toluene on the rat ovary: An ultrastructural study. *Journal of Submicroscopic Cytology and Pathology* 28(4):553–558.

Tardif, R., G. Truchon, and J. Brodeur. 1998. Comparison of hippuric acid and *o*-cresol in urine and unchanged toluene in alveolar air for the biological monitoring of exposure to toluene in human volunteers. *Applied Occupational and Environmental Hygiene* 13(2):127–132.

Taskinen, H., A. Anttila, M.L. Lindbohm, M. Sallmén, and K. Hemminki. 1989. Spontaneous abortions and congenital malformations among the wives of men occupationally exposed to organic solvents. *Scandinavian Journal of Work, Environment & Health* 15(5):345–352.

Taskinen, H., P. Kyyronen, K. Hemminki, M. Hoikkala, K. Lajunen, and M.L. Lindbohm. 1994. Laboratory work and pregnancy outcome. *Journal of Occupational Medicine* 36(3):311–319.

Thiel, R., and I. Chahoud. 1997. Postnatal development and behaviour of Wistar rats after prenatal toluene exposure. *Archives of Toxicology* 71(4):258–265.

Tinston, D.J. 1994. *Perchloroethylene: A multigeneration inhalation study in the rat*. Cheshire, UK: Zeneca Central Toxicology Laboratory.

Torfs, C., E. Katz, T. Bateson, P. Lam, and C. Curry. 1996. Maternal medications and environmental exposures as risk factors for gastroschisis. *Teratology* 54(2):84–92.

Tsukahara, S., D. Nakajima, Y. Kuroda, R. Hojo, S. Kageyama, and H. Fujimaki. 2009. Effects of maternal toluene exposure on testosterone levels in fetal rats. *Toxicology Letters* 185(2):79–84.

Ungvary, G., and E. Tatrai. 1985. On the embryotoxic effects of benzene and its alkyl derivatives in mice, rats and rabbits. *Archives of Toxicology* 8:425–430.

Veulemans, H., O. Steeno, R. Masschelein, and D. Groeseneken. 1993. Exposure to ethylene glycol ethers and spermatogenic disorders in man: A case-control study. *British Journal of Industrial Medicine* 50(1):71–78.

Vinceti, M., C. Malagoli, M. Malavolti, A. Cherubini, G. Maffeis, R. Rodolfi, J.E. Heck, G. Astolfi, E. Calzolari, and F. Nicolini. 2016. Does maternal exposure to benzene and PM_{10} during pregnancy increase the risk of congenital anomalies? A population-based case-control study. *Science of the Total Environment* 541:444–450.

von Ehrenstein, O.S., H. Aralis, M. Cockburn, and B. Ritz. 2014. In utero exposure to toxic air pollutants and risk of childhood autism. *Epidemiology* 25(6):851–858.

von Ehrenstein, O.S., J.E. Heck, A.S. Park, M. Cockburn, L. Escobedo, and B. Ritz. 2016. In utero and early-life exposure to ambient air toxics and childhood brain tumors: A population-based case-control study in California, USA. *Environmental Health Perspectives* 124(7):1093–1099.

Wan, J., and L.M. Winn. 2008. In utero exposure to benzene increases embryonic c-Myb and Pim-1 protein levels in CD-1 mice. *Toxicology and Applied Pharmacology* 228(3):326–333.

Wang, R.S., K. Ohtani, M. Suda, and T. Nakajima. 2006. Inhibitory effect of ethylene glycol monoethyl ether on rat sperm motion. *Industrial Health* 44(4):665–668.

Warren, D.A., L.J. Graeter, S.R. Channel, J. S. Eggers, C.D. Goodyear, K.L. Macmahon, G.L. Sudberry, J.R. Latendresse, J.W. Fisher, and W.H. Baker. 2006. Trichloroethylene, trichloroacetic acid, and dichloroacetic acid: Do they affect eye development in the Sprague-Dawley rat? *International Journal of Toxicology* 25(4):279–284.

Watanabe, A., Y. Nakano, T. Endo, N. Sato, K. Kai, and K. Shiraiwa. 2000. Collaborative work to evaluate toxicity on male reproductive organs by repeated dose studies in rats. 27). Repeated toxicity study on ethylene glycol monomethyl ether for 2 and 4 weeks to detect effects on male reproductive organs in rats. *Journal of Toxicological Sciences* 25(Spec No):259–266.

Welch, L., S. Schrader, T. Turner, and M. Cullen. 1988. Effects of exposure to ethylene glycol ethers on shipyard painters: II. Male reproduction. *American Journal of Industrial Medicine* 14(5):509–526.

Weng, S.P., T.C. Wu, S.U. Chen, J. Wu, C.C. Lin, Y.C. Yang, and P.C. Chen. 2010. The impact of ethylene glycol monomethyl ether on ovarian function may extend to the next generation in female mice: A preliminary study. *Reproductive Toxicology* 29(4):452–457.

White, R., R. Feldman, I. Eviator, J. Jabre, and C. Niles. 1997. Hazardous waste and 19 neurobehavioral effects: A developmental perspective. *Environmental Research* 73:113–124.

WHO (World Health Organization). 2010. *WHO guidelines for indoor air quality: Selected pollutants*. Copenhagen, Denmark: World Health Organization. http://www.euro.who.int/__data/assets/pdf_file/0009/128169/e94535.pdf (accessed August 22, 2018).

Williams, J., J.R. Reel, J.D. George, and J.C. Lamb. 1990. Reproductive effects of diethylene glycol and diethylene glycol monoethyl ether in Swiss CD-1 mice assessed by a continuous breeding protocol. *Fundamentals of Applied Toxicology* 14(3):622–635.

Win-Shwe, T.T., N. Kunugita, D. Nakajima, Y. Yoshida, and H. Fujimaki. 2012. Developmental stage-specific changes in immunological biomarkers in male C3H/HeN mice after early life toluene exposure. *Toxicology Letters* 208(2):133–141.

Windham, G.C., D. Shusterman, S. H. Swan, L. Fenster, and B. Eskenazi. 1991. Exposure to organic solvents and adverse pregnancy outcome. *American Journal of Industrial Medicine* 20(2):241–259.

Wu, K.L., and T. Berger. 2007. Trichloroethylene metabolism in the rat ovary reduces oocyte fertilizability. *Chemico-Biological Interactions* 170(1):20–30.

Xiao, G., C. Pan, Y. Cai, H. Lin, and Z. Fu. 2001. Effect of benzene, toluene, xylene on the semen quality and the function of accessory gonad of exposed workers. *Industrial Health* 39(2):206–210.

Xing, C., F. Marchetti, G. Li, R.H. Weldon, E. Kurtovich, S. Young, T.E. Schmid, L. Zhang, S. Rappaport, S. Waidyanatha, A.J. Wyrobek, and B. Eskenazi. 2010. Benzene exposure near the U.S. Permissible limit is associated with sperm aneuploidy. *Environmental Health Perspectives* 118(6):833–839.

Xu, X., S.I. Cho, M. Sammel, L. You, S. Cui, Y. Huang, G. Ma, C. Padungtod, L. Pothier, T. Niu, D. Christiani, T. Smith, L. Ryan, and L. Wang. 1998. Association of petrochemical exposure with spontaneous abortion. *Occupational and Environmental Medicine* 55(1):31–36.

Yamamoto, S., S. Tin Tin Win, Y. Yoshida, N. Kunugita, K. Arashidani, and H. Fujimaki. 2009. Children's immunology, what can we learn from animal studies (2): Modulation of systemic Th1/Th2 immune response in infant mice after prenatal exposure to low-level toluene and toll-like receptor (TLR) 2 ligand. *Journal of Toxicological Sciences* 34(Suppl 2):SP341–SP348.

Yauck, J.S., M.E. Malloy, K. Blair, P.M. Simpson, and D.G. McCarver. 2004. Proximity of residence to trichloroethylene-emitting sites and increased risk of offspring congenital heart defects among older women. *Birth Defects Research* 70(10):808–814.

Yoon, C.Y., C.M. Hong, Y.Y. Cho, Y. H. Chung, H.K. Min, Y. W. Yun, B.J. Lee, K. H. Yang, Y.S. Lee, and C.K. Kim. 2003. Flow cytometric assessment of ethylene glycol monoethyl ether on spermatogenesis in rats. *Journal of Veterinary Medical Science* 65(2):207–212.

Zahran, S., S. Weiler, H.W. Mielke, and A.A. Pena. 2012. Maternal benzene exposure and low birth weight risk in the United States: A natural experiment in gasoline reformulation. *Environmental Research* 112:139–146.

Zenick, H., K. Blackburn, E. Hope, N. Richdale, and M. K. Smith. 1984. Effects of 1 trichloroethylene exposure on male reproductive function in rats. *Toxicology* 31(3–4):237–250.

Zhou, Y., S. Zhang, Z. Li, J. Zhu, Y. Bi, Y. Bai, and H. Wang. 2014. Maternal benzene exposure during pregnancy and risk of childhood acute lymphoblastic leukemia: A meta-analysis of epidemiologic studies. *PLOS ONE* 9(10):e110466.

8

Outcomes Toward Heritable Effects

The committee's findings for deployment-related exposures, pesticides, combustion products, and solvents, as detailed in Chapters 4 through 7, are summarized here. During the evaluation process, the committee identified important data and knowledge gaps and methodological constraints that hinder an understanding of how veterans' exposures during deployment might affect their children and grandchildren. The committee emphasizes the need to interpret the conclusions in these chapters and also any future research within the broader context of both the veterans' and their descendants' exposures over their lifecourses. In addition to the committee's findings on the basis of the epidemiologic literature, there is a growing body of research on potentially acquired generational effects induced by epigenetic changes. Evidence linking epigenetic changes to health effects in descendants is being developed but is currently insufficient to identify specific associations with the deployment exposures discussed in this report. The committee emphasizes that it reviewed the literature on the exposures indicated in the Gulf War legislation and in other relevant reports (see Chapter 1). However, the literature on each toxicant was not consistent in terms of quantity, quality, or the health effects that were examined and, therefore, the lack of information on some toxicants should not be taken to mean that there are no effects from those toxicants, only that the effects may not have been studied or identified in the published literature.

HEALTH OUTCOMES ASSOCIATED WITH GULF WAR DEPLOYMENT

The committee was charged with summarizing the strength of the scientific evidence regarding exposure to the deployment toxicants identified in the Gulf War legislation (P.L. 105-277 and P.L. 105-368, see Chapter 1) and the reproductive, developmental, and generational effects that may be associated with them, with a particular focus on the health of children of deployed veterans. While both epidemiologic and toxicologic studies were evaluated for health outcomes from the exposures of concern, as described in Chapters 4 through 7, the committee identified categories of association based only on the human data. Mechanistic animal model studies provided additional data that were not available from the human studies. The associations identified by the committee in its review of the literature are provided in Table 8-1 for reproductive effects in men and women and adverse pregnancy outcomes and in Table 8-2 for developmental effects.

TABLE 8-1 Summary of Categories of Association for Reproductive Effects and Adverse Pregnancy Outcomes*

	Categories of Association		
Toxicant	**Sufficient**	**Limited/suggestive**	**Inadequate/insufficient**
Deployment			Reproductive effects in men or women; adverse pregnancy outcomes
Sarin/cyclosarin			Reproductive effects in men or women; adverse pregnancy outcomes
Sulfur mustard		Reproductive effects in men	Reproductive effects in women; adverse pregnancy outcomes
Leishmaniasis	Adverse pregnancy outcomes		Reproductive effects in men or women
Anthrax vaccine			Reproductive effects in men or women; adverse pregnancy outcomes
Depleted uranium			Reproductive effects in men or women; adverse pregnancy outcomes
Pyridostigmine bromide			Reproductive effects in men; adverse pregnancy outcomes
Hexavalent chromium	Reproductive effects in men	Adverse pregnancy outcomes	Reproductive effects in women
Organophosphate pesticides		Reproductive effects in men	Reproductive effects in women; adverse pregnancy outcomes
Carbamate pesticides	Reproductive effects in men		Reproductive effects in women; adverse pregnancy outcomes
Pyrethroids		Reproductive effects in men	Reproductive effects in women; adverse pregnancy outcomes
Lindane		Reproductive effects in women	Reproductive effects in men; adverse pregnancy outcomes
DEET			Reproductive effects in men or women; adverse pregnancy outcomes

TABLE 8-1 Continued

	Categories of Association		
Toxicant	**Sufficient**	**Limited/suggestive**	**Inadequate/insufficient**
Particulate matter	Adverse pregnancy outcomes	Pregnancy-induced hypertensive disorders	Reproductive effects in men or women
Polycyclic aromatic hydrocarbons		Reproductive effects in men; adverse pregnancy outcomes	Reproductive effects in women
Polychlorinated dibenzodioxins/furans			Reproductive effects in men or women; adverse pregnancy outcomes
Exhaust			Reproductive effects in men or women; adverse pregnancy outcomes
Fuels			Reproductive effects in men or women; adverse pregnancy outcomes
Benzene		Reproductive effects in men	Reproductive effects in women; adverse pregnancy outcomes
Toluene			Reproductive effects in men or women; adverse pregnancy outcomes
Xylenes			Reproductive effects in men or women; adverse pregnancy outcomes
Trichloroethylene		Reproductive effects in men; adverse pregnancy outcomes	Reproductive effects in women
Tetrachloroethylene			Reproductive effects in men or women; adverse pregnancy outcomes
Glycols and glycol ethers		Reproductive effects in men	Reproductive effects in women; adverse pregnancy outcomes

* There were no toxicants for which sufficient evidence of a causal association was found between exposure to that toxicant and reproductive effects, nor were there any toxicants for which there was limited/suggestive evidence of no association between exposure and reproductive effects.

TABLE 8-2 Summary of Categories of Association for Developmental Effects*

	Categories of Association		
Toxicant	**Sufficient**	**Limited/suggestive**	**Inadequate/insufficient**
Deployment			Developmental effects
Sarin/cyclosarin			Developmental effects
Sulfur mustard			Developmental effects
Leishmaniasis			Developmental effects
Vaccines			Developmental effects
Depleted uranium			Developmental effects
Pyridostigmine bromide			Developmental effects
Hexavalent chromium	Developmental effects		
Organophosphate pesticides	Neurodevelopmental effects		Other developmental effects
Carbamate pesticides			Developmental effects
Pyrethroid insecticides		Developmental effects	
Lindane			Developmental effects
DEET			Developmental effects
Particulate matter		Respiratory effects; neurodevelopmental effects	Other developmental effects in children
Polycyclic aromatic hydrocarbons		Birth defects; childhood cancer; neurodevelopmental effects; respiratory effects	Other developmental effects
Polychlorinated dibenzodioxins/furans			Developmental effects
Exhaust			Developmental effects
Fuels			Developmental effects
Benzene	Leukemia		Other developmental effects
Toluene			Developmental effects
Xylenes			Developmental effects
Trichloroethylene		Developmental effects	
Tetrachloroethylene		Developmental effects	
Glycols and glycol ethers		Birth defects	Other developmental effects

* There were no toxicants for which sufficient evidence was found of a causal association between prenatal exposure to that toxicant and developmental effects, nor were there any toxicants for which there was limited/suggestive evidence of no association between prenatal exposure and developmental effects.

None of the toxicants examined by the committee were found to have a **causal** relationship with reproductive or developmental effects. The toxicants that were considered to have **sufficient** evidence of an association with reproductive effects were hexavalent chromium (Cr6), carbamate pesticides, and particulate matter (PM). Cr6 exposures were found to be associated with pregnancy loss and broad changes in semen parameters. Carbamate pesticide exposures were found to be associated with reproductive effects in men, and PM exposure was associated with preterm birth and low birth weight.

There was **limited/suggestive** evidence for several toxicants having associations with reproductive effects in either men or women. Male reproductive effects, particularly altered semen parameters, were associated with sulfur mustard, organophosphate (OP) and pyrethroid pesticides, polycyclic aromatic hydrocarbons (PAHs), benzene, trichloroethylene (TCE), and glycols and glycol ethers. Female reproductive effects, specifically changes in endometrial tissue, were associated with lindane. **Limited/suggestive evidence** of associations specific to adverse pregnancy or birth outcomes was found for infection with Leishmaniasis during pregnancy, PAHs, TCE, and glycols and glycol ethers, and pregnancy-induced hypertensive disorders with PM.

Toxicants considered by the committee to have **sufficient** evidence of associations with developmental effects in children were limited to prenatal Cr6 exposure with structural defects and delayed sexual maturation, prenatal exposure to OP pesticides with neurodevelopmental effects, and prenatal benzene exposure with childhood leukemia. Conclusions of **limited/suggestive** evidence of associations with developmental effects were found for pyrethroid insecticide exposures and also TCE and tetrachloroethylene exposures, whereas congenital malformations were associated with glycols and glycol ethers. The committee also found **limited/suggestive** evidence of associations between exposure to PM and PAH and respiratory and neurodevelopmental effects in children, with additional associations between PAH exposure and birth defects and childhood cancer. All these associations are limited to prenatal exposures.

Animal Studies

The committee considered associations between deployment exposures and reproductive and developmental effects on the basis of human data. For some toxicants, human data were lacking, but there was a relative abundance of animal data. The toxicants for which animal data were robust, but a lack of human data precluded the committee from assigning a stronger category of association, are the following:

- Depleted uranium and reproductive effects in males;
- Lindane and reproductive effects in males and developmental effects in offspring;
- Toluene and developmental effects in offspring;
- Xylenes and developmental effects in offspring;
- TCE and reproductive effects in females; and
- Dioxin and reproductive effects in males and females.

On one hand, the use of animal models permits greater control with defined exposures. On the other hand, these models may lack temporal resolution since only specific points in time are considered. Often, they do not model the cumulative effect of exposures to mixtures that are observed in humans. In addition, adsorption, distribution, metabolism, and excretion processes can vary widely between humans and other species, and effects seen in one species might not be seen in another.

SUMMARY OF DATA AND KNOWLEDGE GAPS

The committee's conclusions are limited by the availability of pertinent evidence. In its review of the literature, the committee identified data and knowledge gaps that were used to inform the research agenda detailed in Chapter 9. Some of the priorities for research are discussed below. Data were often not available for an evaluation of the critical windows of exposure for developmental and male and female reproductive effects. Very limited data were found on actual exposure assessment and epidemiological research, the majority of which consisted of civilian-based studies that did not mimic deployment exposures. How these data gaps resulted in a lack of knowledge with which to inform associations between deployment exposures and outcomes is discussed briefly below.

Developmental and Reproductive Effects

Developmental effects were almost exclusively studied with *prenatal* exposures. Studies of *preconception* exposures are virtually nonexistent for all the toxicants reviewed in Chapters 4 through 7. Most of the evidence gathered by the committee was on long-term, continuous occupational and environmental exposures, none of which mimic the potential short-term exposures experienced by veterans during deployment. Such gaps limited the committee's ability to draw conclusions about the potential health effects specific to veterans and their descendants.

The effects of toxicants on female reproductive capacity and function from oocyte to the birth of a child and the ability of that child to reproduce have not been studied in depth. Although effects on sperm have been evaluated for many toxicants, few studies have assessed the reproductive effects in women (Krulewitch, 2016). One area that has been studied in animal models is the apparent link between benzo[a]pyrene (BaP) exposure and effects on endometrial and ovarian function (Li et al., 2017; Luderer et al., 2017).

Unlike Gulf War and Post-9/11 veterans, Vietnam veterans have been extensively studied for the existence of reproductive and developmental health effects. Despite the vast amount of data available from this population, no definitive effects on male or female reproductive endpoints have been identified (NASEM, 2016). The Volume 11 committee acknowledges that limited data on 2,3,7,8-tetrachlorodibenzo-p-dioxin (TCDD) exposures in nonveteran populations show altered semen parameters in men and increased time to pregnancy in women, but those exposures are not similar to what most veterans experienced (e.g., low levels of exposure associated with combustion from burn pits). Although animal studies support specific TCDD effects on reproduction, the effects are highly species-specific, and animal responses do not consistently predict human responses because of differing sensitivities and susceptibilities. Furthermore, previous research has not addressed specific windows of susceptibility for adverse reproductive effects. Therefore, the committee has a residual concern that adverse reproductive effects may occur with different exposure scenarios, and it identifies this area as a major priority for future monitoring and research (see Chapters 9 and 10).

As noted above, many toxicants have been evaluated for their effects on semen. These evaluations typically rely on measurements of physical and morphological sperm parameters, including volume, total count, vitality, motility, and abnormalities (Cooper et al., 2010), but the particular set of measurements used varies across laboratories and studies (Auger et al., 2000). Furthermore, semen parameters are not a good surrogate for determining infertility. As Guzick et al. (2001) concluded, "Threshold values for sperm concentration, motility, and morphology can be used to classify men as subfertile, of indeterminate fertility, or fertile. None of the measures, however, are diagnostic of infertility." Taken together, all of this results in a variability that clouds the relationship between semen parameters and fertility (Khatun et al., 2018; Patel et al., 2017); furthermore, the studies provide no information about the health of a resulting fetus or what long-term clinical outcomes might result from toxic exposures. New and objective omics-based tests—using, for example, RNAs, proteins, and DNA methylation profiles—may provide consistent and standardized analytical methods and measures to help define a suite of parameters that better predict fertility and a father's contribution to the birth and lifecourse of his child. Greater consistency, validity, and biological resolution of measures that are better correlated with clinical outcomes than semen parameters are needed to assess the full impact of toxicants on sperm and male reproduction and their effects on descendants.

The evidence demonstrates the potential risks to children posed by prenatal exposures to toxicants; however, as few female service members are pregnant while deployed in the theater of operation, the applicability of those conclusions to female veterans is unknown. For the few female veterans who were pregnant during deployment—as far back as Vietnam and up to the Post-9/11 era—there has been little follow-up of those pregnancies or of the children.

To understand how prenatal exposures may influence the health of children as they grow, the postnatal environment must also be considered. Prenatal exposures may be modified by postnatal exposures (and vice versa) or, alternatively, by cumulative lifecourse exposures (e.g., throughout pre- and postnatal life). A few of the studies of prenatal exposures discussed in Chapters 4 through 7 assessed the health of the children in their teenage years, but in general the studies have not assessed or controlled for the confounding effects of postnatal exposures on the child's development and health later in life. Important health outcomes that become apparent in adolescence or adulthood (e.g., mental health conditions or illicit drug use with early life exposure to tetrachloroethylene; Aschengrau et al., 2016; Sagiv et al., 2018; and Yang et al., 2016, who assessed children up to age 14) are being studied; however, the link from prenatal exposure to adult disease requires substantial development. Thus, there is a need to assess and adjust for prenatal and postnatal experiences in future studies of preconception exposures and developmental outcomes to be able to differentiate between effects of certain exposures or windows of susceptibility.

Exposure Assessment

In the absence of exposure data, biomarkers may be used as a proxy for exposure assessment. Not all chemical exposures in the human body can be measured with biomarkers, especially a long time after the exposure has taken place, and specificity may be lost. Some exposures can be measured in blood products, but other biomarkers of exposure are better measured in urine or other bodily fluids. And sometimes exposures can be determined only by measuring the breakdown products of the original chemicals—for example, dialkylphosphates (DAPs) as metabolites of OPs—which can lead to a loss of specificity since, for instance, DAPs are nonspecific metabolites of a number of OPs. Additionally, many chemicals have a relatively short half-life in the body and they can be measured only within hours or days after exposure. Therefore, a single measurement may not accurately reflect an exposure that took place over a critical window of development or reproduction, especially if the exposure scenario is variable. For many chemicals there are no laboratory methods to measure them, or the method is not considered to be of sufficient reliability or sensitivity to accurately measure relevant levels of exposure. Thus, exposure assessment especially when conducted after a long period of time—for example, after a member of the military has returned from deployment—can be a major limitation of epidemiologic investigations. Assessment issues are further discussed in Chapter 9. Another challenge is that the effects of multiple, simultaneous, or successive exposures have rarely been studied in human population, yet they more likely reflect the actual exposure scenarios. Deployed military personnel may be exposed to environmental chemicals such as pesticides and PAHs as well as cigarette smoke and nonchemical stressors such as extreme heat, psychological stress, and radiation. Some may act on the same receptors (e.g., nicotine and OPs both act on acetylcholine neurotransmission), raising the possibility that they could enhance toxicity (see Coker et al., 2017; Woods et al., 2017)..

Epidemiologic Analyses

Most of the epidemiologic research reviewed in Chapters 4 through 7 was of environmentally or occupationally exposed populations. In those populations exposure typically occurred continuously, from before conception through the development of health effects during childhood and the entire lifecourse. Veterans' exposures happened during defined time periods, generally several months at a time, and occurred generally with little, if any, direct monitoring. The long-term health risks associated with toxicant exposures over the period of deployment generally have not characterized risks after the exposure ended, with the exception of a few occupational studies. The presentation of long-term health effects may change over time (i.e., it may appear after many years), it may stay the same for some outcomes, or it may decrease over time or be negligible soon after exposure ceases. An overview of epidemiological studies is provided in Chapter 9.

One major limitation of epidemiologic studies is the presence of modifiers of effect. Common modifiers may include lifestyle factors such as cigarette smoking and exercise, diet, a family history of the disease or condition, and sociodemographic characteristics. The difficulty in controlling for modifiers is compounded when multiple generations are evaluated over a long period of time.

The committee's review recognizes the potential for a veteran's preconception or prenatal exposures to result in intergenerational effects, particularly effects in his or her children (the F1 generation). Although transgenerational effects are less certain in humans, some animal studies have found effects in second (F2) and third (F3) generation offspring. The toxicants that have been studied for transgenerational effects in animals include PM, BaP, dioxin, permethrin + DEET, pesticides, stress, and fuels; none of the toxicants of concern for this report have been studied for transgenerational effects in humans (Walker et al., 2018).

Epigenetic Effects

Epigenetic effects resulting from a variety of prenatal exposures to PM, PAHs, polychlorinated dibenzo-p-dioxins/dibenzofurans (PCDD/PCDFs), fuels, Cr6, and pesticides have been observed in various tissues and systems. To date, however, few human studies have included measures of epigenetic alterations. The presence of some epigenetic effects has been shown in toxicological studies of PCDD/PCDFs, BaP, and OP pesticides (Walker et al. 2018) and in human studies—for example, studies of the effects of PM exposure. The epigenetic literature in humans, as illustrated by studies of PM effects, relies on relatively large sets of samples and studies, such as ENVIRONAGE (ENVIRonmental influence ON early AGEing; Grevendonk et al., 2016; Janssen et al., 2012, 2013, 2015); the Children's Health Study (Breton et al., 2016; Salam et al., 2012); PROGRESS (Programming Research in Obesity, Growth, Environment and Social Stressors; Rosa et al., 2017); and MAMC (Metropolitan Area of Mexico City; Alvarado-Cruz et al., 2017). Until recently, the majority of epigenetic studies of PM had not accounted for the variability that arises from the use of heterogeneous cell types in cord blood, placenta, and peripheral blood lymphocyte samples (see Chapter 3). Although epigenetic changes might result in clinically relevant health effects, little is understood about these mechanisms or about how the various changes—and what specific types of changes—modify the presentation of health effects.

The complexity of assessing gene *x* environment interactions increases when exposure to mixtures (Silva da Silva et al., 2015) and the stage of development (Soto-Martinez and Sly, 2010) are considered. A challenge to interpreting results from observational studies is that the estimates of effects are often confounded by other potential modifiers of the epigenome. Potential confounders, such as smoking, have been associated with altered DNA (Jenkins et al., 2017; Knopik et al., 2012) and are often not accounted for in analyses.

Although no human data directly describe the transgenerational effects of these exposures, there is evidence from intergenerational and transgenerational effects in animal studies that prenatal exposures, such as to BaP, can affect the development of reproductive organs and stem cells (EPA, 2017). None of the exposures considered by this committee had been studied for their potential transgenerational effects in humans, although some animal studies are discussed in earlier chapters (PM, BaP, PCDD/PCDFs, the jet fuel JP-8, permethrin + DEET mixture; Walker et al., 2018). However, there is research examining the transgenerational effects of prenatal exposures to some of the environmental stresses and toxicants that are not considered in this report. These studies include the Avon Longitudinal Study of Parents and Children, the Swedish Överkalix cohorts, and studies of the 1944–1945 Dutch famine (Pembrey et al., 2014).

The Volume 11 committee notes that pesticides, including OPs, are routinely tested for reproductive and developmental toxicity in animals and that these studies provide information on intergenerational (F0→F1) effects—that is, the effects of parental exposures in their offspring. However, studies of the transgenerational effects of OPs—that is, the effects in unexposed offspring—have not yet been conducted in animal models. In approaching the issue of pesticide transgenerational effects, the first pesticides chosen for study (e.g., vinclozolin) are well-characterized reproductive toxicants with known genetic or epigenetic effects (Walker et al., 2018). As research progresses, knowledge of the developmental and reproductive toxicity of OPs is likely to guide transgenerational studies in animal models. Nevertheless, in spite of a growing evidence base on the reproductive and developmental toxicity of OPs, such as chlorpyrifos, the exposures most relevant to Gulf War and Post-9/11 deployments—that is, preconception for both men and women and early pregnancy—have not been well studied in human populations.

SUMMARY

Throughout the time the committee spent reviewing and evaluating the epidemiologic and toxicologic literature on deployment toxicants, as described earlier in this chapter, it identified data and knowledge gaps. These gaps included the need for better exposure assessment methods, for identifying the windows of exposure that pose the greatest risk, and for elucidating possible epigenetic effects that may result in heritable effects. Addressing these gaps using both human and animal studies will be a crucial part of helping improve our understanding of generational health effects. Approaches to conducting human studies in veterans and their children and grandchildren are described in Chapter 9, and the use of animal and mechanistic studies is discussed in Chapter 10.

REFERENCES

Alvarado-Cruz, I., M. Sanchez-Guerra, L. Hernandez-Cadena, A. De Vizcaya-Ruiz, V. Mugica, N.A. Pelallo-Martinez, M.D.J. Solis-Heredia, H.M. Byun, A. Baccarelli, and B. Quintanilla-Vega. 2017. Increased methylation of repetitive elements and DNA repair genes is associated with higher DNA oxidation in children in an urbanized, industrial environment. *Mutation Research/Genetic Toxicology and Environmental Mutagenesis* 813:27–36.

Aschengrau, A., P.A. Janulewicz, R.F. White, V.M. Vieira, L.G. Gallagher, K.D. Getz, T.F. Webster, and D.M. Ozonoff. 2016. Long-term neurotoxic effects of early life exposure to tetrachloroethylene-contaminated drinking water. *Annals of Global Health* 82(1):169–179.

Auger, J., F. Eustache, B. Ducot, T. Blandin, M. Daudin, I. Diaz, S.E. Matribi, B. Gony, L. Keskes, M. Kolbezen, A. Lamarte, J. Lornage, N. Nomal, G. Pitaval, O. Simon, I. Virant-Klun, A. Spira, and P. Jouannet. 2000. Intra- and inter-individual variability in human sperm concentration, motility and vitality assessment during a workshop involving ten laboratories. *Human Reproduction* 15(11):2360–2368.

Breton, C.V., J. Yao, J. Millstein, L. Gao, K.D. Siegmund, W. Mack, L. Whitfield-Maxwell, F. Lurmann, H. Hodis, E. Avol, and F.D. Gilliland. 2016. Prenatal air pollution exposures, DNA methyl transferase genotypes, and associations with newborn LINE1 and Alu methylation and childhood blood pressure and carotid intima-media thickness in the Children's Health Study. *Environmental Health Perspectives* 124(12):1905–1912.

Coker, E., R. Gunier, A. Bradman, K. Harley, K. Kogut, J. Molitor, and B. Eskenazi. 2017. Association between pesticide profiles used on agricultural fields near maternal residences during pregnancy and IQ at age 7 years. *International Journal of Environmental Research and Public Health* 14(5):E506.

Cooper, T.G., E. Noonan, S. von Eckardstein, J. Auger, H.W. Baker, H.M. Behre, T.B. Haugen, T. Kruger, C. Wang, M.T. Mbizvo, and K.M. Vogelsong. 2010. World Health Organization reference values for human semen characteristics. *Human Reproduction Update* 16(3):231–245.

EPA (U.S. Environmental Protection Agency). 2017. *Toxicological review of benzo[a]pyrene* [CASRN 50-32-8]. EPA/635/R-17/003Fa. Washington, DC: Integrated Risk Information System, National Center for Environmental Assessment, Office of Research and Development, U.S. Environmental Protection Agency.

Grevendonk, L., B.G. Janssen, C. Vanpoucke, W. Lefebvre, M. Hoxha, V. Bollati, and T.S. Nawrot. 2016. Mitochondrial oxidative DNA damage and exposure to particulate air pollution in mother–newborn pairs. *Environmental Health* 15:10.

Guzick, D.S., J.W. Overstreet, P. Factor-Litvak, C.K. Brazil, S.T. Nakajima, C. Coutifaris, S.A. Carson, P. Cisneros, M.P. Steinkampf, J.A. Hill, D. Xu, and D.L. Vogel. 2001. Sperm morphology, motility, and concentration in fertile and infertile men. *New England Journal of Medicine* 345(19):1388–1393.

Janssen, B.G., E. Munters, N. Pieters, K. Smeets, B. Cox, A. Cuypers, F. Fierens, J. Penders, J. Vangronsveld, W. Gyselaers, and T.S. Nawrot. 2012. Placental mitochondrial DNA content and particulate air pollution during in utero life. *Environmental Health Perspectives* 120(9):1346–1352.

Janssen, B.G., L. Godderis, N. Pieters, K. Poels, M. Kicinski, A. Cuypers, F. Fierens, J. Penders, M. Plusquin, W. Gyselaers, and T.S. Nawrot. 2013. Placental DNA hypomethylation in association with particulate air pollution in early life. *Particle and Fibre Toxicology* 10:22.

Janssen, B.G., H.M. Byun, W. Gyselaers, W. Lefebvre, A.A. Baccarelli, and T.S. Nawrot. 2015. Placental mitochondrial methylation and exposure to airborne particulate matter in the early life environment: An ENVIRONAGE birth cohort study. *Epigenetics* 10(6):536–544.

Jenkins, T.G., E.R. James, D.F. Alonso, J.R. Hoidal, P.J. Murphy, J.M. Hotaling, B.R. Cairns, D.T. Carrell, and K.I. Aston. 2017. Cigarette smoking significantly alters sperm DNA methylation patterns. *Andrology* 5(6):1089–1099.

Khatun, A., M.S. Rahman, and M.G. Pang. 2018. Clinical assessment of the male fertility. *Obstetrics & Gynecology Science* 61(2):179–191.

Knopik, V.S., M.A. Maccani, S. Francazio, and J.E. McGeary. 2012. The epigenetics of maternal cigarette smoking during pregnancy and effects on child development. *Developmental Psychopathology* 24(4):1377–1390.

Krulewitch, C.J. 2016. Reproductive health of active duty women in medically austere environments. *Military Medicine* 181(Suppl 1):63–69.

Li, X., C. Shen, X. Liu, J. He, Y. Ding, R. Gao, X. Mu, Y. Geng, Y. Wang, and X. Chen. 2017. Exposure to benzo[a]pyrene impairs decidualization and decidual angiogenesis in mice during early pregnancy. *Environmental Pollution* 222:523–531.

Luderer, U., F. Christensen, W.O. Johnson, J. She, H.S.S. Ip, J. Zhou, J. Alvaran, E.F. Krieg, Jr., and J.S. Kesner. 2017. Associations between urinary biomarkers of polycyclic aromatic hydrocarbon exposure and reproductive function during menstrual cycles in women. *Environment International* 100:110–120.

NASEM (National Academies of Sciences, Engineering, and Medicine). 2016. *Veterans and Agent Orange: Update 2014*. Washington, DC: The National Academies Press.

Patel, A.S., J.Y. Leong, and R. Ramasamy. 2017. Prediction of male infertility by the World Health Organization laboratory manual for assessment of semen analysis: A systematic review. *Arab Journal of Urology* 16(1):96–102.

Pembrey, M., R. Saffery, L.O. Bygren, and the Network in Epigenetic Epidemiology. 2014. Human transgenerational responses to early-life experience: Potential impact on development, health and biomedical research. *Journal of Medical Genetics* 51(9):563–572.

Rosa, M.J., A. Pajak, A.C. Just, P.E. Sheffield, I. Kloog, J. Schwartz, B. Coull, M.B. Enlow, A.A. Baccarelli, K. Huddleston, J.E. Niederhuber, M.M.T. Rojo, R.O. Wright, C. Gennings, and R.J. Wright. 2017. Prenatal exposure to $PM_{2.5}$ and birth weight: A pooled analysis from three North American longitudinal pregnancy cohort studies. *Environment International* 107:173–180.

Sagiv, S.K., M.H. Harris, R.B. Gunier, K.R. Kogut, K.G. Harley, J. Deardorff, A. Bradman, N. Holland, and B. Eskenazi. 2018. Prenatal organophosphate pesticide exposure and traits related to autism spectrum disorders in a population living in proximity to agriculture. *Environmental Health Perspectives* 126(4):047012-1–047012-9.

Salam, M.T., H.M. Byun, F. Lurmann, C.V. Breton, X. Wang, S.P. Eckel, and F.D. Gilliland. 2012. Genetic and epigenetic variations in inducible nitric oxide synthase promoter, particulate pollution, and exhaled nitric oxide levels in children. *Journal of Allergy and Clinical Immunology* 129(1):232–239.

Silva da Silva, C., J.M. Rossato, J.A. Vaz Rocha, and V.M. Vargas. 2015. Characterization of an area of reference for inhalable particulate matter ($PM_{2.5}$) associated with genetic biomonitoring in children. *Mutation Research/Genetic Toxicology and Environmental Mutagenesis* 778:44–55.

Soto-Martinez, M., and P.D. Sly. 2010. Relationship between environmental exposures in children and adult lung disease: The case for outdoor exposures. *Chronic Respiratory Disease* 7(3):173–186.

Walker, V.R., A.L. Boyles, K.E. Pelch, S.D. Holmgren, A.J. Shapiro, C.R. Blystone, M.J. Devito, R.R. Newbold, R. Blain, P. Hartman, K.A. Thayer, and A.A. Rooney. 2018. Human and animal evidence of potential transgenerational inheritance of health effects: An evidence map and state-of-the-science evaluation. *Environment International* 115:48–69.

Woods, M.M., B.P. Lanphear, J.M. Braun, and L.C. McCandless. 2017. Gestational exposure to endocrine disrupting chemicals in relation to infant birth weight: A Bayesian analysis of the HOME Study. *Environmental Health* 16(1):115.

Yang, A., N.A. Janssen, B. Brunekreef, F.R. Cassee, G. Hoek, and U. Gehring. 2016. Children's respiratory health and oxidative potential of $PM_{2.5}$: The PIAMA birth cohort study. *Occupational and Environmental Medicine* 73(3):154–160.

9

Health Monitoring and Research Programs

Veterans of all eras are concerned that their environmental exposures during deployment may have ramifications for their reproductive health and for the health of their children and grandchildren. The convergence of veteran concerns with the rise of epigenetics has fueled interest in the study of the role of gene *x* environment interactions in mediating adverse reproductive and transgenerational health outcomes. Acknowledging those concerns, the Department of Veterans Affairs (VA) requested that the Volume 11 committee update what is currently known about the reproductive and developmental effects associated with the exposures potentially experienced by Gulf War and Post-9/11 veterans. In addition, VA also asked the committee to identify areas requiring further study in order to assess the potential health effects in the descendants of veterans of any era and to provide guidance on how such research might be conducted. To address the latter task, the committee was requested to do the following:

- develop a framework for a health monitoring or screening program that would be applicable to all veterans and their descendants;
- determine the feasibility of conducting an epidemiologic study on generational health effects in veterans and their descendants; and
- assess the scope and methodology for conducting research, including the use of animal models, on generational health effects.

The committee posits that the implementation of a comprehensive health monitoring and research program (HMRP) that involves veterans, their partners,[1] and their descendants could help to identify areas of priority for VA and provide an appropriate framework for addressing areas of concern in the future. Because a health monitoring program and an epidemiologic research program need to work together to inform each other, this chapter discusses the committee approach to both aspects of an HMRP. Chapter 10 provides guidance and an overview on the basic and translational research studies that can

[1] The committee uses this term to capture male or female spouses, the child's other biological parent, or caregivers who can respond to questions about the child's health and development.

be considered for the study of generational health effects in animal and cellular models. The proposed HMRP should be structured not only to provide a long-term mechanism for health monitoring but also to create the infrastructure and data resources required to design epidemiologic studies to appropriately examine specific veteran and descendant populations for the health outcomes of concern; it should also establish a strong basic and translational research program that can help fill current and future gaps in knowledge. The proposed HMRP should build on the health outcomes identified in Chapters 4 through 7, whether to expand the evidence base for relatively well-studied toxicants (e.g., chlorpyrifos and trichloroethylene) or to identify possible reproductive and developmental effects for poorly studied toxicants (e.g., depleted uranium and jet fuels). It should be tailored to enroll participants who are representative of all conflicts as well as appropriate comparison groups of nondeployed members of the military and civilian populations. By design, the HMRP should create an infrastructure for health monitoring at health care facilities within VA as well as seek participation of health care organizations and providers outside of VA that are involved in providing care to veterans, their partners, and their descendants. This is particularly important given the necessary involvement of partners and children of veterans who may not be receiving care within VA facilities.

Epidemiology studies provide a unique opportunity to study the distribution and determinants of health-related states or events (including disease) and also to apply these studies to the control of diseases and other health problems (WHO, 2018). Epidemiology is often integrated with other scientific disciplines, including biostatistics, the social and behavioral sciences, and environmental health, to study the extent to which a particular exposure might be associated with a health outcome. Epidemiologic studies provide the opportunity for the monitoring and screening of the health of populations over time as well as the testing of hypothesis-driven research to address specific questions—the functions that together constitute an HMRP. These two aspects of epidemiology are not mutually exclusive, but rather work to complement each other and to enhance the value of the research findings. The proposed research program also emphasizes the importance of using experimental animal or cell culture models to help elucidate the biological processes that may be responsible for the generational health effects that appear after deployment exposures (see Chapter 10). As such, specific epidemiology and basic and translational research programs should be established to take advantage of the availability of data collected through the HMRP. Future studies may be nested within the HMRP. These studies may make direct or indirect use of the data collected by the HMRP, identify cases among HMRP participants, or focus on specific exposures or outcomes of interest that have been identified through the HMRP.

Below, the committee provides a framework for the development of an HMRP and ways to optimize current research efforts to conduct longitudinal generational studies. The logistic, organizational, technological, laboratory, and statistical considerations needed to support these efforts are also presented.

OVERVIEW OF VA AND DOD HEALTH CARE SYSTEMS

The Military Health System (MHS) operates within the Department of Defense (DoD) to provide comprehensive health care to active-duty military personnel. The MHS also provides, when space is available, health care to dependents of active-duty service members, to retirees and their dependents, and to some former partners. Such care has been made available since 1966 through TRICARE and its predecessors. In October 2001, TRICARE benefits were extended to retirees and their dependents ages 65 and over. Since 2014 TRICARE has been managed by the Defense Health Agency.

The TRICARE network represents a major component of the MHS. Although TRICARE is sometimes used to describe only purchased care, the committee uses the term in a broader sense: as a wide-reaching health care provider for DoD beneficiaries, including service members, retirees, and their families that delivers direct care through military treatment facilities as well as purchased care through network and nonnetwork civilian health professionals, hospitals, and pharmacies (DoD, 2013). The DoD TRICARE Management Activity contracts with community purchased-care providers when direct-care providers are not available or when supplemental services are required.

In 2013 an estimated 9.4 million beneficiaries were enrolled in the TRICARE system, including 1.37 million active-duty service members, 1.71 million active-duty family members, 170,000 active and inactive National Guard and reserve members, 750,000 family members of National Guard and reservists, and 5.42 million retirees and their family members (DoD, 2018). According to TRICARE Management Activity, the TRICARE network includes 56 hospitals and medical centers and 361 ambulatory health clinics that provide direct care in the MHS, and more than 3,300 network acute-care hospitals and 914 behavioral health facilities provide purchased care (DoD, 2013).

Once a service member separates from the military and becomes an eligible veteran, he or she may receive health care from VA through a network of hospitals, clinics, centers, and long-term care facilities located around the country. VA also has contracts with many health care providers who may treat veterans when they do not have ready access to a VA facility. VA does not typically provide direct health care to veterans' dependents; however, the dependents of veterans who are permanently and totally disabled or who died of a service-connected disability may qualify for CHAMPVA, a health insurance program that relies on private doctors and hospitals for the provision of care. As of 2014, 42% of the total veteran population receives its health care directly from VA or through a VA contract with a private health care provider (Bagalman, 2014).

Although some veterans receive health care within VA, many do not. Veterans who are eligible for VA health benefits are assigned to one of eight priority groups based on need, period of service, and other considerations such as a service-connected disability and being a Medal of Honor recipient (VA, 2018a). Reserve or National Guard members on active duty for training purposes *only* do not meet the basic eligibility requirement. Veterans who are not eligible for VA health care may receive care from a variety of other health care providers outside the VA system. Those outside the VA health care system may be difficult to identify as discussed in the Study Populations section later in the chapter. For example, the 2010 National Survey of Veterans found that fewer than 30% of Vietnam veterans had ever enrolled in VA health care services (Westat, 2010). The health care facilities and providers for veterans and their descendants are essential elements of the HMRP.

FRAMEWORK FOR A HEALTH MONITORING AND RESEARCH PROGRAM

The committee designed a general framework (see Figure 9-1) applicable to any veteran era that can serve as a starting point for a research program. As science evolves, modifications will likely be implemented to improve the framework. An HMRP is an ongoing initiative designed to assess a wide range of health effects in veterans, their partners, and their children and grandchildren, including reproductive and development outcomes. Participants should be assessed periodically using a systematic, longitudinal approach that includes service members and veterans—both men and women—and even those who have yet to join the military. Veterans of the Vietnam War era, the 1990–1991 Gulf War era, and the Post-9/11 era should all be adequately represented.

The framework in Figure 9-1 can be tailored to the specific research questions and the specific veteran cohorts being evaluated, but the basic elements of the framework should remain consistent. To ensure success, a strong program management team will be critical. The lead organization for any given project within the HMRP needs to be specified a priori and the collaborators promptly identified. Inherent in effective program management are communication strategies for both internal and external

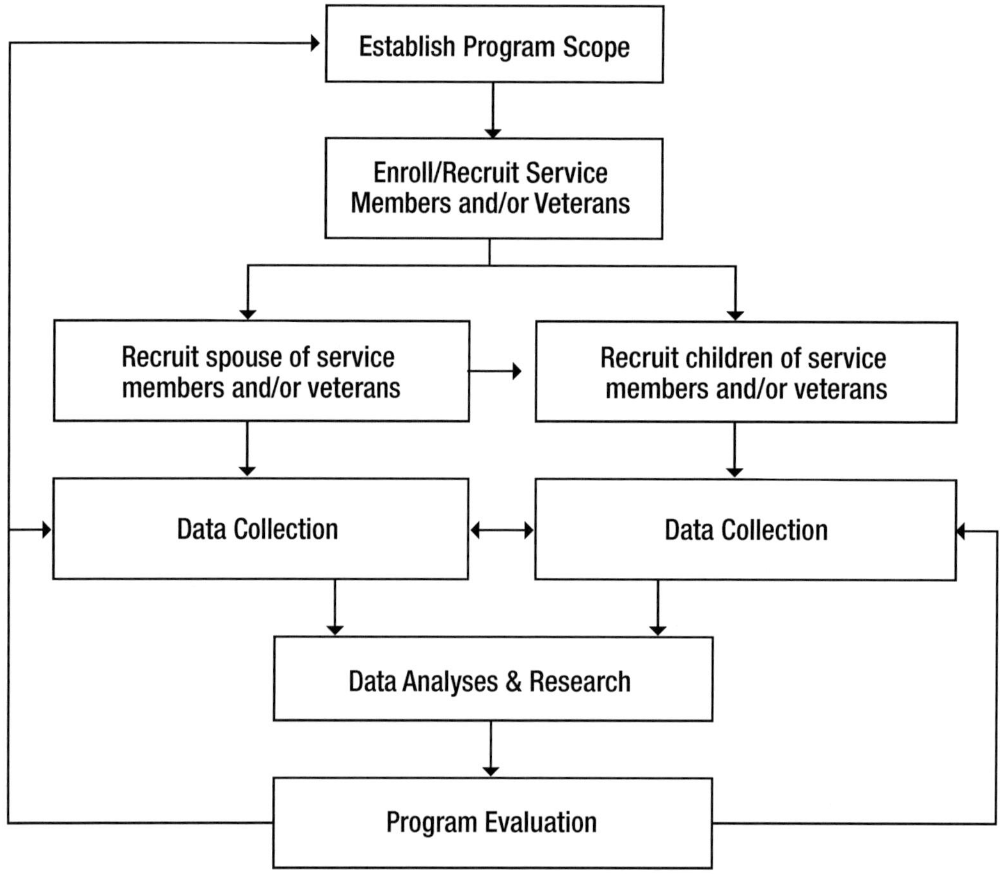

FIGURE 9-1 Framework for an HMRP for service members, veterans, their partners, and their descendants.

audiences (as discussed in more detail later in the chapter), particularly program participants (i.e., service members and veterans, and their descendants) and researchers; the assessment of resources that are available or that will be necessary to conduct the program; the development and implementation of standard operating procedures for data collection, storage, and analysis; and a rigorous process for ensuring that all ethical and legal requirements for human subjects are strictly adhered to. Information technology (IT) will also be an essential aspect of program management since the data to be collected on participants will likely be extensive, as will the links necessary between federal and private (and possibly state) databases. Thus, there is a complexity to VA and DoD health care studies that will require careful scoping and planning in order to conduct the committee's recommended HMRP; this planning should include the specification of methods to track program participants longitudinally in such a way that family-based links can be made and followed.

The program should begin by defining the scope of the health monitoring efforts. This scope will guide the recruitment, enrollment, and engagement of participants—active-duty service members, reservists, veterans, partners, and their descendants—now and in the future, as well as the collection and maintenance of the data for each participant. As these data will not only be electronic but also biological, it will be important for the program to be adequately prepared to receive, catalog, and maintain multiple forms of information. Analyzing data will also require linking databases and statistical software. Biological samples provide one of the keys to understanding a physiological response. Given the essential nature of this component, it will be important to identify appropriate sample collection and storage processing systems and equipment as well as suitable laboratory facilities and biorepositories, and it will be necessary to develop standardized protocols. Among the details of the methodology, emphasis should be placed on the frequency and duration of the monitoring program and also the assessment of any laboratory technologies that might be used in the process.

Publishing program results in a systematic manner, perhaps as a series of papers from program researchers, will ensure that veterans and their descendants are aware of the findings, both positive and negative, that may affect their health and well-being. Furthermore, dissemination to a broader audience, including researchers and the general public, can spur interest in the program and its activities. Finally, the health monitoring effort needs to be evaluated, modified, and updated on a continuing and regular basis, possibly with the oversight of an external advisory board (see Collaboration and Coordination later in this chapter). Without adequate review of all aspects of the program, its resources may not be efficiently used, data collection and analysis may lag, and veterans and their descendants may be participating in a program that does not serve their needs. In the sections below, the committee considers each of these elements in greater detail.

Of critical importance for a successful health monitoring effort will be close and continuous collaboration among and between the various government and private entities that are responsible for the health of veterans and their descendants. As will become evident in the following sections, no one agency is likely to have all the necessary data and resources to implement any part of the program on its own. Therefore, the committee encourages VA, DoD, and the National Institutes of Health (NIH) to work together with other stakeholders, particularly veterans and their families, and with academia to address the veterans' concerns about the possible effects that their war zone exposures may have on their children and future generations.

PROGRAM SCOPE AND STUDY DESIGN

Scope Definition

The first priority of the health monitoring part of an HMRP is to define the program scope, including its goals, priority data measurements, and which health outcomes should be monitored. A second priority might be to decide on the epidemiologic studies that are to be carried out with data from the health monitoring data repositories or that address other critical research questions. The scope of the HMRP will be a major determinant of the overall value of the data and the costs of recruiting and following up on participants over the long term. Establishing the scope of the program and the methodology to be used must be done with care and with input from stakeholders, including veterans and their descendants along with governmental and private entities.

The committee believes that the most effective approach will be to tailor the management of each HMRP for the particular veteran cohort under study. An effective management strategy will require an initial designated lead organization and management team, although the lead organization may change over time as the cohort population evolves or as the research questions change. For example, conducting a study of Vietnam veterans may require VA to serve as the lead organization with support from DoD and other agencies, whereas a study of future veterans may be led by DoD when service members and their families receive care from the MHS and then later transition to VA as service members and their families leave the MHS. Establishing the program scope and goals early in the process will not only provide the overarching framework for the program, but will also help to provide a platform with which to establish communication with veterans and collaborating entities, thus helping to promote clarity and transparency and optimize the use of resources.

One program goal might be to identify the reproductive health effects of veterans that may be the result of specific military exposures, particularly deployments to a war zone. For example, a small health monitoring program is being conducted by the Baltimore VA medical center to assess the health of male Gulf War veterans exposed to depleted uranium through embedded fragments (continuous exposure); however, while the reproductive status of these veterans is being assessed, the health of their descendants is not (McDiarmid et al., 2015).

The program scope should embrace continuous improvement as the program matures and data are analyzed and new health concerns emerge. Focus groups and other exploratory strategies with both veterans and health experts can help identify the specific exposures, health effects, populations, data sets, logistical considerations, and study designs that are most appropriate. These exploratory strategies could answer such questions as:

- Which cohort of veterans is to be studied and why?
- What exposures are most relevant to the specific veteran cohort?
- Are exposures comparable among different cohorts that might help substantiate or provide additional information?
- What does the current scientific and medical literature or other data resources suggest are the health outcomes that should be monitored in veterans and their descendants?
- How long and how often will the monitoring be conducted?
- How and where will biospecimens be collected, processed, catalogued, and maintained?
- What are the deliverables of the program?
- How will success be determined, and what metrics will be used for evaluation?
- What partnerships are needed to carry out the tasks?

Once these and other relevant questions are addressed, pilot studies could be conducted before larger studies are initiated. The committee recommends that VA or other lead organizations design and manage a pilot program that can be used to determine the feasibility of collection strategies, the necessary linkages for the appropriate use of the data, an assessment of response rates among veterans and their descendants, and the testing of whether a survey or other data collection methods can be scaled up and made operable in the field. The results from a pilot program may help to further tailor the scope of the program. The results from the pilot studies should be disseminated to interested parties and the public to provide the basis for a decision on whether to implement a large-scale set of specific studies.

Implementing a pilot study may be the first tier in a multitiered approach to an HMRP. Building on the information gathered in the pilot study, the next tier might encompass a large epidemiologic study that looks more broadly at additional reproductive or developmental health outcomes, a larger cohort of veterans or descendants, or some other variable. Each tier should build on the previous one in terms of scope, study parameters, duration, and resource needs. The committee notes that in Chapter 4, Deployment-Related Exposures, VA and DoD have already conducted epidemiologic studies that may be considered as pilot studies that provide useful information for designing more comprehensive studies. For example, to assess whether exposure to burn pits resulted in adverse birth outcomes, Conlin et al. (2012) used the DoD Birth and Infant Health Registry to identify live infants born to deployed men or women between 2004 and 2007 and categorized veterans as being within a specified distance of a burn pit. This might be considered to be a pilot study. Building on this study, VA and DoD collaborators might follow the infants as they grow and assess long-term effects and distinguish between maternal and paternal exposures. A further tier may be prospective and assess the health of children born to men and women after they return from deployment and even after they leave the military. Again, the cohorts would be categorized as exposed or unexposed to burn pits during deployment. For each tier, feasibility must be evaluated with respect to the strength of the associations being seen in the prior tier and the availability of data and resources to conduct the next tier.

The committee makes no assumptions about VA's goals for an HMRP because the questions to be addressed depend on how VA chooses to prioritize potential deployment-related health effects. For example, questions may be prioritized based on gaps in existing knowledge, concerns raised by veterans, the burden of disease, frequent or widespread exposures, the level of risk or change to be observed, or other issues. Furthermore, it is expected that these goals may change over time as more information on generational effects becomes known. Important to an HMRP is that baseline parameters be established for all participants against which future comparisons can be made. Depending on specific goals, collecting baseline data from active-duty service members may begin when these individuals enter the military and before orders are presented, before and after deployment, or upon the completion of specific assignments. The system should be capable of providing data on the incidence and prevalence of veterans' reproductive health outcomes as well as on the health of their children as they mature. For descendants, baseline data may be collected at birth or after enrollment in the HMRP. For parents who are not active-duty service members or veterans, baseline data may be collected when they enter the program or when they (if women) become pregnant.

Study Design

Various methods can be used to study human health outcomes, including screening, health monitoring, and research. Screening is used to identify the presence of a disease in a target population. The disease is usually known to be an important health problem and one for which there is an effective treatment if detected at an early stage (e.g., screening for colon cancer in individuals 50 years or older) (Andermann et al., 2008). In contrast, health monitoring is the continuous, systematic collection, analysis, and interpretation of health-related data that are needed for the planning, implementation, and evaluation of programs to improve the health of a population. A health monitoring initiative may be used to identify and characterize health problems in a population, to aid in setting priorities for interventions, and to inform future research efforts. Thus, the HMRP outlined here must be distinguished from a surveillance program that passively acquires data and that often lacks participant input. Surveillance programs—such as those that assess health effects in workers who handle hazardous substances—or registries—such as state-sponsored cancer registries that collect data without the active participation of the patients—may be considered as options for assessing veterans' health, but they were deemed by the committee to be unsuitable for the purpose it envisions, although they may be used to provide supplemental information.

An epidemiologic research study addresses a specific hypothesis about whether or how an exposure contributes to the risk of a particular disease or other health outcome. Box 9-1 highlights some existing HMRPs and epidemiologic studies that have assessed health effects in various military and civilian populations and that serve as examples of potential approaches for examining health effects in veterans and generational health effects in their descendants. In addition to the large, longitudinal studies presented in Box 9-1, there are several ongoing studies that may be used by VA and other organizations as examples of how children may be evaluated for health effects as they grow. Several of these studies are discussed in Chapters 5 through 7 and include the assessment of children in eight towns on Cape Cod with drinking water contaminated by tetrachloroethylene (Janulewicz et al., 2008), the Center for the Health Assessment of Mothers and Children of Salinas study in California (Eskenazi et al., 2004), and the Longitudinal Study of Early Development (Stingone et al., 2016). Each of these epidemiologic studies has its strengths and weaknesses and together they illustrate some of the issues that the Volume

BOX 9-1
Selected Examples of Health Monitoring Programs

Veteran Programs

- The Air Force Health Study ("Ranch Hands") of Vietnam veterans, who handled Agent Orange and other herbicides during the Vietnam War.
- Gulf War veterans who have depleted uranium fragments embedded in their bodies and have been studied biennially at the Baltimore VA medical center since 1993.
- The National Health Survey of Gulf War Veterans and Their Families, a longitudinal survey of 30,000 veterans conducted by VA. Three survey waves had been conducted as of 2018. Information is collected on the health of veterans, and three questions in the survey are devoted to the topic of the health of their children. No biological samples have been collected at any time.
- 2009–2011 National Health Study for a New Generation of U.S. Veterans evaluates the impact of deployment and deployment related-exposures on 30,000 men and women veterans of Operation Enduring Freedom/Operation Iraqi Freedom.
- The Million Veteran Program, which is sponsored by VA, collects DNA and other biological samples and also health and exposure information (VA and DoD Resources for Study of Generational Health Effects) from more than 625,000 veterans who use VA health care services.
- The Millennium Cohort Study is the largest prospective health study of service members from all branches of the U.S. military including reservists and National Guard, with more than 200,000 participants, more than 31% of whom are women. Eligible participants are active-duty personnel deployed since 2001 who are then followed after they leave the service or are deactivated. Data are collected via questionnaires and from DoD databases; no biological specimens are collected, and no physical examinations are conducted.

11 committee believes may be addressed by the HMRP framework presented in this chapter. These issues include but are not limited to the following: funding issues (e.g., Air Force Health Study), imprecise or changing program goals (e.g., National Children's Study), poor response rates (National Health Survey of Gulf War Veterans and Their Families), and poor retention rates (Millennium Cohort Study), or they did not collect sufficient data to be applicable to other goals (Millennium Cohort Study). Most of the studies were conducted by one government organization, such as DoD, VA, or NIH, which may make it difficult to leverage resources from other organizations. The committee believes that the HMRP described in this chapter can help overcome some of the challenges inherent in conducting large-scale prospective or retrospective monitoring programs and epidemiologic studies.

There are a number of different epidemiologic study designs which vary in cost, time frame, the selection of study subjects, data collection methods, sample size, causal inference, and feasibility. The choice of study design often depends on the hypothesis being tested and on the study population of interest. The current gold standard for epidemiologic study design is the randomized controlled trial (RCT) in which individuals are randomly assigned to either receive or not receive a given exposure in order to determine whether the exposure increases or decreases the risk of a given outcome. RCTs are

Federal Nonveteran Programs

- The National Health and Nutrition Examination Survey (NHANES) is a population-based survey of a random, nationally representative sample of about 5,000 people each year. The program, conducted by the Centers for Disease Control and Prevention (CDC), assesses the health and nutritional status of adults and children across the United States via a combination of interviews and physical examinations.
- The National Children's Study, sponsored by the National Institutes of Health (NIH), was a national initiative to enroll more than 100,000 children at the time of pregnancy/birth and follow them to adulthood. The program has been revamped with a new 7-year initiative called the Environmental Influences on Child Health Outcomes (ECHO) program.
- The NIH All of Us Research Program, begun in 2016 with $130 million as part of the NIH Precision Medicine Initiative, seeks to enroll 1 million or more participants to enable research for a wide range of diseases, both common and rare, as well as to increase understanding of healthy states. Additionally, a research program of this size will have the statistical power to detect associations between environmental or biological exposures and a wide variety of health outcomes.
- The Behavioral Risk Factor Surveillance System (BRFSS), established in 1984 by CDC, contains information from approximately 400,000 telephone surveys completed annually. Data are collected on individual use of preventive services, health-related risk behaviors, and chronic health conditions and are used to assist with establishing state and local health goals, implementing programs that promote disease prevention, and monitoring for any noticeable trends.

Private Nonveteran Programs

- The Nurses' Health Studies (i.e., Nurses' Health Study I, II, and III) began examining major chronic diseases in women. Begun in 1976, the studies are now in their third generation, with more than 275,000 male and female participants. The "Growing Up Today Study," begun in 1996, includes 16,882 children of participants in the Nurses' Health Study II; a second group of 10,920 children was enrolled in 2007.

commonly used to assess the effectiveness of drugs, but they are difficult to conduct because of their cost, the length of time necessary to see differences in the populations, and, in some instances, the ethical implications of withholding or providing an intervention versus the current standard of care.

Because of these constraints, most epidemiologic studies are observational in nature: that is, the exposures occur through environmental or occupational scenarios or by accident and are therefore not intentional. Most assessment of the effects of deployment-related exposures will be from observational studies. The most commonly used observational studies are cohort studies, case-control studies, and cross-sectional studies. VA has extensive experience in exposure cohort study designs and has used them to assess health outcomes in different cohorts of veterans. For example, VA has conducted three waves for its National Health Survey of Gulf War Era Veterans and Their Families (Dursa et al., 2016), has launched the Health Study for a New Generation of U.S. Veterans, and is currently recruiting participants for its Vietnam Era Health Retrospective Observational Study (VA, 2017a). Each of these cohort studies compares deployed (exposed) veterans with veterans of the same era who did not deploy. Some VA cohort studies stratify veterans based on the number of deployments they have experienced; although veterans of the 1990–1991 Gulf War deployed only once, Post-9/11 veterans have often had more than one deployment.

TABLE 9-1 Epidemiologic Study Designs: Definitions, Advantages, and Disadvantages

Type of Study	Advantages	Disadvantages
Cohort (specifically prospective) Subjects are defined according to their exposure levels and followed over time for outcome occurrence.	• Can evaluate multiple effects of a single exposure • More efficient for rare exposures • Can directly measure incidence • Clear chronological relationship between exposure and outcome	• Expensive • Time-consuming • Inefficient for rare outcomes with long induction or latency periods
Case-control Subjects are defined as cases and controls, and exposure histories are compared.	• Relatively inexpensive • Less time-consuming than cohort studies • Can evaluate the effects of multiple exposures • Efficient for rare outcomes or outcomes with long induction or latency periods	• Subject to recall bias (based on subjects' memory and self-reports) • Inefficient for rare exposures • Difficult to establish clear chronology of exposure and outcome unless it is in a nested design
Nested Case-Control Subjects with a disease and controls are sampled from a larger cohort study with prospective data collection.	• Reduces the number of effects that need to be analyzed, providing cost savings • Not subject to recall bias • Combines the efficiency of a case-control design with the prospective data collection of a longitudinal cohort • Can address exposure timing issues depending on base cohort's design • More expensive than case-control but less expensive than cohort	• Expensive to maintain base cohort • Time-consuming, given that data are prospective
Cross-sectional Examines the relationship between exposure and outcome prevalence in a defined population at a single point in time.	• Less time-consuming than case-control or cohort studies • Inexpensive • Good, quick picture of the prevalence of exposure and prevalence of outcome	• Difficult to determine temporal relationship between exposure and outcome (lacks time element) • May have excess prevalence from long-duration cases (such as cases that last longer than usual but may not be serious)

Table 9-1 lists the advantages and disadvantages of each of the major study designs. Other study designs, such as the case-cohort approach and novel study designs that address lifecourse considerations (see Chapter 3), are less common and are not included in the table. Study designs that have particular relevance for the HMRP include perinatal and birth cohorts such as the National Collaborative Perinatal Project conducted by NIH between 1959–1974, which obtained information on pre- and postnatal child health for 58,000 pregnancies in the United States (NARA, 2015), and high-risk cohorts. High-risk cohorts are selected on the basis of their exposure history, which may be particularly useful for studying veterans and their descendants where one study variable might be a deployment exposure such as hexavalent chromium or sarin compared to a cohort of nonexposed veterans. See *Gulf War and Health, Volume 8* (IOM, 2010) and Buka et al. (2018) for more detailed descriptions of epidemiologic study types and their applications. In the design of a particular study, the collection of covariates that may be assessed as potential confounders, effect modifiers, and mediators for that study need to be considered. The researcher should also consider potential sources of bias and guard against these in the study design. Researchers also need to consider whether and how study participants vary from veterans and descendants who choose not to participate and whether those factors influence the results. Details are provided below.

In addition to the types of epidemiologic studies presented in Table 9-1, ecologic studies may also provide valuable information about the possible health effects of various exposures. In these studies, a population or community is observed, and disease rates and exposures are measured in each of a series of populations. Trends in exposure and disease and their correlation are assessed at the population level. A weakness of the ecologic study design is that it cannot discern whether the exposed individuals are the same as those who get the disease, as there are no measures conducted at the individual level. Ecologic studies may use abstracted data from published statistics and therefore do not require expensive or time-consuming data collection.

STUDY POPULATIONS

An HMRP that includes studies of generational effects requires that an appropriate study population (service members, veterans, descendants, and control populations, if applicable) be identified, recruited to participate in the HMRP, and encouraged to continue their participation over the course of the program and that efficient and effective sampling be conducted from the set of participants. In the sections below, the committee discusses the necessary elements of each of these activities.

Identification

An HMRP cannot be conducted without appropriate definition, selection, and recruitment of veterans, partners, and veterans' children (and where relevant, grandchildren). All these populations will require appropriate participant consent, which may be modeled after the National Health and Nutrition Examination Survey (NHANES), Environmental Influences on Child Health Outcomes (ECHO), or the All of Us studies. Ethical considerations are discussed later in this chapter.

The population of concern (e.g., Gulf War veterans) and the sample to be assessed (e.g., a representative selection of 30,000 Gulf War veterans) will depend on the scope of the HMRP and the questions being asked. The population may range from all veterans, which could be required in order to study a wide range of questions, to smaller groups defined on the basis of various parameters, such as specified times or locations of deployment or exposures or perhaps particular occupations.

It will be necessary to distinguish veterans and their descendants by era. For example, the Vietnam War era is considered to be 1961 to 1975. Vietnam veterans are thus at least 62 years of age, assuming they were at least 18 years old at the time they enlisted or were drafted, and thus they are old enough to have children, grandchildren, and even great-grandchildren. The veterans of the 1990–1991 Gulf War in Iraq are likely to be at least 45 years of age and may have underage children (possibly still in the TRICARE system) and young grandchildren. Post-9/11 veterans may include new enlistees who are as young as 18 years of age, with or without children, but other veterans still serving may be older and may have children, including infants, as well as grandchildren.

DoD conducts regular health surveillance of all military personnel and their dependents through the Defense Medical Surveillance System (DMSS). However, the committee notes that National Guard and reservists who have been federalized and deployed, particularly those who have served in Iraq and Afghanistan since 2001, will not be captured in the DoD MHS after they return home from deployment.

Veterans could be identified using DoD and VA administrative records. One concern is that not all service members represented in DoD databases are represented in VA databases. VA has a congressionally mandated priority system designed to provide health care to those most in need, with eight groups and rankings based on health status, age, and income. As such, not all service members who have a DoD electronic health record (EHR) will necessarily be eligible for care in VA, and even those that are eligible may choose not to receive care at VA health care facilities. Those who do not receive care from VA will not be captured in VA databases. These challenges are compounded by the fact that the MHS records of children of military personnel are not represented in VA medical databases at all. Children born to veterans after they leave the military will also not be in the MHS, further compounding issues concerning the availability of EHRs for veterans' descendants.

Veterans who enter the VA health care system will be easy to capture via VA databases, whereas veterans who do not enter the system may be difficult to locate and may be less inclined to participate. Efforts to identify these men and women may require using other resources such as Social Security records and working with the DoD Defense Manpower Data Center (DMDC) to locate last known addresses. Furthermore, veterans who do not use or are not eligible for the VA system may differ from veterans in the system in important ways such as income and health status. Any such differences should be identified and assessed in any epidemiologic research study.

VA has implemented several programs, particularly registries, to collect health data on defined groups of veterans based on exposure: for instance, the Agent Orange or Airborne Hazards and Open Burn Pit registries. The registries include data on veterans who are not in the VA health care system, but the utility of such registries in investigating exposure–disease relationships is limited (NASEM, 2017).

The focus of an HMRP on assessing reproductive outcomes and generational health effects adds complexity to estimating the size of the population to be monitored. Examples of questions that need to be considered for each HMRP for a veteran cohort include the following:

- What is the size of the veteran cohort that will be representative of all branches of military service?
- What is the appropriate control population and how will they be identified and recruited?
- How many children and grandchildren need to be enrolled for adequate statistical analyses?
- What is the availability of baseline data already collected on all service members?
- Is there a need to oversample women across the branches of military service, and how feasible is it to do so?
- How many pregnancies and births are anticipated for the cohort?
- Do cost or feasibility concerns require that only a subsample of the cohort be studied?
- What are the ethical issues that need to be considered for the veterans and their descendants?

Recruitment and Engagement

In Figure 9-1, the Volume 11 committee provides a framework for assessing the generational health effects in service members, veterans, and their descendants, including men and women who enlist in the military after an HMRP is established. The HMRP begins recruitment at enlistment to provide a baseline, then continues throughout the veterans' lives. This will ensure that a sufficient sample is available with which to observe small effects in veterans and will provide a mechanism to contact dependents (partners and children). The recruitment of veterans, their partners, and their children outside of the military system will pose additional challenges, as discussed below.

To study effects in children and grandchildren, it will be best to recruit, enroll, and collect data from both the partners and the children themselves. Data collected directly from children are important for documenting outcomes and also for assessing risk factors that appear throughout the child's life—for example, with older children, substance use and occupation. Access to the health records of partners will facilitate the study of confounders, such as a partner's occupational exposures, existing health concerns (e.g., obesity, diabetes, cancer), and lifestyle factors such as smoking and nutrition that might affect a pregnancy and the developing fetus. The greater the number of partners and children in the program, the greater the statistical power of the program will be, and the less impact future attrition will have. In the sections below, the committee examines how participants ranging from newly enlisted service members to the children of Vietnam veterans may be recruited into an HMRP.

The Volume 11 committee notes that recruitment and retention are critical aspects of the HMRP. Although the VA has extensive experience in large veteran cohort studies, there have been concerns that the response rate for many of its epidemiologic studies is low. Therefore, the committee suggests that VA explore innovative methods to increase recruitment and retention. It is possible that compensation for completing surveys or providing biospecimens, reimbursement for travel costs to a clinic when necessary, or recognizing HMRP participants in publications such as newsletters may serve as inducements to participate and remain in the program. For example, the *MVP Insider: A Newsletter for Million Veteran Program Participants* highlights stories about individual veterans and why they are participating in the VA Million Veteran Program (MVP). VA or another lead organization will also need to consider whether and how to compensate veterans or their descendants for providing biospecimens, particularly if they are to be collected at medical clinics which may require that veterans or their descendants incur expenses to travel to a clinic. The ability to provide biospecimens through the mail at no cost to veterans and their descendants may also reduce barriers to participation.

Active-Duty Service Members

The Volume 11 committee believes that the most expedient way to observe possible generational health effects associated with military exposures will be to enroll new active-duty service members into an HMRP at the time they enter the military. By enrolling all new recruits, a baseline of health status that includes information on lifestyle and environment can be established prior to any deployment. This preemptive approach will also facilitate the tracking of exposures associated with each deployment or occupational assignment. There is precedent for automatically enrolling and collecting data on military personnel: the DoD Serum Repository collects serum samples from all personnel at regular intervals, for example. Even though the Serum Repository has inconsistent collection procedures (which are being rectified), the availability of these serum samples has been useful in pilot studies (Lushniak et al., 2016). Recruits would receive information on the value of participation in a program that monitors their exposures and health and that of their descendants. Newly recruited participants would be introduced to the concept of monitoring their future reproductive health and the health of future generations and would be informed about the importance of participation by their partners and children. Opportunities to discuss details of the program with partners should be offered. The program would follow service members throughout their military careers to the point of separating from service. If a service member prefers not to participate in the HMRP after having the goals of the program explained, they should be able to decline to participate or to participate at a later date.

Although continued participation in the HMRP would be voluntary once an individual had separated from military service, assessing the long-term sequelae from potential exposures during service requires that there be some sort of follow-up. The importance of such a monitoring program and the value to each participant would be emphasized. Currently there are approximately 2 million active-duty service members, only a portion of whom have been or will be deployed to a war zone or other theater of operation. Given the retention rates of existing programs, the committee considers it likely that a substantial proportion of service members would not agree to be followed indefinitely. However, developing the baseline and other samples would be essential in assessing the effects of any exposure to individuals for which symptoms present after discharge. The need to maximize retention in the HMRP in turn points to the importance of having an overarching communication program so that participating individuals understand the purpose of the program and embrace its goals and potential benefits. A further consideration is that among the veterans who might agree to participate in the HMRP into the future, only a proportion will receive care at VA after they separate from the military; it will be essential to get these individual veterans to agree to permit access to their health care records from private providers.

Veterans

Recruiting veterans from earlier conflicts poses a different set of challenges. Some veterans receive health care within VA, but many do not. As noted earlier, eligibility to receive health care in VA is based on a priority system. Recruiting veterans who are already enrolled in VA does not guarantee that they will participate in ongoing surveys. For example, the annual Survey of Veteran Enrollees' Health and Use of Health Care had a response rate of between 27–36% for 2015 to 2017 using both Web-based and mailed questionnaires (Huang et al., 2017). Veterans who receive care outside the VA system may be difficult to identify and follow, particularly if they move. Veterans who are disabled (not as a result of their military service) or otherwise qualify may be enrolled in Medicaid and those from earlier eras such as Vietnam may be enrolled in either Medicare or Medicaid. Locating those veterans in the Centers for Medicare & Medicaid Services (CMS) system would require cross-referencing the DoD DMDC files with those of CMS, a difficult and time-consuming task. Other approaches may be more fruitful, such as partnering with veterans service organizations (VSOs) for outreach efforts. VSOs may also be helpful as part of a public communication campaign to generate interest and enhance recruitment efforts.

Partners

Establishing a comprehensive HMRP for generational health effects cannot be based on the deployment exposures and reproductive health of active-duty service members and veterans alone. As described in Chapter 2, deployment exposures occur within the larger context of lifecourse exposures; an additional complexity is the fact that any exposures experienced by the child's other parent prior to conception and during pregnancy will also play a role in generational health effects. For this reason, it will be important to recruit and engage the partners of active-duty service members and veterans. Partners of interest would be those who are the other parent, biological or not, of any children born to the active-duty service member or veteran after deployment. Nonbiological parents living with a child may provide information on the child's environment and health as well as on any of their own exposures that may affect the child.

The enrollment of active-duty service members' partners could begin at the time of their entry into the MHS/TRICARE system as a beneficiary, with follow-up for the duration of their eligibility for TRICARE. Only spouses of active-duty service members (whether men or women) are eligible for TRICARE benefits; unmarried partners are not. Special attention and outreach will be needed to identify and recruit the unmarried partners of service members whenever possible. Should a partner for some reason not receive health care through MHS/TRICARE, he or she could be encouraged to provide the necessary information and biological samples. The committee acknowledges that it might be difficult to maintain long-term contact with partners outside the MHS, particularly if the partner is divorced from the service member or is otherwise not covered by the MHS. The need to recruit and maintain partners in the program reinforces the importance of an effective communication strategy that emphasizes the health and well-being of children and future generations.

It will be necessary to develop approaches to identifying and following the nonmilitary parents of children of military personnel over time, regardless of divorce and death, in order to determine preconception and prenatal exposures and to assess such risk factors as lifestyle, occupation, and nutrition that might be related to developmental and health effects in children. After the children reach the legal age of consent, they would provide their own information, as discussed below.

Children and Grandchildren

As the overarching goal of any veteran HMRP focused on generational health effects is to determine if those effects occur in the descendants of active-duty service members potentially exposed to toxicants during deployment, it is critical to follow these descendants for at least two generations—that is, at least through the service members' children and grandchildren. Recruiting children may begin with those who are born to active-duty service members and covered under TRICARE, which would facilitate access to each child's EHR. For example, DoD already has the DoD Birth and Infant Health Registry that may be used to access to these records, as discussed later in the chapter. For the small number of children who have an active-duty parent and who are not covered by TRICARE, DoD should encourage those parents to enroll their children in the HMRP. Additionally, there is a need for VA to identify and recruit children born to veterans after they have separated from the military, regardless of whether the veteran is enrolled in VA services.

The committee notes that birth and health information on an active-duty service member's children, including those born before and after the service member was deployed, will be captured in the TRICARE system. Information on any children born before a service member is deployed would provide a comparison group for any children born after deployment (similar to a case cross-over study design). The HMRP would need to consider that some service members have multiple deployments and that they may conceive one or more children before and after each deployment (and possibly during deployment). Any one of these scenarios would complicate associating exposures across deployments with potential health outcomes in their children: that is, it may be difficult to link a developmental effect to a deployment exposure immediately prior to conception rather than an earlier exposure. Multiple deployments argue for collecting biospecimens from service members before and immediately after deployment to help make such distinctions.

The Volume 11 committee acknowledges that monitoring the health of veterans' children and grandchildren will be difficult. VA (2018a) estimates that there are more than 6 million veteran households with dependent children (and more than 13 million without children). Veterans may elect to continue to provide health information to the HMRP on minor children. However, once children are legally of age, this is no longer possible unless the child or grandchild willingly consents to participate in the HMRP; the adult child may also need to provide consent for the use of previous data and samples collected while he or she was a minor. Thus, continuing encouragement for service members and veterans and their adolescent children to remain in the HMRP will be critical to collecting the data necessary to understand the health effects that may occur as these children grow from infancy through childhood and adolescence and then into adults. Having veterans' children enroll their own children (i.e., the veterans' grandchildren) in the program will be necessary for determining if any adverse health effects are seen in the third generation. For the grandchildren, collecting data (e.g., fertility or pregnancy history and family medical history) from partners who are not biologically related to the veteran would potentially require consent. This would add an additional layer of complexity. Some key considerations in recruiting children into the HMRP are:

- What is the expected number of pregnancies among the male and female registry participants from the time of enrollment until the end of reproductive years? If 10,000 active service personnel were enrolled, what is the reasonable number of pregnancies expected over the next two decades?
- How many children or grandchildren will be required in a birth cohort to provide meaningful data on generational studies? This is dependent on the endpoints of concern and, in particular, on the incidence rates in the population and on retention rates. For example, childhood cancer would require a much larger cohort than an examination of attention deficit–hyperactivity disorder (ADHD) or even autism. Once the number of births projected from the enrolled cohort is determined, what is a reasonable estimate of the number of children who can be monitored prospectively into the future?
- What are the appropriate informed consent strategies and data boundaries during the lifecourse of each participant?
- What are the best approaches for maintaining consent as children age from minors to adults?
- What strategies should be developed for recruiting and gaining consent from adult children and their children after the parent is no longer an active-duty service member?

Sampling of Study Subjects

Sampling is used as a selection process to identify a representative population of the target group because costs can limit the feasibility of carrying out a hypothesis-driven research study in the entire target population. The selection of the study population and comparison population is an important consideration in an epidemiologic study. Different sampling schemes can be used, including a simple random sample, systematic sampling, and stratified sampling. For systematic sampling, individuals are selected from a list at repeated intervals, while for stratified sampling, individuals are first divided into subgroups and then sampled. These methods can often be used to ensure that the study population includes adequate numbers of people or subgroups of people to answer specific health outcome questions. Other methods of sampling include convenience sampling, clustered sampling, snowball sampling, and quota sampling.

Sampling should be done carefully because an improper sampling of a study population can result in selection bias. Selection bias means that the probability of an individual's participation in the study is associated with both the exposure and the outcome. For example, if an investigator sought to obtain a random sample of all military personnel deployed to the Gulf War in 1990, but instead sampled only Air Force personnel, this could result in bias for the particular study under question, as Air Force personnel may have different baseline health/demographic characteristics, exposure levels, exposures to important confounders, and health outcomes than those from other branches of DoD. Biased sampling can lead to biased results in one direction or another (i.e., a false positive or a false negative finding). The tracking of study participants over a period of time should include an analysis of whether the retention rates are nonrandom; if the retention is not random, it can introduce selection bias into the final analysis. For example, if a study of Gulf War veterans was evaluating long-term health effects that were more common in women (e.g., iron deficiency anemia), but had a loss to follow-up rate in which the losses of men and women veterans differed, then the estimates of an association with a deployment exposure that increased the risk of iron deficiency could be significantly biased. This would also be true if the exposure itself caused a health effect that reduced subsequent follow-up. A classic example of this is an exposure in pregnancy that results in an increased risk of early-term spontaneous abortion, an outcome which may occur prior to a woman's awareness of her pregnancy.

Comparison groups may be unexposed military or veteran populations (and their descendants) which would help reduce selection bias for the healthy warrior effect. Whether military, veteran, or civilian, comparison groups should be sampled and surveyed in the same manner (timing and method) as the target population (IOM, 2008). Nevertheless, identifying, recruiting, and retaining HMRP participants will be a substantial task. Researchers need to factor potential loss to follow-up among all HMRP subgroups (e.g., exposed veterans, unexposed, veterans, children) as well as attrition into the determination of how many veterans and their descendants to recruit into the program and recognize that attrition may begin enrollment. Furthermore, there may be phases of the study when loss to follow-up or attrition are more likely to occur such as when service members separate from the military, with the birth of a child, or when a child reaches an age when he or she can decide whether to continue in the program. Consideration also needs to be given to appropriate sampling of minority groups such as women, blacks, Hispanics, and other relevant subpopulations.

Minimizing attrition will be an important aspect of the HMRP. As noted in the later section on Communication, attrition may be reduced by collecting, retaining, and updating participating contact information, sending reminders via the participant's preferred method (email, texts, telephone calls) about follow-up activities, building rapport between participants and researchers, and sharing study findings or new activities with participants on an ongoing basis (Buka et al., 2018).

DATA COLLECTION

Integral to any HMRP is the collection, processing, and maintenance of data from all the participants. An HMRP should be designed to collect data in three key dimensions:

- biological samples to include a person's genome, epigenome, proteome, microbiome, physiology, metabolome/exposome, and health status;
- environmental factors to include exposures to biological, physical, and chemical agents in air, water, and soil; and
- personal and social factors to include occupations, lifestyle habits, education, life events, and neighborhood.

Together these factors constitute the foundation for understanding the impact of potential deployment exposures associated with service on the health of the individual and of his or her descendants. Therefore, collecting data on each of these components is integral to a successful HMRP or epidemiologic study.

The committee encourages HMRP managers to standardize reporting mechanisms, whether for biospecimens or questionnaires and surveys, and to include the resulting information in the individuals' EHRs in order to minimize the reporting burden on both veterans and health care providers as well as to ensure that research can be conducted in a valid way when the HMRP is used as a source of research study populations. The committee notes that an important consideration for any large-scale data collection effort on health effects is a process for validating self-reported health effects and exposure information. Although EHRs are a good source of medical diagnoses, they can be subject to errors in diagnosis and data entry; therefore, an HMRP should include disease diagnosis verification on subsets of participants.

The frequency of monitoring should be increased if exposure to deployment toxicants is suspected on the basis of environmental sampling, and biological samples (e.g., blood, urine, semen) should be collected as close to the time of exposure as possible or at the time of anticipated physiological impact. For women, collecting data after their childbearing years may not be necessary to identify generational effects in descendants. However, data collection for the adult descendants of deployed men and women will be important for understanding developmental impacts on adult disease. The committee envisions the HMRP as providing an opportunity to collect biological, personal, and environmental data for veterans of all eras, which, combined with data from partners, and descendants, could be used to establish a longitudinal program to evaluate transgenerational inheritance.

Electronic Health Records and Other Data Sources

An advantage of the DoD MHS is that some of the critical information that needs to be collected is already found in the EHRs of the service members and, for the most part, of the partners and children who are beneficiaries while the service member is on active duty. The anticipated synchronization of the DoD and VA EHRs may also make it easier to capture health effects for veterans who receive care from VA after they separate from the military.

A service member's EHR can be used to track his or her health from the time of entry into the military until separation. As such, the EHR is a valuable resource for health monitoring which provides baseline data and health effects that may be recorded before (each service member must have a physical prior to deployment) and after a service member deploys. Information from the EHR may also indicate if the service member has reproductive issues before or after deployment as well as how many children the service member had prior to entry into the military and during service.

Numerous data sources for veterans may be accessed as part of the HMRP. These data sources include the DMSS for active-duty service members and the VA EHR for veterans who are separated from the military and are in the VA health care system. The DoD DMDC provides administrative and logistical data (including deployment locations). At present, little information on reproductive effects is collected for male veterans, although male reproductive history is often a bellwether of disease.

VA is encouraged to expand the reproductive effects information that it collects on the veterans in its system. In addition to reproductive effects in male veterans, the EHR should also capture information on pregnancy outcomes or time to pregnancy in the male veterans' partners as well as information on health effects in their children. Information should also be collected on the maternity care that female veterans receive from non-VA providers, including those who are covered by VA benefits if they are eligible for them. This pregnancy health information should be collected from the veteran's EHR since VA tracks this information. Time to pregnancy information could also be helpful if collected in a systematic manner for both men and women. The committee notes that veteran status is not necessarily captured in the medical records of private health care providers, and even if veteran status is noted, the era in which the veteran served and deployment status may not be included. There is a need to recruit and retain non-VA veterans by partnering with private health care providers (e.g., participants in the VA Choice Program) since if only VA health care users were included in a study, selection bias would be a major concern (e.g., biases in age, veteran era, socioeconomic status, and health status).

With regard to children, particularly those born in the TRICARE system, an EHR can provide data on birth outcomes and health status. Many of these data will be contained in the child's medical record, but some health effects may not be captured, such as behavioral and cognitive deficits. Thus, an in-person assessment of the health and development of children and grandchildren should occur at least once during each life stage (e.g., infancy, early childhood, middle childhood, adolescence), and then every 5–10 years or so in adulthood. During these visits, children or their parents (depending on age of the child) might be interviewed, and the children could undergo a brief medical examination (e.g., anthropometry, spirometry, etc.) and a neurodevelopmental assessment (e.g., computerized assessments such as NIH toolbox are possible), with a biospecimen collection as well.

Medical Data Linkages

At present, the medical data linkages between DoD and VA are minimal, largely due to lack of interoperability between the two departments' IT platforms. The DoD EHR is a clinical information management system that provides access to health care records for MHS beneficiaries. Since 2004, DoD has used the Armed Forces Health Longitudinal Technology Application (AHLTA) system for its EHRs.

In contrast, VA uses the Veterans Information Systems and Technology Architecture (VISTA) as its nationwide system for EHRs. VISTA includes more than 180 applications for clinical, financial, and administrative functions within a single integrated database. Of special note is that in June 2017, the Secretary of VA announced that VISTA will be subsumed into the AHLTA system.

The integration of the DoD and VA EHR systems, once it has occurred, may help address data gaps. The Interagency Clinical Informatics Board has endorsed prioritized data domains to support the continuity of care, but to date several domains have no structure to map the data that will be required for the migration of clinical notes stored in the legacy systems. A 2022 completion date has been predicted for the availability of an interoperable DoD and VA EHR system, but the degree to which the DoD/VA system will be interoperable with the EHR systems used by the private sector remains a major unknown.

In order to develop rapid and convenient monitoring of the health of military personnel and veterans that uses real-time hospital discharge or medical data that can be linked with deployment or exposure information captured within the theater of operation, the MHS and VA health care systems must be appropriately linked. Such a link will allow health care professionals and researchers to track veterans longitudinally and to report results in a timely manner.

The Defense Occupational and Environmental Health Readiness System (DOEHRS), a database system managed by the Defense Health Services Systems, includes data in four different categories: industrial hygiene, environmental health, radiation, and general incident reporting. DOEHRS is intended for use by both garrison and deployed operations as the system of record for the individual longitudinal exposure record (ILER). However, as of 2015 DoD did not expect the ILER system to be operative for at least 6 to 8 years (GAO, 2015). For the immediate future, since personalized exposures are not yet available, ILERs will be based primarily on time-weighted average exposure concentrations for a large geographical area. At present the exposure data appears to be limited to chemicals or materials that have been predetermined to be of importance. Until new technologies are developed, this will preclude the identification of potential new threats. Once the system is operational, a veteran's ILER should be available to DoD and VA researchers and help them link veterans' exposures to their symptoms.

More than 50% of military personnel do not enter the VA health care system after they leave the military; instead they enter the private health care system or CMS or else they have no health care. Although HMRP participants may sign medical release forms that allow researchers to access their health care records from multiple private health care providers, the data may be in a format that cannot be efficiently handled, such as existing in different EHR operating systems or as hard copies of test results or as large hospitalization records that to date are available only as paper; the latter may be particularly true for older records, such as health records from the Vietnam War era. The fragmentation of the private health care system in the United States adds to the complexity of designing health monitoring systems for service members and veterans.

HMRP managers will face several hurtles in trying to establish reliable and comprehensive IT systems for collecting and analyzing health data on service members and veterans; including their children and grandchildren will offer even more challenges. Harmonizing or integrating the databases will be difficult if they are incomplete or use coding systems that deviate significantly from those used for data acquisition (e.g., the use of *International Classification of Diseases* [ICD] codes that may not be useful for effects other than diagnoses). It will be necessary to develop database ontologies to harmonize data from different sources in which the same variable may have different names (e.g., sex in one database, gender in another). IT efforts to overcome these challenges to ensure interoperability and that the data are accessible and protected will be critical. As noted, newer medical informatics methods for mining the EHR, including natural language processing, have been shown to be superior to the use of ICD codes in retrieving data from the EHR (Wang et al., 2017).

Surveys

Both DoD and VA have experience using surveys to collect both health status and personal and socioeconomic information from veterans and, in some cases, from their partners. DoD requires that all service members complete a pre-deployment health assessment and as well as post-deployment health assessment and reassessment questionnaires. VA has conducted numerous studies of veterans and of their use of VA services, including the National Survey of Veterans to ascertain who uses VA health care and other services and the 2016 Survey of Veteran Enrollees' Health and Use of Health Care (Huang et al., 2017). VA has also conducted three surveys for the Longitudinal Health Study of Gulf War Era Veterans (in 1995, 2005, and 2012), and in 2016 VA carried out the Vietnam Era Health Retrospective Observational Study (VE-HEROeS), a follow-up study to the 1988 National Vietnam Veterans' Readjustment Study. VA has also conducted separate surveys of women veterans. Several of these surveys have relied on paper documentation, which included the use of mailed invitation letters and surveys to collect participant-specific data. Such an approach is expensive, time-consuming, and inefficient, and generally the response rates have been low (Dursa et al., 2016; NASEM, 2016). VA is moving toward greater use of electronic survey instruments and has used online surveys for epidemiologic studies such as the 2012 Follow-up Study of a National Cohort of Gulf War and Gulf Era Veterans (VA, 2016).

To follow veterans after their separation from active service, it will be necessary to design a systematic process for ongoing data collection from these veterans. The process might include regular, periodic surveys of veterans' and descendants' health status along with permission to access medical records in the event of reported adverse health effects. The committee recognizes that regardless of which veteran cohort is monitored, data collection after a veteran separates from the military may provide a challenge because veterans may receive health care in different places, including DoD, VA, private health care providers, and government providers (e.g., state or local health clinics), or they may not be receiving care at all. Veterans who do receive health care could provide a biological sample at a VA or other medical facility or by mail. Questionnaires could be supplied to primary care physicians (from DoD, VA, or elsewhere), or they may be made available online for the veteran to complete.

Although VA has collected data on veterans' partners, it has not traditionally collected information on the health of veterans' children. The information necessary for an HMRP that assesses generational effects may extend beyond a child's disease status to areas that may not be captured in the health record, such as educational attainment and behavioral concerns. Therefore, other approaches and tools may be required to capture different aspects of children's health outcomes, such as questionnaires, environmental and geographic data collection, and long-term follow-up. The committee encourages VA, in its efforts to capture information on children's health, to collaborate with other organizations, such as the National Institute of Child Health and Human Development, which have more experience with questionnaires and surveys of children and their parents.

New methodologies and efficiencies are available for identifying the population to be sampled, for the issuance of invitations, for the what and how of data collection and analysis, for the use of incentives for recruiting and retaining participants, and for the use of reminders to increase response rates (Toledano et al., 2015). The use of social media may be a novel way to capture cognitive health via games and tests administered via cell phones or other devices as they are developed. Standardized questionnaires will facilitate comparisons across populations.

Biorepository

The utility of DoD and VA biobanks was reviewed in special supplemental issues of the *Journal of Occupational and Environmental Medicine* (Vol. 5, No. 7S, July 2016) and *Military Medicine* (Vol. 180, No. 10, October 2015), both of which described a series of pilot studies that used biological samples for exposure assessments. The biological archives consist primarily of serum collections that have been cross-referenced with other samples to maximize the amount of information associated with any one individual as well as with other datasets (such as DoD Serum Repository, DMDC, and EHR). Of note is that current storage conditions may lessen the potential use of these biological samples in future genomic and epigenomic research.

At a minimum, blood, urine, and semen[2] samples should be collected at entry into the military, prior to each deployment, and after each deployment with the optional collection of saliva and hair. Upon separation from the military, veterans participating in the health monitoring system could be requested to provide additional samples, including hair and saliva, depending on the research questions that are being addressed. The expanded use of omic technologies as they become available may enhance exposure assessment, even those that occur during deployment (Bradburne et al., 2015).

Sample collection from service members should occur at specified intervals from enlistment to separation, perhaps during service members' annual physical (see Table 9-2). Blood samples are now collected by DoD at deployment and then serially every 2 years as part of an HIV screening program; the samples are stored in the DoD Serum Repository.

There is precedent for VA collecting biospecimens from veterans. The VA MVP is assembling a well-curated collection of DNA and other samples paired with health and exposure information (VA and DoD Resources for Study of Generational Health Effects). Veterans using the VA health care system complete surveys about their health and health-related behavior, provide a blood sample, allow researchers to access their VA and VA-linked medical records, and agree to future contact. To date, more than 625,000 veterans have participated in the program (see Leveraging Existing Resources), although complete data are available on fewer than half of them.

It should be noted that a "blood" collection can refer to three types of specimens: whole blood, serum, and plasma. Different types of biomarkers can be measured in each, and ideally all three would be collected.

The biospecimens required to study generational effects should be collected from preconception to birth. The child's health and development should then be monitored postnatally as part of the yearly wellness assessment to at least year 5, at which point the child will generally enter the school system. Health assessments and biological sampling of the child should occur with subsequent follow-up. At a minimum, the follow-up should include visits to a doctor at each life stage (school age, preadolescence, post pubertal and late adolescence, and even into adult life). To capture prenatal exposures, samples

[2] The committee notes that the collection of oocytes from female service members would also be appropriate whenever semen is collected from men; however, it may not be practical or acceptable to do so in most military situations, e.g., prior to deployment.

TABLE 9-2 Veteran Data and Biospecimens to Be Collected for an HMRP

Pre-Deployment	During Deployment	Post-Deployment (days, months, years following deployment)
Military Exposures		
Biomarkers (e.g., blood, urine, semen)	Frequent and consistent exposure assessments of the environment, which may include the collection of additional biospecimens and additional sampling during or following an incident such as the release of chemical warfare agents	Biomarkers (e.g., blood, urine, semen)
Documentation of vaccines	Documentation of vaccines	Documentation of vaccines
Infections (vector borne, bacterial, or viral)	Infections (vector borne, bacterial, or viral)	Infections (vector borne, bacterial, or viral)
Military occupation specialty and any employment prior to joining military	Military occupation specialty	Military occupation specialty and other employment after separation
Exposures Over the Lifecourse		
Dietary and lifestyle data (e.g., smoking, alcohol, use of dietary supplements)	Dietary and lifestyle data (e.g., smoking, alcohol, use of dietary supplements)	Dietary and lifestyle data (e.g., smoking, alcohol, use of dietary supplements)
Measures of mental health (e.g., cognitive issues, depression, anxiety, PTSD)	Measures of mental health (e.g., cognitive issues, depression, anxiety, PTSD)	Measures of mental health (e.g., cognitive issues, depression, anxiety, PTSD)
Health Effects		
Comprehensive assessments of health status (vital signs, weight)	Comprehensive assessments of health status (vital signs, weight)	Comprehensive assessments of health status (vital signs, weight)
Reproductive status and history	Reproductive status and history	Reproductive status history
Socioeconomic Factors		
Demographic data, marital status, education, number and gender of children	Changes to socioeconomic factors (e.g., birth of a child, divorce)	Demographic data, marital status, education, number and gender of children

NOTE: PTSD=posttraumatic stress disorder.

from women should be collected within 5 weeks after conception and upon the child's birth or as soon as possible thereafter. The obstacles to blood draws, saliva, and even urine collection in very young children need to be considered. Capturing as many life stages as possible would enable researchers to encompass all the periods in which an immediate generational response may present, for example, within the first trimester when most birth defects appear and potentially are diagnosed.

Preconception samples from veterans may also be available from the DoD Serum Repository, but these could be supplemented with samples from those couples who seek fertility care. Additional opportunistic samples that are indicative of early development may be available when assisted reproductive technology (in vitro fertilization) is used.

Exposure Assessment

The primary reason to distinguish among veteran cohorts is that deployment exposures and health outcomes or status may be vastly different from one cohort to another. For example, many Vietnam veterans were exposed to a number of herbicides that included the contaminant 2,3,7,8-tetrachlorodibenzo-p-dioxin (TCDD, or dioxin), although there is little information on the actual exposures that veterans experienced during the war, and these herbicides were not used in subsequent conflicts. Veterans of the 1990–1991 Gulf War and the Post-9/11 conflicts in Afghanistan and Iraq had different exposures, which included severe dust storms, burn pits, and chemical warfare agents (e.g., sarin at the Khamisiyah munitions depot in Iraq, and for Gulf War veterans, burning oil wells in Kuwait).

Deployment and occupational exposures may result in or contribute to a biological response and the manifestation of adverse health effects in not only the veterans but also their descendants. Exposure to stressors—nutritional, psychological, physical, radiological, and chemical—during the preconception period and in utero may affect the health of descendants. In addition to the more typical stressors associated with veterans, the stressors may also include vaccines, infectious diseases, smoking, and drug and alcohol use.

Currently, one major limitation of conducting a study using available data on veterans is the lack of adequate exposure information. Validated individual measures of exposure are not available for veterans of any era, and estimates of exposure often rely on self-reported information or military records (e.g., whether a veteran was deployed to a base that had an operating burn pit, or associating exposures with a specific military occupational specialty code). Few environmental sampling studies have been conducted (e.g., see IOM, 2011). The Volume 11 committee recognizes that it may be impossible to determine veterans' deployment exposures retroactively. Therefore, to better identify deployment exposures in the future, two different types of studies might be helpful. One series of studies would describe the quality (i.e., reliability and validity) of both retrospective and prospective exposure assessment data available for the toxicants of interest for a given veteran cohort—for instance, air sampling at burn pits for Post-9/11 veterans—and make recommendations about the use of such data in future studies. This type of study might demonstrate that some exposures are measured so poorly that future studies of these exposures would be of questionable value. In such situations, cohort studies of deployed versus nondeployed veterans may be the best assessment of exposure. A second series of studies could identify the extent and combinations of exposure to toxicants of interest. Such descriptive epidemiology studies of exposure prevalence, timing, frequency, and combinations might inform future studies to identify mixture effects among veterans in different exposure scenarios.

Exposure misclassification is possible when relying on self-reports of exposure or when measurements of exposure are not available. For example, Gulf War veterans who were originally determined to have been exposed to chemical warfare agents at the Khamisiyah munitions depot in Iraq on the basis of environmental modeling were later reclassified as unexposed when the model was corrected. Misclassification may also occur if a veteran is unaware of what toxicants he or she was exposed to in a certain situation, such as what materials were being disposed of in a burn pit. Exposure misclassification may be reduced by using more than one source of information to assess exposure, such as environmental sampling and an inventory of toxicants that were used. As noted in the 2011 National Academies (IOM, 2011) report on the health effects associated with exposure to burn pits

> Compared with personal monitoring, use of environmental concentrations loses information because personnel at a given site may experience varied levels of exposure based on their activities, personal characteristics, and day-to-day differences in ambient pollutant concentrations; use of environmental concentrations assumes personnel are exposed to the average exposure at each site. Any approach that blurs the distinction between individual exposures while maintaining the collection of individual health outcomes will reduce the estimated variation in exposure and lead to exposure misclassification of some individuals. These issues bias the study, increasing the chance that any association between exposure and health outcome will not be detected.

Role of Partners and Descendants in an HMRP

Partners

The participation of partners will be critical to the success of an HMRP designed to study health outcomes in the children, grandchildren, and future generations of veterans. To monitor the effects of preconception or prenatal exposures, it will be essential for the HMRP to also enroll the partners (men and women) of the service members, whether active-duty or veterans. Biological samples from male partners of study participants that may be used to assess the genetic and chemical risk factors for reproductive and developmental effects include blood and urine samples, which can be linked to the timing of other required pregnancy specimen collections, and a semen sample when pregnancy is first suspected or, at the latest, during the first month of pregnancy. From female partners, the specimens to be collected include blood and urine and cord blood obtained at the time of birth and a heel stick (blood spot) sample from the newborn, which is collected as part of all newborn screening programs. Other information to be collected from partners includes the same lifecourse exposure data collected for service members and veterans, occupational and recreational/environmental exposures, a comprehensive assessment of health status (e.g., vital signs, weight, presence of disease), and a reproductive history.

Optimally, if both parents are members of the military, their health records will be in the MHS, and both will agree to the use of their health information for the monitoring program. Although the DoD EHRs may include health information for partners if they are beneficiaries, it may be difficult to obtain health information for those individuals who do not use TRICARE. Issues of consent may also arise if the parents are not married, get divorced while in TRICARE, or otherwise have objections to the HMRP.

Descendants

Obtaining health effects information from the children of service members and veterans will be challenging, but various approaches may be used to reduce the burden of sample collection. Data collection will depend on whether a parent is active-duty, enrolled in VA, or a civilian in another health care system. Medical data for children who are TRICARE beneficiaries will be available through the MHS until they are no longer eligible for TRICARE, either because they are no longer dependents of a military parent or because their parents have separated from the military. The TRICARE system can provide information on a child's birth and health as long as the child is covered. Should a child leave the TRICARE system, further monitoring will be challenging, especially if the child receives health care from private providers. The child/adult would need to authorize the release of his or her medical information. With the proper permission, health information from pediatric visits might be obtained.

In addition to retrieving the information from a child's medical record, it will also be useful to collect and store a child's blood spot taken at birth, which can be used for genomic testing and other omics testing. Deciduous, or "baby," teeth might also be collected from those children ages 5–12 years who were in utero at the time of maternal deployment in order to reconstruct exposures in pregnancy. New technologies have been developed that can reconstruct certain chemical exposures (e.g., metals) experienced in pregnancy and early childhood from deciduous teeth (Andra et al., 2016). Table 9-3 identifies the data and biospecimens that should be collected for an HMRP from children and grandchildren.

Several health outcomes should be assessed for veterans' children—specifically, prenatal and neonatal health (e.g., fetal growth, preterm birth, birth defects, sex ratio); neurodevelopment; growth (e.g., weight, height, head and waist circumference); metabolic, endocrine (e.g., thyroid hormone), and immunologic function; respiratory health; reproductive health (e.g., age of onset of puberty and menopause, fertility); behavioral health (e.g., depression, anxiety, and other mental health disorders), and chronic disease in childhood and adulthood (e.g., cardiovascular and metabolic diseases, cancer). Many of these endpoints are routinely collected as part of standard medical care. For example, it is usual for states to conduct a neonatal screen for thyroid-stimulating hormone, in which case it is important to ensure that the authorities record the actual level and time of postnatal collection and not just whether the level was normal. Grandchildren should also be assessed for these outcomes, if possible. For practical purposes, the diseases of childhood will be easier to study than the adult-onset diseases in any generational research

TABLE 9-3 Descendant Data and Biospecimens to Be Collected for an HMRP

Birth	Childhood	Adolescence	Adulthood
Growth (e.g., weight, height, head circumference) Anogenital distance Vital signs (e.g., Apgar) Biomarkers (e.g., cord blood, blood spot) State mandated neonatal screen Feeding (e.g., breast-feeding)	Growth (e.g., weight, height, waist circumference) Vital signs (e.g., blood pressure) Neurodevelopment Biomarkers (e.g., blood, urine, hair) Baby teeth Behavioral health Physical health and chronic illnesses School performance Physical activity and diet	Growth (e.g., weight, height, waist circumference) Vital signs (e.g., blood pressure) Neurodevelopment Biomarkers (e.g., blood, urine, hair) Onset of puberty Other reproductive status Physical health and chronic illnesses Lifestyle (e.g., smoking, drugs) and diet Behavioral health School performance	Growth (e.g., weight, height, waist circumference) Vital signs (e.g., blood pressure) Neurodevelopment Biomarkers (e.g., blood, urine, hair) Semen/oocytes Reproductive status (fertility, time to pregnancy, number of children, etc.) Physical health and chronic illnesses Lifestyle (e.g., smoking, drugs, diet, physical activity) Behavioral health Education and socioeconomic information

since waiting for the F1 or F2 generation to age into adulthood will delay the results. In addition, the field is still too young to clearly delineate which health outcomes are likely to be generationally transmitted.

Veteran subpopulations, such as children born to women who became pregnant while deployed or to veterans who had specific hazardous duties or exposures, should be studied more extensively. Collections of data on pregnancy complications (e.g., gestational diabetes and hypertension disorders of pregnancy such as preeclampsia) and birth outcomes (e.g., low birth weight, preterm birth, birth defects, sex ratio, thyroid levels) will be important. The grandchildren of the veterans should also be followed in order to ascertain their health and development.

DoD currently collects data on all births covered by TRICARE. For VA, it might be possible to capture pregnancies and birth with periodic surveys of veterans. In addition to the blood spot that the committee suggests be collected at birth and be maintained by the states' newborn screening programs, and in addition to any project-specific aliquots, other additional biological samples (e.g., saliva or meconium collected from offspring) would depend on the specific goals and questions asked. Other data resources for children's health, such as state and DoD registries of birth defects and cancer registries and also national vital statistics for birth and death certificates, should be considered.

DATA ANALYSES

Studies looking for associations between veterans' exposures and specific outcomes in those veterans and their children should be focused on and driven by exposures that were incurred during deployment (suspected or measured), by the emerging literature on genetics and epigenetics, and by the reproductive and developmental effects identified in Chapters 4 through 7. The analytic techniques that can be used in assessing generational health outcomes include epidemiologic studies and experiments with animal and cellular models; these techniques are briefly described below.

It is essential that the analysis include certain critical elements: proper adjustments for confounders; consideration of mediators and modifiers; identification of appropriate comparison groups; timeliness of the analysis and its reporting; and making the data used in the analysis accessible to outside researchers for their evaluation and further analysis. Each of these elements is discussed below.

The amount of information that will be collected for such an analysis will be substantial, and it will continue to grow as veterans and their descendants age. Current statistical methodology and computing resources permit the screening of a large number of health outcomes in order to determine whether particular diseases are over-represented in the descendants of veterans.

VA or other organizations maintaining the HMRP will need a systematic process for analyzing the data and disseminating results. Technical personnel should regularly review the data to ensure its quality and optimize its effectiveness. VA, DoD, and other collaborators should work together to standardize the data-reporting tools and the analytic programs to be used by each organization to collect, store, and present the information. HMRP data should be analyzed and the results should be reported on a regular basis to aid in the detection of even subtle changes in health over time. For example, DoD regularly analyzes DMSS data and reports on various health statistics of service members in its *Medical Surveillance Monthly Report*.

Where HMRP data suggest an association, more in-depth investigations in the form of hypothesis-driven epidemiologic studies should be considered to verify or further explore the association. Animal or cellular models may also be used to examine the potential mechanisms and biological underpinnings of the findings.

The data collected as part of the HMRP should be made available for extramural research, but it will also be crucial to include appropriate human subject protection as part of the standardized data access; this can be done by making the data available through such resources as dbGAP, a NIH database developed to archive and distribute the data and results from human studies on genotype and phenotype interactions. In addition, the NIEHS Children's Health Exposure Analysis Resource (CHEAR) seeks to provide the "extramural research community access to laboratory and data analyses that add or expand the inclusion of environmental exposures in children's health research" (NIEHS, 2018) (see Box 9-2). Allowing outside investigators to address additional research questions makes the task of conducting a myriad of potential analyses much more manageable. Analyses by outside investigators may target areas of research not yet prioritized by VA, such as rare diseases. The results from such analyses may help redirect the priority health outcomes selected; the methods used to assess exposures, outcomes, or confounders; and additional research priorities for VA and DoD.

Biospecimen and Environmental Analyses

Blood must be processed shortly after collection in the case of both serum and plasma, as freezing a whole blood sample and processing later would destroy the integrity of the serum/plasma due to hemolysis. Infrastructure to process samples shortly after collection will be needed. Spot cards may be an alternative for some measures, but their applicability is not universal.

The committee notes, however, that sera may not be adequate for detecting many of the biomarkers of exposure, response, and susceptibility. Some chemicals or their metabolites are best measured in different biological matrices. For example, exposure to chlorpyrifos might be determined by measuring its metabolite 3,5,6-trichloro-2-pyridinol in urine, whereas organochlorine pesticides such as lindane

BOX 9-2
The Children's Health Exposure Analysis Resource (CHEAR)

CHEAR's goals are to provide researchers with tools to expand the number of studies in children that include environmental exposure analysis, to implement the exposome concept in children's health studies, to create a public resource of children's exposures across the country, and to develop data and metadata standards for the environmental health sciences community. To accomplish these goals, CHEAR has three units:

- The **National Exposure Assessment Laboratory Network** provides access to state-of-the-art infrastructure for the analysis of biological samples as well as for understanding the biological responses associated with those exposures.
- The **Data Repository, Analysis, and Science Center** provides a repository for all data and support for statistical analysis and interpretation. It will also lead the development of community-based data standards and support the development of technologies and metadata standards.
- The **Coordinating Center** provides administrative management of the resource, an interface with the research community, and an index of additional exposure analysis tools not included within the CHEAR infrastructure.

SOURCE: NIEHS, 2018.

would best be measured in serum and dioxins in adipose tissue. Thus, it is important that at least blood and urine be collected for each veteran; blood samples alone will not be sufficient for some toxicants.

A further consideration in biospecimens analysis is the need to conserve individual specimens while still being able to use them for research assays. One approach to this is to use specimen pooling. In case-control studies, cases and controls may be separately pooled to permit an estimation of individual-level exposure effect using modified logistic regression analysis. This approach allows the study of biomarkers while reducing assay costs. Saha-Chaudhuri and Weinberg (2013) have demonstrated how pooling specimens can also be used to screen for discrete exposure effects such as time to pregnancy, although they acknowledge that the approach may produce slightly biased odds ratios. Pooling also helps permit sampling when individual samples may be at or below the level of detection, which may be particularly important when assessing veteran biospecimens for toxicants such as dioxins, although this approach is not recommended for use when more than half of the samples are below the level of detection (Mumford et al., 2006). Schisterman and Vexler (2008) have proposed a combined design, which uses pooled and unpooled biospecimens to capture the strengths of the different sampling strategies and overcome limitations such as levels of detection.

Driven by such issues, the sample-processing and analytic capabilities used to develop biomarkers are advancing at a rapid pace. The capacity to generate a wealth of data is growing at an exponential rate, and this information is being integrated into various precision medicine initiatives, including the NIH All of Us program. Calls to incorporate exposome analyses (i.e., untargeted chemical screens using high-resolution mass spectrometry) as a discovery approach to understanding deployment exposures have already been made (Accardi et al., 2016; Liu et al., 2016; Walker et al. 2016). These specimens can be used to carry out a comprehensive screen of biological systems.

To identify emerging health problems as well as to pinpoint the possible generational effects associated with various exposures, omics data generated from biospecimens can, in the context of the child's and the parents' health status, provide a resource with which to evaluate biomarkers of exposure and mechanisms of action and to develop a personalized response profile. The committee recognizes that the number of complete sets of data on children is likely to be limited, certainly in the early years of any HMRP. But as the program matures, particularly for Post-9/11 veterans and future veterans, these data could provide a robust resource that is well-suited to the growing omics field of personalized and precision medicine.

Because it is not clear which health effects are most likely to be generationally transmitted, a broad spectrum of health effects will need to be assessed. Recent advances in phenomics—the study of all health outcomes—may be adapted in a future HMRP. Hebbring (2014) suggests that phenome-wide association studies that use electronic medical record systems to conduct a genotype-to-phenotype approach when studying human disease may be a complementary approach to genome-wide association studies. Phenomic advances in image analysis, the use of machine learning to process biological lab data, and the use of natural language processing to perform computational searches of the EHR may be key to reducing the number of phenotypes to be studied to a more manageable number.

Regardless of their deployment or occupational status, humans are affected by environmental exposures from countless sources during their lifetimes, including parental exposures that may occur even before the conception of an individual. Accordingly, one must not only consider exposures that occur during deployment, including multiple deployments to the same or different locations, but also take into account how previous or subsequent exposures throughout a lifetime affect a person's health and that of subsequent generations. Some environmental exposures, such as tobacco use, may cause adverse effects, but many exposures will not—or they may even be beneficial (e.g., vitamins, medicines). As a result, deployment-related exposures cannot be examined in isolation; rather, they must be considered in the context of the many other exposures that occur over the lifecourse. For example, if the veteran is a smoker, what effect might smoking have on the veteran's response to an additional exposure such as particulate matter during a dust storm in Iraq? Thus, it becomes difficult to know with certainty whether a health effect can be attributed to an exposure during deployment or to an exposure prior to or after deployment or to a combination of all three. Furthermore, as is evident from prior *Gulf War and Health* volumes, a toxicant may be associated with multiple health outcomes making it difficult to attribute any given health effect to a single toxicant. For example, polycyclic aromatic hydrocarbons (PAHs) have been associated with reproductive effects in men as well as adverse pregnancy outcomes. Because so little is known about the generational effects of deployment-related exposures, it is difficult to answer questions about how exposures over the lifecourse, including deployment exposures, may affect subsequent generations. However, the use of appropriate epidemiological methods and robust data could assist in determining the associations between potential deployment-related exposures and the health effects across multiple generations.

A well-conducted epidemiologic study will need estimates of environmental exposures during deployment, including during incidents of special concern such as the demolition of the Khamisiyah weapons depot. This will require the use of state-of-the-art exposure assessment methods. For example, recently developed wearable monitoring devices could be employed by either all deployed personnel or to a generalizable subset. Wearable devices are a rapidly evolving field; thus, the program should stay abreast of developments as they occur because improvements over current methods are likely to arise. As observed at Khamisiyah in 1991, researchers need to be aware of the limits of the detection of exposures and where additional methods for detecting exposures should be deployed. This is particularly important for exposures such as Khamisiyah where the exposure was to a chemical warfare agent where air sampling at the time of the demolition or shortly afterward would have helped to determine the extent and severity of the sarin plume and thus the number of service members who were potentially exposed. Such monitoring by DoD can facilitate risk communication and help identify a cohort of exposed individuals. For most veterans, however, exposures will need to be modeled from environmental data, lists of chemicals used on-site, and other geospatial information. Other deployment exposures that should be captured include the use of pesticides (such as permethrin-impregnated uniforms), the application of chemical agent-resistant coatings, and the use of weapons containing depleted uranium. The 2000 NRC report *Strategies to Protect the Health of U.S. Deployed Forces: Analytical Framework for Assessing Risks* provided a risk assessment framework that might be used by DoD to assess threats to service members by establishing strategic baseline preparations based on military activities (rather than on specific threats), characterizing activities during deployment (including environmental sampling and information on unit activities), and monitoring veterans for effects from those activities after deployment.

Statistical Considerations

Applying the results of a health monitoring effort to the design and implementation of an epidemiological research study requires that the researchers have the appropriate sample size so that the study has sufficient power to detect an effect. Without a sufficiently large population, it is difficult for researchers to know if their study will answer the questions they developed when establishing the goals of the study. The size of the health monitoring effort, the amount of data collected on the specified populations (including comparison groups), and the manner in which exposures are measured or estimated and health outcomes assessed will all contribute to determining the statistical methodology used for the epidemiologic research study, including sample size and power.

Sample Size and Power

Choosing a targeted sample size is an important step in designing a hypothesis-driven epidemiologic study. Sample-size calculations are based on the expected magnitude of the difference between the exposed and unexposed groups, the relative sizes of the groups to be compared, and specified levels for type I error (the error of rejecting the null hypothesis when it is true) and type II error (the error of failing to reject the null hypothesis when the alternative hypothesis is true). To calculate the minimum required sample size, the number of subjects per group must be multiplied by the number of groups used for comparison (IOM, 2008). Although not specific to a reproductive or developmental effect, a prior Institute of Medicine (IOM) committee (IOM, 2008) did calculate sample sizes for a statistically significant difference in mean serum creatinine concentration, a biomarker for renal injury, between depleted uranium-exposed and -unexposed subjects, setting a type I error (that is a false positive) at 5% and the power at 80%. To detect a risk ratio of 1.50, approximately 9,000 participants (1,760 exposed and 7,038 unexposed) would be required.

A sample size that is too small will not provide estimates that are precise enough to reliably answer the questions of interest, whereas a sample size that is too large may not make optimal use of time and resources. Sample size is often chosen on the basis of a power calculation. The power of a study is the probability that it can detect an association between an exposure and an outcome if there really is such an association. If the statistical power is high, the probability of concluding that there is no association when in fact such an association does exist goes down. In clinical trials, a power of at least 80% is typically required; however, this threshold should depend on context. Knowing the power of a study helps with the interpretation of negative results.

To perform a power calculation and use it to determine the sample size needed to achieve a given level of power, three critical inputs are needed: (1) the size of effect that is to be detected (intuitively, to detect a smaller effect with high power, a larger sample size is needed); (2) the variability of the outcome—for example, the standard deviation of the outcome variable in the population (i.e., with higher variability, a larger sample size is needed); and (3) the range of the exposure (i.e., with a smaller range, it is harder to detect effects of the exposure, and a larger sample size is again needed). Reviews of power calculations and sample size determination are provided by Hajian-Tilaki (2011), Lenth (2001), and Liu et al. (2005).

In cohort studies, many exposures and outcomes may be of interest, and the power will differ for each exposure/outcome combination. It may then be advisable to assess power calculations for a few representative exposure/outcome combinations. The needed sample size will be larger if the researcher wants to gain information about specific subpopulations, such as those carrying certain genotypes, and for the power calculations to be correct, these subpopulations will need to be defined and fixed before the study is conducted. Thus, it may be advisable to expand targeted sample sizes to compensate for exposure-classification issues, attrition of subjects by dropout, other losses to follow-up, and deaths of veterans and their descendants over the lengthy follow-up period.

When planning a generational cohort study, there are additional considerations for power calculations that will need to be taken into account. Since the initial sample size needs to be determined based on the generation receiving the initial exposure, one needs to consider what the effect of the initial exposure will be on the survival and fecundity of subsequent generations in order to estimate the sample size that will be available for subsequent generations, given the initial generation sample size. The committee is not aware of any substantial research on this topic, and further research would be valuable.

Bias

An important contribution of statistical theory to epidemiology is a method to understand the statistical uncertainty associated with effect size estimates. In particular, this theory provides an approach to computing the expected values and standard errors of estimates. By increasing the sample size, estimates can be made to approach the population quantity being estimated. However, the theory assumes that there is no bias or systematic error in the approach. In the presence of bias, this theory is no longer valid. When an estimate of an effect size is consistently different from the actual effect size in the population of interest, regardless of the sample size, the estimate is said to be biased. For example, consider a survey that seeks to measure the proportion of individuals in a population with hypertension. Due to a flaw in the methodology, older individuals are more likely to be included in the sample. This would result in a biased estimate: no matter how large the sample size for the study, the study would be expected to produce a higher estimate than the real proportion of the population with hypertension.

Reducing bias is therefore an important part of epidemiologic studies. Bias can arise from a number of sources. Below the committee describes some common examples: selection bias, information bias, confounders, mediators, and effect modifiers.

Selection Bias

As noted in Chapter 2 and in the section on Sampling of Study Populations earlier in this chapter, bias can result when study participants are selected in such a way that they do not represent the target population or if the probability of selection is related to exposure or disease status. This may be due to a poor definition of the eligible population or a failure to obtain a random sample. This is an important consideration when surveying veterans or any volunteer population where those who agree to participate may be different from those who decline to participate. For example, VA has determined that male veterans who use VA benefits tend to be older than those who do not (64 versus 57 years of age), whereas among female veterans, VA beneficiaries are slightly younger than non-beneficiaries (46 versus 48 years of age) (VA, 2017b). Furthermore, veterans who are more concerned about their children's health, possibly because the child has a health problem, may be more inclined to participate in an HMRP than veterans with healthy children (i.e., a volunteer bias). Other types of selection bias include nonresponse bias and the healthy-warrior effect, which is similar to the healthy-worker effect. Such biases can be acknowledged and adjusted for in the statistical analyses of study data.

In some cases, selection bias can be introduced if subject inclusion correlates with disease and exposure. For example, autistic children might be excluded from an analysis that required a blood-based biomarker. Newer technologies—such as blood spot–based biomarkers and volumetric absorptive microsampling (a technology that enables quantitative blood volume collection from a capillary prick)—will reduce, but probably not eliminate, selection bias from biomarker sample collection. Both the MVP (discussed later in the chapter) and the proposed HMRP will collect extensive demographic data on correlates of exposure such as socioeconomic status, location of residence, education levels (see Tables 9-2 and 9-3), and disease. Modern methods of EHR mining, such as machine learning–based methods, will allow more complete covariate and phenotype data to be collected. In all cases when studies are conducted on subsets of cohort subjects, investigators may compare the included versus excluded groups using sensitivity analyses to determine whether there is selection bias. With respect to measurement error, the committee recommends that researchers consult the growing body of literature on applicable measurement corrections (e.g., Bennett et al., 2017; Keogh and White, 2014).

Information Bias

When a study misclassifies the exposure, outcome, or both, it is said that there is *information bias*. These errors can occur either differentially or non-differentially. For non-differential misclassification, an error in the measurement of the exposure or outcome has occurred evenly across these two groups. With differential misclassification, an error in the measurement has occurred in the exposure group that differs according to the outcome or else an error in measurement has occurred in the outcome that differs between the members of the exposed and unexposed groups. These different types of misclassification result in different forms of bias. Other types of information bias include recall bias and interviewer bias.

Confounders

In epidemiological studies, there are variables that can be associated with both the exposure of interest and the outcome of interest. When not considered in the study, these factors can lead to bias. For example, cigarette smoking could be a confounder of a particular association of interest, such as ambient air pollution and respiratory conditions, because cigarette smoke contains constituents of air pollution and can cause adverse respiratory effects. In this case, if the analysis does not take into account individuals' cigarette smoking, it can end up overestimating or underestimating the association of interest. Because of this, it is essential that confounders be measured and adjusted for in the statistical models in order to reduce bias and obtain valid estimates of the association of interest. Much work has been dedicated to issues of validity in epidemiologic studies.

Mediators

These variables are often confused with confounders because they are associated both with exposure and with outcome. But unlike confounders, mediators are on the pathway between the exposure and the outcome and are part of the reason the exposure causes the outcome. These variables are therefore not confounders, but rather are considered to be mediators of the exposure-outcome association. Mathematically, they would behave similarly to confounders in a regression analysis. Special statistical methods are used to address mediators. Multiple mediators can be on a given pathway of interest. Information on mediators can be highly informative and can provide key information about the mechanisms involved in a given exposure-outcome association, especially in the context of generational health effects. However, limitations in the power of the analysis or in the data can make it difficult to detect mediators.

Effect Modifiers

Variables that modify the association between an exposure and an outcome of interest are defined as effect modifiers. In biological terminology, synergism and potentiation are two concepts that are similar to effect modification. In effect modification, the association between the exposure and the outcome is amplified in the presence of another variable. For example, it may be hypothesized that posttraumatic stress disorder (PTSD) could be an effect modifier of the effect of ambient PAHs on asthma. In this case, individuals who have PTSD and who are exposed to PAHs are much more likely to develop asthma than individuals who are exposed to PAHs but who do not have PTSD. Because the effect modification says something about the biology underlying the exposure and the outcome, findings are reported stratified by the modifier. Often, effect modification is used synonymously with interaction. In statistical models, interaction terms can account for the presence of effect modification. Effect modification is different from confounding. It provides important information about potentially vulnerable or resilient populations because it relates to the exposure and outcome associations. To avoid a biased sample, it is necessary to account for such interactions in the data.

Directed acyclic graphs (DAGs) require that the temporal relationship of covariates be considered as well as whether the covariates are confounders or mediators of the association of interest. Over extended periods of time, it may be difficult to determine whether a variable is a fixed confounder or mediator. This is particularly true when considering research questions that involve multiple generations. Even in cases where a shorter period of time is considered for the mediating mechanism, such as maternal exposure during deployment and fetal growth, it is important to note the non-static nature of the exposures and time-varying confounders as they relate to the outcomes of interest. In this example, there may be uncertainty about the impact of confounding on the associations of interest. As such, DAGs should be used with caution in situations with multiple variables.

Appropriate statistical methods should address the temporality of exposure and its potential confounders and mediators as it relates to a given outcome across the lifecourse. As the field of generational health effects develops, it will likely require both current methods, such as the use of DAGs, and new statistical approaches that have yet to be developed (Hernan and Robins, 2018; Pearl et al., 2016). Statistical methods for mediation analysis distinguish between pre-exposure confounders and potential post-exposure mediators. Instead of adjusting for the post-exposure variable as one would for a confounder, the variable is treated as an intermediate outcome in the analysis. Reviews of considerations and methods for mediation analysis and of the analysis of post-exposure variables are provided by Bellavia and Valeri (2018), Rosenbaum and Rubin (1984), Taguri et al. (2018), Ten Have and Joffe (2012), and VanderWeele (2015).

Challenges with Mixtures

As discussed in Chapter 2, a major challenge in assessing the effect of human exposure to a specific chemical agent is that humans are usually exposed to many environmental agents at once and these exposures are often highly correlated (i.e., colinear). Many health effect studies focus on a single agent or else consider simple two-agent interactions. However, the results of such studies can be very misleading when the agent is highly correlated with multiple biologically active agents. An example of this would be the way that exposures to ambient particulate matter may be highly correlated with exposures to NO_2 because they are both components of fossil fuel combustion. The complexity of assessing mixtures, particularly poorly defined mixtures such as combustion products and their implications for epidemiologic studies of veterans was discussed in the IOM report on the long-term health effects of exposure to burn pits (IOM, 2011).

Several methods have been developed for dealing with exposures to mixtures. Billionnet et al. (2012) reviewed the statistical methods used to assess the health effects associated with the multiple chemicals that constitute air pollution and other researchers have explored the challenges of assessing exposures to mixtures for epidemiological studies. Braun et al. (2016) acknowledge that measuring exposure to a mixture requires the accurate measurement of the individual components of the mixture, which may be difficult given within-person variability and misclassification of exposures, reverse causality due to pharmacokinetic factors, and the validity of the biomarker for assessing exposure over time. Nevertheless, it may be possible to identify and prioritize important mixtures which pose greater risks or are more common in certain situations (e.g., the mixture of pyridostigmine bromide, permethrin, and DEET that along with stress are used to mimic Gulf War exposures suspected of causing Gulf War illness). The committee recognizes, however, that there are no standard analytical methods for the mixtures that may be encountered during deployment. Braun et al. (2016) present several methods to quantify the association between individual exposures and health effects and apply those to mixtures, examine interactions between chemicals in a mixture, and assess the cumulative chemical exposures with a health effect by quantifying the "summary effect of a class or multiple classes of exposure."

New methods and statistical approaches may also be useful when assessing mixtures. Hamra and Buckley (2018) state that the research question to be answered by the assessment of a mixture will drive the parameterization of the exposure variables. The committee encourages VA to follow scientific advances in mixture assessment, including both measuring environmental concentrations of individual components of mixtures as well as new techniques for sampling mixtures themselves and new toxicologic information on the effects of mixtures in animal models (see Chapter 10). Some of the issues with assessing exposure to Gulf War mixtures in animal models of Gulf War illness are reviewed in *Volume 10*, Chapter 5, Animal Studies (NASEM, 2016).

LEVERAGING EXISTING RESOURCES

Thus far, the committee has laid out the basic elements of an HMRP. These elements may be perceived as establishing a contemporary gold standard for answering questions about generation health effects. But the committee realizes that time and resources are finite, and while it may be possible to implement parts of the proposed health monitoring effort and hypothesis-driven epidemiologic studies, it may be more feasible and expedient to leverage ongoing programs such as the VA MVP. Regardless of the approach used, the utility of the results of any program will hinge on the availability and quality of the data on the veterans' exposures and of the data on their health and the health of their partners and descendants. In the sections below, the committee provides guidance on how VA and DoD might improve the collection of information to determine possible generational health effects using existing infrastructure. The committee examined a number of ongoing research programs from the perspective of which offered the best opportunity for answering questions about the health of veterans' descendants. These research programs include the VA-sponsored MVP and the DoD-sponsored Millennium Cohort (MilCo) and MilCo Family Study as well as the DoD Birth and Infant Health Registry.

Million Veteran Program[3]

The Million Veteran Program is a VA initiative aimed at developing a better understanding of how genes affect health, with the ultimate goal of improving health care for male and female veterans of any era as well as for the general population. The MVP was established in 2011 to serve as a resource for precision medicine by collecting biological samples that may be used to develop prevention interventions, diagnostic tools, and treatments to improve health care. Although the goal of the MVP is to have a representative sample of all veterans who use VA health care across the nation, participation in the program is voluntary and by invitation only (i.e., not a self-selected population). As of October 2017, 49% of the 625,000 veterans enrolled in the MVP were from the 1961–1975 Vietnam era, 23% served from 1975 to 1990, 23% served from 1990 to 2001 (of whom 5% are Gulf War veterans), and 12% have served since 2001 (of whom 6% are Operation Enduring Freedom/Operation Iraqi Freedom veterans). Veterans currently enrolled in the VA health care system complete surveys about their health and health-related behavior, provide a blood sample, allow researchers to access their VA and VA-linked medical

[3] References: https://www.research.va.gov/mvp/veterans.cfm#6; https://www.nih.gov/sites/default/files/research-training/initiatives/pmi/pmi-presentation-million-veteran-program-cohort-example-large-scale-health-system-based-cohort.pdf; and https://www.nihcollaboratory.org/Pages/GR-Slides-09-09-16.pdf.

records, and agree to future contact (VA, 2017c). Data for the MVP can be extracted from VA clinical and administrative databases, including the National Patient Care Database, VA Managerial Cost Accounting National Data Extracts, the Corporate Data Warehouse (Health Data Repository), Medical Domain Web Services, the Patient Care Services Clinical Data Warehouse, the Veteran Informatics and Computing Infrastructure, the Veterans Health Administration Support Service Center, the VA Cancer Registry, and the VA Vital Status File. VA has recently partnered with the Department of Energy (DOE) for the MVP's Computational Health Analytics for Medical Precision to Improve Outcomes (CHAMPION) initiative. The goal of the initiative is to bring the Department of Energy's state-of-the-art expertise and capabilities in a secure computing environment to analyze large amounts of health care and genetic data from VA and other federal sources, beginning with MVP data (VA, 2017c).

From male veterans the MVP questionnaire collects basic information on reproductive health, fertility, and the number of children they have fathered. More detailed information is collected from female veterans, including age at menarche, age at menopause, reproductive health (hysterectomy, ovary removal), and fertility; the use of contraceptives, hormone replacement therapy, and fertility treatments; and details about pregnancies (number, stillbirths and miscarriages, age at first and last births, and breast-feeding). Women are also asked about the birth weight of their first child, but no other data are gathered on the health status of the veterans' children.[4]

The only biological specimen that is collected is a blood sample that is processed into plasma, buffy coat, and DNA. Samples are to be stored indefinitely under liquid nitrogen unless the veteran withdraws from the program and the samples are destroyed.

The strengths of the MVP study are its large sample size, the fact that it uses a representative sample of the VA population, its collection of blood samples and establishment of the genetic biorepository, its ability to link together and merge other VA databases, its collection of vital statistics data, and its use of a physical examination. The MVP can be an important resource for the study of inter- and transgenerational effects because participating veterans are willing to be contacted again in order to provide additional information on the course of each generation.

The MVP is the largest existing VA genomic biobank with sufficient data depth to be used to assess genetic susceptibility to certain exposures, particularly those that can be measured in plasma samples, such as exposures to lindane and dioxins. Its DNA resource could be used to assess genome methylation status with the goal of identifying DNA methylation patterns that arise following chemical and other exposures. This is a potential way to reconstruct past exposure such as is currently done with the methylation patterns in the aryl hydrocarbon receptor repressor gene to identify smoking status. As of 2015, genotyping data were available on 199,348 veterans in the program (92% men), of whom 77% were white, 13.5% were black, the remainder were "other" or not reported (Gaziano et al., 2016).

Augmenting the MVP could make possible the study of multiple generations. The committee identified several strategies that could be adopted, including conducting regular participant and offspring follow-up sessions. Information on parental reproductive history, such as time to pregnancy (fecundability) and clinical infertility, might also be collected. The frequency of this follow-up would be determined by logistic and economic factors, but the committee suggests that information on children be collected at least once in every life stage, as outlined in the section on Health Outcome Data on Children and Grandchildren. Data from annual medical visits to primary care providers could be merged with the MVP data. Biological samples (e.g., urine, saliva, and blood) from the children and grandchildren might be collected and stored for future use.

[4] Personal communication from Victor Kalasinsky, Office of Research and Development, VA, October 17, 2017.

Because the MVP does not include veterans who do not use the VA health care system, information on how MVP participants differ from veterans who do not use VA (demographics, deployment, and military characteristics) would add to the usefulness of information on veterans that do use it and would strengthen MVP estimates of health risk for all veterans. The committee is encouraged by the way in which VA and the NIH All of Us program entered into a partnership for leveraging data collection, and the committee expects that this partnership will provide a sound mechanism for helping VA collect data on veterans who do not use the VA health care system and for recruiting those veterans into an HMRP.

If such additions were made to the MVP, the data could be used for a variety of future epidemiologic and other experimental research studies. Because the MVP records can be linked to deployment history and other military exposures, adopting the committee's recommendation to include enhanced exposure data collected during military service in a veteran's ILER would allow researchers to conduct nested case-control studies on, for example, the prevalence of a reproductive health outcome in veterans.

Millennium Cohort

In response to concerns about the health effects of deployments following the 1990–1991 Gulf War, Congress and IOM recommended that DoD conduct prospective epidemiological research to evaluate the impact of military exposures, including deployment, on the long-term health outcomes of veterans. DoD responded by establishing the MilCo, the largest prospective health study service ever conducted with members from the Army, Navy, Air Force, Marine Corps, and Coast Guard; at present it has more than 200,000 participants, with more than 31% of them women (Smith, 2009).[5] The study is being conducted by the Naval Health Research Center. The eligible population consists of active-duty personnel deployed since 2001 in support of the operations in Iraq and Afghanistan, including reservists and National Guardsmen; participants are followed after they leave the service or are deactivated.

MilCo contains data collected via questionnaires and from DoD databases. No biological specimens are collected, and no physical examinations are conducted. The questionnaires have self-reported outcomes, and participants are asked to complete them every 3 years through 2022. The questionnaire covers the following topics: general health (functional status, including physical and mental; well-being; height and weight); health behaviors (alcohol and tobacco use, eating behaviors/disorders, sleep duration and quality, physical activity); health conditions and symptoms (provider-diagnosed medical conditions); physical symptoms (e.g., pain, headaches, fatigue, shortness of breath, cough, forgetfulness); mental health (PTSD, depression, anxiety); pregnancy and infertility; potential exposures (combat experiences; injuries, including head injuries; motor vehicle accidents; burn pits/smoke; chemicals/pesticides/depleted uranium; assault, sexual and physical; adverse childhood experiences); and military life (deployments; military occupation specialty; perception of the military; status, active duty, reserve/National Guard, separated/retired).

Health data from the questionnaires can be linked to the DMSS and the DMDC for demographic, deployment, and occupational data. Service data, including deployment dates and locations, are supplied by the DMDC, and environmental exposure data for Army personnel are described in U.S. Army Public Health Command reports. Self-reported exposures are incorporated from the pre- and post-deployment health assessments.

The strengths of MilCo include its large sample of military personnel, including those specifically deployed to war zones, and its use of regular follow-up surveys to monitor for the onset of new health problems. Although the data are collected by questionnaire, this is not a weakness for social/behavioral/

[5] See https://www.millenniumcohort.org/about (accessed June 13, 2018).

dietary and environmental factors, many of which cannot be measured by biomarkers. In addition, questionnaire data on chemical exposures are collected prior to the development of health effects in the participants' children, which may reduce recall bias. The cohort may therefore play a critical role in evaluating the role of these types of exposures during deployment as predictors of inter- and transgenerational health effects from deployment.

A limitation of the MilCo is its lack of biospecimens and physical examinations. Selection bias is also a potential issue because military personnel who choose to participate may differ from nonparticipants in various ways. In addition, those who continue to participate may differ from those who drop out (e.g., those with medical issues may be retained, but healthy individuals may drop out). Mortality rates also need to be carefully considered in the interpretation of findings. Other limitations to using the MilCo data include: lack of confirmation of self-reported medical issues for participants who are not active-duty, allowing for disease misclassification; and exposure misclassification is also possible as individual exposure information is not available.

DoD has extended the MilCo to include the partners and children of MilCo participants in the Millennium Cohort Family Study (the Family Study). In the section below, the committee discusses modifications to the Family Study that would aid in studying the generational effects of deployment.

Millennium Cohort Family Study

The Family Study is a DoD-sponsored research project nested within MilCo that is intended to study the impact of deployment on family functioning. The participants are partners of service members from the Army, Navy, Air Force, Marine Corps, and Coast Guard who have served since 2000 and are enrolled in MilCo. The Family Study began in 2011 and is intended to follow partners for 21 years or longer, regardless of whether their marriage to the service member continues. Follow-up surveys are conducted every 3 years. The surveys collect information on partners' physical and mental health, their reports of their children's physical and mental health and functioning, and family functioning. As of 2014, 9,921 partners of MilCo participants had enrolled in the Family Study, with 8,152 children represented as well. Male partners make up 12% of the participants, and 63% of all participants have children.[6]

Parents report on their children's health concerning physician-diagnosed conditions, behavioral problems, and the use of medical, psychological, and social services. The screening questionnaire for behavioral problems among children ages 3 to 17 years includes the Strengths and Difficulties Questionnaire. Additional health data on the children are obtained from DoD sources, including the Birth and Infant Health Registry (described in the next section), and medical and pharmaceutical records from military medical facilities and civilian facilities covered by TRICARE.

The Volume 11 committee finds that there are both strengths and limitations to this study. The strengths of this study are that it actively enrolls partners and children, collects some health information on children, and follows children regardless of whether their parents remain on active duty or separate from the military and regardless of whether the partners separate. The main limitations of this study are that physical exams are not conducted, nor are biospecimens collected. Furthermore, it does not include partners and children of service members who are not MilCo participants. In addition, a child's behavior is based on only the SDQ screener, which does not allow for the assessment of cognition and other aspects of neurodevelopment.

To enhance the value of the Family Study for investigating generational health effects, the committee has several suggestions. First, it would be advantageous to have MilCo data link with other resources,

[6] See http://www.familycohort.org/whatsnew (accessed May 10, 2018).

such as biospecimens collected as part of the DoD Serum Repository and VA health care records, for continued follow-up. These links would facilitate conducting in-depth investigations of possible associations between deployment exposures and health outcomes. A linkage to DoD and VA medical records would also allow other health outcomes to be assessed and self-reported outcomes to be validated.

Second, because the Family Study is relatively small, with only about 10,000 partners, the committee suggests increasing the sample size; this would permit researchers to look for rare outcomes in children about which veterans are concerned. As an example, if a relatively rare outcome in the offspring such as cleft palate (incidence ~1 in 1,000 births) or childhood cancer (incidence ~18 in 100,000 births) were to be assessed, it would be difficult to identify any such outcomes in the current study population.

Third, the follow-up of the children is limited to questionnaires completed by a parent. The committee suggests that an in-person evaluation be conducted with a brief medical exam (e.g., anthropometry, blood pressure, spirometry in older children) and a developmental examination (a computerized assessment could be done with older children using, e.g., the NIH Toolbox).

In addition, participant permission should be obtained to store and access biospecimens collected as part of routine health care visits. For example, urine samples and blood samples are routinely collected during most pregnancies, but after clinical tests are completed, they are discarded. The committee recommends that the residual sample be aliquoted and saved for those receiving care through TRICARE facilities. These samples would be extremely valuable to use in studying the genetics and epigenetics of participants and in examining prenatal exposures. Parental permission could be obtained to acquire a punch sample from newborn screening cards for genetic information and for assessing in utero exposures. Finally, permission should be obtained to merge data from other state registries, including neonatal screening data (e.g., neonatal thyroid hormone), birth defects and cancer registries, educational records (e.g., state examinations), child special services (e.g., for autism), and other vital statistics data such as the DoD Birth and Infant Health Registry as described below.

DoD Birth and Infant Health Registry

In response to the growing number of women on active duty and the diverse hazardous exposures associated with military service, DoD created the Birth and Infant Health registry in 1998, housed at the Naval Health Research Center in San Diego, to address women's reproductive health concerns, primarily birth defects. The registry collects comprehensive health care data on live births and infant health outcomes through the first year of life for infants born to TRICARE beneficiaries. Recorded outcomes include preterm birth, pregnancy outcomes, birth weight, growth problems in utero and in infancy, and birth defects. The population-based electronic surveillance system, which contained more than 1.6 million births as of 2017 (NHRC, 2017), draws from hospitalizations at military medical facilities (including those overseas), outpatient encounters at DoD facilities, and civilian medical encounters paid for by TRICARE; the system is supplemented by case validation. Links to demographic and military service information, including information on occupational and military exposures, are available through DMDC (Conlin et al., 2012; Ryan et al., 2001).

The strengths of the registry include its ability to link with other DoD databases and the large number of births that are recorded in it. A limitation of the registry is its lack of a mechanism for following children after 1 year of age even if they continue to be in the TRICARE system or for following children under 1 year if their parents separate from the military. The registry does not capture the children of military personnel who receive care through other insurers, and, finally, the registry does not capture data on pregnancy terminations, miscarriages, or stillbirths (Ryan et al., 2001). Both of these are limitations.

The registry, linked to health care data supplied by TRICARE and the MHS, could be used to compare health conditions in children beyond the first year of life and make comparisons based on known exposures or occupations of the parent. For example, surveillance data from the registry describing pregnancy outcomes and birth defects among women of childbearing age have been published (Bukowinski et al., 2012; Conlin et al., 2012). Several published studies, as discussed in Chapter 4, have described birth outcomes in female veterans who were exposed to burn pit emissions or who received vaccines during their pregnancies (Conlin et al., 2012, 2013, 2015, 2017).

The committee suggests that other useful studies would be feasible with this database. For example, the health status of children conceived within a specific time frame relative to a service member's return from deployment—say, 90 days for men to cover one spermatogenesis cycle—could be compared with the health status of children of nondeployed service members. Or, children who were conceived shortly before or during deployment, as determined from their mother's administrative data, could be followed to ascertain their health status, at least while in the TRICARE system.

Other Resources

As noted earlier in the chapter, in addition to the programs discussed above, there are a number of large-scale health-monitoring and epidemiologic studies that may be useful for answering questions about the reproductive health of veterans and the health of their children. The committee believes that these programs and studies, while not sufficient to answer those questions on their own, may provide ancillary resources for VA and DoD efforts. In addition, they also demonstrate the many advantages and challenges faced by VA and other researchers when studying cohorts of veterans. They include

- **The National Health Survey of Gulf War Era Veterans and Their Families** compares the mental and physical health status of a cohort of 15,000 Gulf War veterans from each branch of the military, including active-duty, reserve, and National Guard, with 15,000 of their nondeployed military peers. Three phases of the study have been conducted: 1995 (n=11,441; response rate not reported), 2005 (n=9,970; response rate 34%), and 2012–2013 (n=14,252; response rate 50%). A questionnaire package was mailed to invitees with follow-up reminder postcards; computer-assisted telephone interviewing calls were made to veterans who had not responded. Respondents received $10. Data collected included sociodemographic information health information on chronic medical conditions, chronic fatigue syndrome-like illness and unexplained multi-symptom illness, mental health, health behaviors, general health, functional health, women's health, use of complementary and alternative medicine, and VA health care utilization and satisfaction (VA, 2016).
- **The National Health Study for a New Generation of U.S. Veterans** began as a pilot study in 2009 with data collection concluding in 2010. The goal of the study was to assess the health of Post-9/11 veterans, help identify VA health services that veterans may need, and improve the quality of care offered by VA (VA, 2018b). About 30,000 veterans who were deployed to Iraq and Afghanistan were randomly selected from DoD records and compared with 30,000 veterans who served elsewhere during the same time. More than 20,500 veterans participated in the study with representation from active-duty, reserve, and National Guard members; women comprised 20% of the participants. Data collection included questionnaires with topics that focused on health risk behaviors, health conditions, general health, health care utilization, and potential exposures. No biological samples were collected; however, medical records were reviewed for about 2,000 veterans.

- **The Vietnam Era Health Retrospective Observational Study (VE-HEROeS)** is designed to evaluate the current health and well-being of 43,000 veterans who served in Vietnam, in the Blue Water Navy, and those who served elsewhere from 1961 to 1975. Veterans' health will be compared with about 11,000 civilians within the same age groups who never served in the military. Special emphasis is given to assessing any neurologic conditions and hepatitis C infections. Participants complete a questionnaire pertaining to military service, general health, aging, and lifestyle. Data for this study are still being analyzed as well as a review of medical records for participants (VA, 2017a).
- **The Armed Forces Health Surveillance Branch** conducts medical surveillance of and for the U.S. service members. It has four components:
  - Data Management and Technical Support, which manages the databases to conduct surveillance and analysis of health-related information of U.S. service members.
  - Epidemiology and Analysis includes the DMSS, which contains up-to-date and historical data on diseases and medical events (e.g., vaccines, hospital visits) and longitudinal data on more than 7 million personnel and deployments, including pre- and post-deployment health assessments; and the Department of Defense Serum Repository, which contains more than 62 million serologic specimens.
  - Global Emerging Infections Surveillance develops, implements, supports, and evaluates an integrated global emerging infections surveillance and response system.
  - Integrated Biosurveillance supports many worldwide biosurveillance and public health activities to improve force health protection.
- **The Air Force Health Study,** begun in 1979, was a longitudinal, prospective cohort study of more than 2,700 men who had participated in Operation Ranch Hand, the wartime herbicide spraying in Vietnam. Participants were followed for approximately 20 years, and they received up to six intensive physical examinations that included clinical measurements and observations, the collection of serum and other biological samples, and responses to questionnaires addressing health, lifestyle, socioeconomic status, employment, families and offspring, and potential sources of environmental exposures (Styka and Butler, 2015).

The DoD Serum Repository, the Joint Pathology Center Biorepository, and the Air Force Health Study all maintain biospecimens of military personnel or veterans. The National Health Survey of Gulf War Era Veterans and Their Families and the Health Study for a New Generation of U.S. Veterans and their follow-up survey have longitudinal designs, representative samples, and questions about reproductive health. DMSS is a set of relational databases that integrate service members' deployment, health, and exposure data for DoD health surveillance purposes.

PROGRAM MANAGEMENT

Program management is a critical, integral, and continuous function of any HMRP that includes epidemiologic studies. Addressing the many complementary requirements and opportunities of an HMRP will require the identification of lead organizations to design and implement the overall program and specific research studies. This lead organization may be VA, DoD, NIH, or another organization, such as an academic research center or consortium. Close coordination and collaboration among the program partners is critical for accountability.

Once the lead organization for the HMRP has been identified, an organizational structure of the program that includes partners and collaborators along with the responsibilities for each partner will need to be delineated. The chains of command, personnel, and lines of communication will need to be agreed upon. The strengths and limitations of each collaborator will need to be weighed so that activities are assigned to the most appropriate affiliate. The strengths of the partners may include the availability of subject matter experts, access to relevant data or records, and strong IT capabilities (e.g., DOE). Limitations might reflect the lack of a legislative mandate to participate in the program, financial constraints, and a lack of familiarity with program data requirements, each of which can be understood and addressed through a true multi-organization, cross-country collaborative effort among all participants.

Collaboration and Coordination

The development and implementation of an HMRP to assess generational health effects in veterans and their descendants will require the joint efforts of a number of governmental and nongovernmental organizations. Although the statutory language in P.L. 114-315 Section 362 implies that VA will lead the effort to conduct the HMRP, the scope of the mandate will require well-focused collaborative efforts to achieve success. Although VA may lead the assessment of reproductive effects in veterans, it has limited experience in monitoring the health of nonveterans, especially children. VA will need to work closely with other organizations, public and private—and potentially other countries—to implement a program that includes assessing the health of descendants and partners in order to avoid duplicating resources or parts of programs to minimize costs while maximizing benefits.

Collaborators and affiliates for the HMRPs might include DoD; DOE; the Department of Health and Human Services, including NIH (e.g., National Institute of Child Health and Development and the National Institute of Environmental Health Sciences [NIEHS]) and the Centers for Disease Control and Prevention; the Agency for Toxic Substances and Disease Registry (ATSDR); states' departments of health, including newborn screening and vital statistics; VSOs; foundations with an interest in the health and well-being of service members, veterans, and families (e.g., the Robert Wood Johnson Foundation, Henry M. Jackson Foundation); and academic institutions, all of which may provide guidance on, and resources for, specific aspects of the HMRP. Furthermore, it may be advantageous to consider working with large health care organizations in the private sector, as it is likely that many veterans and their children and grandchildren may receive medical care from such providers. The collection of health data, access to those data, and the sharing of information among collaborators and affiliates and with the public would be addressed by the HMRP management team. In addition, VA may want to consider working with other countries, such as the United Kingdom or Australia, that were part of the coalition forces that fought in the Gulf War and the Post-9/11 conflicts. Service members from those countries had many exposures similar to U.S. forces and they have the advantage of national health systems that include all citizens, including veterans and their descendants. The United Kingdom Medical Research Council and Wellcome Trust established the UK Biobank prospective cohort in 2002 to help investigate risk factors for the major diseases of middle and old age. The biobank recruited more than 500,000 men and women ages 40–69 years between 2006–2010 and their health is being followed long term (Collins, 2012). Should veteran status be included, this might provide a valuable resource even for U.S. researchers.

Each collaborator and affiliate should bring different yet complementary strengths and resources to the program. For example, VSOs may be able to reach out to their members to encourage participation and retention in the program and to assist in the dissemination of surveys. Their expertise in crafting surveys and identifying research priorities should also be solicited. They may also serve as a staging platform for the collection of biological specimens such as blood, saliva, and urine samples. Academic institutions, particularly those affiliated with medical centers, may provide guidance concerning program design, the selection of biomarkers, statistical and bioinformatics assessments, and innovative approaches for data collection and analysis, in addition to access to experts in reproductive and child health and genetics and epigenetics. State health departments and other state programs may provide access to state registries and other data, whereas local city and county agencies can provide supportive efforts.

In P.L. 114-315, Section 633, Congress called on the Secretary of VA to establish an "Advisory Board On Research Relating To Health Conditions Of Descendants Of Veterans With Toxic Exposure While Serving In The Armed Forces." The Advisory Board is to "advise the Secretary in the selection of a research entity or entities under section 634, advise such entity or entities in conducting research under such section, and advise the Secretary with respect to the activities of such entity or entities under such section." The committee is to be composed of 13 members with expertise in birth defects, developmental disabilities, epigenetics, public health, reproduction, environmental exposure assessment, the science of toxic substances, and medical and research ethics. The Volume 11 committee strongly endorses the creation of such a term-limited rotating advisory board to energize the HMRP. Such an advisory board may serve as a catalyst for promoting collaboration and coordination among participants, including both governmental and nongovernmental organizations. To ensure interoperability, this oversight body can provide critical feedback for each veteran cohort–specific program as it is established and can ensure periodic evaluations so that progress toward program goals is monitored and necessary adjustments to the program are implemented in a timely manner. As cohorts are delineated, membership on the oversight committee should adapt to meet the needs of the program. This would inform the rotation of, and membership to, the Scientific Advisory Board on Research Relating to Health Conditions of Descendants of Veterans with Toxic Exposure While Serving in the Armed Forces. For example, an advisory board may recommend new biomarkers of effect as they come into use or provide input on specifics for the number of veterans or their descendants that will need to be included in each cohort-specific program.

Data Resource Needs

The data resources that will be required to conduct a comprehensive and longitudinal HMRP will be substantial. The committee considers that, at a minimum, the lead and collaborating organizations should have access to distributed IT systems capable of handling a large amount of data. When an interface with other IT systems is necessary, program managers will also need to ensure that the appropriate data privacy safeguards are in place, including processes to ensure compliance with the Health Insurance Portability and Accountability Act (also known as HIPAA). The "NIH Security Best Practices for Controlled-Access Data Subject to the NIH Genomic Data Sharing (GDS) Policy" (NIH, 2018a) is one resource for guidance on ensuring the security of human data from which the specifications could be drawn. Other resource needs include personnel (e.g., scientific, technological, administrative, logistical), facilities, and equipment.

The committee considers IT to be one of the pillars of the HMRP. Independent of the particular veteran cohort to be studied, the data needs of the program will be voluminous, and the management of these data will be critical to all aspects of the program. The extensive interoperable database created during the course of the program data collection will likely include, for example, detailed data from DoD regarding deployments, dependents, medical care, occupation and duties; VA medical data; contact information; updated dependent information; biospecimen data (collection dates, status, location, etc.); genomic data; and responses to surveys. Thus, the scope of the technological requirements for the HMRP will include substantial storage capabilities; linkage of EHRs for veterans and their descendants as they move from DoD to VA and other health care providers; and maintenance of a secure cloud by

IT specialists who can work with program managers and analysts to support databases, interfaces, websites, and other electronic information exchange platforms. This integral component that will ensure the veracity, accessibility, and usefulness of the data collected. Furthermore, processes and protocols to protect sensitive personal information will be essential to ensure secure data collection, maintenance, and use. Although the committee realizes that VA and DoD already maintain extensive and well-protected databases on veterans and service members, the necessary collaborations will require that each partner (e.g., NIH, private foundations, state cancer registries) has data privacy safeguards and appropriate IT capabilities in place. Some aspects of medical data linkages for DoD and VA were discussed earlier.

COMMUNICATION

Communication activities will be essential for a successful HMRP and its associated epidemiologic studies. As described above in Collaboration and Coordination, lines of communication and authority will need to be established among the HMRP collaborators and affiliates. The HMRP will need to communicate effectively with all stakeholders, the general public, Congress, and other researchers. This can be achieved as the HMRP management team formalizes bidirectional communication networks with veterans and their descendants. This communication pathway should engage veterans in a dialogue and involve them in the program from start-up to evaluation.

Return of Results

Researchers and veterans and their families together should develop clear guidelines on the communication of individual and group-level study results since these results may have marked ramifications for each participant. For example, researchers and veterans and their families together should consider what health or developmental information should be returned to individuals, carefully weighing the benefits versus the risks of receiving this information. In most cases, individuals should be able to opt in to or opt out of receiving individual-level results. It should also be determined a priori what information will be given back to health care providers with the individual's permission and which data will under law need to be reported to authorities (e.g., suspected child abuse or neglect or reportable diseases), and under what criteria. In addition, the overall study results should be regularly reported to participants, and the best vehicle for this report should be discussed with participant groups. The return of results is governed by well-established principles of ethical conduct in research, and some of these key elements are discussed below within the context of the proposed HMRP to evaluate reproductive and generational health effects.

Veterans and Their Descendants

Achieving high levels of participation (recruitment and retention) in the HMRP will require purposeful, consistent, and comprehensive communication among the leadership of the HMRP, the U.S. military, and the veteran populations and their descendants. A communication strategy should be developed early that will include the recruitment and enrollment of service members and veterans and their descendants into the program. As noted earlier, the strategy will need to facilitate the retention of HMRP participants through the ongoing reporting of results to stakeholders. Transparency and the inclusion of the public will be essential attributes of the program. DoD, VA, and other collaborators should have a well-developed and validated communication mechanism for engaging service members and their children in the MHS. Engaging children from an early age using age-appropriate methods may encourage their participation as they mature and after their parents separate from the military or no longer receive TRICARE coverage. These attitudes may also translate to the children's children—that is, the veteran's grandchildren—as it becomes part of a family tradition. Given that many children of military parents join the military themselves, this may be an important group to identify and engage to assess for generational effects.

The committee suggests that in order to better recruit and retain participants, activities that have been demonstrated to be successful by other longitudinal studies should be considered, modified, and adopted as appropriate by the HMRP. For example, participants in the National Children's Study felt pride in identifying themselves as part of the study cohort, and their interest was encouraged with such meaningful incentives from the researchers as networking, priority newsletters, and the occasional special event that prompted group recognition of the participants' continuation in the program. The Nurses' Health Study Growing Up Today Study (GUTS), has employed newsletters, emails, and birthday cards to promote a sense of community and create a sense of added value in belonging to the program among participants. Communication with the participants of the HMRP will have to be in multiple forms (e.g., social media, Internet, mailings, media, and messaging) that reflect the preferred methods of communication for different groups of participants, factoring in considerations such as age, which often predicts social media usage.

The use of electronic surveys for collecting information and the ability to rapidly analyze that information is essential. For example, to reduce the time and effort for data collection on the part of both the HMRP staff and the program participants, the program could quickly disseminate reminders and notices regarding the availability of surveys to large numbers of recipients by using electronic databases such as voter rolls to locate the descendants of veterans. The MilCo program offers a good example of how electronic surveys and data analysis can be used with a veteran population. Interactive websites, mobile apps, electronic reminders, and other electronic approaches may optimize veteran and public interest in and response to the program.

Communication campaigns must be tailored to the target constituency. For example, Vietnam and Gulf War veterans and their adult descendants may respond better to the use of telephone landlines and the U.S. Postal Service than to electronic forms of communication, including texting, emails, and social media campaigns, which may be of more appeal to Post-9/11 veterans. This should also be a consideration for reaching out to the children and grandchildren of the veterans. Mass media communications such as brief public television announcements and AM/FM radio might also be helpful in some instances. The program must keep pace with new trends in technology that will most likely reach the early adopters—the children and grandchildren of the veterans—who will be a key group in the generational and transgenerational study.

In-person meetings might be held at VSO facilities, if appropriate, or at local VA medical facilities, including Vet Centers, around the country. Virtual connectivity would allow veterans and family members to engage if they are unable to attend in person. The use of VA facilities might serve the dual purpose of engaging HMRP participants and familiarizing the veterans with VA if they have not already been receiving VA medical care. HMRP staff needs to be culturally aware of the veteran communities with whom they are trying to engage. Messages may need to be in the language the veteran uses at home, such as Spanish or Vietnamese. Public advertisements might also be needed to inform veterans and the public about the program. Regular updates on the implementation of the HMRP need to be presented in an array of national scientific meetings in addition to meetings attended by military and veteran populations.

As noted earlier, the return-of-results policy developed for the HMRP can be based on recently developed protocols by the All of Us research program. This is an important issue for any longitudinal study, and documents are being developed for communicating child health outcomes by the NIH ECHO consortium.

Other Key Stakeholders

Information about the HMRP needs to be disseminated and to reach all stakeholders, such as members of the scientific community, health care systems, government officials, veterans and their descendants, and the general public, as discussed above. Communication among governmental and nongovernmental agencies will need to be efficient and effective in order to ensure that program goals are achieved. A biennial report detailing what has been discovered, the status of recruitment efforts, and participation statistics might be an effective communication mechanism for enhancing public awareness of the program. Publicity and media releases might include widely accessible videos, such as podcasts and TED Talks.

A comprehensive and user-friendly webpage for the HMRP would be an important communication tool for all stakeholders as well as a way of preparing for the future with virtual reality and other forms of media that are being developed and gaining audiences as communication media. VA is familiar with designing such webpages for stakeholder information such as the one for the MVP.[7] Information on the webpage could be divided into information useful for the veterans and their descendants, for researchers, and for the general public, yet still remain accessible to all. New research may be highlighted; new procedures or surveys may be announced; basic background information on toxicants and their effects may be explained; and appropriate links to other agencies with additional information, such as ATSDR, could be provided with annotation.

PROGRAM EVALUATION

A well-conducted HMRP would include an iterative evaluation process and guidance from a veterans advisory committee and scientific advisory board to provide important feedback on priorities and evaluation metrics. For example, as the program matures and information is analyzed, it will likely be necessary to adjust the data collection efforts to capture new exposures for veterans and to more closely examine outcomes in descendants. As new sampling techniques and instruments become available for environmental toxicants, it may be advantageous to collect new or different types of information on deployment exposures. As the science of omics advances, it may become easier to identify biomarkers of exposure or biomarkers of effect and susceptibility in both veterans and their descendants. Furthermore, as more information is gathered, it may become evident which exposures and effects are most likely to be associated with each other, and this would allow HMRP leadership to narrow or broaden the scope of the program.

The scope and complexity of the program and the research to be proposed will require repeated feedback from researchers and veterans and their descendants to help modify the HMRP to address new information and processes. Such evaluations should be conducted on a regular basis with a mechanism for communicating with program administrators, researchers, and the public. VA is already familiar with many aspects of program evaluation, particularly those related to improving patient care. Should the need arise, there are other organizations that have developed relevant metrics that may be used by VA and its collaborators in assessing the value of the program to governmental organizations as well

---

[7] See https://www.research.va.gov/MVP/veterans.cfm (accessed February 7, 2018).

as to veterans and their descendants; one example is the *Partnerships for Environmental Public Health Evaluation Metrics Manual* from NIEHS (2012).

To ensure a successful program there will also be a need to regularly assess the efficiency of the HMRP's processes, its methods to recruit and retain participants, and the appropriateness of its data collection efforts. Those challenges and limitations that are identified throughout the process should be used to inform and modify the HMRP. For example, if administrators notice a particularly low participation rate for a certain demographic group, efforts should be made to adjust recruitment efforts in a timely manner.

ETHICAL CONSIDERATIONS

There are important ethical considerations in designing and conducting an investigation on the health of veterans, their partners, children, and grandchildren. Voluntary participation in the HMRP requires developing informed consent procedures as defined in protocols reviewed and approved by the institutional review boards of the lead and collaborating institutions. Such procedures typically follow the ethical principles identified in the Belmont Report of beneficence, justice, and respect (HEW, 1979). VA and DoD have already applied these principles in the MVP, MilCo, and other comparable programs. However, the recruitment, engagement, and participation of the children and grandchildren of veterans will involve unique considerations and challenges. The structuring of such programs could benefit from the procedures developed by other initiatives, such as the NIH National Children's Study and the ECHO and All of Us studies.

While the goal of studying veterans and their partners and descendants is to generate knowledge concerning the health outcomes of these individuals as shaped by the veterans' deployments, additional knowledge may be gathered that can improve personalized medicine and be generalized to the broader U.S. population. It is essential to secure voluntary informed consent from adults who clearly understand their involvement and the risks and benefits associated with participation. Whether and how individual and group results will be returned to them should be apparent to the participants. If results, particularly those for individuals, are to be provided to participants, they should be presented in a manner that promotes the health of the recipient. Providing results to individual participants may be difficult for the proposed HMRP, given the need for proxy consents for studies across multiple generations and the fact that much of the research to be conducted is being developed upon a very limited database that may not allow for a clear explanation of risks and benefits for participants. As such, additional levels of scrutiny will be required to assess the level of risk inherent in any one study developed under the HMRP umbrella as well as the benefits to be derived in the short term and across multiple generations. A key question to be addressed will be how the risks and benefits to participants and their descendants, as determined from the HMRP, will be communicated to them.

The participation of children and grandchildren, especially those who are minors, will require special considerations. Because children are considered uniquely vulnerable research subjects, important decisions will need to be made about what will be studied; whether there will be particular risks inherent in the research that must be shared with the children's parents or guardians; whether the children are old enough to provide oral or written assent themselves; and what results will be shared with parents and clinicians or educators and how they will be shared. The researcher should also consider the intended and unintended consequences of the findings and which options will be made available should negative health outcomes be identified when remediation at this time is not possible. If recontact is not possible, the disposition of any associated data has to be considered with the utmost care. Careful consideration must also be given to the possible perception by authorities that the children of veterans might be treated as a "captive population" with restricted opt-out options. It will also be important in instances when multiple follow-ups are necessary to consider how frequently adults and children are asked to re-consent or re-assent.

The legality of proxy consents for a child in the case of procedures that are not related to the child's need for medical diagnosis or treatment will also be critical factors. Furthermore, the participation of children with preexisting conditions and the options for the return of results along with the choice to receive or not receive certain types of information are but a few of the many ethical considerations that will require careful review and consideration by VA and collaborating organizations. Thus, efforts must be made to develop studies that can be justified for specific populations, with appropriate safeguards and oversight and clear and definable benefits, especially as the children mature and begin to participate in decisions in situations where the risks and benefits to them may not be entirely clear.

When the child is of age to provide assent, the purpose and the procedures of the study should be described to the child in a developmentally appropriate manner. When the child reaches adulthood, he or she may be required to consent to the use of all previous data and samples collected when the child was a minor. This will require a special consenting procedure and the need to retain detailed contact information for recontact. If recontact is not possible, the disposition of any associated data has to be carefully considered. Sponsoring organizations will have to address issues related to inter-institutional variation in human subject procedures, the utility of centralized human subjects protocol review (with a central institutional review board), and alternatives for the completion of face-to-face, mail, telephone, or electronic consenting. Many advances have been made in this regard during the course of the implementation of several large-scale national initiatives by both VA and DoD.

The opportunity for and interest in genetic testing research as part of the proposed HMRP deserves special comment as it presents unique ethical challenges, especially those related to the testing of asymptomatic children, familial identity, incidental findings, variants of unknown significance, and carrier status, to list a few difficult issues. Several authoritative reviews and guidelines are available that can be used to guide efforts (e.g., HEW,1979; NIH, 2018b; WHO, 2011). This can be a particularly sensitive area in situations where the investigation identifies genetic risks for which no clear intervention is available. In the context of investigations conducted over a lifetime and into future generations, the risk-benefit considerations of genetic testing will be influenced by the timing of disease onset and the availability of treatments. Similar issues arise from the collection of stem cells from parents and children and the possible future use of these specimens by participants, their family members, and society at large.

The practice of protecting human participants in research has evolved, and it is expected that ethical practices in human subject research will continue to do so as new adverse events, advanced methodologies, and altered philosophies concerning the protection of human subjects emerge. Clearly, the challenge for policy makers and researchers at VA, DoD, and collaborating organizations will be to develop an HMRP that minimizes risk, provides acceptable risk-benefit ratios to participants, and ensures the engagement of parents and children over time in studies likely to generate valuable findings. In the end, VA and veterans must weigh the risk of conducting and participating in such research against the risk of not seeking answers. Only VA, in consultation with veterans and their descendants, can make this decision.

SUMMARY

Designing, implementing, maintaining, and evaluating a program to conduct research to identify current or possible health effects in veterans' descendants is a substantial task, but many new technologies and methods are available to facilitate such a program, and the committee believes that it is an important undertaking. Understanding the possible generational health effects that may result from

BOX 9-3
Critical Features of and Challenges to an HMRP

- Identifying, recruiting, and retaining a representative cohort of male and female veterans, nonveteran spouses, children, and grandchildren;
- Obtaining and managing informed consent from eligible participants and from minors as they progress toward adulthood;
- Measuring exposures to toxicants and toxicant mixtures during deployment and nondeployment;
- Measuring nonmilitary life exposures to potential toxicants;
- Measuring personal behavior characteristics that may impact outcomes of interest;
- Accurately identifying and characterizing prenatal and natal gestational events and birth defects;
- Extracting deployment and health data from DoD and VA records and health data from other health care providers;
- Periodically collecting standard health measures during military service for veterans and for nonveteran spouses, children, and grandchildren over a period of decades;
- Creating a biorepository that includes blood, urine, semen and oocytes, and other biospecimens;
- Identifying relevant biomarkers and applying them to banked specimens; and
- Securely storing vast amounts of data over decades and performing complex data analyses that include adjustments for multiple modifiers and sources of confounding.

veterans' exposures during deployment begins with determining, to the extent possible, which toxicants they encountered. Newer technologies that can screen thousands of chemicals in biological samples combined with biobanks may provide an important new method for determining the relevant environmental exposures. Furthermore, developments in high-throughput computing and informatics can strengthen such a program's ability to zero in on the most relevant health outcomes. At present, the answers to which environmental exposures and which health outcomes are most related to transgenerational inheritance are largely speculative, but advances in bioassays, computer science, and study design should help in addressing these issues, as long as they are rigorously employed. This information on exposures and outcomes should be complemented with the concurrent collecting of biological samples from service members and veterans. As children are born following their parents' deployment, they too may be monitored during their lifetimes to determine what, if any, health effects they may have compared with children of veterans who were not deployed.

An HMRP with a structured data collection and analysis protocol is an ideal approach for framing research questions that may be addressed by epidemiologic studies. By building on existing health monitoring and epidemiologic research programs such as the DoD MilCo and the VA MVP, and taking advantage of access to databases such as the DoD Serum Repository and the DoD Birth and Infant Health Registry, it should be possible to reduce costs, expedite data collection, and provide access to already-engaged study populations.

An HMRP with epidemiologic studies will require efficient program management and access to a variety of resources. In particular, it will be critical for the program to have sufficient IT capabilities combined with linked medical records from DoD and VA and potentially other participants. With a sustained commitment from governmental and other organizations, the generational health effects that may stem from veterans' exposures experienced while defending their country may be illuminated.

The critical features of any HMRP devoted to veterans and their descendants are described above and listed in Box 9-3. Such a program could feasibly encompass any theater of operation, ranging from humanitarian disaster relief to a direct combat mission. A coordinated health monitoring system is needed to address these important questions. This HMRP will integrate and expand existing and future information across the multiple levels of decision making in order to generate timely and actionable knowledge for individual veterans and their children, VA, DoD, and Congress.

REFERENCES

Accardi, C.J., D. I. Walker, K. Uppal, A.A. Quyyumi, P. Rohrbeck, K.D. Pennell, C. T. Mallon, and D.P. Jones. 2016. High-resolution metabolomics for nutrition and health assessment of Armed Forces personnel. *Journal of Occupational and Environmental Medicine* 58(8 Suppl 1):S80–S88.

Andermann, A., I. Blancquaert, S. Beauchamp, and V. Déry. 2008. Revisiting Wilson and Jungner in the genomic age: A review of screening criteria over the past 40 years. *Bulletin of the World Health Organization* 86(4):241–320.

Andra, S., C. Austin, and M. Arora. 2016. The tooth exposome in children's health research. *Current Opinion in Pediatrics* 28(2):221–227.

Bagalman, E. 2014. *The number of veterans that use VA health care services: A fact sheet.* CRS Report 7-5700. Washington, DC: Congressional Research Service. R43579.

Bellavia, A., and L. Valeri. 2018. Decomposition of the total effect in the presence of multiple mediators and interactions. *American Journal of Epidemiology* 87(6):1311–1318.

Bennett, D.A., D. Landry, D.J. Little, and C. Minelli. 2017. Systematic review of statistical approaches to quantify, or correct for, measurement error in a continuous exposure in nutritional epidemiology. *BMC Medical Research Methodology* 17:146–168.

Billionnet, C., D. Sherrill, I. Annesi-Maesano, and GERIE study. 2012. Estimating the health effects of exposure to multi-pollutant mixture. *Annals of Epidemiology* 22(2):126–141.

Bradburne, C., D. Graham, H.M. Kingston, R. Brenner, M. Pamuku, and L. Carruth. 2015. Overview of 'omics technologies for military occupational health surveillance and medicine. *Military Medicine* 180(10 Suppl):34–48.

Braun, J.M., C. Gennings, R. Hauser, and T.F. Webster. 2016. What can epidemiological studies tell us about the impact of chemical mixtures on human health? *Environmental Health Perspectives* 124(1):A6–A9.

Buka, S., S.R. Rosenthal, and M.E. Lacy. 2018. Epidemiological study designs: Traditional and novel approaches to advance life course health development research. In *Handbook of Life Course Health Development*, edited by N. Halfon, C. Forrest, R.M. Lerner, and E.M. Faustman. 10.1007/978-3-319-47143-3 (accessed July 18, 2018).

Bukowinski, A.T., C. DeScisciolo, A.M.S. Conlin, M.A.K. Ryan, C.J. Sevick, and T.C. Smith. 2012. Birth defects in infants born in 1998–2004 to men and women serving in the U.S. military during the 1990–1991 Gulf War era. *Birth Defects Research (Part A): Clinical and Molecular Teratology* 94:721–728.

Collins, R. 2012. What makes UK Biobank special? *The Lancet* 379:1173–1174.

Conlin, A.M., C. DeScisciolo, C.J. Sevick, A.T. Bukowinski, C.J. Phillpis, and T.C. Smith. 2012. Birth outcomes among military personnel after exposure to documented open air burn pits before and during pregnancy. *Journal of Occupational and Environmental Medicine* 54(6):689–697.

Conlin, A.M., A.T. Bukowinski, C.J. Sevick, C. DeScisciolo, and N.F. Crum-Cianflone. 2013. Safety of the pandemic H1N1 influenza vaccine among pregnant U.S. military women and their newborns. *Obstetrics and Gynecology* 121(3):511–518.

Conlin, A.M.S., A.T. Bukowinski, and G.R. Gumbs. 2015. Analysis of pregnancy and infant health outcomes among women in the National Smallpox Vaccine in Pregnancy Registry who received anthrax vaccine adsorbed. *Vaccine* 33(36):4387–4390.

Conlin, A.M.S., C.J. Sevick, G.R. Gumbs, Z.G. Khodr, and A.T. Bukowinski. 2017. Safety of inadvertent anthrax vaccination during pregnancy: An analysis of birth defects in the U.S. military population, 2003–2010. *Vaccine* 35(34):4414–4420.

DoD (U.S. Department of Defense). 2013. *TRICARE management activity FY 2013 military construction, defense-wide.* Chief, Acquisition and Management Office.

DoD. 2018. *Patients by beneficiary category.* https://www.health.mil/I-Am-A/Media/Media-Center/Patient-Population-Statistics/Patients-by-Beneficiary-Category (accessed June 22, 2018).

Dursa, E.K., S.K. Barth, A.I. Schneiderman, and R.M. Bossarte. 2016. Physical and mental health status of Gulf War and Gulf era veterans. *Journal of Occupational and Environmental Medicine* 58(1):41-46.

Eskenazi, B., K. Harley, A. Bradman, E. Weltzien, N.P. Jewell, D.B. Barr, C.E. Furlong, and N.T. Holland. 2004. Association of in utero organophosphate pesticide exposure and fetal growth and length of gestation in an agricultural population. *Environmental Health Perspectives* 112(10):1116–1124.

GAO (U.S. Government Accountability Office). 2015. *Defense health care: DOD needs to clarify policies related to occupational and environmental health surveillance and monitor risk mitigation activities*. GAO-15-487. Washington, DC: U.S. Government Accountability Office.

Gaziano, J.M., J. Concatoc, M. Brophy, L. Fiore, S. Pyarajana, J. Breeling, S. Whitbourn, J. Deena, C. Shannona, D. Humphries, P. Guarino, M. Aslan, D. Anderson, R. LaFleur, T. Hammond, K. Schaaf, J. Moser, G. Huang, S. Muralidhar, R. Przygodzki, and T.J. O'Leary. 2016. Million Veteran Program: A mega-biobank to study genetic influences on health and disease. *Journal of Clinical Epidemiology* 70:214–223.

Hajian-Tilaki, K. 2011. Sample size estimation in epidemiologic studies. *Caspian Journal of Internal Medicine* 2(4):289–298.

Hamra, G.B., and J.P. Buckley. 2018. Environmental exposure mixtures: Questions and methods to address them. *Current Epidemiology Reports*. https://doi.org/10.1007/s40471-018-0145-0 (accessed August 5, 2018).

Hebbring, S.J. 2014. The challenges, advantages and future of phenome-wide association studies. *Immunology* 141(2):157–165.

Hernan, M.A., and J.M. Robins. 2018. *Causal inference*. https://www.hsph.harvard.edu/miguel-hernan/ causal-inference-book (accessed July 27, 2018).

HEW (U.S. Department of Health, Education, and Welfare). 1979. *The Belmont report: Ethical principles and guidelines for the protection of human subjects of research*. Washington, DC: Office of the Secretary, The National Commission for the Protection of Human Subjects of Biomedical and Behavioral Research. April 18.

Huang, G., S. Kim, J. Gasper, Y. Xu, T. Bosworth, and L. May. 2017. *2016 survey of veteran enrollees' health and use of health care: Main results report*. Prepared for the Department of Veterans Affairs. Rockville, MD: Westat.

IOM (Institute of Medicine). 2008. *Epidemiologic studies of veterans exposed to depleted uranium*. Washington, DC: The National Academies Press.

IOM. 2010. *Gulf War and health, volume 8: Update of health effects of serving in the Gulf War*. Washington, DC: The National Academies Press.

IOM (Institute of Medicine). 2011. *Long-term health consequences of exposure to burn pits in Iraq and Afghanistan*. Washington, DC: The National Academies Press.

Janulewicz, P.A., R.F. White, M.R. Winter, J.M. Weinberg, L.E. Gallagher, V. Vieira, T.F. Webster, and A. Aschengrau. 2008. Risk of learning and behavioral disorders following prenatal and early postnatal exposure to tetrachloroethylene (PCE)-contaminated drinking water. *Neurotoxicology and Teratology* 30(3):175–185.

Keogh, R.H., and I.R. White. 2014. A toolkit for measurement error correction, with a focus on nutritional epidemiology. *Statistics in Medicine* 33(12):2137–2155.

Lenth, R.V. 2001. Some practical guidelines for effective sample size determination. *The American Statistician* 55:187–193.

Liu, A., E.F. Schistermann, M. Mazumdar, and J. Hu. 2005. Power and sample size calculation of comparative diagnostic accuracy studies with multiple correlated test results. *Biometrical Journal* 47(2):140–150.

Liu, K.H., D.I. Walker, K. Uppal, V. Tran, P. Rohrbeck, T.M. Mallon, and D.P. Jones. 2016. High-resolution metabolomics assessment of military personnel: Evaluating analytical strategies for chemical detection. *Journal of Occupational and Environmental Medicine* 58(8 Suppl 1):S53–S61.

Lushniak, B., T.M. Mallon, J.C. Gaydos, and D.J. Smith. 2016. Utility of the Department of Defense Serum Repository in assessing deployment exposure. *Journal of Occupational and Environmental Medicine* 58(8S):S1–S2.

McDiarmid, M.A. 2015. Biologic monitoring and surveillance results for the Department of Veterans Affairs' depleted uranium cohort: Lessons learned from sustained exposure over two decades. *American Journal of Industrial Medicine* 58:583–594.

Mumford, S.L., E.F. Schisterman, A. Vexler, and A. Liu. 2006. Pooling biospecimens and limits of detection: Effects on ROC curve analysis. *Biostatistics* 7(4):585–598.

NARA (U.S. National Archives and Records Administration). 2015. *National Collaborative Perinatal Project, 1959-1974*. https://www.archives.gov/research/electronic-records/nih.html (accessed September 17, 2018).

NASEM (National Academies of Sciences, Engineering, and Medicine). 2016. *Gulf War and health, volume 10: Update of health effects of serving in the Gulf War, 2016*. Washington, DC: The National Academies Press.

NASEM. 2017. *Assessment of the Department of Veterans Affairs Airborne Hazards and Open Burn Pit Registry*. Washington, DC: The National Academies Press.

NHRC (Naval Health Research Center). 2017. *Research and development focus areas*. https://www.med.navy.mil/sites/nhrc/Pages/Research-and-Development-Focus-Areas.aspx?Category=MILITARY-RANDDFOCUS (accessed June 4, 2018).

NIEHS (National Institute of Environmental Health Sciences). 2012. *Partnerships for environmental public health evaluation metrics manual*. NIH Publication No. 12-7825. Research Triangle Park, NC: National Institute of Environmental Health Sciences.

NIEHS. 2018. *Children's Health Exposure Analysis Resource (CHEAR)*. www.niehs.nih.gov/research/supported/exposure/chear/index.cfm (accessed June 29, 2018).

NIH (National Institutes of Health). 2018a. *NIH security best practices for controlled-access data subject to the NIH genomic data sharing (GDS) policy*. https://osp.od.nih.gov/wp-content/uploads/ NIH_Best_Practices_for_Controlled-access_Data_Subject_to_the_NIH_GDS_Policy.pdf (accessed June 22, 2018).

NIH. 2018b. *NIH human subjects policies and guidance*. https://humansubjects.nih.gov/nih-human-subjects-policies-guidance (accessed July 22, 2018).

NRC (National Research Council). 2000. *Strategies to protect the health of deployed U.S. forces: Analytical framework for assessing risks*. Washington, DC: The National Academies Press.

Pearl, J., M. Glymour, and N. Jewell. 2016. *Causal inference in statistics: A primer*. Chichester, UK: Wiley.

Rosenbaum, P.R., and D.B. Rubin. 1984. Reducing bias in observational studies using subclassification on the propensity score. *Journal of the American Statistical Association* 79(387):516–524.

Ryan, M., M. Pershyn-Kisor, W. Honner, T. Smith, R. Reed, and G. Gray. 2001. The Department of Defense Birth Defects Registry: Overview of a new surveillance system. *Teratology* 64:S26–S29.

Saha-Chaudhuri, P., and C.R. Weinberg. 2013. Specimen pooling for efficient use of biospecimens in studies of time to a common event. *American Journal of Epidemiology* 178(1):126–135.

Schisterman, E., and A. Vexler. 2008. To pool or not to pool, from whether to when: Applications of pooling to biospecimens subject to a limit of detection. *Paediatric and Perinatal Epidemiology* 22:486–496.

Smith, T. 2009. The US Department of Defense Millennium Cohort Study: Career span and beyond longitudinal follow-up. *Journal of Occupational and Environmental Medicine* 51(10):1193–1201.

Stingone, J.A., K.H. McVeigh, and L. Claudio. 2016. Association between prenatal exposure to ambient diesel particulate matter and perchloroethylene with children's 3rd grade standardized test scores. *Environmental Research* 148:144–153.

Styka, A. N., and D. A. Butler. 2015. The Air Force Health Study Data and Specimens as a Resource for Researchers. *Military Medicine* 180(10 Suppl):79–84.

Taguri, M., J. Featherstone, and J. Cheng. 2018. Causal mediation analysis with multiple causally non-ordered mediators. *Statistical Methods in Medical Research* 27(1):3–19.

Ten Have, T.R., and M.M. Joffe. 2012. A review of causal estimation of effects in mediation analyses. *Statistical Methods in Medical Research* 21(1):77–107.

Toledano, M.B., R.B. Smith, J.P. Brook, M. Douglass, P. Elliott. 2015. How to establish and follow up a large prospective cohort study in the 21st Century—Lessons from UK COSMOS. *PLOS ONE* 10(7): e0131521.

VA (U.S. Department of Veterans Affairs). 2016. *Health study of Gulf War era veterans*. https://www.publichealth.va.gov/epidemiology/ studies/gulf-war-longitudinal-study.asp (accessed September 11, 2018).

VA. 2017a. *VE-HEROeS: Studying the Health of Vietnam Veterans*. https://www.publichealth.va.gov/exposures/publications/agent-orange/agent-orange-summer-2016/ve-heroes.asp (accessed August 30, 2018).

VA. 2017b. *VA Utilization Profile FY 2016*. National Center for Veterans Analysis and Statistics. https://www.va.gov/vetdata/docs/QuickFacts/VA_Utilization_Profile.pdf (accessed September 7, 2018).

VA. 2017c. *Million Veteran Program*. https://www.research.va.gov/MVP (accessed September 19, 2018).

VA. 2018a. https://www.va.gov/HEALTHBENEFITS/apply/veterans.asp (accessed September 14, 2018).

VA. 2018b. *Health Study for a new generation of U.S. veterans*. https://www.publichealth.va.gov/epidemiology/studies/new-generation/index.asp (accessed September 11, 2018).

VanderWeele, T.J. 2016. Mediation analysis: A practitioner's guide. *Annual Reviews in Public Health* 37:17–32.

Walker, D. I., T. Mallon, P.K. Hopke, K. Uppal, K.Y.-M. Go, P. Rohrbeck, K.D. Pennell, and D.P. Jones. 2016. Deployment-associated exposure surveillance with high-resolution metabolomics. *Journal of Occupational and Environmental Medicine* 58(8):S12–S21.

Wang, M., A. Cyhaniuk, D.L. Cooper, and N.N. Iyer. 2017. Identification of patients with congenital hemophilia in a large electronic health record database. *Journal of Blood Medicine* 8:131–139.

Westat. 2010. *National Survey of Veterans, Active Duty Service Members, Demobilized National Guard and Reserve Members, Family Members, and Surviving Spouses. Final report*. Deliverable 27. Prepared for the U.S. Department of Veterans Affairs. Rockville, MD: Westat.

WHO (World Health Organization). 2011. Standards and operational guidance for ethics review of health-related research with human participants. Geneva, Switzerland: World Health Organization.

WHO. 2018. *Epidemiology*. http://www.who.int/topics/epidemiology/en (accessed June 4, 2018).

10

Pathophysiologic Research

The study of generational health effects is a complex, evolving, and fast-paced area of research. Understanding the heritability of the health effects that may result from environmental exposures, particularly those that may occur in a war zone, requires a holistic approach involving multiple avenues of research to address data gaps and expand our knowledge of the mechanisms of inheritance that may affect future generations. The Volume 11 committee believes that to assess the potential long-term generational health effects of deployment exposures, a range of basic research using animal and cellular or mechanistic models will be necessary to complement the health monitoring plan and epidemiologic studies discussed in Chapter 9, thus encompassing a state of the science transgenerational study. This basic and translational research can help elucidate the genetic and epigenetic mechanisms that may be responsible for generational health effects in humans.

The Volume 11 committee recognizes that many of the research efforts described in this chapter cannot be undertaken by a single organization. The required competencies will be spread across numerous organizations, from governmental organizations to academic institutions and private entities. Whenever appropriate, the opportunities for collaboration and coordination across organizations should be explored and embraced. Two collaborations are exploring children's health or the epigenetic markers of exposure. One is the National Institute of Environmental Health Sciences' (NIEHS's) Children's Health Exposure Analysis Resource (CHEAR), an "extramural research community access to laboratory and data analyses that add or expand the inclusion of environmental exposures in children's health research" (NIEHS, 2018). The second is the Toxicant Exposures and Responses by Genomic and Epigenomic Regulators of Transcription (TaRGET) II Program, sponsored by NIEHS, that seeks to explore changes in "epigenomic marks across target tissues/cells (those adversely affected by environmental exposures) and surrogate tissues/cells (those that are easily accessible and reflect the environmental exposures) using mouse models of environmentally relevant exposures" (Wang et al., 2018). Other consortia that are working to understand the human epigenome include the National Institutes of Health Roadmap Epigenomics Mapping Consortium that aims to develop a "public resource of human epigenomic data to catalyze basic biology and disease-oriented research" and that has mapped the epigenomes of more than 100 types of cells and tissues (NIH, 2018), and the International Human Epigenome Consortium that has a goal of understanding "the extent to which the epigenome has shaped human populations over generations and in response to the environment" (IHEC, 2018). The Department of Veterans Affairs, the Department of Defense, the National Institutes of Health, and other government agencies are part of the Armed Forces Institute of Regenerative Medicine (AFIRM) network which is seeking to develop advanced treatment options for severely wounded service members using an interdisciplinary, multi-institution approach (MRMC, 2018). These and other such consortia and networks provide examples of mechanisms for taking advantage of new and existing research resources.

This chapter outlines some of the data and knowledge gaps of the molecular, biochemical, cell, and tissue basis for generational effects. It also identifies mechanistic (including in vitro models using human tissues) studies in animal models of human health outcomes that might help to fill data gaps and improve our understanding of how deployment exposures affect the health of veterans and their descendants.

UTILITY OF ANIMAL STUDIES

During its review of the epidemiologic and animal toxicology literature described in Chapters 4 through 7, the Volume 11 committee identified research on generational health effects from exposures that are potentially relevant to Gulf War and Post-9/11 veterans, such as organophosphate pesticides. The committee also observed many data gaps in the research on the effects of the veterans' exposures on their children, with even less known about effects on grandchildren. As was shown in Chapter 8, determining whether a veteran's exposure to a toxicant causes health effects in his or her descendants is a complex problem. Researchers are beginning to search for human generational health effects and to devise the lengthy and costly epidemiologic studies needed to properly detect this phenomenon. Although targeted studies are being designed, it may be years or even decades before the effects (if any) of parental exposures become evident in a subsequent generation. Furthermore, health monitoring programs and epidemiologic studies may not capture rare events that occur in only a few descendants, that result from a narrow range of exposures (e.g., at very high or low doses), or that occur only in those instances where specific genetic profiles interact with specific exposures. To address these and the many other complexities inherent to human studies, medical researchers can turn to basic research to provide critical information on the heritability of the health effects of parental exposures across generations and the genetic and epigenetic mechanisms that may be involved.

Studies in model systems—in vitro systems that use cells and tissues as well as whole animals—where both genetics and exposures can be controlled, and generational animal studies that can be conducted in days or months rather than in the years and decades required for human studies, are powerful research approaches that can complement and inform human studies. Such studies may detect subtle effects and can follow genetic or epigenetic changes at the molecular, cellular, and whole-animal levels, including effects on germ cells.

No individual study in a model system is adequate to identify or define human risk; such studies must be complemented by an understanding of the similarities and differences between species in their biology and their responses to a toxicant. Furthermore, the results of health effects studies in model organisms must be extrapolated to humans if they are to be used to enhance our understanding of the reproductive, developmental, or generational effects of toxicant exposures across the exposure → effect → outcome continuum. Understanding the range of biological diversity across species can help with this extrapolation. For example, it has been shown that the gene for the aryl hydrocarbon receptor that mediates dioxin toxicity exhibits differences in sensitivity between mouse strains, between rats and mice, and between the model species and humans. Understanding these differences makes it possible to estimate human risk from rodent studies. For example, in its assessment of dioxins, the U.S. Environmental

Protection Agency (EPA) stated that "animal data show a wide range of species sensitivity to dioxin for a given developmental or reproductive endpoint" (EPA, 2012). For some endpoints, data show that human sensitivity is comparable to that of experimental animals (e.g., semen morphology), but for other endpoints, humans are insensitive compared to other species (e.g., cleft palate) (EPA, 2012). Although mice and rats are the most commonly used species, there can be differences in the response among different species and strain of these model animals. For example, Fischer 344 and Wistar rats exposed to trichloroethylene during gestation had an increased risk of decreased fetal weight, live birth weights, and postnatal growth, but Sprague Dawley rats did not (EPA, 2011). More expedient organism models, such as fruit flies, round worms, and zebra fish, are more easily used to examine system- or organism-wide effects and potential target tissues of effect, but they may not fully mirror the effects in humans.

LIFECOURSE EXPOSURES

To help distinguish between the effects of specific deployment exposures and the effects of other lifecourse exposures on veterans and their descendants, it is necessary to develop a better understanding of how the exposures and their timing (e.g., the age of exposed individuals or pregnancy status) affect an individual's genome and the epigenome (see Figure 9-1). Other questions include how such genetic and epigenetic alterations are inherited through the germ line and how exposure-related adverse health outcomes are defined and identified in subsequent generations. It is in these areas where basic research may be most valuable, as it provides a unique opportunity to uncover the targets and mechanisms of action and to link exposures to adverse outcomes in a causal way. Model organisms are well suited for conducting studies of toxicants across multiple generations because investigators are able to carefully control for other variables, such as diet, that can also influence effects.

Thus, the Volume 11 committee gives high priority to a basic research program that examines all aspects of the exposure → effect → outcome continuum and, where possible, that does so in an integrative manner. This research might begin with identifying targets and mechanisms in order to identify biomarkers of exposure and effect for a toxicant; exploring factors that underlie individual variation in response to exposures, such as the impact of sex differences on response to a toxicant; and identifying which cell types (e.g., somatic cells, eggs, sperm) are most susceptible to specific exposures. This research should also include developing the following: fit-for-purpose models and reagents for generational studies; genetically engineered induced pluripotent stem cells (iPSCs); validated models (both animal- and cell-based) that are most appropriate for studying specific exposures; and methods and databases for acquiring, curating, and analyzing the resulting datasets. Each of these areas for basic research on lifecourse exposures is described below.

- **Biomarkers** The identification, development, and validation of biomarkers of exposure, effect, and susceptibility, including "omics" biomarkers (RNA, DNA, proteins, metabolites, and lipids). Foundational work for such biomarker studies will also be needed and may include studies to explore how a particular agent may affect the genome/epigenome and manifest as adverse health effects in descendants. Studies using human materials (e.g., urine), animal models (mammalian and nonmammalian animals such as mice and *Caenorhabditis elegans*, respectively), and appropriate cell-based (e.g., iPSCs) systems would all reasonably be expected to contribute to the development of biomarkers of exposure and to our mechanistic understanding of multigenerational inheritance and of adverse reproductive and developmental health effects.

  The derivation of an individual cell type from a person's own iPSCs would enable a direct personalized assessment of changes to that person's genome. At the time of a person's enlistment into the military or prior to deployment, iPSCs could be collected from tissue biopsies (e.g., skin, bone marrow, or adipose tissue), and stored for later analysis (Ohnishi et al. 2012). When required, cells could be differentiated—for example, into the particular cell type that is affected in the individual being examined—and then tested directly. The use of iPSC makes it possible to model an individual's response to a toxicant, with the advantage of directly testing the effect of exposure on a cell type and having a specific genotypic response for that individual. Reducing this process to routine practice and automating it would require substantial development, but it would provide personnel with baseline genomic information upon which an effect could be tested or confirmed.

- **Target cells** Understanding which cells and organs are vulnerable to specific exposures, how cell type influences genetic/epigenetic changes induced by specific exposures (i.e., which cells and tissues are at risk), and which tissues and organs exhibit an alteration linked to adverse health outcomes in descendants. Studies in this area might focus on the timing of the epigenetic programming of gametes to determine windows of susceptibility for generational effects; fundamental molecular and cell-based studies to elucidate the mechanisms underlying epigenetic reprogramming or other pathways for generational inheritance; studies of the combined effects of stress or heat exposure with specific toxicants or mixtures of toxicants or deployment-related mixtures; and studies using surrogate tissues such as blood, saliva, urine, or sperm to inform the exposures, mechanisms, and outcomes in target tissues and organs. Research efforts in this area should coordinate with and be informed by ongoing studies being conducted by the TaRGET consortium and the other consortia working on mapping the human epigenome.
- **Data analysis and experimental design** Development of best practices for designing robust generational studies across the exposure → effect → outcome continuum, including analysis of complex data sets generated by high-content omics technologies (e.g., the ENCODE consortium[1]) and those derived from observational studies in humans, which must include consideration of their many potential confounding variables. Within the context of assessing lifecourse exposures, confounders may include the following: single exposures to mixtures of toxicants, other exposures experienced by individuals over their lifecourse (e.g., occupational, recreational), potential lack of specificity in biomarkers used to measure specific exposures, and a potential inability to link the biomarker to an adverse health outcome in either the exposed parent or the child. Accounting for these confounders can best be accomplished with robust analytical tools. With the help of such tools, the joint influences of these variables can be identified and parsed so as to clarify the influence of the variable of interest. These new methods include neuronal nets, machine learning, and artificial intelligence to develop and validate statistical methodology and software—as well as platforms, pipelines, and databases—to analyze and substantiate the data. The computational studies that follow will inform and ensure reproducibility of studies designed to address these knowledge gaps.
- **Sex-specificity** The identification of—and discovery of the mechanisms responsible for—sex-specific differences in sensitivity to specific exposures, in effects on the genome and epigenome, and in adverse health outcomes on reproduction and in descendants. Studies that would be considered responsive to these research needs could include, for example, a comparison of the

[1] ENCODE (the Encyclopedia of DNA Elements) is a program supported by the National Human Genome Research Institute to identify and characterize all functional elements of the human genome and to support the development of new technologies for high-throughput data (https://www.genome.gov/10005107/the-encode-project-encyclopedia-of-dna-elements; accessed June 13, 2018).

effects of an exposure on male versus female germ lines and the use of sex-specific iPSCs to uncover germ-cell determinants of susceptibility and generational inheritance.

DATA GAPS TO BE ADDRESSED

Chapters 4 through 7 described the evidence for the reproductive and developmental effects of deployment-related exposures that could occur in veterans or their offspring. Because there were so few studies in veterans themselves and virtually no new studies of their children, the Volume 11 committee considered other studies of humans exposed to the agents of concern, such as occupational and residential cohorts. Summary data presented in Tables 8-1 and 8-2 show that for the majority of agents of concern, there is inadequate/insufficient evidence linking exposures to reproductive or developmental effects or establishing the absence of such a linkage. Therefore, more data are needed to make casual inferences linking exposures to adverse outcomes. Responsive studies should focus on deployment-specific exposures (single-agent or mixtures), although reproductive or multigenerational studies using surrogate exposures may be adequate if they sufficiently address the research needs identified in this report. The knowledge gaps related to the adverse reproductive effects in veterans and developmental effects in offspring of these exposures include the following:

- **Windows of susceptibility** It is understood that exposures across the lifecourse have the potential to cause adverse health effects in exposed individuals. What is less clear is whether exposures at certain times during an individual's life are more able to affect subsequent generations than exposures at other times. Thus, research is needed to identify the times at which exposures have the greatest potential to affect subsequent generations. A related issue is whether the effects of exposures differ between men and women. Because germ-cell maturation differs between the male and female germ line, it is possible that exposures during deployment will affect generational inheritance differently for men and women. Male veterans whose partners conceive will potentially have preconception exposures, whereas female veterans may have preconception exposures or exposures during early pregnancy (i.e., the first trimester, as it is unlikely that female veterans would have deployment exposures later in pregnancy) or both. Thus, it is important to delineate those times during the lifecourse when there is susceptibility to specific exposures and whether those times correspond to windows of susceptibility for modifying the genome/epigenome in a way that will affect the next generation and possibly the generations after that. Unlike human epidemiologic studies, basic research in animal models provides an accessible model for precisely identifying the windows of susceptibility. However, caution must be exercised when designing the experiments and interpreting the results because the reproductive and developmental cycles in different species do not have a one-to-one correspondence with human reproductive and developmental cycles. Thus, it is critical to select the animal model and the timing of the exposure to reflect the reproductive or developmental effects of concern. Research into which effects or mechanisms define these windows of susceptibility will also be important.
- **Dose–response** Although there are few measurements of deployment exposures from Vietnam, the Gulf War, or even the Post-9/11 conflicts, dose–response studies can help identify effects that may result from a range of exposures. The studies can also help elucidate information on how the agent is metabolized in the body. For agents that bioaccumulate, such as dioxins that accumulate in adipose tissue, determining exposure may not be a straightforward measurement.

The half-life of an agent in the body is also important. Agents that are metabolized quickly, such as organophosphate pesticides, may be difficult to detect in the body or in urine after the exposure ceases, making biomarkers of exposure elusive. Such difficulties are compounded when studying the internal dose to a fetus or germ cells.

- **Acute versus chronic exposures** The length, location, duties, and number of deployments that a veteran experienced will vary depending on the veteran's service branch, military occupation specialty, particular war zone (e.g., Vietnam, Gulf War, Post-9/11), and mission. Some exposures may be acute (e.g., a 1-day exposure to sarin from the demolition of the Khamisiyah munitions depot), others may be chronic (e.g., occupational exposures, such as fueling vehicles or cleaning equipment with solvent), and others may be intermittent (such as exposures to the black smoke from the burn pit at Joint Base Balad). At this time, the environmental measurements of the agents of concern during each deployment are minimal. Animal studies will be particularly helpful in determining the possible long-term reproductive and generational effects from acute versus chronic and intermittent exposures, as data for human exposures are, for the most part, not available. These limitations were evident in much of the epidemiology and basic research cited in Chapters 4 through 7.
- **Mixtures** How exposures to mixtures—mixtures of chemicals as well as co-exposures to chemicals and other environmental factors, including stress—affect reproductive and generational outcomes is another important knowledge gap. As described in Chapter 2 under Committee's Approach, identifying mixtures and their variations is a significant data gap for distinguishing the effects of deployment exposure from lifecourse exposures in both veterans and their descendants. Many deployment exposures are mixtures, such as the smoke from burn pits, and these exposures may be compounded by frequent exposures to other mixtures such as pesticides in and around living quarters, or to individual toxicants such as pyridostigmine bromide. Although they are not specific to reproductive or developmental effects, animal studies have attempted to replicate deployment exposures to mixtures, such as to a combination of permethrin, DEET, and pyridostigmine bromide, in an effort to produce the symptoms of Gulf War illness. Numerous organizations have active programs that seek to understand how best to assess the toxic effects of mixtures. However, the bulk of the research on mixtures has focused on effects in the exposed individual with little information on inter- or transgenerational effects. While progress is being made in this area, much work remains to be done.

EFFECTS OF GENETIC AND EPIGENETIC ALTERATIONS ON DESCENDANTS

Both genetic and epigenetic alterations induced by environmental exposures can cause changes that result in reproductive, developmental, or generational effects. Although a few of the toxicants considered in this report are known to be reproductive or developmental toxicants or mutagens (e.g., benzene), for none of them is there strong evidence that they affect germ cells and cause developmental effects in offspring when one parent or the other was exposed to the toxicant prior to conception (see Tables 8-1 and 8-2). What effects occur in parental germ cells, what happens after the exposure ceases, and whether and how lifecourse events compound epigenetic alterations are some of the knowledge gaps related to the nature of these alterations, as discussed below.

- **Heritable transmission** A critical knowledge gap continues to be the nature of the heritable factor (e.g., DNA, histone modifications, RNA) that is perturbed by specific exposures and responsible for generational transmission. The types of studies that can address this knowledge gap include mechanistic studies using cell-based models or human tissues (e.g., blood, semen, saliva, and urine) or multigenerational animal model studies to understand how deployment-related exposures affect DNA, histone modifications, and RNA. Other important studies are genetic/epigenetic studies using comprehensive, unbiased next-generation approaches with state-of-the-art techniques for genomic, epigenomic, chromatin conformation, and transcriptional profiling as well as proteomic and other omics technologies. Studies in model organisms on the early detection and reversibility of exposure-related epigenetic alterations and adverse health outcomes should also be encouraged, as such interventions would be very valuable if they could be developed and applied to humans to mitigate or prevent the adverse outcomes associated with deployment-related exposures.

- **Persistence** The committee uses the term "persistence" to refer to how long effects are maintained after the discontinuation of exposure. Alterations that remain after the exposure ceases can occur in germ cells or somatic cells in other target tissues and can result in an adverse phenotype across generations. There is a need to identify persistent alterations that are relevant (i.e., casually linked) to the generational inheritance of effects. In the case of human studies, it will be important to collect baseline or background biological samples from veterans (e.g., semen) to make sure that such alterations were not present before the exposure.
- **Gene *x* environment (G*x*E) interactions** In ways both subtle and obvious, the response to environmental exposures is determined not only by the nature of the exposure itself but also by the genetics and epigenetics of the exposed individuals—what is often termed gene *x* environment interactions. Similar interactions also occur at the level of the epigenome (epigenome *x* environment; E*x*E interactions), as allele specificity and DNA polymorphisms can modulate the vulnerability of neighboring epigenetic marks to deployment-related exposures. It will be important to undertake both G*x*E and E*x*E studies in order to understand how these interactions influence generational inheritance and also to carry out specific studies aimed at providing actionable information, including the identification of P450 and other genetic polymorphisms that modulate the risks to specific exposures and generational inheritance by altering chemical metabolism.
- **Modifiers** The impact of modifiers such as stress, obesity, drugs, or diet on the type or persistence of genetic and epigenetic changes. For example, it is important to understand the role that modifiers such as stress or the immune system's response to vaccines and novel antigens play in shaping responses to deployment exposures. This should be considered as a function of age-related methylation that is known to represent developmentally programmed changes that occur throughout the genome and the accumulation of random changes as the epigenome drifts. Epigenetic drift, the gradual change away from baseline, reflects the fidelity of maintaining the epigenetic marks (Issa, 2014). Together, the age-related methylation and accumulation of random changes constitute environmental deflection that can alter the physiological outcome of the other G*x*E modifiers (Kochmanski et al., 2017).

INTER- AND TRANSGENERATIONAL HEALTH EFFECTS

As summarized in Chapter 8, the reproductive and developmental health outcomes that may be associated with parental deployment exposures include the following:

- behavioral and neurological dysfunction in offspring associated with maternal exposure to organophosphate pesticides;

- birth defects associated with maternal exposure to polycyclic aromatic hydrocarbons and glycol ethers;
- persistent respiratory diseases such as asthma associated with maternal exposure to particulate matter (PM);
- childhood leukemia associated with parental exposure to benzene; and
- adverse reproductive and pregnancy outcomes (not limited to infertility) associated with several of the agents of concern, including hexavalent chromium, PM, several pesticides, and glycols and glycol ethers.

Chapter 8 also identified several toxicants—for example, depleted uranium, solvents, and lindane—for which the animal data showed reproductive or developmental effects but few data existed to support similar findings in humans. While there is a growing human and animal evidence base on the reproductive and developmental effects of many of the toxicants of concern to exposed men and women and their children, there is still relatively little information on the specific effects of veterans' exposures on their children, grandchildren, and great-grandchildren. Animal models will be particularly useful to begin to address these knowledge gaps. They can provide information on the biological plausibility of deployment-related health outcomes and insights into the mechanisms that underlie such effects through several different types of studies.

- **Transgenerational studies in animal models** Generational studies that focus on meiotic inheritance will need to be done on the various exposures of concerns, and they will need to assess the impact of the generational inheritance variables discussed above (e.g., persistence, G*x*E interactions). Conducting multigenerational studies in animals poses a number of challenges. The typical generational animal studies required by regulatory agencies to protect human health expose animals to a toxicant throughout the entire study period, and each generation is exposed. These studies are not particularly helpful for trying to determine the types of generational effects that might manifest in offspring following parental exposure during deployment. In such cases typically the father would have been exposed before the conception of the child, or the mother would have been exposed before conception or during the early prenatal period, or perhaps both. Generational animal studies should look at parental exposure (and gestational exposure of the offspring), but the effects should also be studied across multiple generations, at least to the F2 (for paternal exposures) and F3 (for maternal exposures) generation, in order to study potential transgenerational effects among offspring which would have not had any exposure to the agent (see Figure 3-2 in Chapter 3).

  It is also essential in animal studies to take sex into account as a biological variable for both parental exposures and offspring effects. Therefore, mechanistic studies on multigenerational inheritance should focus on toxicant exposures (preconceptional or affecting the parental or offspring germ cells) that yield a reproducible phenotype in the offspring or subsequent generations, coupled with an examination of alterations associated with these exposures in germ cells or in the offspring (or both) or modifications caused by the surrounding environment (i.e., lifecourse exposures).

  Importantly, epigenetic alterations induced by environmental exposures may be further modified postexposure (e.g., erased or altered by subsequent environmental exposures), and often the adverse effects of these perturbations are only revealed in response to later life environmental exposures (Walker and Ho, 2012). For example, early life exposures to exogenous estrogens cause reprogramming of the prostate epigenome. In the case of androgen-responsive genes that are reprogrammed, the effect of epigenetic changes induced by early life exogenous estrogen exposure is seen only when the reprogrammed animals are exposed to exogenous androgen later in life. In these animals, the reprogrammed androgen-responsive genes exhibit an exaggerated response to testosterone, becoming more highly expressed than those in control animals and promoting the development of prostate tumors (Wang et al. 2016). This makes clear the potential for the post-deployment environment to influence whether future generations exhibit an adverse health effect that is related to parental deployment exposures and, importantly, the possibility that adverse health effects could "skip" a generation if lifetime exposures do not act to reveal those effects. Accordingly, animal studies that examine the effects of the postexposure environment (e.g., lifestyle, diet, drugs, occupational exposures) on epigenetic reprogramming and multigenerational inheritance should be encouraged.

Also of importance is the sex-specificity of epigenetic reprogramming by environmental exposures and also of multigenerational inheritance. Elucidating the role of sex will require studies on how both maternal and paternal lineages are affected by environmental exposures, how subsequent genetic and epigenetic alterations can be passed through the germ line, and whether both male and female offspring are affected by the alterations. For example, males may be at a greater risk of neurological deficits than females following prenatal exposure to certain organophosphate pesticides (Furlong et al., 2017).

- **Impact on reproductive function** Examples of studies to address how deployment-related exposures may affect reproductive outcomes include studies of toxicant effects on sexual performance, research on ovulatory cycles and parturition, and the screening of semen samples beyond fertility measures to identify potential markers of reproductive and generational effects. Other studies might explore the disease processes for polycystic ovary syndrome, endometriosis, and sexual dysfunction.
- **Identification of adverse phenotypes** Little is known regarding how a deployment-related exposure would manifest as a generationally heritable adverse phenotype. Knowledge gaps include whether there is a correlation between exposure-related adult effects and manifestations in subsequent generations and whether the adverse effects seen in the offspring of exposed veterans are indeed caused by specific deployment-related exposures. Thus, there is a pressing need for identifying robust phenotypes for use in tracking multi- and transgenerational effects, both to facilitate model organism studies and for translation to humans. Such phenotypic assessments would also be key for obtaining evidence of persistent epigenetic alterations of gametes that are linked to adverse outcomes in offspring.

SUMMARY

There are many data and knowledge gaps preventing a clearer understanding of how deployment exposures can affect children or descendants that can be addressed by basic research. In some cases it may be advantageous to conduct animal and mechanistic research rather than epidemiologic studies or a health monitoring program, given the ethical, time, and resource constraints inherent in human research. However, an expanded understanding of how deployment exposures can affect the health of veteran's children or other descendants will require an integrated approach informed by health monitoring, epidemiological studies, and basic research. The committee strongly believes that such an understanding will be facilitated by consistent and multifaceted collaborations among a variety of research institutions, both governmental and nongovernmental, that seek to improve the health of veterans and their descendants.

REFERENCES

EPA (U.S. Environmental Protection Agency). 2011. *Toxicological review of trichloroethylene*. Washington, DC: U.S. Environmental Protection Agency.

EPA. 2012. *EPA's reanalysis of key issues related to dioxin toxicity and response to NAS comments, volume 1*. EPA/600/R-10/038F. Washington, DC: U.S. Environmental Protection Agency.

Furlong, M.A., A. Herring, J. P. Buckley, B.D. Goldman, J.L. Daniels, L.S. Engel, M.S. Wolff, J. Chen, J. Wetmur, and D.B. Barr. 2017. Prenatal exposure to organophosphorus pesticides and childhood neurodevelopmental phenotypes. *Environmental Research* 158:737–747.

IHEC (International Human Epigenome Consortium). 2018. http://ihec-epigenomes.org (accessed September 6, 2018).

Issa, J.-P. 2014. Aging and epigenetic drift: A vicious cycle. *The Journal of Clinical Investigation* 124(1):24–29.

Kochmanski, J., L. Montrose, J.M. Goodrich, and D.C. Dolinoy. 2017. Environmental Deflection: The Impact of Toxicant Exposures on the aging epigenome. *Toxicological Sciences* 156(2):325–335.

MRMC (U.S. Army Medical Research and Materiel Command). 2018. *What is the Armed Forces Institute of Regenerative Medicine?* www.afirm.mil (accessed June 21, 2018).

NIEHS (National Institute of Environmental Health Sciences). 2018. *Children's Health Exposure Analysis Resource (CHEAR)*. www.niehs.nih.gov/research/supported/exposure/chear/index.cfm (accessed June 21, 2018).

NIH (National Institutes of Health). 2018. *NIH Roadmap Epigenomics Mapping Consortium*. http://www.roadmapepigenomics.org (accessed September 6, 2018).

Ohnishi, H., Y. Oda, T. Aoki, M. Tadokoro, Y. Katsube, H. Ohgushi, K. Hattori, and S. Yuba. 2012. A comparative study of induced pluripotent stem cells generated from frozen, stocked bone marrow- and adipose tissue-derived mesenchymal stem cells. *Journal of Tissue Engineering and Regenerative Medicine* 6:261–271.

Walker, C.L., and S.M. Ho. 2012. Developmental reprogramming of cancer susceptibility. *Nature Reviews Cancer* 12(7):10.1038/nrc3220.

Wang, Q., L.S. Trevino, R.L. Wong, M. Medvedovic, J. Chen, S.M. Ho, J. Shen, C.E. Foulds, C. Coarfa, B.W. O'Malley, A. Shilatifard, and C.L. Walker. 2016. Reprogramming of the epigenome by MLL1 links early-life environmental exposures to prostate cancer risk. *Molecular Endocrinology* 30(8):856–871.

Wang, T., E.C. Pehrsson, D. Purushotham, D. Li, X. Zhuo, B. Zhang, H.A. Lawson, M.A. Province, C. Krapp, Y. Lan, C. Coarfa, T.A. Katz, W.Y. Tang, Z. Wang, S. Biswal, S. Rajagopalan, J.A. Colacino, Z.T.-Y. Tsai, M.A. Sartor, K. Neier, D.C. Dolinoy, J. Pinto, R.B. Hamanaka, G.M. Mutlu, H.B. Patisaul, D.L. Aylor, G.E. Crawford, T. Wiltshire, L.H. Chadwick, C.G. Duncan, A.E. Garton, K.A. McAllister, TaRGET II Consortium, M.S. Bartolomei, C.L. Walker, and F.L. Tyson. 2018. The NIEHS TaRGET II Consortium and environmental epigenomics. *Nature Biotechnology* 36(3):225–227.

11

Moving Forward

The *Gulf War and Health* series has examined the health outcomes associated with numerous harmful exposures, intentional and unintentional, to which Gulf War and Post-9/11 veterans may have been exposed during their deployments to the Persian Gulf region and Afghanistan. Some volumes in the series also evaluated the prevalence of health outcomes among veterans who deployed to the Persian Gulf region compared with veterans who did not deploy or deployed elsewhere. Each of the volumes in the series, when appropriate, attempted to ascertain which, if any, adverse reproductive effects might be occurring in male and female veterans and, when data were available, which health effects might be occurring in their children. However, none of the previous volumes considered windows of exposure during the prenatal and, particularly, the preconception periods. Generally, although deployed Gulf War veterans were more likely to self-report sexual difficulties than their nondeployed counterparts, no other adverse reproductive or developmental effects were reported in veterans or their children (NASEM, 2016a). As such, none of the *Gulf War and Health* volumes have specifically addressed whether generational health effects are attributable to a toxicant, other potentially harmful exposures, or deployment in general. The most recent volume in the *Veterans and Agent Orange* series drew attention to the possibility that exposure to dioxin, present in the herbicides sprayed in Vietnam during the war, might result in adverse health effects in the children of veterans (NASEM, 2016b). Given those concerns, coupled with the concerns of Gulf War and Post-9/11 veterans about the long-term effects of their deployment exposures on their reproductive function and on the health of their children, the Department of Veterans Affairs (VA) and Congress requested that the National Academies of Sciences, Engineering, and Medicine examine what the scientific and medical literature says about generational health effects and, importantly, how current knowledge gaps may be addressed. This volume specifically summarizes the science and provides guidance for the development of future programs that can help to fill those gaps.

In Chapters 4 through 7, the Volume 11 committee reviewed the literature on 24 toxicants or groups of toxicants and other related harmful exposures with a specific focus on reproductive and developmental health outcomes. For most exposures, there was little or no information on specific effects in veterans, so the committee relied on studies that examined other exposed populations, such as occupational or residential cohorts, in order to reach conclusions about the strength of the association between exposures and effects. It is important to note that studies of nonveteran populations raise questions regarding the comparability of both the study population and their exposures as they relate to veterans' experiences and their deployments. This was apparent for toxicants such as dioxins and pesticides where the preponderance of the evidence is for occupational (e.g., pesticide sprayers) and residential exposures, and not related directly to the military experience. Nevertheless, the committee is confident that nonveteran studies can help identify relevant toxicants and related exposures that need to be prioritized for future research efforts, as discussed in the following sections.

As the committee reached its conclusions regarding the categories of association for each toxicant or group of toxicants or for other exposures, it became evident that there were three areas with a substantial dearth of information. Those areas are:

- the effects that may occur in germ cells, embryos, fetuses, neonates, infants, or children following preconception exposures;
- the long-term health outcomes in children who have been prenatally exposed to potentially harmful substances; and
- the occurrence, if any, of adverse effects in grandchildren and subsequent generations as a result of veterans' deployment exposures.

In addition, compared with studies on male reproduction, there are relatively few studies on the effects of the toxicants of concern on female reproduction. Even for exposures with a relatively robust human literature, the vast majority of information on developmental effects in embryos, fetuses, and children is based on prenatal—not preconception—exposures. In light of the Department of Defense (DoD) requirement that pregnant service members be removed from deployment as soon as possible after the pregnancy is known, preconception exposures may be more common or likely to cause problems than prenatal exposures for deployed women. For male veterans, all exposures would be considered preconception.

Several of the toxic exposures reviewed by the committee, including solvents, pesticides, and polycyclic aromatic hydrocarbons (PAHs), have been associated with health effects in children following prenatal exposures. One difficulty in assessing these studies is that no matter how much care is taken when measuring the levels of the toxicants or their metabolites in the mother's urine or blood, the exposure of the children to the toxicants may have extended beyond their mother's pregnancy and into their infancy and childhood. Such exposures early in childhood not only add complexity to the interpretation of findings but also can have significant impacts on the child's health. However, some studies have continued to follow children exposed prenatally to a number of toxicants (e.g., pesticides and tetrachloroethylene), and this provides an unparalleled opportunity to monitor health outcomes throughout the children's lifecourse.

These and other data gaps highlight the need for programs to monitor veterans prior to, during, and following deployment and to assess their children (and subsequent generations) periodically to determine what, if any, health effects they are experiencing and whether those effects might be associated with their parents' deployment exposures. To achieve this, the committee provided a framework for the creation and implementation of a health monitoring and research program (HMRP) for veterans and their children and grandchildren as well as guidance on epidemiologic studies that might further enhance our understanding of the association between a veteran's deployment exposures and health outcomes in their children and grandchildren. Recognizing that even a concise epidemiologic study might take several years to produce meaningful results and that conducting prospective generational studies will require even more time, the committee also provided a research agenda addressing the genetic and epigenetic changes that underpin generational effects. That research agenda includes using animal models, target tissues, and cells, including induced pluripotent stem cells, to model observed exposures in parallel with the epidemiologic studies in order to move the science of generational health effects forward in a more expeditious and effective manner.

The proposed HMRP would establish a process for identifying service members and their families and a framework upon which specific research studies could be developed in the future. This program would also provide access to information on veterans' military exposures (both suspected and measured); the reproductive health of the veterans and their spouses; pregnancy outcomes; and neonatal, infant, and child health outcomes. These data would allow VA to evaluate the occurrence, distribution, and overall trends of reproductive effects in veterans as well as any relevant health outcomes in their descendants, which in turn would allow researchers to investigate the biological mechanisms and epidemiologic associations of health effects and veterans' exposures. Importantly, the committee foresees that this information will be of value not only to veterans and their children but also to the general public, given that many of the exposures, as noted earlier, are not unique to deployment but are also representative of occupational and residential exposures and, in some instances, of daily living.

There is evidence of direct reproductive and developmental effects that are related to deployment exposures, especially pesticides, particulate matter (PM), and solvents (see Tables 8-1 and 8-2). Although evidence of heritable generational effects is lacking in humans, basic research studies have provided evidence for the biological plausibility of many of the observed findings. The direct or indirect effects of prenatal exposures on the somatic cells of the embryo or fetus—that is, all the cells in the body other than reproductive cells—can lead to reproductive and developmental effects, but these should not be confused with effects on the germ cells that produce the sperm and oocytes which combine to form an embryo, for it is these changes that may give rise to transgenerational health effects. Toxicants and harmful exposures that directly or indirectly affect reproduction and development act through a variety of pathways, whereas, based on current knowledge, the toxicants capable of inducing generational effects are limited to genetic and epigenetic mechanisms in germ cells. These generational effects in turn alter normal embryonic development in ways that modify the genetic programming of one or more cell types to alter the organism's further development. Some research has examined possible genetic and epigenetic changes in the placenta, the developing embryo, maternal blood, or cord blood as a result of deployment-related exposures, such as to PM or benzo[a]pyrene (see Chapter 6). The relationship of those changes to health outcomes, such as birth weight, has also been explored in some detail and was discussed in earlier chapters of this report. However, the committee did not identify any studies that assessed whether deployment-related exposures produced genetic or epigenetic effects in the germ cells of prenatally exposed children. This dearth of information is an important finding, because changes in the germ cells in exposed offspring represent a major pathway for the occurrence of generational inheritance of health outcomes.

A literature review by Walker et al. (2018) found that most deployment exposures of interest for this report have not been studied for potential transgenerational effects in humans. However, some toxicants, such as dioxins and permethrin in combination with DEET, have been studied in animal models. Any experimental study on chemical exposure should be combined with stress (physical or psychological) to better simulate deployment exposure scenarios.

As the committee completed its review of the epidemiologic and toxicologic literature on the Gulf War and Post-9/11 toxicants, developed a framework for an HMRP and future epidemiologic studies, and laid out an agenda for basic research on generational effects, several scientific priorities became evident. Addressing these priorities will be critical to implementing a functional and useful HMRP and a concrete agenda for answering questions about the reproductive, developmental, and generational health effects of deployment exposures; if these priorities are not addressed, it would compromise the effectiveness and success of the proposed HMRP. These priorities are listed below and discussed in the sections that follow:

- **The collection, storage, and maintenance of comprehensive baseline and longitudinal data and biospecimens from veterans, their partners, and their descendants;**
- **A detailed characterization and assessment of exposures during and after deployment; and**
- **The development, evaluation, standardization, and interoperability of biomarkers of exposure, susceptibility, and biological effects.**

COLLECTION OF BASELINE AND LONGITUDINAL DATA

An accurate assessment of changes in health status requires baseline data against which future data can be compared in order to properly evaluate patterns and outcomes. Thus, to determine whether any health outcomes in veterans and their children are potentially associated with the veterans' deployments, it is essential that a properly curated and maintained database be created. The database should contain baseline exposure and health information for all new incoming service members, including biological specimens—at a minimum, blood and urine as well as sperm for men and, where feasible, oocytes for women—collected at the time of entry into the military and also before deployment. At times when it proves too difficult to collect blood and urine samples—for example, in a war zone—saliva or buccal swabs may be collected instead. The resulting extensive collection of pre-deployment data and specimens will require significant and extensive coordination, as detailed elsewhere in this volume, but it is a crucial requirement that medical staff and investigators establish a reference framework against which post-deployment exposures and health status can be evaluated.

As discussed in Chapter 9, one practical option would be to build upon the existing DoD Serum Repository. DoD already collects serum for every service member at the time of entry into the military and then every 2 years while on active duty, as well as before and after deployment. At present there are about 60 million sera samples that have been collected from about 10 million service members representing all the branches of the military and including both men and women (Lushniak et al. 2016). A well-coordinated and systematic expansion of this biobank would provide an extremely valuable resource for DoD, VA, and affiliated stakeholders. At a minimum, DoD should continue to biobank and process samples so that a longitudinal profile encompassing the baseline health status and pre- and post-deployment exposures of service members can be established. As elaborated in Chapter 9, the existing biobank could be expanded to include the collection of sperm and oocytes following defined protocols for sample collection and storage and to acquire samples immediately after a specific "incident" of potential concern.

The committee strongly believes that although the current collection of blood and urine will help with eventual exposure assessments, collecting baseline semen samples will be crucial for understanding the impacts of veterans' exposures on their children and grandchildren. The effects of exposures on semen have been suggested as an important sentinel of environmental exposures (Montano et al., 2017); these exposures may also have impacts on the fertility of the exposed male veterans and, possibly, health effects in his offspring. Given the reports of decreasing rates of fertility in industrialized nations that have been associated with reduced semen quality, which in turn has been associated with increasing levels of environmental pollution, this issue is of significant public health relevance (Mima et al., 2018). As such, a robust, accessible, searchable, and well-curated biorepository could help provide valuable data for answering future questions about exposure–disease associations, deployment exposures, and susceptibility to disease.

As the number of women entering the military and being deployed continues to grow, concerns regarding the possible health effects of those deployment exposures on female germ cells (oocytes) also escalate. These concerns gain added significance when one considers that women are born with a finite number of germ cells which are available throughout their reproductive period. Although the collection of oocytes when women enter the military is desirable, the committee recognizes that such biospecimens are difficult to obtain. The opportunistic collection of oocytes is feasible and might be accomplished as part of fertility preservation.

As with veterans, sample collections from infants and children will provide a baseline that can be used to create a longitudinal record of changes as a child grows. The committee suggests that blood spots be collected at birth and be maintained by the states' newborn screening programs and that additional biological samples (e.g., saliva or meconium), also be collected from offspring to address specific goals of the HMRP. Blood and urine samples may be collected on a periodic basis from older children as well.

PRIORITIZATION OF EXPOSURES

Not all deployment exposures are equal. Some exposures during deployment may be similar to those experienced by the veteran as part of his or her military occupation specialty—diesel exhaust, for example—while others may be unique to the deployment experience, such as combat stress, chemical warfare agents, and the regular use of pesticides. Some exposures may be of particular concern because veterans are more likely to be exposed to them at higher concentrations, at a heightened frequency, or for longer periods of time than would be the case in most other occupational settings—PM and some solvents are examples—or because the substances have significant toxicity, as is the case with sarin or hexavalent chromium.

Both the overall evaluation completed by the committee and the conclusions it reached about exposure–effect associations are based on data from a wide range of exposure scenarios and populations that were not equivalent to the deployment exposures experienced by service members or veteran populations. Therefore, the committee strongly recommends that such exposures should be studied specifically in active-duty service members and in veterans in order to confirm that the associations are valid for those populations.

As discussed in Chapter 9, DoD should conduct more systematic exposure monitoring using the most appropriate, state-of-the-art analytic technologies whenever service members encounter extraordinary exposures such as sarin or depleted uranium—that is, exposures that are clearly not considered to be routine during deployment or occupational activities and for which the long-term health consequences are considerably less well characterized. The Volume 11 committee reiterates the concerns of earlier Gulf War and Health committees about the lack of precise exposure information for veterans or information on exposures at military locations, such as the Khamisiyah munitions depot containing sarin that was below the detection levels of the personal monitors yet still produced symptoms, or installations with burn pits. This uncertainty about exposures continues to significantly hamper the ability of DoD and VA to characterize hazards and to determine whether deployment exposures reached high levels of concern. The paucity of exposure data for individuals and aggregate data for military units means that future assessments will have to rely on qualitative assessments that compare "deployed versus nondeployed" rather than on precise monitoring data. The limitations of this approach are clearly substantial and greatly detract from the effectiveness with which the findings can be interpreted and followed in future investigations. Nevertheless, the committee is encouraged by steps that are being taken to improve exposures assessments during deployment. For example, DoD conducted real-time personal breathing zone sampling of U.S. Air Force security personnel at Bagram Airfield in Afghanistan to determine pollutant levels associated with a burn pit and an incinerator. SKC Deployable Vapor samplers and SKC Deployable Particulate samplers were used to collect both breathing zone sampling and ambient air samples for 24 hours beginning with the start of each work shift at multiple sites at the airfield (Blasch et al., 2016). Similar approaches may be used in other deployment situations and military installations. This was demonstrated when the oil fields in Kuwait were set ablaze in the first Gulf War. Air monitoring of soil and air and biomonitoring of 22 service members were conducted. Blood samples were assessed for changes in PAH-DNA adducts as biomarkers of exposure. This demonstrated the feasibility of environmental monitoring when a potential threat is known (Poirier et al., 1998).

Ideally, all substances that lie at the intersection of high likelihood of exposure and great inherent toxicity would be considered a high priority for monitoring and for research on their reproductive and developmental health outcomes and toxicity. However, because the reproductive, developmental, and generational effects of many toxicants are generally not well understood, particularly in humans, it is not possible at this time to identify those particular toxicants that pose the greatest risk to veterans, their descendants, or both. A list of toxicants for which the committee concluded there is limited/suggestive or sufficient evidence of association with reproductive and developmental effects in humans is presented in Tables 8-1 and 8-2. Following those tables is a short list of toxicants for which robust animal data, but few human data, are available. Of note is that hexavalent chromium; benzene; organophosphate, carbamate, and pyrethroid pesticides; PM, PAHs; polychlorinated dibenzodioxins and furans; trichloroethylene and tetrachloroethylene; and glycols and glycol ethers all warrant further immediate research, as risks have been indicated for each. Research on generational effects from exposure to these chemicals should also be assigned top priority. Preemptively, where little or no human data are available, broad cellular, animal, and literature screening programs for early indications of concern are warranted. Compounds for which a concern is identified could then be directly assessed using biobanked resources.

DEVELOPMENT OF BIOMARKERS

Concurrent with the effort to measure veteran's exposures during deployment, there should be research into the identification of biomarkers for those exposures, biomarkers of susceptibility, and biomarkers of various effects, including those specifically designed to evaluate reproductive effects in veterans and developmental effects in embryos, fetuses, and children. The committee notes that the assessment of generational effects will require the development of sensitive and meaningful epigenetic markers as well as biomarkers of susceptibility.

There are existing federal programs focused on biomarker research that may facilitate VA and DoD efforts in this endeavor. For example, the National Institute of Environmental Health Sciences (NIEHS) Toxicant Exposures and Responses by Genomic and Epigenomic Egulators of Transcription (TaRGET) II consortium is focused on the development of epigenetic biomarkers in animal models. These biomarkers of exposure, susceptibility, and effect will also need to discriminate with some degree of certainty, when feasible, between adverse deployment exposures and exposures that occur throughout the veteran's lifetime as well as the lives of his or her children and grandchildren. Of particular relevance to this report is that the consortium will be collecting and analyzing target and surrogate tissues over the lifecourse following perinatal, peri-adolescent, or adult exposure to tetrachlorodibenzo-p-dioxin and to air pollution in the form of $PM_{2.5}$ (Wang et al., 2018).

The NIEHS Children's Health Exposure Analysis Resource (CHEAR) described in Chapter 9 (see Box 9-2) is another example of efforts to develop and disseminate data on children's exposures and provide a public resource for environmental health studies (NIEHS, 2018). Depending on the half-life of the toxicant and the timing of sample collection, biomarkers of exposure may be assessed using high-quality assays, including untargeted chemical analyses. Laboratory approaches for exposomic analysis often combine targeted and untargeted methods, with the targeted analysis providing a more accurate quantification of the untargeted screen (Cajka and Feihn, 2016; Feihn, 2016). The CHEAR program is scheduled to be converted in 2019 to a human health exposure analysis resource which will include adults. CHEAR is also at the forefront of developing untargeted chemical assays that screen hundreds to thousands of chemicals in biological samples. Untargeted chemical testing screens are based on high-resolution mass spectrometry (HRMS) and are a newer approach to assessing chemical exposures. Such assays can be used to discover which exposures from deployment are candidates for inter- and transgenerational inheritance effects. Targeted assays are more precise quantitatively, but they measure only one or a small number of chemicals in a panel.

Untargeted assays screen thousands of chemicals at once, and while they are less quantitative, they provide a more comprehensive view of the totality of chemicals within a biological sample. Untargeted assays allow researchers to discover important chemicals that drive health effects rather than subjectively choosing chemicals to test based on the published literature and available assays. No single platform captures all metabolites and exogenous chemicals, and most laboratories use multiple platforms. Gas chromatography (GC) coupled with HRMS is ideal for exogenous chemicals (Dennis et al., 2017; Feihn 2016), but methods that use both GC and liquid chromatography would be more comprehensive. Of note is that untargeted assays can capture both endogenous metabolites and exogenous chemicals (Michely et al., 2018), affording added value as measures of exposure response and exposure. A number of programs are developing assays for high-dimensional untargeted multi-chemical screens, including the Emory University HERCULES Research Center, the Mount Sinai Institute for Exposomics, the NIEHS CHEAR program, the West Coast Metabolomics Center at the University of California, Davis, and the National Institutes of Health's Common Fund Metabolomics Program, among others. Using untargeted assays to assess thousands of chemical signatures at a time in such biological samples as urine or plasma can help identify candidate chemical exposures that may play a role in transgenerational inheritance. This approach would be the current state of the art, and it is expected that methods for both the assay and its associated bioinformatics will change and improve dramatically in the coming years, as this is an area of rapid scientific advancement.

DoD has already funded research using untargeted assays to assess exposures during deployment (Accardi et al., 2016; Jones et al., 2016; Walker et al., 2016), including for military personnel exposed at burn pits (Mallon et al., 2016), thus illustrating its interest in this line of research. Such work should be relatively easy to leverage for the HMRP proposed here and represents a logical and natural synergistic extension of the overall effort. The committee envisions that untargeted assays will be increasingly used to screen for chemical exposures during deployment and that this work will lead to the establishment of a program in exposomics[1] within the DoD and VA research portfolios. Pilot studies assessing burn pit exposures in Iraq and Afghanistan have suggested that the DoD Serum Repository is a useful

[1] *Exposomics* is a scientific discipline focused on the measure of all the exposures throughout a lifetime (the exposome), beginning at birth and including environmental and occupational sources, and on how they relate to health. The goal is to understand how exposures from our environment, diet, lifestyle, etc., interact with individual characteristics (i.e., genetics, physiology, and epigenetics) to affect health. The measurement of the exposome relies on internal and external exposure assessment methods. Internal exposure assessment methods frequently rely on omics approaches and biomarkers to quantify internal dose and biological effects (NIOSH, 2014).

resource for identifying nonroutine exposures using omics approaches, particularly those encountered during deployment, and that untargeted screens are now being used (Lushniak et al., 2016; Mallon et al., 2016). For example, serum microRNAs from the DoD Serum Repository are being explored as a novel biomarker of deployment exposure to dioxins (Woeller et al., 2016).

Biomarkers of exposure, susceptibility, and effect will also need to discriminate with some degree of certainty, when feasible, between adverse deployment exposures and exposures that occur throughout the veteran's lifetime as well as the lifetimes of the veteran's children and grandchildren.

FUNDING

As the population of veterans and their descendants continues to grow, the importance of a consistent and committed funding stream for the HMRP and its underlying basic research cannot be overemphasized. The costs of designing and conducting a HMRP for any veteran cohort will be substantial, as already demonstrated by the cost of similar programs. For example, the National Children's Study, which attempted to examine the health of 100,000 children, had an estimated 7-year total field cost in the range of $1.3 billion to $1.6 billion (NRC/IOM, 2013). The Air Force Health Study (see Box 9-1), funded directly by Congress as a line item in the DoD budget appropriation, cost approximately $143 million as of 2006 to study more than 2,000 Ranch Hand and control veterans, including the collection of data on almost 10,000 pregnancies (IOM, 2006). The study also followed more than 20,000 Vietnam veterans for almost 25 years to gather health outcomes and mortality data.

While the programmatic costs of a HMRP, including future epidemiologic and basic research studies, may be substantial, the costs of the some of the underlying technologies have plummeted. For example, the cost of whole-genome sequencing has rapidly decreased—from an estimated $3 billion for the first human genomes sequenced in 2003 to about $1,000 per individual recently, with the cost continuing to trend downward toward the predicted $100 personal genome (NHGRI, 2018). This cost savings has expanded the use of gene sequencing for medical diagnosis and treatment to the point that this practice is now routine in many clinical medicine facilities (Krier et al., 2016). For example, sequencing is now routinely used in many cases of cancer therapy to predict response and optimize treatment (NCI, 2018), and its use has extended to personalized precision medicine, including applications in the neonatal intensive care unit (Farnaes et al., 2018; Rehm, 2017) as well as into wellness programs (Patel et al., 2013). Untargeted chemical assay costs are also declining and have been estimated to be as low at $125 per sample (Walker et al., 2016). While the effort to decode a human genome previously required substantial infrastructure, it has now been miniaturized to the size of a flash drive using nanopore sequencing technology (Jain et al., 2018). This presents a new set of opportunities for its use in research (both human and animal), clinical practice, and the theater of operation. The committee finds that the costs of an HMRP and the associated basic research efforts will be offset, at least in part, by an increased ability to identify and respond to early medical needs with treatments, interventions, and prevention.

FEASIBILITY

The Volume 11 committee concludes that new large-scale HMRPs and epidemiologic studies designed specifically to address the question of whether descendants of deployed veterans are at increased risk of adverse health effects compared with descendants of nondeployed veterans will be an ambitious undertaking. While it will be possible to generate valuable information for veterans and their descendants from this effort, several important outstanding issues need to be addressed to optimize the timing of future investments. These include the following:

- **An integrated electronic health record system** The need to have a fully integrated electronic health record (EHR) system between DoD and VA cannot be overstated; the committee is encouraged that VA and DoD are working toward that end. An integrated electronic health record system is needed not only to improve the transition of veterans from one health care system to the other, but also to improve access to longitudinal health data, particularly those that relate to reproductive and birth health. Access to electronic health data will also be essential for the large number of veterans who receive care at ancillary facilities or outside the VA system.
- **Improved exposure monitoring** The lack of exposure monitoring during deployments, whether at the individual or the military unit level, precludes an adequate assessment of the nature, duration, and frequency of deployment exposures. This limitation is exacerbated by the lack of information on lifecourse exposures and toxicological information as this relates to the complex chemical mixtures often encountered during environmental and occupational exposures.
- **Collecting data on descendants** It will be important but also challenging to capture health information on veterans' partners and their children and grandchildren from health systems that are often fractured and location-specific. Countries with nationalized health care systems, such as Australia, Canada, Scandinavia, and the United Kingdom, have better infrastructure to properly follow children and obtain longitudinal data and biospecimens with which to conduct studies such as those proposed in this volume.

At present, there are numerous resource, methodologic, and organizational considerations that must be addressed across several governmental agencies—and likely private organizations as well—in order to implement a large-scale study of the magnitude envisioned and recommended by the Volume 11 committee. Some of the critical considerations for implementing and sustaining an HMRP are the following:

- sustained funding;
- legal mandates for and potential obstructions of participation by relevant government agencies such as the Social Security Administration, the Department of Health and Human Services, and DoD;
- the availability and expertise of adequately trained personnel;
- the level of technologic competencies, including an integrated EHR and data systems;
- ready accessibility to well-curated data, including biorepositories;
- maintenance of the confidentiality of human health data;
- logistical barriers to identifying descendants of veterans;
- ethical considerations regarding investigations that include parents and children; and
- the development and implementation of appropriate risk and health communication strategies between and among organizations as well as with veterans and their families.

As a result of these considerations, among many others, the committee proposes that a more practical and expedient approach to examining generational health effects may be to leverage ongoing veterans' health research programs, such as the Million Veteran Program and the Millennium Cohort Study. Such an approach would greatly benefit from past investments and take advantage of existing infrastructure to address some of the critical issues identified in this report. These programs, as detailed in Chapter 9, have already enrolled large cohorts and are linked to a variety of rich big data sources, and some of them already have in place protocols for the collection of biological specimens and the participation of partners and children.

The Volume 11 committee believes that the feasibility of an HMRP and accompanying research agenda will be substantially improved by implementing the tiered approach described in Chapter 9. Building on the committee's conclusions regarding the strength of the associations between exposures to the toxicants of interest and the reproductive and developmental effects described in Chapters 4 through 7, VA and collaborators may design a pilot HMRP to test hypotheses about associations that appear to be most important. Concurrently, those associations should also be explored by complementary animal studies to refine the scope of the problem and help to identify relevant biomarkers of exposure and effects. Results of the pilot program results would feed into an expanded HRMP encompassing potentially more participants, more data collection and analysis, and more detailed evaluation of effects. An iterative evaluation process would provide necessary course correction throughout the life of the HMRP to ensure that the program is meeting its goals and providing value to the participants.

SUMMARY

The available scientific and medical data on generational health effects associated with environmental and occupational exposures in humans are extremely limited. However, interesting and compelling findings from investigational studies in laboratory animals and in experimental model systems provide suggestive evidence that generational effects as a result of exposures associated with deployment, the military experience, or life in general are biologically plausible. On the bases of the available evidence, the Volume 11 committee concludes that systematic health monitoring coupled with epidemiologic and laboratory-based investigations are warranted and should be implemented. Although the scientific evidence is not yet sufficient to predict with confidence which exposures are most likely to result in genetic or epigenetic disturbances in a veteran's somatic or germ cells that can compromise reproductive or generational health outcomes, progress is being made, and the mechanisms of generational inheritance are being explored. Thus, targeted epidemiologic studies combined with research using experimental models of epigenetic inheritance should be developed and promoted. Such programs can take advantage of the existing research infrastructure to establish whether adverse effects occur in the children of male and female veterans and whether these outcomes are related to their military service and, particularly, to their deployments.

As emphasized earlier, addressing the priorities outlined in this volume will require substantial resources, long-term commitment by DoD and VA and other governmental organizations, and considerable engagement by past, current, and future veterans and their families. While carrying out these priorities will be challenging, the committee firmly believes that there are actions that VA, working in partnership with DoD and other key stakeholders, partners, and collaborators, can take now and in the near future to address important health questions related to the health and well-being of future generations.

The committee commends the efforts of VA and Congress to address veterans' concerns about generational health effects and cautions all involved that developing an increased understanding of these critical issues will be a long and complex undertaking. The committee also believes that the results and deliverables that arise from such an investment will ultimately be rewarded with new knowledge of veterans' exposures, their reproductive health, and the health of their children and grandchildren. Importantly, the knowledge and understanding derived from these investments will be relevant to the health of all Americans now and for generations to come.

REFERENCES

Accardi, C.J., D.I. Walker, K. Uppal, A.A. Quyyumi, P. Rohrbeck, K.D. Pennell, C.T. Mallon, and D.P. Jones. 2016. High-resolution metabolomics for nutrition and health assessment of Armed Forces personnel. *Journal of Occupational and Environmental Medicine* 58(8 Suppl 1):S80–S88.

Blasch, K.W., J.E. Kolivosky, and J.M. Heller. 2016. Environmental air sampling near burn pit and incinerator operations at Bagram Airfield, Afghanistan. *Journal of Occupational and Environmental Medicine* 58(7S):S38–S43.

Cajka, T., and O. Fiehn. 2016. Toward merging untargeted and targeted methods in mass spectrometry-based metabolomics and lipidomics. *Analytical Chemistry* 88(1):524–545.

Dennis, K.K., E. Marder, D.M. Balshaw, Y. Cui, M.A. Lynes, G.J. Patti, S.M. Rappaport, D.T. Shaughnessy, M. Vrijheid, and D.B. Barr. 2017. Biomonitoring in the era of the exposome. *Environmental Health Perspectives* 125(4):502–510.

Farnaes, L., A. Hildreth, N.M. Sweeney, M.M. Clark, S. Chowdhury, S. Nahas, J.A. Cakici, W. Benson, R.H. Kaplan, R. Kronick, M.N. Bainbridge, J. Friedman, J.J. Gold, Y. Ding, N. Veeraraghavan, D. Dimmock, and S.F. Kingsmore. 2018. Rapid whole-genome sequencing decreases infant morbidity and cost of hospitalization. *Genomic Medicine* 3(1):10.

Fiehn, O. 2016. Metabolomics by gas chromatography-mass spectrometry: The combination of targeted and untargeted profiling. *Current Protocols in Molecular Biology* 114:30.4.1–30.4.32.

IOM (Institute of Medicine). 2006. *Disposition of the Air Force Health Study*. Washington, DC: The National Academies Press.

Jain, M., S. Koren, K.H. Miga, J. Quick, A.C. Rand, T.A. Sasani, J.R. Tyson, A.D. Beggs, A.T. Dilthey, I.T. Fiddes, S. Malla, H. Marriott, T. Nieto, J. O'Grady, H.E. Olsen, B.S. Pedersen, A. Rhie, H. Richardson, A.R. Quinlan, T.P. Snutch, L. Tee, B. Paten, A.M. Phillippy, J.T. Simpson, N.J. Loman, and M. Loose. 2018. Nanopore sequencing and assembly of a human genome with ultra-long reads. *Nature Biotechnology* 36(4):338–345.

Jones, D.P., D.I. Walker, K. Uppal, P. Rohrbeck, C.T. Mallon, and Y.M. Go. 2016. Metabolic pathways and networks associated with tobacco use in military personnel. *Journal of Occupational and Environmental Medicine* 58(8 Suppl 1):S111–S116.

Krier, J.B., S.S. Kalia, and R.C. Green. 2016. Genomic sequencing in clinical practice: Applications, challenges, and opportunities. *Dialogues in Clinical Neuroscience* 18(3):299–312.

Lushniak, B., T.M. Mallon, J.C. Gaydos, and D.J. Smith. 2016. Utility of the Department of Defense Serum Repository in assessing deployment exposure. *Journal of Occupational and Environmental Medicine* 58(8S):S1–S2.

Mallon, C.T., M.P. Rohrbeck, M.K. Haines, D.P. Jones, M. Utell, P.K. Hopke, R.P. Phipps, D.I. Walker, T. Thatcher, C.F. Woeller, C.P. Baird, H.B. Pollard, C.L. Dalgard, and J.C. Gaydos. 2016. Introduction to Department of Defense research on burn pits, biomarkers, and health outcomes related to deployment in Iraq and Afghanistan. *Journal of Occupational and Environmental Medicine* 58(7S):S3–S11.

Michely, J.A., M.R. Meyer, and H.H. Maurer. 2018. Power of Orbitrap-based LC-high resolution-MS/MS for comprehensive drug testing in urine with or without conjugate cleavage or using dried urine spots after on-spot cleavage in comparison to established LC-MSn or GC-MS procedures. *Drug Testing and Analysis* 10(1):158–163.

Mima, M., D. Greenwald, and S. Ohlander. 2018. Environmental toxins and male fertility. *Current Urology Reports* 19(7):50.

Montano, L., P. Bergamo, M.G. Andreassi, and S. Lorenzetti. 2017. The role of human semen as an early and reliable tool of environmental impact assessment on human health, spermatozoa. In R. Meccariello (ed.). *Spermatozoa: Facts and perspectives*. Rijeka, Croatia: IntechOpen. Pp. 173–202. https://cdn.intechopen.com/pdfs/59074.pdf (accessed July 10, 2018).

NASEM (National Academies of Sciences, Engineering, and Medicine). 2016a. *Gulf War and health, volume 10: Update of health effects of serving in the Gulf War, 2016*. Washington, DC: The National Academies Press.

NASEM. 2016b. *Veterans and Agent Orange: Update 2014*. Washington, DC: The National Academies Press.

NCI (National Cancer Institute). 2018. *Tumor DNA sequencing in cancer treatment*. www.cancer.gov/about-cancer/treatment/types/precision-medicine/tumor-dna-sequencing (accessed July 10, 2018).

NHGRI (National Human Genome Research Institute). 2018. *The cost of sequencing a human genome*. www.genome.gov/27565109/the-cost-of-sequencing-a-human-genome (accessed June 29, 2018).

NIEHS (National Institute of Environmental Health Sciences). 2018. *Children's Health Exposure Analysis Resource (CHEAR)*. www.niehs.nih.gov/research/supported/exposure/chear/index.cfm (accessed June 29, 2018).

NIOSH (National Institute for Occupational Safety and Health). 2014. *Exposome and exposomics*. www.cdc.gov/niosh/topics/exposome/default.html (accessed July 10, 2018).

NRC/IOM (National Research Council/Institute of Medicine). 2013. *Design of the National Children's Study: A workshop summary*. Washington, DC: The National Academies Press.

Patel, C.J., A. Sivadas, R. Tabassum, T. Preeprem, J. Zhao, D. Arafat, R. Chen, A.A. Morgan, G.S. Martin, K.L. Brigham, A.J. Butte, and G. Gibson. 2013. Whole genome sequencing in support of wellness and health maintenance. *Genome Medicine* 5(6):58.

Poirier, M.C., A. Weston, B. Schoket, H. Shamkhani, C.F. Pan, M.A. McDiarmid, B.G. Scott, D.P. Deeter, J.M. Heller, D. Jacobson-Kram, and N. Rothman. 1998. Biomonitoring of United States Army soldiers serving in Kuwait in 1991. *Cancer Epidemiology Biomarkers and Prevention* 7(6):545–551.

Rehm, H.L. 2017. Evolving health care through personal genomics. *Nature Reviews Genetics* 18:259.

Walker, D.I., T.M. Mallon, P.K. Hopke, K. Uppal, Y.-M. Go, P. Rohrbeck, K.D. Pennell, and D.P. Jones. 2016. Deployment-associated exposure surveillance with high-resolution metabolomics. *Journal of Occupational and Environmental Medicine* 58(7S):S12–S21.

Walker, V.R., A.L. Boyles, K.E. Pelch, S.D. Holmgren, A.J. Shapiro, C.R. Blystone, M.J. Devito, R.R. Newbold, R. Blain, P. Hartman, K.A. Thayer, and A.A. Rooney. 2018. Human and animal evidence of potential transgenerational inheritance of health effects: An evidence map and state-of-the-science evaluation. *Environment International* 115:48–69.

Wang, T., E.C. Pehrsson, D. Purushotham, D. Li, X. Zhuo, B. Zhang, H.A. Lawson, M.A. Province, C. Krapp, Y. Lan, C. Coarfa, T.A. Katz, W.Y. Tang, Z. Wang, S. Biswal, S. Rajagopalan, J.A. Colacino, Z.T.-Y. Tsai, M.A. Sartor, K. Neier, D.C. Dolinoy, J. Pinto, R.B. Hamanaka, G.M. Mutlu, H.B. Patisaul, D.L. Aylor, G.E. Crawford, T. Wiltshire, L.H. Chadwick, C.G. Duncan, A.E. Garton, K.A. McAllister, TaRGET II Consortium, M.S. Bartolomei, C.L. Walker, and F.L. Tyson. 2018. The NIEHS TaRGET II Consortium and environmental epigenomics. *Nature Biotechnology* 36(3):225–227.

Woeller, C.F., T.H. Thatcher, D. Van Twisk, S.J. Pollock, A. Croasdell, P.K. Hopke, X. Xia, J. Thakar, P.J. Sime, T.M. Mallon, M.J. Utell, and R.P. Phipps. 2016. MicroRNAs as novel biomarkers of deployment status and exposure to polychlorinated dibenzo-p-dioxins/dibenzofurans. *Journal of Occupational and Environmental Medicine* 58(7S):S89–S96.

Appendix A

Committee Biographical Sketches

Kenneth S. Ramos, M.D., Ph.D., PharmB. (NAM), is the associate vice president for precision health sciences, the interim dean of the University of Arizona College of Medicine, the executive director of the Center for Applied Genetics and Genomic Medicine, and a professor of medicine at the University of Arizona Health Sciences. Dr. Ramos is a leading expert in the study of the molecular mechanisms of environmental injury and the genetic and epigenetic determinants of environmental disease. A major focus of his research is the study of mammalian retroelements and endogenous retroviral-like sequences and their role in human pathogenesis. He completed undergraduate studies in pharmaceutical sciences at the University of Puerto Rico, a Ph.D. in biochemical pharmacology at the University of Texas at Austin, and undergraduate and graduate medical studies with a focus on internal medicine and pulmonary medicine at the University of Louisville. Dr. Ramos is the 2008–2009 president of the Society of Toxicology and has served on numerous National Academies committees, including the committees responsible for the *Veterans and Agent Orange: Update 1996* and *Update 1998* reports, and he chaired the 2016 Update report. He has also served as a member of the National Research Council's Committee on Application of Toxicogenomics Technologies to Predictive Toxicology, Committee on Emerging Issues and Data on Environmental Contaminants, and Committee on Application of Genomic Signatures: A Workshop. He is currently serving on the Roundtable on Public Interfaces of Life Sciences and is co-chair of the Committee on Sustainable Infrastructures for Public Communication of the Life Sciences: A Workshop. Dr. Ramos was designated an associate of the National Academy of Sciences in 2008 and elected to the National Academy of Medicine in 2015.

Tracy L. Bale, Ph.D., is a professor of pharmacology and the director of the Center for Epigenetic Research in Child Health and Brain Development in the School of Medicine at the University of Maryland, Baltimore. She completed her Ph.D. at the University of Washington in the Department of Pharmacology and her postdoctoral work at the Salk Institute with Dr. Wylie Vale. Her research focuses on understanding the role of stress dysregulation in neurodevelopmental and neuropsychiatric diseases and the sex differences that underlie disease vulnerability, using mice as the model organism. Dr. Bale's laboratory has initiated multiple lines of investigation that examine the timing and sex-specificity of early life events promoting disease susceptibility, the maturation of central pathways during key periods of development, and the epigenetic mechanisms involved in long-term effects following stress exposure. Her expertise is in developing models of parental stress and the germ cell epigenetic mechanisms involved in the intergenerational programming of neurodevelopment. She serves on numerous advisory committees, panels, and boards, served as the chair of the Neuroendocrinology, Neuroimmunology, Rhythms, and Sleep Center for Scientific Review study section, and has been a reviewing editor at the *Journal of Neuroscience* for the past 6 years. She has been the recipient of several awards for her research in this area, including the Richard E. Weitzman Memorial award from the Endocrine Society, the Medtronic Award from the Society for Women's Health Research for improvement of women's health, and recently the Daniel H. Efron award from the American College of Neuropsychopharmacology.

John R. Balmes, M.D., is a professor of medicine in the division of occupational and environmental medicine at the University of California, San Francisco, and also a professor of environmental health sciences at the University of California, Berkeley. Dr. Balmes studies the respiratory health effects of various air pollutants. He has a particular interest in occupational respiratory disease. He has investigated the acute effects of inhalation exposures to ambient air pollutants in his human exposure laboratory at San Francisco General Hospital and the chronic effects of such exposures in epidemiological studies with collaborators at the University of California, San Francisco, and the University of California, Berkeley. Dr. Balmes also is investigating genetic determinants of responses to air pollutants and has been the physician member of the California Air Resources Board since 2008. He was a member of the Institute of Medicine's Committee on the Long-Term Health Effects of Exposure to Burn Pits in Iraq and Afghanistan and Committee on the Review of the Department of Labor's Site Exposure Matrix (SEM) Database. Dr. Balmes received his M.D. from the Icahn School of Medicine at Mount Sinai.

Brenda Eskenazi, Ph.D., is a professor of epidemiology at the University of California, Berkeley, School of Public Health. She is also the director of the Children's Center for Environmental Health and is the chair of community health and human development. Her research interests are in the effects of environmental exposures (such as pesticides, lead, solvents, dioxin, and tobacco smoke) on reproductive, perinatal, and children's health as well as the reproductive and development effects of environmental toxicants on fetal and child health and reproductive health in men and women and also reproductive and pediatric epidemiology. Dr. Eskenazi was a member of the National Academies of Sciences, Engineering, and Medicine's Board on Children, Youth and Families and served on the National Research Council's Committee to Review California's Risk Assessment Process for Pesticides. She received her M.A. in psychology from Queens College and her Ph.D. in neuropsychology from the City University of New York.

Elaine M. Faustman, Ph.D., is a professor in environmental and occupational health sciences in the School of Public Health at the University of Washington. She is the director of the Institute for Risk Analysis and Risk Communication, the Center for Child Environmental Health Risks Research, and the Pacific Northwest Center for Human Health and Ocean Studies. Dr. Faustman is a developmental and reproductive toxicologist with an interest in biological monitoring and modeling. Her published research is on children's environmental health, in vitro toxicology, and the effect of pesticides, drugs, and food additives and contaminants on children's health. Her current research focuses on the neurodevelopmental toxicity of metals and pesticides, gene expression analyses as early biomarkers of effect, and the mechanisms of methylmercury-induced developmental toxicity. Dr. Faustman was the chair for the National Research Council (NRC) report on developmental toxicology and has previously served as a member of the NRC's Committee on Toxicology and other NRC committees. She received her Ph.D. in toxicology from Michigan State University.

Mari S. Golub, Ph.D., is an adjunct professor emerita with the Department of Environmental Toxicology at the University of California, Davis. Her research focuses on developmental neurotoxicity, with an emphasis on the behavioral assessment of brain function. She uses mouse and nonhuman primates to study the influence of nutrition, drugs, and chemicals on brain development. She also conducts risk assessments for the California Environmental Protection Agency (CalEPA). Dr. Golub recently retired from the California Office of Environmental Health Hazard Assessment at CalEPA where she performed risk assessments in the area of developmental and reproductive toxicology. She received her Ph.D. from the University of Michigan.

Rafael A. Irizarry, Ph.D., is a professor of biostatistics in the Department of Biostatistics and Computational Biology at the Dana-Farber Cancer Institute at Harvard University. Dr. Irizarry's research interests focus on applied statistics, epigenetics, cancer genomics, and high-throughput technology. He was a member of the National Research Council planning committee on Training Students to Extract Value from Big Data: A Workshop. Dr. Irizarry received his Ph.D. in statistics from the University of California, Berkeley.

Tamarra James-Todd, Ph.D., M.P.H., is the Mark and Catherine Winkler Assistant Professor of Environmental Reproductive and Perinatal Epidemiology at the Harvard T.H. Chan School of Public Health, an associate epidemiologist at Brigham and Women's Hospital, and an instructor in medicine at Harvard Medical School. She is an epidemiologist with a research expertise in reproductive and developmental outcomes following exposure to environmental risk factors. She has conducted epidemiologic research on perinatal and reproductive health outcomes in Kuwait (the TRACER study) and has assessed the impact of environmental endocrine disruptors on women's reproductive outcomes. Dr. James-Todd has also examined the impact of in utero exposures and long-term chronic disease risk. She received her Ph.D. in epidemiology from Columbia University and M.P.H. in international health from the Boston University School of Public Health.

Stephen A. Krawetz, Ph.D., is the Charlotte B. Failing Professor of Fetal Therapy and Diagnosis and the associate director of the C.S. Mott Center for Human Growth and Development in the Department of Obstetrics and Gynecology and Center for Molecular Medicine and Genetics, Wayne State University School of Medicine, Detroit, Michigan. He is the founding editor-in-chief of *Systems Biology in Reproductive Medicine*. He received his Ph.D. in biochemistry from the University of Toronto and then trained as an Alberta Heritage Foundation for Medical Research postdoctoral fellow with Gordon Dixon at the University of Calgary. He has published more than 200 manuscripts detailing the regulation of gene expression by chromatin structure, emphasizing human spermatogenesis and its application to personalized medicine. Over the past two decades, his group established that the fitness of the paternal contribution reflects the relative diversity of sperm RNAs that continually respond to the environment. They showed that at fertilization the spermatozoon delivers a cadre of unique RNAs to the oocyte. These RNAs may provide an essential component to early paternal genome reprogramming, acting as genetic and epigenetic impactors of the fetal onset of adult disease. They provide a personalized time stamp of the physical and reproductive health of the father, providing the opportunity to develop a personalized blueprint promoting the birth and healthy life of his children.

Linda A. McCauley, Ph.D., FAAN, RN (NAM), is a professor in and the dean of Emory University's Nell Hodgson Woodruff School of Nursing. Dr. McCauley has special expertise in the design of epidemiological investigations of environmental hazards and is nationally recognized for her expertise in occupational and environmental health nursing. She is a national leader in the area of research on environmental exposures such as pesticide exposures among minority communities. Her work aims to identify culturally appropriate interventions to decrease the impact of environmental and occupational health hazards in vulnerable populations, including workers and young children. Dr. McCauley was previously the associate dean for research and the Nightingale Professor in Nursing at the University of Pennsylvania School of Nursing. She received a bachelor of nursing degree from the University of North Carolina, a master's in nursing from Emory, and a Ph.D. in environmental health and epidemiology from the University of Cincinnati. She became a member of the National Academy of Medicine in 2008 and has served on numerous Institute of Medicine committees, including for the Update 2006 and Update 2008 in the *Veterans and Agent Orange* series. She is currently a member of the National Academies of Sciences, Engineering, and Medicine's Board on Population Health and Public Health Practice.

Jacob D. McDonald, Ph.D., is a senior scientist and the vice president of applied sciences at Lovelace Respiratory Research Institute. He serves as the chief science officer for Lovelace Biomedical, the commercial services arm of Lovelace. Dr. McDonald's core expertise is in toxicology (emphasis in respiratory), analytical chemistry, and risk assessment. Dr. McDonald previously served on the National Research Council's Committee to Review the Army's Enhanced Particulate Matter Surveillance Project Report and the Institute of Medicine committees on the Long-Term Health Effects of Exposure to Burn Pits in Iraq and Afghanistan and on the Acute Exposure Guidelines Levels for Selected Chemicals. He earned a Ph.D. in environmental chemistry and toxicology from the University of Nevada.

Dylan S. Small, Ph.D., is a professor in the department of statistics at the Wharton School at the University of Pennsylvania. His research interests include causal inference, the design and analysis of experiments and observational studies for comparing treatments, longitudinal data, measurement error, and applications of statistics to public health, medicine, and public policy. He is the editor of the journal *Observational Studies*. Recently, he was a member of the National Research Council Panel on Research Methodologies and Statistical Approaches to Understanding Driver Fatigue Factors in Motor Carrier Safety and Driver Health. Dr. Small received his Ph.D. in statistics from Stanford University.

Jacquetta Trasler, M.D., Ph.D., is a James McGill Professor in Pediatrics, Human Genetics and Pharmacology and Therapeutics at McGill University and a senior scientist at the Research Institute of the McGill University Health Centre (RI-MUHC). Dr. Trasler has mentored a number of trainees and served as the director of pediatric research at the RI-MUHC (2008–2015) and the McGill University M.D./Ph.D. Program (1999–2007). Her research interests focus on epigenetics and the molecular and developmental regulation of gene expression in the germ line and early embryo. More specifically, she studies DNA methylation and genomic imprinting and the molecular and cellular targets for drug effects on germ cells and embryos. Ongoing studies include the effects of drugs, diet (folate), and assisted reproductive technologies on the epigenome of germ cells and embryos and the implications for transgenerational passage of epigenetic defects.

Cheryl Lyn Walker, Ph.D., is the director of the Center for Precision Environmental Health at Baylor College of Medicine, where she holds the Alkek Presidential Chair and is a professor in the departments of molecular and cell biology and medicine. She also directs the National Institute of Environmental

Health Sciences' (NIEHS's) Center for Translational Environmental Health Research and serves on the board of scientific advisers for the National Cancer Institute. Dr. Walker is an international leader in environmental carcinogenesis and the elucidation of molecular mechanisms of disease. Her studies on the role of the epigenome in gene–environment interactions have yielded significant insights into mechanisms by which early life exposures influence health and disease across the lifecourse. Her work has also led to the discovery of new tumor suppressor functions in the cell and a dual role for the cell's epigenetic machinery in regulating both chromatin and the cytoskeleton. She has been recognized with the Dallas–Ft. Worth Living Legend Faculty Achievement Award in Basic Research from MD Anderson Cancer Center, the Cozarrelli Prize from the National Academy of Sciences, the 2015 Outstanding Distinguished Scientist Award from Sigma Xi, and the 2016 Leading Edge in Basic Research Award from the Society of Toxicology. Dr. Walker is a fellow of the Academy of Toxicological Sciences and the American Association for the Advancement of Science and in 2016 was elected to National Academy of Medicine. She is a past-president of the Society of Toxicology, past-president of Women in Cancer Research of the American Association for Cancer Research, and has participated on committees for the Institute of Medicine and the National Research Council. Dr. Walker earned her Ph.D. in 1984 in cell biology from the University of Texas Southwestern Medical School, with additional postdoctoral training as a staff fellow at NIEHS.

Carol S. Wood, Ph.D., is a staff scientist in the Environmental Sciences Division of Oak Ridge National Laboratory. She has more than 20 years of experience as a toxicologist, with extensive work in risk assessment for inhalation/pulmonary effects and the oral toxicity of heavy metals, pesticides, and industrial chemicals. She has worked on acute exposure guideline levels and provisional advisory levels, in which health-based exposure levels were developed for priority toxic chemicals. These projects often used toxicokinetic data and physiologically based pharmacokinetic models for extrapolation from animals to humans. She served on the board of directors for the American Board of Toxicology from 2014 to 2017. Her research experience and interests include models of developmental, reproductive, and neurotoxic outcomes from environmental contaminants. Dr. Wood has served on the Institute of Medicine's Committee on the Review of Clinical Guidance for the Care of Health Conditions Identified by the Camp Lejeune Legislation and the National Research Council's Committee on Spacecraft Exposure Guidelines. She earned a Ph.D. in toxicology from Oregon State University in 1993 with emphasis in developmental and reproductive toxicology.

Robert O. Wright, M.D., M.P.H., is Ethel H. Wise Professor of Pediatrics and the chair of the Department of Environmental Medicine and Public Health at the Icahn School of Medicine at Mount Sinai. His research interests focus on effect modifiers of metal toxicity, including gene–environment interactions and the role of toxic stress in neurodevelopment and fetal growth. The role of epigenetic biomarkers in reproductive health is a particular interest. He founded the Programming Research in Obesity, Growth, Environment and Social Stressors in 2006 in Mexico City. Dr. Wright is a pediatrician with clinical fellowship training in emergency medicine and medical toxicology. He also completed research fellowships in environmental epidemiology and genetic epidemiology. He is the director of the Lautenberg Laboratory for Environmental Health Sciences at Mount Sinai as well as the Mount Sinai CHEAR (Children's Health Exposure Analysis Resource) lab hub. He has served as a member of the National Research Council's Committee on Inorganic Arsenic and Committee on the Superfund Site Assessment and Remediation in the Coeur d'Alene River Basin. Dr. Wright received his M.D. from the University of Michigan, completed his pediatrics residency at Northwestern University, and received his M.P.H. in epidemiology and biostatistics from the Harvard School of Public Health.

Appendix B

Glossary

Acetylation: Describes the reaction that introduces an acetyl group onto a protein, such as a histone.

Allele: Human genes occur in pairs, one on each chromosome of a chromosome pair. Each gene of the pair is called an "allele." Although each allele specifies the same gene, alleles can differ slightly from each other and give rise to proteins that may differ in form and significance. For instance, in the case of some flowers, the allele on one chromosome may produce a red petal color and the other a white petal color.

Amino acid: A set of 20 different molecules used to build proteins. Proteins consist of one or more chains of amino acids called polypeptides. The sequence of the amino acid chain causes the polypeptide to fold into a shape that is biologically active. The amino acid sequences of proteins are encoded in the genes.

Apoptosis: Series of biochemical reactions occurring in a cell whereby cells undergo a process of self-destruction; also known as programmed cell death or cell suicide.

Bases: The basic building blocks of DNA and RNA. The bases used to make DNA are adenine (A), cytosine (C), guanine (G), and thymine (T). In RNA, the base uracil (U) takes the place of thymine. Bases are attached to a phosphate group and a sugar molecule (either ribose in RNA or deoxyribose in DNA) to build DNA or RNA.

Blastocyst: A distinct stage of embryo development when the undifferentiated cells of the zygote implant in the uterine lining and differentiate into two cell types: the inner cell mass that will develop into the fetus, and the trophectoderm that will develop into the placenta.

Carrier: An individual who carries and is capable of passing on a genetic mutation associated with a disease and may or may not display disease symptoms. In some cases, carriers are associated with diseases inherited as recessive traits, whereby an individual having one normal allele and one mutated allele does not have the disease. For such recessive traits, in order to have the disease, an individual must inherit mutated alleles from both parents. Because carriers of recessive alleles may not display the disease, two "normal" appearing carriers may produce children with the disease.

Cell: A fundamental unit of life comprised of a membrane-encapsulating cytoplasm and genetic material (DNA or RNA) contained in a nucleus. First discovered by Robert Hooke in 1665 in cork, then in living plant tissue using an early microscope rebuilt after Anton van Leeuwenhoek's microscopes.

Cell cycle: The orderly sequence of events in which a cell duplicates its contents, including its genetic material, and divides into two cells.

Cell fate: The final cell type that an undifferentiated cell is destined to become. Usually refers to the outcome of cell differentiation during the process of development.

Cell nucleus: Membrane-bounded organelle common to all eukaryotic cells that contains and separates the genetic material (DNA and associated proteins organized into chromosomes) from the remainder of the cell (the cytoplasm).

Chromatin: In the nucleus of each cell, DNA is packaged into chromatin made up of DNA tightly coiled many times around proteins called histones that support its structure.

Chromosome: A structure visualized during cell division containing condensed chromatin and its associated genes as the unit of inheritance. Humans have 46 chromosomes, 22 pairs of autosomes (the non-sex chromosomes), and the sex chromosomes either XX (females) or XY (males).

CpG: Cytosine-adjacent-to-guanine amino acid sites in the human genome.

Developmental origins of health and disease (DOHaD): The theory that environmental exposures early in life can have lasting effects on health and susceptibility to disease into adulthood. Sometimes referred to as Fetal Origins of Disease Hypothesis or Barker Hypothesis.

Developmental toxicity: The ability of a toxicant to cause an adverse effect in a developing organism. Examples of developmental toxicants include chemicals such as diethylstilbestrol, lifestyle factors such as alcohol, and drugs such as retinoic acid.

Differentiation: Process whereby cells/tissues become more specialized during embryonic development.

DNA: Deoxyribonucleic acid, the genetic material of most organisms. It is made of a double-helically coiled sugar-phosphate backbone, held together by organic base pairs (adenine with thymine; guanine with cytosine). This generates two complementary strands of base-pairs. The entire sequence of the human genome contains billions of base-pairs.

DNA adduct: A chemical covalently bound to a DNA base, such as benzo[a]pyrene, which can cause a DNA mutation, and which is frequently used as biomarkers to reflect exposure, as the presence of such an adduct reflects prior exposure to that chemical.

DNA damage: Any damage to DNA, which if unrepaired can cause defects such as mutation, chromosome breakage, or loss of portions of chromosomes.

DNA methylation: The reversible addition of a methyl (CH¬3) group to the DNA. It usually occurs at DNA cytosine nucleotides followed by guanosine (C-phosphate-G; CpG) and generally (but not always) functions to represses gene expression.

DNA methyltransferases (DNMT): Enzymes that catalyze the transfer of a methyl group to DNA from S-adenosylmethionine.

DNA sequence: The sequence of bases in 5'→3' direction (printed left to right) along a strand of DNA. There are four organic bases: adenine (A), thymine (T), guanine (G), and cytosine (C), which define the sequence in a single strand DNA. The DNA sequence of a gene will determine the amino-acid composition of a protein.

DNA structure: The physical shape of DNA molecules, such as coiling into tight loops or other shapes, can determine how, where, and when genes are expressed.

Embryo: A term used to describe the early life stage of a developing organism after fertilization. In humans, the embryo begins after fertilization of an oocyte by a sperm cell and persists up until week 14 of pregnancy.

Embryogenesis: The formation and development of an embryo, referring to early pregnancy beginning with fertilization of an oocyte by sperm.

Embryonic stem (ES) cells: ES cells are self-renewing cells isolated from the vertebrate inner cell mass of a developing embryo. As ES cells are totipotent they are capable of differentiating into any somatic cell or tissue, but they also preserve their capability to remain within the developmental pathway of germ cells. Thus, they are part of the germ line.

Embryotoxicity: The toxic effect of a substance on an embryo in the first period of pregnancy, between conception and the fetal stage. Effects may include malformations and variations, malfunctions, altered growth, prenatal death, and altered postnatal function.

Environmental deflection: The cumulative effect of environment mediated change away from baseline epigenetic drift.

Enzyme: A protein that facilitates (catalyzes) a specific biochemical reaction. Many enzymes work together to build up and break down biomolecules within the cell. Enzymes drive key processes such as DNA replication, the addition of epigenetic marks on chromatin, and transcription of DNA into RNA and translation of RNA into proteins.

Epigenetic code: In addition to the genetic code of DNA that specifies how genes are made into proteins, the epigenetic code specifies, via DNA methylation and histone modifications, which genes are turned on (transcribed) and which genes are turned off.

Epigenetic drift: The stochastic accumulation of changes in the epigenome associated with age.

Epigenetic inheritance: The transmission of epigenetic information from a dividing cell to its daughter cells. In the case of epigenetic alterations, such alterations may occur in one cell and be inherited by daughter cells after cell division—this is referred to as mitotic inheritance; when the alterations occur in the germ line of a parent, the changes may be passed down to offspring (and possibly subsequent generations)—this is referred to as meiotic (or generational) inheritance.

Epigenetic marks: Chromatin features that govern gene expression and are not part of the genetic code. These include methylation of DNA and covalent modification of histone proteins. The primary histone modification that is considered an epigenetic mark is methylation, although other modifications, such as acetyl, ubiquitin, phosphate, and poly(ADP)ribose, are sometimes also grouped in this category. Importantly, alterations induced by environmental exposures, both DNA and histone methylation, can be passed down from mother to daughter calls after cell division, or if they occur in the germ line, from parent to offspring (and possibly subsequent generations).

Epigenetic reprogramming: In biology, epigenetic reprogramming refers to changes in patterns of epigenetic marks, such as DNA or histone methylation. This can refer to the normal process of erasure and reestablishment of epigenetic marks that occurs after fertilization, or the response to environmental exposures that perturb normal epigenetic programming, resulting in establishment of an abnormal epigenetic program.

Epigenetics: This term is most commonly taken to refer to processes responsible for heritable changes in gene expression that do not result from change in actual gene sequences.

Epigenome: The epigenome refers to the entirety of the epigenetic marks of chromatin, analogous to the "genome" which refers to all the genes of an organism. Within a single organism, while virtually all cells have the same genome, different cell types have distinct epigenomes that specify which genes are turned on or off to determine each cell type.

Epigenome environment interaction (E*x*E): When the response to an environmental exposure is a combination of both the exposure and the epigenome of the exposed cell/individual. This ExE interaction can occur, for example, if the epigenome itself is the target of the exposure and/or if the pattern of gene expression determined by the epigenome modifies the response to the environmental agent.

Epimutations: A heritable change in gene activity that is not associated with a DNA mutation but rather with gain or loss of DNA methylation or other heritable modifications of chromatin.

Estrogen: A female steroid hormone produced by the ovaries and, in lesser amounts, by the adrenal cortex, placenta, and male testes. Estrogen helps control sexual development, including the physical changes; influences ovulation in the monthly menstrual cycle; lactation after pregnancy; aspects of mood; and the aging process.

Fertilization (conception): The process of sexual reproduction when the fusion of gametes (sperm and oocyte) initiate the development of a new individual organism.

Fetotoxicity: Toxic effects on the fetus in the later period of pregnancy after organogenesis.

Folate: Vitamin B9; is needed by the body to synthesize, repair, and methylate DNA and histones; alcohol consumption can lead to folate deficiency.

Gamete: A reproductive germ cell—an egg cell in the female or sperm in the male. Reproductive germ cells are haploid (that is, they carry only 23 chromosomes (only one chromosome from each of the 22 pairs plus one sex chromosome, X or Y).

Gametogenesis: The process by which diploid (46 chromosomes) precursor cells undergo meiotic division to become haploid (23 chromosomes) gametes.

Gene: The smallest unit of heredity, usually that portion of DNA that encodes a protein.

Gene expression: The transcription of genes to form RNA. This process represents one of the critical processes to translate genetic information into functional components of the cell, such as via production of messenger RNA (mRNA) and ribosomal (rRNA) and ultimately proteins.

Gene silencing: Refers to the outcome of epigenetic modification(s) that turns a gene off so that it is not transcribed into RNA.

Gene transcription: A cell uses a gene as a template to make a transcript (also called an mRNA molecule); this transcript will be further processed and then be translated to make a protein.

Generational health effect: Describing health effects of an exposure to a past (parental) generation that manifests in subsequent generations, such as children or grandchildren.

Generational inheritance: Refers to effects inherited by subsequent generations; may be intergenerational or transgenerational.

Genetic code: Three bases in a DNA or RNA sequence called a codon, each of which specifies for 1 of the 20 amino acids (e.g., the bases ATG specify the amino acid methionine) in a protein. Genes are frequently tens of thousands of base-pairs long, with every three bases of the DNA sequence coding for the amino acids that are used to make the protein.

Genome: All the DNA in an organism or cell, especially with reference to the total sequence of nucleotide bases, or "letters" of the genetic code.

Genome environment interaction (G*x*E): When the response to an environmental exposure is a combination of both the exposure and the genome of the exposed cell/individual. This often occurs when a particular genotype changes the way an environmental chemical is metabolized (making it more or less potent), or how DNA damage by an environmental exposure is repaired (increasing or decreasing mutation frequency). G*x*E interactions explain how human populations with the same environmental exposure will respond differently to that exposure due to genetic heterogeneity in the population.

Genotype: The complete genetic makeup of an individual organism that is determined by the specific variants (i.e., alleles) of each gene carried by the individual. Differences in alleles among individuals can account for the differences in phenotype, and response to environmental exposures, observed among those individuals.

Germ cell: Oocyte (egg) of females or spermatocyte (sperm) of males. A kind of cell that is part of the germ line and is involved in the reproduction of organisms.

Germ line: The series of germ cells each descended from earlier cells in the lineage of germ cells, containing the genetic material to be passed to successive generations.

Heterogeneity: A quality describing diverse, dissimilar, and not uniform components.

Heterozygous: Carrying two different variants (i.e., alleles) of a given gene.

Histone modification: The addition or subtraction of any one of several chemical groups to an individual amino acid of a histone. These modifications can include acetylation, methylation, phosphorylation, and ubiquitination (among others).

Histones: Proteins upon which chromatin is tightly wound and that function to package and organize DNA in the nucleus, termed a nucleosome. Epigenetic modifications occur on both the DNA strand and the histone proteins that make up a nucleosome.

Implantation: The stage of pregnancy at which the embryo adheres to the wall of the uterus in order to receive oxygen and nutrients from the mother, usually between 6 and 12 days after ovulation. At this stage of prenatal development, the embryo is called a blastocyst.

Imprinting: A phenomenon by which certain genes are epigenetically marked to identify the parent of origin of each allele (i.e., from the mother or the father). In general, imprinting serves to direct the expression of only one allele, either from the mother or father, and silence the other allele, so that the gene is expressed in a parent-of-origin fashion. For example, for certain genes only the copy inherited from the father will be expressed while the gene from the mother is silent.

Induced pluripotent stem cells (iPSCs): Pluripotent stem cells derived from adult cells, such as embryonic cells or skin cells, that can be "reprogrammed" to give rise to many cell types. This technology is important to the fields of personalized and regenerative medicine, and to understanding the patient-specific underpinnings of disease.

Inner cell mass (ICM): Cells of the blastocyst, surrounded by the trophectoderm, which will develop into a fetus.

Intergenerational inheritance: Generally used to describe the effects of events affecting parents (e.g., in response to an environmental exposure) that manifest in subsequent generations (children, grandchildren, etc.). Such inheritance is thought to occur via events affecting the germ line or on the developing embryo and its germ line (which will eventually produce grandchildren).

Meiosis: The formation of egg and sperm cells by which diploid (46 chromosomes) cells undergo DNA replication, followed by two rounds of cell division, producing four haploid (23 chromosome) gametes.

Meiotic inheritance: The transmission of genetic and epigenetic information through the germ line.

Messenger RNA (mRNA): Key intermediary molecule generated when a gene is expressed (i.e., when the information encoded in the gene is converted into a protein product by the cell); mRNA levels for a gene are used as an indicator of how "active" the gene is (i.e., how much of the protein is produced).

MicroRNA (miRNA): Single-stranded, non-protein-coding RNAs about 21–24 nucleotides in length expressed in plants and animals. They bind to their target gene's 3' untranslated region and generally block transcription or promote mRNA degradation.

Mitochondria: Structures within cells that generate most of the cells' energy through the production of adenosine triphosphate (ATP), a molecule that provides the energy needed for many key metabolic reactions.

Mitochondrial genome: A circular molecule of double-stranded DNA in the mitochondria that is 16,569 base-pairs long and contains 37 genes coding for 2 rRNAs, 22 tRNAs, and 13 polypeptides.

Mitosis: The cellular process that replicates chromosomes and produces two identical nuclei in preparation for cell division, followed by the equal division of the cell nuclei and other cell contents into two daughter cells.

Mitotic inheritance: The transmission of genetic and epigenetic information daughter cells during cell division (mitosis).

Mutagenicity: Ability of a physical, chemical, or biological agent to induce (or generate) heritable changes (mutations) in DNA. Often mutations change, or result in loss of, function of a gene, and if inherited, can change phenotype and/or cause disease.

Mutation: A change in the DNA base pair sequence at a particular locus in an organism. The term is used specifically to indicate point mutations (change in a single base), but is often loosely used to include other alterations such as chromosomal changes, including translocations, deletions, and inversion of larger DNA segments. Many physical (i.e., radiation) and chemical (i.e., benzo-[a]-pyrene) agents, as well as normal biological processes (i.e., reactive oxygen species formed during cellular metabolism) and transposable DNA elements can cause mutations.

Noncoding RNA (ncRNA): RNA molecules that are not used as a template to produce proteins, for example, microRNA.

Nucleosome: A nucleosome is a section of DNA that is wrapped around a core of proteins (histones); it is a fundamental subunit of chromatin. Each nucleosome is composed of a little less than two turns of DNA wrapped around a set of eight histones (a histone octamer).

Nucleus: The organelle-compartment of a eukaryotic cell that contains DNA organized into chromosomes; separated from the cytoplasm by double membrane perforated by nuclear pores.

Omics: The fields of study in biology ending in -omics, including genomics, proteomics, and metabolomics. Omics aims to collectively characterization the biological molecules that translate into structure, function, and dynamics of an organism.

Oocyte (ovocyte or egg): A female gametocyte or germ cell that divides twice by mitosis and meiosis into two other oocytes or into two ootids. It is involved in reproduction.

Organogenesis: The phase of embryonic development when cellular differentiation occurs and the internal organs are formed.

Oxidative stress: An imbalance between oxidants (e.g., reactive oxygen species [ROS]) and antioxidants that can lead to excessive oxidation and cell damage.

Pathophysiology: The processes and mechanisms operating in an organism that lead to or accompany a disease state.

Phenotype: The observable structural or functional characteristics of an individual organism that result from the interaction of its genetic makeup (i.e., genotype) with environmental factors.

Piwi-interacting RNA (piRNA): A class of small noncoding RNA molecules that form complexes and interact with piwi proteins (regulatory proteins involved in stem cell differentiation). piRNA complexes have been linked to gene silencing of retrotransposons and other genetic elements in germ line cells.

Placenta: Temporary membranous vascular organ that develops in mammals when young are developing in the womb. It attaches to the fetus via the umbilical cord and is expelled after birth.

Polymorphism: The presence of two or more variants (i.e., alleles) of a gene or other DNA sequence in a population.

Primordial germ cell: Precursor cells to gametes. These cells are designated in early embryo development and migrate to the developing ovaries or testes to develop into oocytes or sperm.

Progesterone: Progesterone is a female steroid hormone that is secreted by the corpus luteum, a temporary endocrine gland that the female body produces to prepare the endometrium for the potential of pregnancy after ovulation.

Protamine: A small protein found in the nucleus that replaces histones during spermatogenesis and play a role in the condensation and stabilization of DNA in the formation of sperm.

Protamine compaction: The process by which protamines compact DNA during spermatogenesis.

Protein: A polypeptide chain or complex of polypeptide chains, each consisting of a long string of amino acids. Amino acid sequences are specified by the underlying DNA sequence of the gene that encodes that protein.

Reactive oxygen species (ROS): Highly reactive oxygen–containing free radicals that are generated during oxidative metabolism. ROS can react with and damage lipids, proteins, and DNA in cells, causing oxidative stress. Common ROS include hydrogen peroxide, superoxide radicals, and hydroxyl radicals.

Repetitive elements: Patterns of bases in DNA or RNA that are repeated throughout the genome that can have structural and regulatory impact on DNA. More than two-thirds of the human genome consists of repetitive elements.

Reproductive toxicity: The ability of a toxicant to interfere with normal reproduction function, resulting in adverse effects on sexual function and fertility in adult males and females.

Retrotransposon: DNA segment that can duplicate itself and thus multiply in the genome; during this process, the original DNA sequence first copies itself into RNA and then back into DNA, which is then incorporated back into the genome; retrotransposons make up a substantial portion of the genome.

Ribonucleic acid (RNA): A nucleic acid that is generally single stranded and plays a role in transferring information from DNA to the protein-forming system of the cell.

Somatic cell: Any cell of the body, except germ cells.

Sperm: A male reproductive (germ) cell.

Spermatocytes: A male gametocyte derived from a spermatogonium, and gives rise to haploid spermatids through meiosis, which in turn give rise to mature sperm cells. Spermatocytes are found in the male gonads of sexually reproducing organisms. In humans, they are found in the seminiferous tubules of the testis.

Spermatogenesis: The process occurring in the male gonad of sexually reproducing organisms wherein the undifferentiated male germ cells develop into spermatocytes, which then transform into spermatozoa. It occurs in the male testes and epididymis in a stepwise fashion. The entire process can take approximately 64 days.

Stem cell: Primal undifferentiated cells that retain the ability to differentiate into other cell types.

Targeted chemical screening: Analyses for sets of preselected compounds determined to be important. Methods used to identify these substances are based on known chemical properties, such as their fragmentation profile and retention time. Quantification is achieved by comparing molecular characteristics with internal standards of known concentration. They are the gold standard exposure biomarker when measuring exposure to chemicals that are biologically relevant.

Teratogenicity: The ability of a substance to produce a permanent abnormality in structure or function, restriction of growth, or death of the embryo or fetus. Teratogens can produce a congenital malformation (a birth defect). Teratogens include radiation, maternal infections, chemicals, and drugs.

Testosterone: Male sex hormones produced in a testis that help to develop and maintain secondary sexual characteristics and are required for spermatogenesis.

Toxicant: Any substance that can have a toxic effect, including synthetic, biologic, or naturally occurring substances. Toxicants can be poisonous.

Transcription: Biochemical process in which an intermediary molecule called messenger RNA is generated based on the genetic information of the DNA.

Transfer RNA (tRNA): A kind of RNA molecule, about 76 to 90 nucleotides long, that translates the code carried by mRNA to into an amino acid to be synthesized into a protein.

Transgenerational inheritance: Parent-to-child inheritance of an environmentally induced genetic or epigenetic change, without direct exposure of the child. The term "transgenerational" is often used broadly to describe all environmental effects that can be transmitted from one generation to the next, However, it is important to distinguish parental (or **intergenerational**) effects, such as the impact of in utero exposure to particular nutritional, hormonal, or stress/toxin environments on the developing embryo and its germ line (which will eventually produce grandchildren), from truly transgenerational effects that are found in generations that were not exposed to the initial signal or environment that triggered the change.

Translation: The process of making proteins based on genetic information encoded in messenger RNA.

Transposable element (transposon): Sequences of DNA that move around to different positions within the genome of a single cell. The process is called transposition. DNA transposons move by a cut-and-paste mechanism, while replicative transposons usually move via RNA intermediates.

Trophectoderm (trophoblast): The cells forming the outer layer of a blastocyst, which provide nutrients to the embryo and develop into the placenta.

Untargeted chemical screening: Analyses used to screen for hundreds to thousands of compounds using high-resolution mass spectrometry methods coupled to gas chromatography or liquid chromatography. The overall chromatogram contains reproducible features that represent thousands of chemical constituents of the sample, but the identity of the vast majority of the compounds represented by the chromatogram are unknown. Statistical methods allow researchers to use features of the chromatogram in analyses without knowing the compound's identity to narrow research efforts. While less quantitative, untargeted assays capture a greater breadth of compounds than targeted assays and allow for the discovery of new chemicals that are biologically relevant. Once a compound is identified in an untargeted assay as biologically relevant, targeted assays for that chemical are developed.

Zygote: A cell formed by the fusion of two gametes, that is, fertilization. Its genome is a combination of the DNA in each gamete.